www.wadsworth.com

wadsworth.com is the World Wide Web site for Wadsworth and is your direct source to dozens of online resources.

At *wadsworth.com* you can find out about supplements, demonstration software, and student resources. You can also send email to many of our authors and preview new publications and exciting new technologies.

wadsworth.com
Changing the way the world learns®

Related Titles

Clinical Psychology

Casebook in Child Behavior Disorders, Second Edition
Christopher A. Kearney

Clinical Psychology, Sixth Edition
Timothy A. Trull & E. Jerry Phares

Abnormal Psychology: An Integrative Approach, Third Edition
David H. Barlow & V. Mark Durand

Essentials of Abnormal Psychology, Third Edition
V. Mark Durand and David H. Barlow

Casebook in Abnormal Psychology, Second Edition
Timothy A. Brown and David H. Barlow

Behavior Management

Behavior Modification in Applied Settings, Sixth Edition
Alan Kazdin

Behavior Modification: Principles and Procedures, Second Edition
Raymond Miltenberger

Special Education

Special Education in Contemporary Society: An Introduction to Exceptionality
Richard M. Gargiulo

Understanding Child Behavior Disorders

FOURTH EDITION

Donna M. Gelfand

Clifford J. Drew

THOMSON

WADSWORTH

Australia • Canada • Mexico • Singapore • Spain
United Kingdom • United States

THOMSON
WADSWORTH

Psychology Editor: *Marianne Taflinger*
Assistant Editor: *Jennifer Wilkinson*
Editorial Assistant: *Nicole Root*
Marketing Assistant: *Laurel Anderson*
Project Manager, Editorial Production: *Trudy Brown*
Print/Media Buyer: *Vena Dyer*
Permissions Editor: *Bob Kauser*
Production Service: *Lifland et al., Bookmakers*
Text Designer: *Ellen Pettengell*

Photo Researcher: *Quica Ostrander*
Copy Editor: *Jane Hoover*
Illustrators: *Jay Alexander, Gayle Levee, Gail Magin*
Cover Designer: *Lisa Henry*
Cover Image: © *Jesse Fleetwood, a participating artist of VSA arts*
Compositor: *UG / GGS Information Services, Inc.*
Text and Cover Printer: *Phoenix Color Corp.*

For more information about our products, contact us at:
Thomson Learning Academic Resource Center
1-800-423-0563
For permission to use material from this text,
contact us by:
Phone: 1-800-730-2214
Fax: 1-800-730-2215
Web: http://www.thomsonrights.com

ExamView® and ExamView Pro® are registered trademarks of FSCreations, Inc. Windows is a registered trademark of the Microsoft Corporation used herein under license. Macintosh and Power Macintosh are registered trademarks of Apple Computer, Inc. Used herein under license.

Library of Congress Control Number: 2002110769

Student Edition with InfoTrac College Edition:
ISBN 0-15-508480-1
Student Edition without InfoTrac College Edition:
ISBN 0-534-24776-8

Wadsworth/Thomson Learning
10 Davis Drive
Belmont, CA 94002–3098
USA

Asia
Thomson Learning
5 Shenton Way #01-01
UIC Building
Singapore 068808

Australia
Nelson Thomson Learning
102 Dodds Street
South Melbourne, Victoria 3205
Australia

Canada
Nelson Thomson Learning
1120 Birchmount Road
Toronto, Ontario M1K 5G4
Canada

Europe/Middle East/Africa
Thomson Learning
High Holborn House
50/51 Bedford Row
London WC1R 4LR
United Kingdom

Latin America
Thomson Learning
Seneca, 53
Colonia Polanco
11560 Mexico D.F.
Mexico

Spain
Paraninfo Thomson Learning
Calle/Magallanes, 25
28015 Madrid, Spain

Brief Contents

Contents

Part I Foundations

Chapter 4

Assessment and Classification of Child Behavior Disorders 78

In the Beginning: "What's Wrong?" "He'll Grow Out of It." 78

Part II Adversity in Children's Lives

Chapter 5

Drugs and Social Issues 103

In the Beginning: How Many Kids Use Drugs? 103

Chapter 6

Abuse, Neglect, and Children's Rights 123

Part III Emotional Disorders

Chapter 7

Anxiety, Posttraumatic Stress, and Obsessive-Compulsive Disorders 152

Part IV Behavior and Conduct Disorders

Chapter 10

Conduct Disorder and Related Conditions 215

Part V Conditions That Affect Learning and Academic Performance

Chapter 11

Learning Disabilities 238

Part VI Pervasive Developmental Disorders and Schizophrenia

Part VII Mental and Physical Health: New Roles for Psychologists

Preface

Everyone reading this book probably has some personal interest in the topic of children's behavior disturbances, how they develop and how they can be overcome. Perhaps you are a parent and your child is having trouble, you work with special-needs children, or you are considering a career in one of the helping professions serving children and families. Or childhood adjustment problems may strike even closer to home. Many people who have had personal experience with behavioral problems when they were young wonder why this happened to them and would like to learn more. This book is for all of you.

As instructors, we find that classes on children's psychological and educational problems tend to draw students who feel passionately about protecting children and improving treatment services for them and their families. We share this commitment and believe that the search for solutions to such problems should be one of society's major goals. This book offers a guided tour of the many childhood conditions considered to be disorders of some type, whether they are called behavioral, psychological, social-emotional, or mental disorders. This may not sound like a pleasant tour, and in some respects, it isn't. It is sometimes upsetting to study the discrimination suffered by children who are different from the others and whose behavior is considered deviant in some way. But there is much progress from the times, centuries ago, when children with behavior disorders were considered clowns and fools or, worse yet, were shunned, punished, or abandoned because they were a burden. So, much of the news is optimistic and reports enlightenment and progress in helping disturbed children.

Unifying Themes Add Meaning

We aim to present more than just a collection of facts about an assortment of unrelated psychological disorders. Scattered facts lack meaning and are difficult to remember. Like all good stories, ours is tied together by several major themes used throughout the book:

- Research protects children.
- Children develop in contexts, not in isolation.
- Behavior has biological and genetic roots.
- Development is fundamental.

These statements may not mean much to you at first, but they convey a great deal about the field of child psychopathology, which is the study of psychological disorders (sometimes called disorders for short). We believe that familiarity with these major themes will increase your appreciation for the science of child psychopathology and help you realize that it is a unified field of study.

Focus on Research Contributions

Let's examine the book's four themes again in more detail and see why each is important. "Research protects children" is much more than a catchy motto. It is impossible to understand child psychopathology without the aid of trustworthy research. Before the era of psychological research based in careful, objective data acquisition, most people thought they knew how to treat children, but they were simply wrong much of the time, and there was no way to correct them. Children's inability to behave properly was attributed to evil influences, willfulness, and other punishable offenses, rather than being seen as a possible sign of mental disorder. Imagine a child with ADHD (attention-deficit/hyperactivity disorder) trying to control himself unsuccessfully in the strict schools and churches of the past. Ineffective, harsh discipline was administered for behaviors that children could not control. In today's world, research and clinical practice go hand in hand as we study the reasons for youngsters' problems scientifically. Research aids treatment also. Skeptical health insurance companies and social services agencies refuse to pay for treatments that have not proved effective in rigorous scientific tests. Research can and does protect the interests of children.

Focus on Social and Cultural Contexts

What does it mean to say that children develop in contexts? Briefly, this expresses the principle that to understand a child's behavior, it is necessary to take into account the many factors operating in the child's world. By the term *contexts,* we mean the family and parenting practices, the teachers and the school, the child's siblings and playmates, the neighborhood, the customs of an ethnic group, and even broad cultural and national influences on children's development. Too often, people are given credit for their successes and criticized for their failures, when much of the responsibility is beyond their control and belongs to their families, schools, churches, friends, and other social influences. The theme that children develop in contexts reminds us that development is a complex process involving many people, times, and places. We cannot understand development if we concentrate on just the child alone. Behavior has many and deep social roots.

Advances in Biological Science

Rapid progress in genetics, biochemistry, and physiology has revealed a greater biological contribution to human psychological development than previously imagined. Scientists have made significant advances in tracing some types of mental retardation to genetic abnormalities. Other mental disorders show family hereditary patterns, although the exact mechanisms of genetic action remain unknown. We present the latest, most trustworthy information on genetics and the biological bases of behavior throughout this book.

Understanding Child Development

When studying abnormal child behavior, you will encounter terms that refer to child development, such as developmental psychopathology, developmental psychopharmacology, and others. The word *development* or *developmental* indicates that the subject matter deals with the processes of growth and change at different periods throughout life. Infants and teenagers are vastly different on many dimensions. Some problems wane, while others intensify with age. Other problems persist, but appear to change form, with different symptoms over time. This book stresses the developmental features of the entire range of child behavior disorders. Children are not all alike developmentally, and their differences must be recognized and accommodated.

We hope that our four themes help add meaning to the coverage of the many, very diverse disorders described in this book. For some disorders, research has been particularly influential in improving services; for others, the influence of context or development may predominate. Some disorders are known to have physical causes, but others seem to arise from various environmental and biological sources. Some children's disorders respond well to drug therapy, and others poorly. But we hope to highlight the overall importance of research, social contexts, biological influences, and developmental factors in the study of children and their difficulties.

Logical but Flexible Organization

Instructors have their own preferences for the order in which they present topics in their classes. We like the individual approach, and this book's chapters can be covered in any order the instructor prefers. However, chapters are grouped logically to include topics that are most closely related:

I. The first group, Foundations, includes Chapters 1 through 4, covering an introduction to the field, explanatory theories, research principles, and classification and assessment issues.

II. Adversity in Children's Lives is the organizing topic for Chapter 5 on drug use problems and associated social conditions and Chapter 6 on child abuse, neglect, and children's rights.

III. Emotional disorders are covered in Chapter 7 on anxiety disorders and related problems and Chapter 8 on depression and mood disorders.

IV. Behavior and conduct disorders are covered in Chapter 9 on attention-deficit/hyperactivity disorder and Chapter 10 on conduct disorder, delinquency, and other externalizing disorders.

V. Learning and academic performance difficulties are described in Chapter 11 on learning disabilities and Chapter 12 on mental retardation.

VI. Pervasive developmental disorders and schizophrenia are discussed in Chapter 13, which covers autism, childhood schizophrenia, and similar conditions.

VII. Health-related psychological disorders such as eating, sleep, and elimination disorders are covered in Chapter 14, while Chapter 15 considers the range of prevention and treatment approaches and their growing effectiveness.

New and Noteworthy in This Edition

Previous users of this book will notice extensive changes and improvements in this edition, ranging from the writing style to the coverage. The level and tone of the writing is livelier, more student-friendly, and less formal and scientific than in previous editions, without sacrificing content. More case material is presented, and each chapter opens with a section entitled "In the Beginning," a description of a child or group of children, which is referred to throughout the chapter and discussed at the end to help students integrate what they learned. Applying principles, research, and controversies to the case of a particular child or group helps students understand the material at a deeper level and makes it more memorable. Some chapters begin and end with a dramatic research finding, which is used in the same instructive way as a case description.

The new DSM-IV-TR edition is used, and diagnostic criteria are described in brief, understandable form. Events reported in newspapers and television news programs are featured and analyzed. The tragic events of September 11, 2001 enter into our discussion of posttraumatic stress disorder, and we analyze news reports of school shootings and effective racism and violence prevention programs. In all cases, we rely on professional interpretations and research findings to interpret events in the news.

We present glossary term definitions in a new way. To promote use of the definitions without disturbing the flow of reading, we have presented the defined terms in bold type. Readers can look up boldfaced terms in the glossary at the end of the book. Terms used in several chapters can be looked up directly without any need for cross-referencing.

InfoTrac® College Edition is a widely used online database that students find to be helpful and easy to negotiate as they write papers and give presentations. We list at the end of each chapter relevant search terms for InfoTrac College Edition and encourage stu-dents to explore this flexible teaching aid. Wadsworth offers free access to InfoTrac College Edition to instructors and purchasers of this textbook.

Another new feature in this edition is In Focus, a set of study questions accompanying headings in each chapter and highlighting major points in the text so that students can test their understanding as they read. Answers to all the In Focus questions appear at the end of each chapter, providing a convenient, easy-to-use self-test. Instructors can include In Focus questions in brief quizzes to check that students are current in their reading and understand the material. The In Focus questions can also be used in longer examinations.

Our coverage of child and adolescent substance use and abuse is the most up-to-date and extensive of any textbook in print. We combine it with coverage of family and social conditions that lead to drug use and psychopathology. Throughout the book, we stress the many roots of child behavior disorders and the need for public policy reform to reduce the prevalence of these disorders. New and abundant research on anxiety and depressive disorders persuaded us to devote an entire chapter to each of these types of disorders. Also, ADHD and its treatment now appear in a separate chapter, as does conduct disorder. Assessment and diagnosis are now combined in one chapter to stress their close connection. Some older theories of etiology have been replaced by newer ones, such as attachment theory, developmental psychopathology, and object relations theory. Biological bases of disorder receive new emphasis in Chapter 2 and throughout the book. This new coverage reflects advances in research and theory in the field.

Most of all, we try to convey the vitality, importance, and contributions of the field of abnormal child psychology without minimizing the problems and complexities. As authors, we try to be open, evidence-oriented, tough-minded, and idealistic. We are committed to a humanitarian cause, but require solid and convincing evidence for or against our positions. And that is the attitude we hope our book will inspire.

Aids for the Instructor

The textbook package offers three instructional aids free to instructors: a print Instructor's Manual with Test Bank, computerized test creation software

(ExamView®), and lecture outlines in Microsoft® PowerPoint®. The print Instructor's Manual with Test Bank includes chapter outlines, key terms, ideas for instruction, annotated video lists, website references, multiple-choice test items, and short answer test items. The test items are also available in ExamView. This easy-to-use assessment and tutorial system allows instructors to create, deliver, and customize tests (both print and online) in minutes. ExamView offers both a Quick Test Wizard and an Online Test Wizard that guide instructors step-by-step through the process of creating tests, while the unique "WYSIWYG" capability allows them to see the test being created on the screen exactly as it will print or display online. Instructors can build tests of up to 250 questions using up to 12 question types. Using ExamView's complete word-processing capabilities, they can enter an unlimited number of new questions or edit existing questions.

Acknowledgments

We are grateful to William R. Jenson, our long-time co-author of the previous editions, for completing a draft of Chapter 4, Classifying and Assessing Disorders, before withdrawing from participation in this edition. He shared the preparation of that chapter with Dr. Daniel Olympia, also on the faculty of the Department of Educational Psychology at the University of Utah. Clifford Drew then assumed sole responsibility for the editing and writing of the finished chapter in addition to his own chapters. To recognize the contributions of all three writers, they are named as authors at the beginning of Chapter 4. We are happy to have the opportunity to draw upon the assessment expertise of our colleagues in educational psychology in this way.

Changes in corporate ownership allowed us to take advantage of Bradford Potthoff's editorial talent and experience only in the initial phases of planning. Brad's belief in our project gave us support at a critical time, and the book is better because of his contributions. Our major development editor is Marianne Taflinger, whose wisdom, inventiveness, and humor guided us expertly through the throes of production. As experienced book authors, we appreciate Marianne's capable hands, and enjoy working with her.

We relied heavily on the advice of the keen-eyed users who served as reviewers of this book. All of the reviewers added nuggets of useful advice, and all were unsparing but considerate in their reviews. We acknowledge and thank the following colleagues:

Eric Cooley, Western Oregon University
David Crystal, Georgetown University
Jeffrey Danforth, Eastern Connecticut State University
Mark Koorland, Florida State University
Jeanne McIntosh, DePaul University
Lee Rosen, Colorado State University
Susan Scharoun, Le Moyne College
Sean Ward, Le Moyne College

We also would like to thank the following undergraduate and graduate students:

Ginger Apling, DePaul University
Leah Brzezinski, DePaul University
Shannon Edison, University of Guelph
Lauren Gaskill, DePaul University
Polly Gipson, DePaul University
Anastasia Liosatos, DePaul University
GiShawn Mance, DePaul University

We especially thank the children and families who appear in the case descriptions throughout this text. Many of these are descriptions of real people with real problems, but with their identity concealed. Others are disguised descriptions of people we have worked with or combined descriptions of several cases, which conceal individual identities and highlight features of a disorder. But in all instances, the children who experience disorders and their families are the heart of this book, and they keep the human element first and foremost in our minds.

The students in our classes are our best critics and the ones who most appreciate a good textbook. They detect errors that have escaped numerous readings by authors, editors, and colleagues, and we greatly appreciate their discernment and candidness. They keep us striving for excellence.

As always, Sid and Linda kept us going. Perhaps next to spouses of long-distance truckers, husbands and wives of writers spend the most time alone and unacknowledged. At least they know we are at home because they can hear the computer keyboard clicking. Sid and Linda—you never fail us, and we appreciate you more than ever.

Introduction to Abnormal Psychology of Childhood

In the Beginning

Bonnie's "Nerves"

Bonnie was a 15-year-old Caucasian girl in the 9th grade . . . her problem was that she would get nervous about everything, particularly things at school and doing anything new. When asked to give an example, Bonnie told the interviewer that her father wanted her to go to camp this summer, but that she did not want to because of her "nerves." During the course of the interview, it became clear that Bonnie's anxiety stemmed from a persistent fear of social situations where she might be the focus of other people's attention. For example, Bonnie reported that she felt very self-conscious in the mall and constantly worried about what others might think of her.

The interviewer asked Bonnie about a variety of situations that are frequently feared or avoided by teenagers with social anxiety. For almost every situation, Bonnie reported at least some level of fear and avoidance. Bonnie stated that she was very fearful of such situations as eating in public, using public restrooms, being in crowded places, and meeting new people. She claimed that she would almost always try to avoid these situations. . . . When Bonnie had a panic attack, the following symptoms would usually accompany her intense fear: accelerated heart rate, chest discomfort, shortness of breath, hot flashes, sweating, trembling, dizziness, and difficulty swallowing. Bonnie also reported that she would often get headaches and stomachaches when she was anticipating a situation that she found difficult. Although Bonnie often had panic attacks, the interviewer determined that her attacks always occurred during, or in anticipation of, difficult social situations. (Brown & Barlow, 2001, pp. 37–38)

Bonnie's fear of facing social evaluations is not uncommon, but its intensity and generality are. She was panicky about many too many harmless situations for far too much of the time, and her problems were increasing. As this chapter will show, instances of psychopathology such as Bonnie's are often exaggerations of common reactions that have become painful enough to interfere with everyday activities. Fortunately, Bonnie's parents spotted her problems as increasingly incapacitating, so they obtained a professional evaluation. She was diagnosed with social phobia (generalized) and also had a single episode of mild major depression.

INTRODUCTION

Child psychopathology may not be the best name for our field, especially for anyone trying to give a lecture. Try saying "child psychopathology" over and over as fast as possible, if you want a real tongue twister. Although this scientific term is a mouthful, its meaning is vastly important. Child psychopathology is a dynamic, rapidly changing field devoted to the study, prevention, and treatment of children's disturbed behavior. Many students are drawn to this area of study because children are appealing and it is natural to want to help them overcome their psychological problems. Many find it intriguing to learn why children become disturbed and fulfilling to master the techniques of assessment and treatment. Large numbers of Americans choose to work with children and families or contribute their time as volunteers.

However, the field of child psychopathology is built on more than just good intentions. Educators, health practitioners, caseworkers, and therapists undergo long and demanding training programs in which they learn about child development and abnormal psychology and acquire specialized knowledge in their disciplines. The ability to understand and advance the study of children's abnormal behavior requires some knowledge of many fields, including clinical, cognitive, physiological, genetic, and developmental science. Research training guards prospective helpers and their clients from being misled by attractive-sounding fads. It is always possible, even probable, that the new, miraculously effective treatment everyone is talking about is only an illusion. To actually help troubled children, it is necessary to detect and dismiss the baseless treatments and apply only the rigorously tested and proven ones.

Specialized research knowledge enables people to detect impressive-sounding but unsubstantiated claims that receive sensational press coverage. Consider the following actual headlines. How could someone tell which ones represent genuine scientific advances and

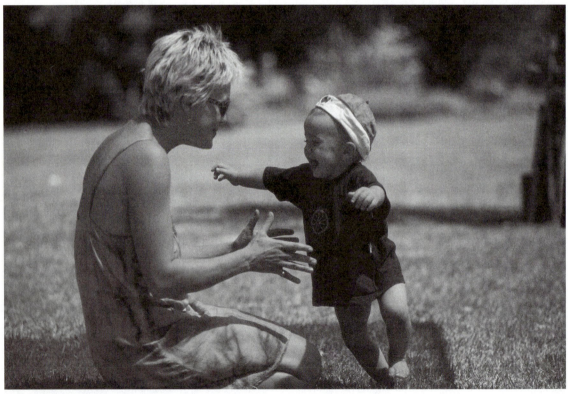

Most adults find babies naturally appealing, which optimizes positive interactions.

which are overstatements of actual findings or, worse, ill-founded pseudoscience?

- Studies show normal children today report feeling more anxiety than child psychiatric patients in the 1950s.
- Child abuse "rewires" brain, produces adult problems.
- Mother and teen conversations can prevent harmful college drinking behavior.
- Environment may hamper inner-city children's development more than *in utero* cocaine exposure.
- Musical training during childhood may influence regional brain growth.

In fact, all of these headlines were drawn from legitimate research studies. However, as is typical of many news reports, some of these are purposely dramatic, giving readers the impression that a major problem has just been uncovered or a fantastically effective treatment discovered, which occurs only rarely. As we shall see in the course of this book, science is incremental, progressing a bit at a time, and replication of findings is essential. That is, many similar studies must produce the same finding before it can be confidently accepted. We attempt to present the science of child psychopathology as it exists at the moment when this book went to press, pointing out major new developments, discussing how they add to previous knowledge, and saying what additional information is needed in order to understand and treat emotional illnesses.

THEMES OF THIS BOOK

IN FOCUS 1 ▶ Identify the difficulties in predicting which children will develop psychological problems and which will not.

This book focuses on four major themes:

- Research protects children.
- Children develop in contexts, including family, neighborhood, and cultural settings.
- Behavior has biological and genetic roots.
- Development is fundamental.

Here is what we mean by these "headlines." Like most of our professional colleagues, we are convinced that *research protects children*. Well-designed and conducted research allows us to base our treatment interventions on objective, controlled studies rather than on informal observations by therapists who strongly believe in their treatments or on other possibly biased sources. Research is a major theme that pervades nearly every chapter of this book. If you think research is boring, you will be surprised at the ingenuity and helpfulness of the studies we cite and how surprising and enlightening some of the findings can be. We hope to convince you of the advantages of the scientific approach as you read our book. But, above all, research on psychopathology helps children by revealing the sources of their illnesses and sorting out the effective interventions from those that represent a fad or an ill-founded belief.

Children's lives are so complex and they undergo so many changes as they grow that it is difficult to tell why some of them develop few problems despite difficult circumstances, while others in similar situations are plagued by difficulties. Headlines, such as the one above about mother and teen conversations preventing excessive college-age drinking, may give the false impression that a problem has a single cause. This is not the view of the authors of that study and is far from correct. The field of developmental psychology stresses that there may be and often are multiple causes of a particular psychological problem. As an example, it is easy to think of several possible causes for heavy drinking, such as attending a college noted for heavy drinking, having close family members with alcohol problems, responding to advertising promoting alcohol, or drinking to counteract stress. One or more of these may be more responsible for excessive drinking than the lack of certain conversations between a mother and teenager. And if such conversations do relate to the teenager's later drinking, is that because of the conversations themselves or the fact that they signify a close and confiding mother-child relationship? The study of child psychopathology is a complicated business, in which there are few clearly right or wrong answers, and causation of psychopathology is extraordinarily difficult to trace.

We also hope you will remember another theme of our book: *Children develop in contexts*. Few adjustment problems arise from the child in isolation, but instead develop as a result of influences in the child's home, family, neighborhood, and school. Cultural customs and values can affect the prevalence of children's emotional problems, as can natural disasters and political events such as terrorist attacks or economic reces-

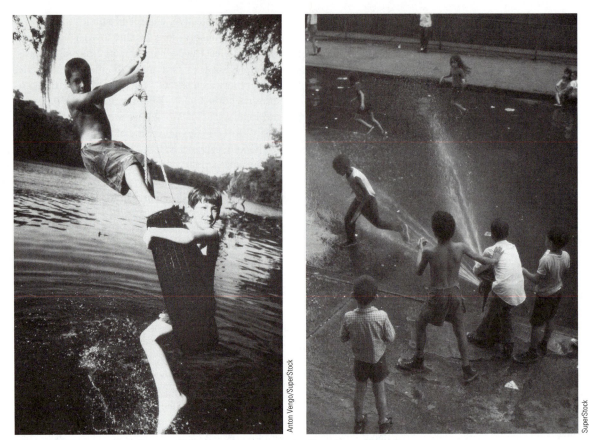

Anton Vengo/SuperStock

SuperStock

Different contexts, such as farms and city streets, provide contrasting play and learning opportunities.

sions. The availability, profitability, and popularity of illicit drugs and the scope of drug addiction in the United States provide a good example of how the national and cultural context fosters serious problems for children. Members of marginal social groups lacking in education and power can acquire wealth, influence, and status through the highly profitable drug trade but not through filling the few legitimate unskilled jobs that mostly do not pay a living wage. The drugs themselves appeal strongly to young people who seek the thrills of chemically induced highs and experience stress relief and escape from humdrum lives. But in the process, they may become addicted. This same sequence of events happens with so many adolescents and young adults that illicit drug use and addiction cannot be attributed to the personal weaknesses of the users.

As we show in Chapter 5, widespread and dangerous drug misuse is probably the result of many social factors. Research has identified risk factors including poverty, family strain and breakdown, discrimination, greedy dealers, fads in preferred substances, misuse of prescription drugs, unwise and ineffective laws and law enforcement tactics, and the lack of appealing recreational and employment opportunities for young people. In other words, many intractable social problems combine to lead huge numbers of American children and adults to use illegal substances. Different combinations of these potential causes could affect different children, but the result, illegal drug use, could be the same. This has been called the principle of **equifinality**—that is, different beginnings can lead to similar outcomes in children's lives (see Figure 1-1). A related principle, called **multifinality,** states that simi-

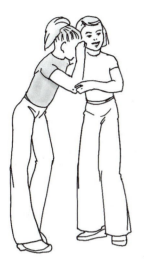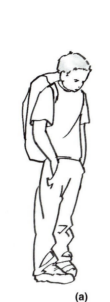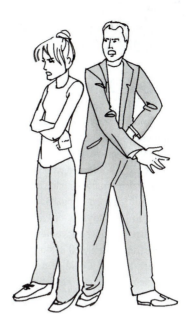

(a)

(b)

Figure 1-1 Equifinality and Multifinality

(a) Equifinality holds that various factors can lead to similar outcomes for children. Here, family troubles and peer rejection could each contribute to a boy's depression. (b) Multifinality holds that similar early experiences can lead to different behaviors in different children. For example, family violence could produce depression in one child and conduct disorder in another.

A Severely Abused Child

It was not until her nearly blind mother fled from her abusive husband to seek help for herself and her daughter that the world found out about Genie. Genie was 13 years old when she was discovered, but social services caseworkers at first thought that she was a much younger child, because she was so tiny and wasted. She also appeared to be severely retarded and unable to talk. Her lack of toilet training, silent tantrums, and strange repetitive movements suggested a psychotic condition. But probably all of these handicaps came from her father's keeping Genie in near complete isolation and confinement 24 hours a day. Himself a recluse, the father fashioned a harness to keep Genie restrained on a potty seat in a back bedroom during the day and in a mummy-like sleeping bag on the floor at night. He beat her viciously if she made any sounds. It is hard to understand why anyone would do such things, but the mother reported that her husband believed that Genie was mentally retarded. Two of their other babies had died earlier under what later seemed to be suspicious circumstances involving the father. He apparently did not abuse one favored child, Genie's brother.

Despite all of this neglect and extreme abuse, Genie did not die, but later became the object of intense scrutiny by linguists, psychologists, psychiatrists, social workers, physicians, and others who hoped to demonstrate that the effects of mistreatment could be reversed. Many different theories suggested equally different remedies, and Genie received intense treatment. The linguists recorded Genie's every syllable, the psychologists and psychiatrists attempted to have her bond to parent surrogates, and many experts visited her each day. She made progress in speaking, but her speech remained fragmentary and primitive. Eventually, she became toilet trained and stopped smearing herself and objects around her with her mucous. Her public masturbation decreased. She became emotionally attached to several people and showed a lively sense of humor and a talent for drawing. But Genie remained a very troubled and limited young woman, at least in part because of the severe abuse she experienced for so much of her childhood.

Sources: Curtiss (1997); Rymer (1993).

---

lar early experiences can lead to different outcomes for different children (Cicchetti & Cohen, 1995). For example, one child might respond to stern physical discipline with obedience and a growing conviction that strictness is right and proper, while a more autonomous child might react with hatred and rebellion. A related principle, **inequality,** is that early experiences can be unequal in potency. Stronger, longer, and more pervasive early experiences typically affect children more than do weaker, more passing ones. A child who is badly maltreated by several caretakers is much more likely to be affected by it than a well-cared-for child who has one unfortunate experience with a particular adult. (See Genie's Story.)

These complicated relationships between early experiences and later characteristics give headaches to professionals who try to advise people on how to be good parents. Very often, such professionals find themselves telling parents, "It depends." The age, sex, and personality of the child, the parent-child relationship, and the skill and warmth of the parent all matter, as does the powerful peer group. And *culturally pervasive childhood experiences* mold many children's characters in similar ways. Circumstances that many children experience, such as widespread availability and use of psychoactive drugs, being victimized by bullies at school (see Jack's Story), an economic depression, or repeated exposure to extreme violence on TV, can be expected to shape the lives of entire generations. When you see a high or increasing prevalence of a certain type of problem throughout a region or nation, it is wise to ask about cultural forces that might underlie the problem.

You may have noticed that some of the headlines cited earlier refer to biological processes, such as physical abuse "rewiring" the brain, *in utero* cocaine

Is Bullying Abnormal?

His mother thinks that Jack was destined to become a bully, and she has given up trying to reform him now that he is 12. Jack is heavy and tall for his age and seems engaging, with his freckles, curly ginger hair, and direct gaze. But even as a baby, Jack was a difficult child, crying and raging whenever he could not get his own way and demanding attention all the time. It seemed as though they were in the emergency room all the time because of Jack's accidents. Jack donned a towel as a Superman cape and hurled himself off the second-story deck, drank household cleaner on a dare from his brother, and rode his bicycle pell-mell off the dock and into the lake. His adventures got him a succession of abrasions, burns, and broken bones, but he survived and seemed to get tougher from all the hard knocks. Maybe he got it from his father, a testy, hard-drinking, drug-using roofer, who got into fights, sometimes physical ones, on the job and when drinking at bars. Jack Senior bullied his wife and children, and Jack Junior treated his classmates in the same way, threatening to beat them up if they didn't let him go first in line, or simply because he was meaner than the other children and could get his way with them. He and two pals were the scourge of the elementary school, and he had been excluded from school a number of times without any noticeable result. His dad was proud of him for standing up for himself and refusing to take insults, but everyone else expected to see Jack Junior in serious trouble with the law before too long.

How did this happen to Jack and his family, and what could be done to prevent a bad problem from worsening? Research reveals several common elements in the backgrounds of hostile and aggressive children (American Psychological Association, 1993):

- A difficult, tempestuous temperament from early infancy
- A father who is aggressive and violent and trains his son to act the same way
- A defeated mother who is unable to control her son and husband (or a mother who is also extremely aggressive and antisocial)
- Classmates who give in to bullying
- Teachers who cannot prevent bullying

SOURCE: American Psychological Association (1993).

---

exposure affecting development, and regional brain growth being influenced by music. Such news stories emphasize another theme of this book—*behavior has biological and genetic roots*. Advances in neuroscience are rapidly changing the field of child psychopathology, thus expanding our understanding of brain-behavior links. Few people realize that this is not a one-way process: Experience changes brain function just as brain function underlies experience and behavior. Examples of this complex interaction between physiological processes and psychological and behavioral ones appear throughout this book, beginning in Chapter 2. Today, more than ever before, students of psychopathology need some background in biological science simply in order to keep up with advances in developmental and abnormal psychology.

The book's final theme, *development is fundamental*, advocates learning about human development. It is common knowledge that children's cognitive, social, and physical abilities are limited at birth and develop as they mature. Children's perceptions, language abilities, and memory are different from those of adults. Yet this simple truth is often overlooked in the study of abnormal child behavior. Even the experts too often assume they know exactly how children think and feel and do not attempt to verify their opinions through careful research. Children are not just miniature versions of adults, and you cannot understand their normal or disturbed behavior from limiting your research to adults. That "adultcentric" approach has been tried and has failed many times in the past, when theorists or clinicians tried to reconstruct what happened during a patient's childhood to

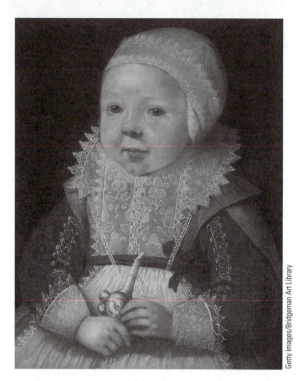

Hundreds of years ago, children in Europe were dressed much like adults. Some of their playthings were similar to those of children today, however; note the combination rattle and teething implement held by this child.

Getty Images/Bridgeman Art Library

produce mental disorder later in life. Even the great Sigmund Freud erred in believing that he could deduce what his adult patients must have experienced when they were young. Some of them described having been sexually abused as children, but Freud originally thought these reports were fictitious, based on distorted, neurotic thought processes. He later decided that the women's reports of incest and other sexual abuse could have been accurate, after all. Despite his brilliance and clinical perceptiveness, Freud could not reconstruct a childhood experience based on an adult patient's recall.

We now recognize, from decades of research, that children's memories of events are quite unreliable when they are less than 2–3 years old and improve markedly after that. This early weakness in autobiographical memory means that it is essential to independently confirm preschoolers' reports of events, such as of being physically or sexually abused, with other witnesses' accounts or physical evidence. Actually, very young children can remember events under some circumstances. Even infants can remember how to do simple nonverbal motor tasks over intervals from 2 days to 10 weeks, with older infants remembering the tasks longer than younger ones (Rovee-Collier, 1999). For example, babies were trained to kick a leg in order to pull a ribbon that operated a colorful mobile or depress a lever to move a toy train. The infants remembered how to do these tasks even after a significant delay. Visual and motor memory is necessary to perform these tasks. Nevertheless, it is not clear that they could remember and describe what they did in words later, when they had learned to speak. So it is possible that very young children remember events nonverbally, but cannot describe them in words.

Developmental differences must also be considered in the psychopharmacological (drug) treatment of children. For many years, prescription drugs were developed for and used mainly with adults and not children, who comprised a commercially smaller market. The customary practice among physicians has been to use drug hand-me-downs with children, using particular medications that have been found to be effective with adults. Many medications that researchers found to be effective with adults have been tried and then widely used with children without adequate testing. Tricyclic antidepressants such as imipramine have often been used to treat juvenile depression, but they are much less effective for this purpose than they are with adults (Geller, Reising, Leonard, Riddle, & Walsh, 1999). Fortunately, some newer antidepressants for adults, the selective serotonin reuptake inhibitors (SSRIs), are proving effective for children's depression, as we describe in Chapters 8 and 15. In fact, almost all psychoactive drug treatments that were developed for adults have been freely prescribed for children, in the hope that their effects would transfer to the younger age group. If so, it would not be necessary to go through the costly process of developing and testing a special group of medications for younger patients. Most, but not all, of the drugs developed for adults are safe for children but may not be effective, since the child's developing nervous system can react differently than the adult's mature system. Here again, two of our themes are relevant: *Research protects children* and *de-*

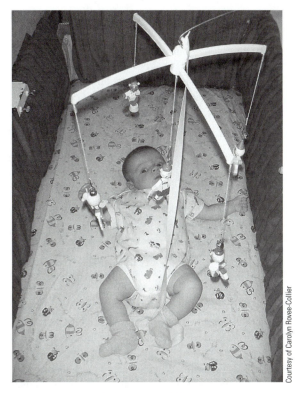

Even young babies learn to control their environments. Because the action produces an interesting visual display, this 3-month-old kicks his legs more often when the overhead mobile is activated by a ribbon attached to his ankle than when the ribbon is not attached.

velopment is fundamental. Research protects children from ineffective, potentially harmful treatments, and research results with adults cannot be assumed to automatically apply to children, who are at a different stage in development.

Throughout this book, we will point out the relevance of the four themes for understanding the origins, nature, and treatment of the different varieties of childhood adjustment problems. The themes are also important for understanding the process of developing and testing diagnostic criteria, assessment procedures, and preventive and treatment interventions. Our work is informed and enriched by a common commitment to research, understanding the role of social and cultural contexts, biological bases of psychological functioning, and the crucial role of the child's developmental level.

WHAT IS CHILD PSYCHOPATHOLOGY?

IN FOCUS 2 ▶ Identify the major criteria used to identify abnormal behavior in children.

If you work in child assessment and treatment, you will encounter the same reaction over and over. Your neighbor, friend, or casual acquaintance will say, "You're a child psychologist. I'll bet you'll want to study my children!" or "Oh, oh, a child psychologist. We'd better watch out what we say around you." These are simply jokes in most cases, but they reveal an uneasiness and uncertainty about what is normal or not and a concern about whether their children have problems requiring treatment. Almost all parents have qualms such as these at one time or another while their children are growing up. So exactly what are parents concerned about? How do we tell whether a child's behavior is normal?

A large part of this book is devoted to child assessment and diagnosis, that is, the determination of whether a child's behavior meets the criteria established for one or more mental disorders. The diagnostic standards are purposefully very stringent, so only a few individuals meet them and are given a psychiatric diagnosis. This means that most, but not all, of the jocular parents we meet have children whose behavior may be bothersome, but is far from diagnosable. Parents are uneasy because they don't know when their child's troublesome behavior crosses the line and should be considered abnormal. In truth, there is no such line. There is no universally accepted clear distinction separating normal from abnormal behavior. Even the diagnostic criteria presented in the *Diagnostic and Statistical Manual of Mental Disorders*, 4th Edition, Text Revision (DSM-IV-TR) represent agreements and compromises reached by panels of experts, sometimes after considerable debate (American Psychiatric Association, 2000).

To complicate matters, many childhood disorders are more quantitatively than qualitatively different from normal conduct. As an example, many children are aggressive, some are bullies, and many tell lies at least occasionally, but a child must have these problems to an exaggerated degree in order to be diagnosed with conduct disorder. If children fail to meet every one of the recognized diagnostic criteria for a particular disorder, their behavior then falls within the wide normal range. Many children pass in and out of meeting the formal criteria for conduct disorder at different points during childhood. Essentially, these youngsters may be difficult and aggressive, but they do not have a mental disorder. In fact, they may grow up to be productive and successful adults whose confrontational manner may serve them well in occupations such as law enforcement, professional sports or coaching, or trial law.

A good rule of thumb is that concerned parents should consider getting a professional consultation if the child's behavior causes serious problems in school performance or in getting along with others; that is, if it interferes with normal functioning. Another clue is the distress caused to the child or others, with greater and more continual distress indicating a behavioral disorder. However, parents and teachers will not be happy to know that a great many behaviors are marginal, not clearly normal or abnormal, and so their questions will not receive a definitive answer. Fortunately, the same types of psychological treatments that relieve diagnosed disorders also work well with more minor, or subclinical, problems. These interventions are described in Chapter 15 and throughout the book in the chapters devoted to specific disorders.

In the next subsection, we describe everyday subclinical behavior disturbances that occur commonly among children of different ages. Then, in later chapters, we present the more serious syndromes included in the official diagnostic manuals used by mental health professionals. One of the most important, most basic questions in child clinical psychology is how to determine whether a child's behavior is within the wide range of normal limits or is so unusual and troubled that it meets diagnostic criteria for a disorder.

- First, in order to be diagnosable, the child's actions or emotions must be painful or objectionable to himself and others. The behavior *causes distress* of some type to the child or others.
- Second, the behavior *interferes with the child's everyday functioning* at school, at home, or in other contexts. A child who remains at home because she is too afraid and anxious to leave and attend school has a psychological disorder of the internalizing type. Another child who is excluded from school because he bullies and hits smaller children is a candi-

date for diagnosis with an externalizing type of disorder. There are many different ways in which a troublesome behavior pattern can impede a child's performance, but whatever the situation, a clinical problem has a significant effect on functioning.

- A third consideration is a behavior's *cultural or social appropriateness*. A behavior that is highly socially or culturally inappropriate might be considered a disorder if it does not represent an understandable form of defiance or a joke or mocking someone. For example, highly disturbed people with thought disorders sometimes are so disturbed that they neglect simple hygiene, so they might wet themselves rather than use a bathroom. They may also suffer from hallucinations and yell at imaginary people even though they are not on drugs. When these actions are not culturally acceptable, they probably indicate a mental disorder. Bizarre acts this extreme are relatively easy to identify as abnormal in people of any age or culture. However, some behaviors that appear unusual to people of one culture are not at all unusual in another, which creates confusion. For example, ethnic Japanese people tend to laugh nervously when they are uneasy or embarrassed. This reaction is confusing to Europeans who may inadvertently say something to embarrass Japanese people and then inexplicably be laughed at. Europeans and Americans don't typically laugh in these situations, so they could incorrectly interpret anyone who does as showing inappropriate affect and even as potentially disturbed. Cultures are distinguished by social codes that dictate whether a person looks directly at another in a conversation, whether a child can address an adult directly or must show respect by remaining silent, whether marriages are arranged or are decided on by the bride and groom, whether women can show their hair in public, and countless other examples. It is easy to think of situations in which cultural practices are highly restrictive and conflict with individuals' freedom of expression and belief. Nevertheless, for the most part, following the acceptable practices of one's culture is considered an essential part of individual adjustment.

In addition to the three general criteria used to identify a behavior pattern as abnormal (causing distress, interfering with functioning, and being culturally or socially inappropriate), several more specific aspects of the behavior and the child must be considered. First, the clinician must consider *the child's age and developmental level* in order to interpret the child's behavior.

Normal Behavior Is Age-Appropriate

A child's age is crucial to deciding whether her behavior is normal. Behavior that is usual and acceptable at one age may be highly deviant at another. A normal infant's wariness of strangers and crying and protesting about even brief separations from her mother would be very abnormal in an older child. Similarly, adult behaviors such as using alcohol, smoking, and staying out late at night would be considered unacceptable in a 9-year-old. So developmental norms frequently are

used to decide whether a particular child's behavior is normal or not. Highly prevalent behavior may not be desirable behavior, but it is still normal. If a large proportion of high school students cheat on exams, it would be incorrect and unfair to say that a particular student is disturbed simply because he cheated on an exam, as objectionable as that behavior might be. This is why the familiar adolescent's excuse that "everyone is doing it" holds a germ of truth. Behaviors that are statistically frequent may be deplorable, but generally cannot count as clinically deviant.

The importance of understanding the principles of human development cannot be overemphasized. Clinicians must be familiar with the behavior patterns of children of different ages in order to say whether a particular youngster's actions are normal or not. As just mentioned, many behaviors that concern parents and teachers occur in a large proportion of children at

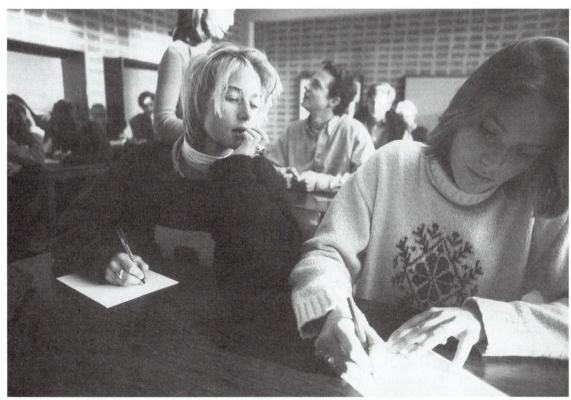

Some undesirable behaviors such as cheating are widespread among schoolchildren. The girl on the left hopes to improve her test score by copying the answers of her classmate.

Ghislain & Marie David de Lossy/Getty Images

Table 1-1 Problem Behaviors Characteristic of Children and Youth at Various Ages

Age Range	Problem Behaviors
$1\frac{1}{2}$–2 years	Temper tantrums, refusal to do things when asked, demanding attention constantly, overactivity, specific fears, inattentiveness
3–5 years	Temper tantrums, refusal to do things when asked, demanding attention constantly, overactivity, specific fears, oversensitivity, lying, negativism
6–10 years	Temper tantrums, overactivity, specific fears, oversensitivity, lying, school achievement problems, jealousy, excessive reserve
11–14 years	Temper tantrums, oversensitivity, jealousy, school achievement problems, excessive reserve, moodiness
15–18 years	School achievement problems, skipping school, cheating on exams, depression, drinking, smoking, drug misuse, early sexual activity, trespassing, shoplifting and other minor law violations

a particular age, and so must be considered statistically normal, even if undesirable. Table 1-1 presents some troublesome but normative behaviors found in many children at different ages. These behaviors resemble potentially abnormal characteristics, but however bothersome they are, they are also common, typically occurring in 30% or more of all children.

Even though problem behaviors like those in Table 1-1 are not of a magnitude to constitute a disorder, some are not benign and can escalate into diagnosable conditions. After a period of experimentation, children simply discontinue some of these problem behaviors, especially if the episodes are mild and managed well by parents and teachers. Other behaviors are not initially serious, but become so if not handled well. This is especially true for aggression and noncompliance, which may appear in children as young as 2 years and persist into elementary school in many children (Luby & Morgan, 1997). Early disruptive behavior naturally draws counteraggression and punishment by others, and thus increases the risk of persistent problems (Patterson, Forgatch, Yoerger, & Stoolmiller, 1998).

Similarly, unusual anxiety in young children can become persistent, leading to social and physical withdrawal, which interferes with school performance (Ialongo, Edelsohn, Werthamer-Larsson, Crockett, & Kellam, 1995). So, although some early problems of subclinical severity continue and worsen, most simply dissipate over time. Next, we briefly review the typical, everyday problems of children at different ages.

Common Problems of Preschool Children

Everyone has heard about "the terrible twos," a time between the ages of $1\frac{1}{2}$ and 3 years when a formerly cheery toddler can develop negativism, temper tantrums, and general contrariness. This behavioral change is common, but not inevitable. Mothers and other caretakers report that at least half of toddlers have frequent temper tantrums and often disobey. In addition, many demand constant attention and protest loudly to attract their parents' attention when they are ignored. Students with young children know that it is difficult to find an uninterrupted time to study at home with their preschoolers. When they open their books and begin reading, their kids do ingenious things to get their attention: sitting beside them and pretending to read aloud, yelling "Watch me!" while they try to do somersaults, or claiming to be hungry, thirsty, bored, or otherwise needy. Many toddlers also seem to have trouble paying attention. Fortunately, tantrums, destructiveness, bullying, and lying decrease markedly as children grow older. Yet, many kindergarten children, especially boys, continue to throw tantrums and exhaust adult caregivers with their incessant activity. Other preschool children are overly sensitive to minor slights, shy, and withdrawn and develop specific fears, such as fears of animals, the dark, storms, and injuries (Gullone, 1999). Already in the first three years of life, two major types of abnormal behavior are appearing: externalizing problems of the aggressive, overactive, antisocial type, and internalizing problems such as anxiety, depression, fears, obsessive-compulsive behavior, and physical complaints with psychological features (see Figure 1-2). Externalizing and internalizing problems are not incompatible and sometimes affect the same child at the same time, in which case they are called co-occurring (or comorbid) disorders. Both internalizing and externalizing disorders continue to be prevalent in older children and adolescents and constitute the major classification types of adult psychopathology.

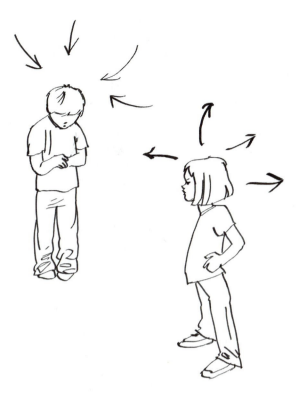

Figure 1-2   Internalizing and Externalizing Problems
The boy expresses his distress as internalizing symptoms of depression, fear, and anxiety. The girl's externalizing behavior is directed outward as attacks on others.

Common Problems of 6- to 12-Year-Olds

Perhaps because these behaviors are disruptive in the classroom, elementary school teachers most often complain about their students' overactivity, temper tantrums, lying, and oversensitivity. It is not surprising that so many children are thought to have attention-deficit/hyperactivity disorder (ADHD), since rambunctious activity and inattention are common in the classroom, particularly among boys. Many children seem to become less energetic as they grow older, and teachers more effectively control their behavior in the classroom, so overactivity is less of a problem in the later elementary grades. At the same time, excessive reserve, oversensitivity, and temper outbursts are common, and more children begin to suffer from moodiness and mood swings. What do they worry about? Mostly, children's worries have a realistic basis, but are exaggerated because children

lack necessary information and judgment. School-age children are concerned about their grades, their parents' health, getting injured or being rejected by the other children, and appearing foolish. And since they hear upsetting news stories of murders and attacks, they become concerned about the threats of violent crime, war, terrorist attacks, or some natural disaster such as a flood that might leave their family homeless (Silverman, La Greca, & Wasserstein, 1995; Weems, Silverman & La Greca, 2000). A large number of children, about 10–20% of them, develop a phobia or intense, unmanageable anxiety of some type (Barrios & Dell, 1998; Beidel, 1991).

The number of children suffering from the more serious *diagnosable* mental disorders is around 20%, according to the U.S. Surgeon General (2000). The huge number of children with problems explains why the need for educational services for children with learning-connected disabilities greatly outpaces the growth in school enrollment (U.S. Department of Education, 2000). The prevalence of mental disorders in children and adolescents is roughly the same as in adults (Shaffer et al., 1996). It appears that far from enjoying a protected existence, as many adults imagine they do, children on the whole are no happier or better protected from mental illness than adults.

In addition to behavioral disturbances, many children have academic achievement problems. On the Hawaiian island of Kauai, the entire population of young people was extensively studied for many years. More than half of the 10-year-old boys and more than a third of the girls were found to have serious academic achievement problems (Werner & Smith, 1992). Many received unsatisfactory or failing grades in basic skills such as reading or arithmetic or were placed in remedial classes. Academic problems such as these are more common in low-income groups with many families below the poverty line. In addition, cultural factors must be considered. Native Hawaiian children are particularly likely to have school achievement troubles, perhaps because their traditional customs stress cooperative learning in small groups of children rather than in teacher-instructed classes. This aspect of their culture conflicts with the more impersonal, individually competitive, and adult-directed atmosphere of most schools (Tharp, 1993, 1994). Other cultural groups with traditional expectations and practices at odds with those in regular classrooms include some American Indian tribes, African Americans, and Hispanic Americans, all of which benefit from educational practices that are more compatible with their traditions than are the usual schoolroom routines (Tharp, 1994). However, similar types of achievement problems appear to some degree in nearly all U.S. schools and among all cultural groups. Large numbers of elementary school children need help to overcome both academic and social problems.

Common Problems of Adolescents

IN FOCUS 3 ▶ Discuss the pros and cons of the argument that adolescence is a time of identity crisis and rebellion.

American teenagers have a bad reputation. Adults tend to dismiss adolescents' virtues and complain about their shortcomings, when they attend to issues affecting teenagers at all. These negative views of teenagers are reflected in news broadcasts, most of which concern adults. The few programs that present stories about youth often feature those who are violent criminals or victims of crimes or accidents (Gilliam & Bales, 2001). Viewers come to associate teens with images of violence, injury, and crime. News accounts of teens who work hard, share, and help are rare in comparison. When interviewed, many adults say they believe that teens today are less moral and ethical than those of past generations, although all available evidence contradicts this negative view (Gilliam & Bales, 2001). Parents and others who have close contact with teenagers are less likely to accept this wholesale criticism of youth, but do not question it because they believe the young people they know are exceptions to a general decline in character. Such strong negative stereotypes make it difficult for many adults to assess the actual characteristics of teenagers.

Actually, adults have always been ready to see adolescents as more conflicted, emotional, and rebellious than they were when young. Memory favors our own positive self-perceptions, so we are likely to conclude that we were exemplary but the current generation represents a decline. Mental exaggerations of the virtues of former generations were evident as early as classical Greece, when Plato referred to youth as a drunkenness of the spirit leading, of course, to impulsivity, lack of responsibility, and moral and ethical

shortcomings. A similar, but more temperate, opinion appears in the writings of the 20th-century psychoanalysts Anna Freud and Erik Erikson, who picture adolescence as troubled. Psychoanalysis portrays middle childhood (from about 6 to 10 years of age) as a latency period of quiet intellectual and social development, which at puberty gives way to emotional turbulence and personality turmoil. Erikson's (1956) influential concept of the **identity crisis** portrays adolescence as a time of stress and strain during which problem behavior is common but of little permanent consequence.

Although many personality theorists accept Erickson's formulation that adolescence involves a crisis, other authorities portray identity formation as gradual and often uneventful (Grotevant, 1998). Contrary to popular belief, most adolescents state that they respect and admire their parents, want to be like them, and get along well with adults (Allen, Hauser, Bell, & O'Connor, 1994). So the older generation's bad opinion of teens is largely mistaken, and national databases reveal that "youth today are at least as healthy or healthier than their parents' generation" (Youniss & Ruth, 2000).

Nevertheless, adolescents, like other age groups, have their problems. A majority of them experiment with alcohol and drugs, and many are involved in petty crimes, such as vandalism and shoplifting. Their love of excitement and novelty lead them to reckless acts (Arnett, 1995), some of which are self-destructive and illegal. Adolescents may become sexually active but engage in unprotected sex, from which they may contract sexually transmitted diseases, including HIV (Panchaud, Singh, Feivelson, & Darroch, 2000). Young women in the United States are more likely to become unmarried mothers than are young women in comparable countries (Singh & Darroch, 2000). Young people under the age of 21 account for a disproportionate number of all arrests, about 30% (U.S. Department of Justice, 2000). And this crime statistic is an underestimate, since many additional youthful crimes go undetected. These facts seem to support the "evil teenager" stereotype, but in reality most of these illegal acts are minor, involving disorderly conduct, theft of small items, and status offenses illegal only for minors, such as underage drinking, curfew violation, and running away from home.

This survey of age-related problems shows that some problems are so common at particular ages that it would be illogical to consider them pathological unless they are unusually severe and incapacitating. Clinicians and teachers find that some knowledge of child development is essential in order to avoid identifying age-typical difficulties as true disorders. As Figure 1-3 illustrates, youngsters tend to develop age-typical types of problems, which may differ for girls and boys.

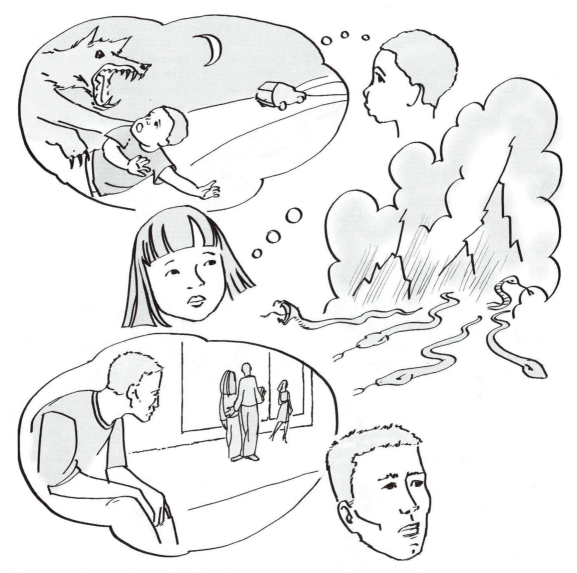

Figure 1-3 Common Fears of Childhood
Younger children fear dogs and other animals, the dark, and separation from parents. Older children and adolescents fear appearing foolish and being unable to perform socially or academically. As they grow, children overcome some fears but develop others, particularly evaluation apprehension.

Sex Differences in Problem Behavior: Boys Will Be Boys

IN FOCUS 4 ▶ Which problems are more prevalent in each sex during childhood and adolescence? Is either sex more troubled than the other?

Research confirms the popular belief that boys are more aggressive than girls. That is, boys are more likely to taunt, hit, and bully others, throw things, destroy property, use a weapon in a fight, and generally act in ways that hurt people. Between the ages of 9 and 17, boys are more likely than girls to behave aggressively and to commit property offenses (destructiveness and frequent lying) and status offenses (age-inappropriate acts such as smoking). And the sex differences in aggression widen during childhood and adolescence, when males become much more aggressive than females (Lahey et al., 2000). The emergence of marked sex differences in aggression during this period could represent the effects of physical maturation, intensification of sex-role socialization, or perhaps both factors (see Chapter 10 for a discussion of

etiology of aggression). The odds are 9 to 1 that a child or teenager who commits violent or aggressive acts is a male (Keenan & Shaw, 1997; Offord et al., 1987).

If boys are more physically aggressive, are girls kinder, gentler, and more compassionate? This tends to be the case, but there are exceptions. One antisocial behavior that does not appear more often in either sex is oppositional behavior during the childhood and teen years (Lahey et al., 2000). Most girls are as likely as most boys to argue with their parents, defy them, deliberately annoy people, blame others for their own errors, and be spiteful, vindictive, resentful, and angry. Nobody is perfect.

Boys also show more attention problems and hyperactive behavior (including ADHD) than girls. ADHD can appear alone or combined with antisocial behavior. Male antisocial behavior tends to be more persistent across the life course and is often combined with hyperactivity-inattention or ADHD, poor peer relations, impulsiveness, and mild cognitive and academic impairment (Aguilar, Sroufe, Egeland, & Carlson,

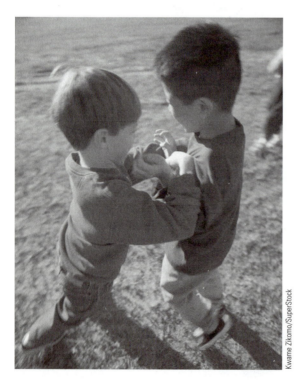

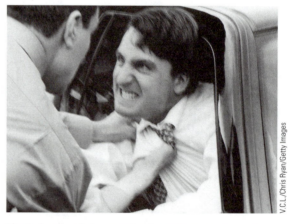

Physical and verbal aggression is common among young boys on the playground, and it can continue into adulthood—for example, as road rage.

2000; Rutter & Sroufe, 2000). This combined antisocial syndrome is dangerous because, if untreated, it can escalate into serious adult criminal offenses.

Female depression rates escalate during later adolescence and continue to be higher into adulthood (Peterson, 1993; Rutter & Sroufe, 2000). Younger boys and girls are equally likely to be diagnosed with depression, but starting in the mid-teens, girls' depression rates soar to twice those of boys. This gender difference in depression continues throughout most of adulthood (American Psychiatric Association, 2000). Chapter 8 offers further discussion of this disorder.

In adolescence, girls increasingly develop eating disorders such as anorexia nervosa (self-imposed starvation and compulsive overexercise) and bulimia nervosa (alternate gorging of excessive amounts of food and purging involving vomiting or laxatives). These eating disorders are described in Chapter 14. Although some boys develop eating disorders, as many as 95% of the victims are female, perfectionistic, and overly concerned about their appearance (American Psychiatric Association, 2000). Many people have developed theories about why these devastating disorders appear in adolescence and why their prevalence is increasing. Some writers believe that impossible standards for female beauty are responsible; others point to possible physical changes around the time of puberty or perhaps a fear of sexual maturation that stimulates fasting to retain a childlike body. Like many other types of disorders, eating disorders are not yet well understood.

Research on sex differences in adjustment problems suggests that there is no simple answer to the question of whether girls or boys are more troubled. The answer depends in part on the nature of the problem and the age of the children. For example, there are no sex differences in depressive disorder rates for children, but very large differences during later adolescence, when depression selectively strikes girls. Further, although boys are more aggressive and have up to 10 times more conduct problems than girls (Keenan & Shaw, 1997; Offord et al., 1987), there is equality between the sexes when one form of externalizing, antisocial behavior is considered—oppositional behavior. As many parents know, girls can be fully as oppositional and defiant as boys. Like many other issues in child psychopathology, gender differences are

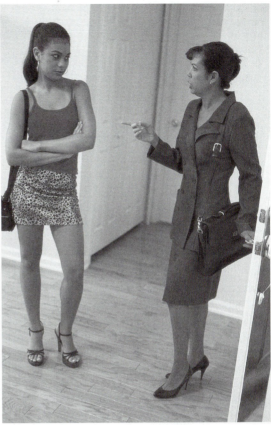

Most girls are less physically aggressive than boys, but they can be just as defiant and oppositional.

much more complex and more dependent on child age and family circumstances than is evident at first.

To evaluate the validity of psychological and physical tests, Meyer and his colleagues (2001) pooled all of the available research findings on many variables, including gender. The resulting correlations ranged from zero, indicating no relationship, to low correlations, such as .09 between children's cognitive performances and their sugar consumption, to a strong correlation of .67 between male gender and adult height (see Table 1-2). Arm strength was also greater in males than females. But not far behind in magnitude, at .42, was the correlation between female gender and self-reported empathy and nurturance. Note that some of these correlations were based on self-reports, rather

Table 1-2 How the Sexes Do and Don't Differ: Some Variables That Relate to Gender

Observed risk-taking behavior (males are very slightly higher)	.09
Self-reported assertiveness (males are significantly higher)	.32
Self-reported empathy and nurturance (females are higher)	.42
Arm strength of adults (men are stronger)	.55
Height of U.S. adults (men are taller)	.67

SOURCE: Meyer et al., 2001.

NOTE: Correlations are statistics that can range from .00, indicating no relationship, to 1.00, for a perfect relationship. Zeros are common, and perfect correlations of 1.00 almost never occur, in part because it is difficult to measure variables accurately.

than objective observations of prosocial behavior, which might have been different. The other correlations between gender and behavior were smaller, with a medium-sized correlation of .32 between being male and seeing oneself as assertive. In comparison, receiving some type of psychological, educational, or behavioral treatment correlated with measured improvement at a lower level, .23. *Observed* risk-taking behavior did not differ between the sexes. Apparently there are equivalent numbers of male and female risk takers. These figures suggest that when all published studies are combined, behavioral gender differences are unimpressive, with two exceptions. Males *say* they are the more assertive sex, and females *say* they are more empathetic and nurturant. These self-perceptions may or may not translate into actual behavior.

Role of Adults' Expectations and Experience: Babies Shouldn't Cry

Child protective service workers encounter the following situation repeatedly: A mother goes to work, leaving her baby in the care of her boyfriend. Hours later the infant is seen in the emergency room for injuries that look suspiciously like physical abuse. The boyfriend explains that the baby cried for hours, wailed louder when he tried to comfort her, and finally "fell" down the stairs. A judge later sentences him to jail for child abuse. The man may never before have assaulted anyone seriously, so why did he violently attack a defenseless baby? Some child abusers seem unable to realize that babies cannot think and react similarly to adults. These people have unrealistic expectations about young children's ability to endure hunger, thirst, or pain stoically, in silence. Many of these abusers are men who are unwillingly thrust into the role of babysitter, which they consider demeaning. They have no training and little experience in caring for young children and believe that babies cry out of willfulness or malice toward them personally. They believe punishment is called for, never realizing that crying is the only way a preverbal child can communicate distress. Most victims of physical abuse are infants and toddlers whose distress is misinterpreted as willful disobedience and mishandled by stressed, angry, and inexperienced adults. This tragic misunderstanding of how babies behave contributes significantly to child abuse. This example accentuates that anyone who assesses children, especially infants and toddlers, must be as familiar with child development as with adult psychopathology and should have formal training in working with children. This is increasingly the case in mental health services, with more mental health professionals specializing in clinical work with children and families.

Adults are more likely to be accurate in classifying a child's behavior as normal or deviant if they are familiar with the particular child they assess and can observe her closely for weeks or months at a time. Adults who know children and see them every day, such as parents and teachers, notice the more subtle psychological problems such as fears, phobias, and mood disorders. These often subtle emotional problems are less apparent to adults who do not interact with the children regularly.

Which Problems Are More Persistent?

IN FOCUS 5 ▶ Describe the personal and family factors that help children to avoid or overcome adjustment problems.

A key question is whether or not children will outgrow their behavior problems. Other people usually reassure worried parents that their kids will grow out of it and no professional consultation is necessary. They dismiss the parents' concerns as exaggerations and advise them that if they don't make too much of it, the child's problem will blow over. Many times, this well-meant reassurance is correct; in other cases, the problem persists and perhaps worsens. The answer to the question, of course, is a weak sounding "maybe." A child's behavior problem may disappear, because the outcome of childhood disturbance depends on many things, including problem type, severity, appearance in many settings (generality), the family and social environment, and the child's other strengths or weaknesses. A list of persistent and transitory childhood characteristics appears in Table 1-3.

Let's consider the factors that relate to the continuity or discontinuity of disordered behavior:

- The *type of problem* matters; for example, children diagnosed with conduct disorder are at particular risk for continued problems. About half of them engage in criminal behavior and drug abuse during adolescence, and as many as 85% of them grow up to face chronic unemployment, perhaps because their hostility and suspicion alienate coworkers,

Table 1-3 Persistence of Childhood Characteristics

Persistent Characteristics

Self-confidence and sociability

Intellectual interests, achievement motivation

Preference for sex-typed rather than opposite-sex activities

Clinically significant depression

Obsessional, recurrent thoughts and compulsive rituals

Developmental disorders such as autism, psychotic reactions

Highly aggressive, antisocial, illegal, defiant behavior

Academic underachievement and other school problems

Unpopularity linked with aggression

Negative self-image, strong inferiority feelings, tension, physical complaints

Marked mental retardation

Sexual assaultiveness in adolescent males

Severe or numerous adjustment problems

Transitory Characteristics

Nonsevere shyness and social withdrawal

Anxiety, fears, and phobias, except for agoraphobia (terror about leaving the house), which is more persistent

Chronic nervous habits such as nail biting

Sleep disturbances and minor eating problems, except for obesity or anorexia (self-starvation), which persist

bosses, and customers. Adults who had conduct disorders as children often have continued interpersonal problems. Plagued by unstable personal relationships, these adults are impulsive and physically aggressive, and they may abuse their spouses (Lahey, Waldman, & McBurnett, 1999).

- *Severe and more persistent problems* are not easily or quickly overcome. The more severe the adjustment problem, the more likely it is to last, either in the original form or as new, but related problems. Severe mental retardation, developmental delay, autism, childhood-onset schizophrenia, eating disorders, and other major problems are particularly difficult, but not impossible, to overcome. Sometimes, children suffer from a number of adjustment problems and develop a mental disorder in adolescence or adulthood. For example, people who develop schizophrenia often have a troubled psychological history. Schizophrenia is a complex set of related disorders, which involves delusions, hallucinations, and disorganization, and other disturbances such as emotional flatness, incoherent speech, periodic mutism, and profound lethargy. One would expect that such symptoms would be preceded by profound childhood disturbance, but that is not necessarily the case. Instead, the preschizophrenic child may have problems in concentrating, sleeping, and completing schoolwork and may begin to avoid people. That is, the child's problems persist and worsen, and new types of problems appear. So problem persistence does not necessarily mean that exactly the same types of problems continue. Instead, new symptoms such as epileptic attacks, delusions, or hallucinations can emerge, while the person continues to be disturbed.

- Problems that *occur in more than one setting*, such as at school, at home, and in the neighborhood, are often more serious and lasting that those that are confined to a single place and group of people. These multicontext problems represent a *general orientation or set of attitudes* directed to self and others. For example, a child may have a hostile, oppositional attitude combined with a feeling of being picked on; another child may show extreme timidity and lack of self-confidence together with feelings of anxiety and depression. These pervasive attitudes are more persistent and difficult to combat than an otherwise adequately adjusted youngster's isolated problem such as a specific fear or a violent dislike of a certain person.

- *Children's personal strengths and characteristics* enable them to overcome stress and adapt well. Children who are physically healthy, do well in school, and have many friends are less likely to develop incapacitating psychological disorders than those who are stressed, ill, unpopular, and academically challenged. However, the lives of even the advantaged children can be disrupted by traumatic events. Children may have to endure their parents' acrimonious divorce, severe family money problems, an unwilling move to an undesirable neighborhood, and serious illness. Some situations are so bad that most children experiencing them develop physical or mental health difficulties of some type, at least temporarily. Even then, the children differ in how well they adjust to bad times. Children with calm, easygoing temperaments fare better than those who are difficult and irritable, in part because the former attract more supportive responses from others (Smith & Prior, 1995; van den Boom & Hoeksma, 1994). Intellectual ability and good school performance also help, perhaps because more successful students get more recognition and support from teachers.
- *A close, confiding relationship with at least one parent and a secure attachment to a parent* provide a haven for the child, even in dire circumstances (Smith & Prior, 1995). An attachment relationship is vital to a child in infancy, and a secure, trusting relationship to a primary caregiver is an advantage throughout life.
- *A caring adult* who provides warmth and guidance even when parents are neglectful or absent is a positive influence (Werner & Smith, 1992; Zimmerman & Arunkumar, 1994). This could be another family member (commonly a grandparent), a close family friend, or even a neighbor. But children need some caring adult in their lives.

Sometimes problems are overwhelming and cannot be counteracted by even the most resourceful child or supportive family, as with the September 11, 2001 terrorist attacks that killed so many people. No one is completely invulnerable to tragedies. But the greater the number of positive features in the child's life, the more optimistic the forecast for his adjustment. Many times, adversity teaches children skills in living, especially if they have help and guidance from caring adults. The right guidance at the right time helps children prevent or overcome their adjustment problems.

RESOURCES FOR PARENTS AND TEACHERS

Today's parents and teachers have access to excellent, research-based professional advice on the early detection of budding adjustment problems and the proper ways to manage them. Some general resources can help adults understand children's difficulties and get a general idea about whether a child should be referred for assessment and possible treatment. Such advice is available in the form of self-help books and on the Internet. Some Web sites feature chatrooms for parents of children affected by particular disorders. Books for parents are published by the American Psychological Association, the American Academy of Child & Adolescent Psychiatry, Research Press (a commercial publisher specializing in behavioral management), and other recognized presses and professional associations. An excellent Internet resource is the Child & Family WebGuide (http://www.cfw.tufts.edu) sponsored by Tufts University, which features Web sites that offer the most credible research-based information. The American Psychological Association's Com-

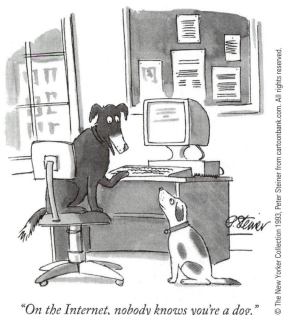

"On the Internet, nobody knows you're a dog."

Back to the Beginning

Help for Bonnie

Many youngsters suffer from at least some symptoms of social anxiety, but few develop a case as serious as Bonnie's. Many children discover that participating in enjoyable social situations reduces their apprehension, and they naturally become more socially skilled as they grow. In a way, Bonnie resembled a much younger, less socially skilled child emotionally, which highlights this book's developmental theme that people's judgments of whether behavior is normal are based partly on a child's age and maturity level. The intensity of Bonnie's anxiety left no doubt that she had a psychological disorder, and her parents gave up on simply trying to reassure her, since that obviously did not work.

Bonnie's future was uncertain before she entered a cognitive-behavioral treatment program for adolescents with social phobia. The sessions included small groups of teenagers and helped them to identify the situations they avoided and how they interpreted them as dangerous and menacing. They learned to detect their automatic thoughts about catastrophes and how to challenge these thoughts and replace them with plans for mastering feared situations. They learned good skills, such as facing the person you are talking to, looking the person in the eye, and smiling, and they learned how to praise themselves for doing so. They rehearsed difficult social interactions with their groups and were helped to participate in real social situations at school. Gradually, Bonnie began to successfully eat meals in public, order pizza over the telephone, play her flute for a small group, and participate in class at school (although this caused her some apprehension). Most of all, Bonnie and her parents learned that problems like hers can be overcome and should she develop similar problems in the future, she can get therapy and relief.

---

mittee on Children, Youth, and Families also has a Web site (http://www.apa.org/pi/cyf), which offers information and advice in both electronic and printed form. The advent of the Internet technology means that copious amounts of information and advice about child development and parenting are available. Unfortunately, much of this advice is offered by unknown sources that lack credibility, but appear expert simply because they seem to have knowledge about mental health and are on the Internet. Look for the name of the Web site sponsor or manager. Be cautious, especially if the Web site requires a membership fee or features a particular medication, clinic, or type of treatment.

SUMMARY

This book's four major themes are: Research protects children, children develop in contexts, behavior has biological and genetic roots, and development is fundamental. What we mean by these statements is that the best assessment, prevention, and treatment practices are based on sound, objective research, rather than on popular but poorly founded beliefs. So we stress research and what it can do to promote children's welfare. We examine children's lives in context—within their families, at their schools, in their neighborhoods, and in their cultures. Further, genetic and biological factors interact with environmental conditions to influence children's development, so we devote much of this book to this crucial interaction. And one cannot study children without attention to the changes they go through during development. Children's characteristics are not stable or fixed, but are in the process of growth and transformation. In this process, they develop age-typical problems, which can be either internalizing or externalizing in type. Typical internalizing problems include shyness, specific fears, depressed mood, social withdrawal, and physical complaints with psychological components. These internalizing problems can appear even in infants and toddlers, as can attachment problems. Externalizing problems such as oppositional behavior, defiance, temper tantrums, aggression, property destruction, and lying can also begin in the first 3 years of life, but are more typical of school-age children.

Problems of clinical proportions exceed age-typical problems in their severity and persistence. If a child's difficulty is so severe that it interferes with academic performance, school attendance, or social relationships, the child may have a diagnosable mental disorder. This is particularly likely if the problem creates distress for the child or others, most often the parents and teachers. Additional cues that the child may have a disorder are usually noted by adults who know the child well, can tell whether the problem is persistent, and can determine whether it is age-typical or not. Also, the child's behavior may be termed abnormal if it is inappropriate for the child's social group, culture, and gender. The more persistent problems with poorer prognoses include severe antisocial and aggressive behavior, severe autistic and other pervasive developmental delay disorders, and profound mental retardation. In general, the more severe disorders are the most difficult to treat successfully. Fortunately, these conditions are rare. Diagnosing children's psychological disorders is not easy because development brings dramatic behavioral changes and there is no clear and universally shared distinction between typical and atypical behavior.

⏻ INFOTRAC COLLEGE EDITION

For more information, explore this resource at http://www.infotrac-college.com/Wadsworth. Enter the following search terms:

developmental psychology
developmental psychopathology
antidepressant medications
diagnostic criteria
co-occurring (or comorbid) disorders
identity
sex differences
attention-deficit/hyperactivity disorder (ADHD)
childhood schizophrenia

IN FOCUS ANSWERS

IN FOCUS 1 ▶ Identify the difficulties in predicting which children will develop psychological problems and which will not.

- Different beginnings can lead to similar problems (equifinality).
- Similar early experiences can lead to different outcomes (multifinality).
- Some influences are stronger and more pervasive than others (inequality).

IN FOCUS 2 ▶ Identify the major criteria used to identify abnormal behavior in children.

- Is painful to self and others
- Interferes with everyday functioning
- Is culturally or socially inappropriate
- Is inappropriate to child's age and developmental level

IN FOCUS 3 ▶ Discuss the pros and cons of the argument that adolescence is a time of identity crisis and rebellion.

- Psychoanalytic theorists thought adolescents experienced identity crises.
- However, most teens are close to their parents and get along well with adults.
- The drug culture and teens' thrill-seeking can get them into trouble, but not as much as adults fear.

IN FOCUS 4 ▶ Which problems are more prevalent in each sex during childhood and adolescence? Is either sex more troubled than the other?

- Boys are more physically aggressive and have attention-deficit/hyperactivity disorder more often.
- Adolescent girls are more depressed and have more eating disorders.
- Overall, neither sex is more psychologically disturbed than the other.

IN FOCUS 5 ▶ Describe the personal and family factors that help children to avoid or overcome adjustment problems.

- A calm, easygoing temperament that attracts support from others
- Academic and intellectual ability
- Close relationship with a parent or substitute

In the Beginning

Understanding June

Nearly everyone who knows her has an opinion about why June cannot read and write as well as her classmates, despite her caring parents and stable, middle-class home. June is in the 6th grade, but complains that the work is too hard for her. She claims the teacher is mean and says she just cannot do the assignments. Recently, she has begun to lie about having done her homework, and other girls suspect that she has stolen money from their purses at school. But June's main problem is her schoolwork. It takes her forever to read the simplest text, and she can't make herself stay up late and get up early enough to complete Mrs. Turner's assignments. Mrs. Turner doesn't see herself as mean or overly demanding. She is concerned that June seems so defeated and hostile and is falling farther and farther behind in school. She thinks June's problem is a neurologically based learning disability and has advised June's parents to have her tested. Mr. and Mrs. Adams don't know what to think. Neither of them had any trouble with schoolwork, and they are very concerned when June won't even try. They were shocked that June lied about completing her work, and they think it's mostly an attitude problem, perhaps learned from other kids. They particularly blame the loud and defiant girl next door. They hope their pep talks will finally take hold and inspire June to work harder and act more maturely. There has never been an Adams child who did not succeed in school, her mother has told June many times. Her parents sometimes wonder whether June is a true Adams, because she is so different from all the other family members. They remember she had a fussy, difficult temperament even as a baby.

June's case illustrates several of the major explanations of disordered behavior. The teacher's interpretation is that the problem is biological, perhaps hereditary. Consequently, the best treatment could be both chemical (appropriate medications) and instructional (a structured program to teach June how to improve her reading and writing). In contrast, June's parents believe that social influences such as undisciplined classmates produced June's problems. June herself also traces her difficulties to the social environment, but she blames strict, overly demanding teachers and her disapproving parents rather than her peers. There is a lot at stake in identifying the best explanation of June's learning problems: Each one dictates a different type of treatment, and it is important that June's schoolwork improve quickly, before she enters a more demanding middle school.

INTRODUCTION

Theories of child psychopathology are well-developed and formal written explanations of how and why children become disturbed. Many psychological theories explicitly trace disorders to events that occurred early in life, such as the child's disrupted emotional attachments to the mother. Biological explanations of psychopathology may go back even further and identify genetic or hormonal abnormalities during prenatal development that predispose a child to particular mental illnesses. Still other theories emphasize the power of current social influences, such as attention, power, and approval, as factors that maintain abnormal behavior patterns. There are many possible causes of psychological disorders, and different theories emphasize biological and psychological-social factors to varying extents. Theoretical explanations gain acceptance to the extent that they predict research findings, identify groups at risk for developing problems, and yield interventions that can prevent or reduce suffering. In short, good theories are useful.

In this chapter, we present some of the major approaches to child psychopathology, indicate their strengths and limitations, and illustrate how each one would help explain the troubled behavior of a particular girl named June.

BRAIN AND BEHAVIOR: THE NEUROSCIENCE OF DISORDERS

If her teacher is correct, June's problems have mainly a physical cause—a genetic predisposition toward developing learning disabilities, a biochemical dysfunction, or some other structural or functional cause. When people explain a child's personality by saying that the child has always had a difficult or easy temperament or closely resembles some relative, they are using a biological model of problem etiology (problem origins). The neuroscience model points to genetic abnormality or some brain or nervous system dysfunction as the primary underlying cause of certain types of psychological disorders. Many people find biological explanations to be more compelling than psychological ones. Perhaps this is because nonscientists have the mistaken opinion that biological models are more understandable and verifiable than environmental explanations of behavior. Another possible reason is that biological models tend to exonerate the family, particularly its handling of the child, as the cause of the problem. Parents, teachers, and others cannot reasonably be accused of causing a problem that has a physical basis unconnected with how they cared for the child.

Genetic Basis of Psychological Disorders

IN FOCUS 1 ▶ Identify four types of abnormality in normal gene replication that can cause physical or mental problems.

As will be apparent from this brief description of the neuroscience underlying abnormal behavior, we still know very little about the genetic basis that predisposes individuals to develop behavioral disorders. The connections between genes and abnormal behavior are unbelievably complicated and often misunderstood. For example, people do not inherit psychological disorders directly. What people actually inherit is the DNA that makes up their genes, rather than behavior itself. Genes encode proteins involved in the development and regulation of neural circuits governing behavior. After conception, the environment assumes major importance in development. By *environment*, we mean all the physical and psychological surroundings in which the child develops. So, for the most part, abnormal behavior is not inherited; instead, genes may confer the tendency toward developing a certain type of disorder under particular environmental conditions. That is, genetic effects are probabilistic because genes statistically increase the odds of developing a disorder rather than being deterministic (invariably and directly causing a disorder). Whether a genetic tendency to problem development eventually results in the disorder is determined by many things, most especially the child's environment. Stress, ill health, poverty, and neglect may greatly increase the chances of a child's developing a disorder to which she is genetically predisposed.

Acceptance of genetic explanations of family resemblances in personality traits or psychological disorders requires a leap of faith, because the hard, objective evidence is still lacking. Genetics is a well-funded, rapidly developing research field, so our understanding of genetic factors in mental disorders is certain to improve in the next several years. We will see later how behavioral genetics studies of twins and other relatives demonstrate the role of genes in psychological disorders.

> What we commonly call the mind is a set of operations carried out by the brain. The actions of the brain underlie not only relatively simple motor behaviors such as walking or eating, but all the complex cognitive actions that we believe are quintessentially human, such as thinking, speaking, and creating works of art. As a corollary, all the behavioral disorders that characterize psychiatric illness— disorders of affect (feeling) and cognition (thought)—are disturbances of brain function. (Kandel, 2000, p. 5)

Brain development begins during fetal life and continues for years after birth. During this sensitive formative period, the central nervous system is particularly vulnerable to injury, disease, and harmful teratogens (toxic substances). As a result, nervous system functions continue to be susceptible to damage or delay during infancy and early childhood. However, children's brain functions are very resilient and show impressive recovery from the effects of disease and damage. Environmental influences are also important during early life, since they can affect neurological functioning through nutritional deprivation, diseases, and highly excessive or deficient levels of stimulation. Individual children and adults differ in how well they cope with illness, neglect, and abuse, depending partly on genetic factors and partly on their experiences. Close and complex relationships between a child's genetic endowment, physical health, and environment govern development. Nature (biological factors) and nurture (physical and psychological environmental factors) act in conjunction with each other, influence each other, and cannot really be separated.

June's teacher might be correct to say that June's learning disability has a physical basis, but she would be wrong to overlook the importance of psychological factors. June's misbehavior might be learned, perhaps in response to subtle mishandling by her parents or from that ungovernable girl next door, and she could respond powerfully to social controls, such as how other people inadvertently reinforce her undesirable behavior. Actually, whether her behavior ultimately turns out to be more biologically or more socially based, June could still respond positively to psychological interventions, medications, or a combination of both. That is, the type of treatment intervention need not directly parallel the cause of the problem in order to be effective. Particularly revealing is how June reacts to the attention she gets for acting out. Does she regularly receive praise for sticking at her schoolwork when it is hard for her, or must she resort to whining and refusing to work in order to attract attention to herself? Do her parents typically criticize her no matter what she tries to do, or do they encourage her attempts to improve? We will return to the discussion of June's situation later. First, let's examine some of the biological processes that help explain children's psychological problems.

Some Basic Concepts of Genetics

At the outset, we present a brief review of some of the basic concepts used in the study of genetics, including the nature of genes and their actions. This discussion requires introducing some vocabulary terms and concepts used in neurobiology and psychopathology.

Using powerful microscopes, scientists can see and count the human chromosomes taken from body cells, and they can even see the physical damage to chromosomes that produces some disorders, such as Down syndrome. Chromosomes are made up mainly of DNA (deoxyribonucleic acid), a complex molecule containing the genetic information. Double strands of a DNA molecule, twisted together, resemble a spiral staircase or a twisted ladder and are often described as a *double helix* (see Figure 2-1). Normal human body cells have 46 chromosomes arranged in 23 pairs. The pairs contain one chromosome from the person's father and one from the mother. One pair, the sex chromosomes, determines the individual's gender and gender-related traits, and the remaining 22 pairs control different aspects of the complex processes of development.

A gene is a segment of DNA that contains the information for one trait or aspect of development. In the simplest case, a single defective dominant gene can produce a trait regardless of the influence of the other, recessive, gene of the pair. This is what occurs for certain characteristics such as color blindness. In contrast, recessive genes prevail only if both genes of a pair are recessive, as is the case for the genes deter-

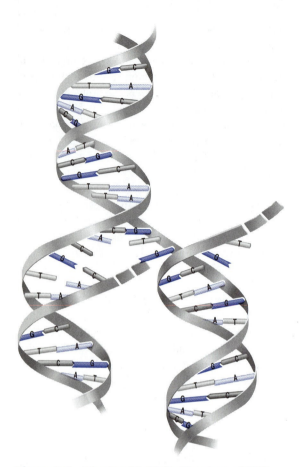

Figure 2-1   The Double Helix Structure of DNA
The DNA "ladder" splits down the middle. The rungs of the ladder are composed of paired chemical structures known as bases: adenine (A) with thymine (T), and cytosine (C) with guanine (G).

mining blue eye color. Some problems can be traced to sequences of genes on the chromosome that are disarranged or replicated an unusual number of times in the process of duplication or to gene pairs that fail to divide completely. Genes also differ in **penetrance,** or the degree to which they produce observable physical and behavioral characteristics. Some, such as those determining eye color, are difficult to counteract by any known environmental manipulation, while others, such as those determining height, can be radically affected by nutrition and other environmental factors.

Research indicates that most personality characteristics and psychological disorders with high **heritabil-**

ity reflect the actions of many genes, each contributing a little to the characteristic or disorder, rather than just one gene. This is a **polygenic model,** in which multiple genetic abnormalities are usually required for a person to develop a disorder. Some physical diseases are also polygenic in nature, including diabetes, epilepsy, and coronary heart disease. The combination of the operation of multiple genes and the differing penetrance levels of genes makes it difficult to trace a possible genetic basis for many types of psychopathology. There have been many false leads and prematurely announced findings that could not be replicated. It was once believed that bipolar (manic-depressive) mood disorder could be attributed to a specific gene, but later research failed to confirm this finding (Kelsoe, 1997). Bipolar disorder and most other behavior disorders are likely to stem from the cumulative action of many genes, each adding a small portion of the effect.

Heredity plays an obvious role in characteristics such as hair and eye color, height, and skin pigmentation, and genes are important in the appearance of some cancers and other physical diseases. Consequently, people may leap to the conclusion that heredity is so powerful that it explains normal personality variations and disordered behavior as well. In fact, except for a few serious and progressive neurological disorders (Huntington's chorea, Tay-Sachs disease) and some types of mental retardation (Down syndrome, fragile X syndrome), there is little or no accepted evidence of a genetic basis for behavior disorders. Or perhaps it would be better to say that we currently lack evidence concerning genetic influences on the types of disorders discussed in this book. However, the rapid advance of genetic research may someday yield explanations of psychological disorders.

> One of the most important messages of genetic research has been that genetic influences are probabilistic and not deterministic, and that environmental factors are broadly speaking of roughly equal importance. (Rutter & Sroufe, 2000, p. 270)

Behavioral Genetics

The field of **behavioral genetics** aims to discover the contributions of genes to many human behaviors, ranging from everyday characteristics, such as temperament, to psychological disorders, such as depression or conduct disorder. Behavioral geneticists study similarities in the most closely related individuals (identical twins, who share 100% of their genes) and in first-degree relatives, such as parents and their children or siblings who are not identical twins (who share 50% of their genes). Sometimes these groups are compared with less closely related people and with samples of unrelated people. Since identical twins are identical genetically, it would seem that their shared behavioral characteristics can be attributed to their shared genetic makeup. Adoption studies are particularly important, since they can reveal whether the behavior patterns and problems of adoptive children more closely resemble those of their biological parents or their adoptive parents. Behavioral geneticists have studied pairs of twins reared together or separated soon after birth. If genetic factors underlie disorders, when one twin has a disorder, so should the other twin. Also, there should be higher rates of the disorder among the biological relatives of the separated adopted twins than among the adoptive families who reared them. In contrast, higher rates of shared behavior problems among adopted children and their adoptive families would point to aspects of child rearing in problem development.

Twin studies have revealed that genes underlie family similarities in many skills and behaviors. For example, research suggests that the heritability of general mental ability (as shown in ability to do schoolwork) is relatively high (McClearn et al., 1997). This means that there is probably a sizable genetic effect on mental abilities as measured by intelligence tests and other cognitive tests. The concordance rate of a trait is determined by measuring how often one member of a pair of twins has the trait when the other member also has it. That is, if both twins always share the trait of high intelligence when one twin is highly intelligent, the concordance rate for intelligence is 100%. When identical twins have significantly higher concordance rates than fraternal twins, the trait in question is presumed to be highly genetically determined. The pairs of identical twins studied by McClearn's group had a 62% concordance rate for general mental abilities, which was much higher than the concordance rate for the fraternal twins studied. Of course, this leaves a significant role for the environment in determining mental ability.

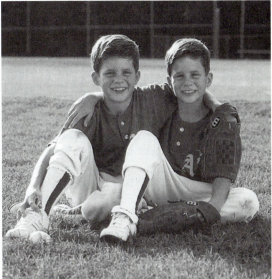

Identical twins may look so much alike that they are mistaken for each other, even by close friends and family members. Their social environments are the most similar for any pairs of siblings, which may account for some of their behavioral similarity.

Evaluation of Genetic Models of Abnormality

Critics have complained that environmental similarities could explain many of the behavioral resemblances of twins, particularly identical twins, who share the most similar environments, from the time of conception onward. Perhaps a stronger test is provided by comparing sets of identical and fraternal twins, some of whom are adopted and others are not. If genes determine personality, identical twins reared apart should have more similar personality traits than fraternal twins reared apart. It is difficult to find a large enough group of twins reared apart to conduct this type of research, but psychologists at the University of Minnesota have done so and have reported remarkable personality similarities among adult identical twins separated at birth (Hur, Bouchard, & Eckert, 1998; Newman, Tellegen, & Bouchard, 1998). These investigators estimate that the heritability of traits such as shyness or social sensitivity is between .30 and .50, which indicates that genetic factors account for approximately half of the person's shyness or social sensitivity. They describe amazing correspondences between the life choices of some identical twins reared apart from infancy to the time when the study brought them together. For example, some separated identical twins independently selected the same occupation, married women with the same first name, selected the same name for one of their children, named their dogs the same, had the same hobbies, and had similar decorations in their houses. No, there are no genes for selecting mates, names, or hobbies, but the researchers drew the conclusion that people with identical genes may be drawn to the same activities, occupation, and life-style.

Unfortunately, the researchers in the Minnesota study did not provide a detailed list of the dissimilarities of identical twins, reared either together or apart. That list should also be quite long, and there should be some remarkable similarities in the independent choices of less closely related pairs such as fraternal twins, non-twin siblings, and unrelated people. One cannot claim uncanny resemblances between identical twins reared apart without presenting comparative data on the number of similarities between fraternal twins reared apart, both types of twins reared together, and non-twin siblings reared together and apart.

Behavioral geneticists offer another intriguing alternative genetic explanation of social behavior. Suppose the effect of genes is indirect. What if genes affect behaviors that shape a person's social environment, which then affects his or her behavior? The resulting social context could promote some behaviors (e.g., high activity, hostility, or nurturance) and discourage others, appearing to be a case of simple environmental control. So a very smart, active, vigorous child would look and act appealing. This appealing child would inspire many more people to approach, interact with him, and teach him various skills (affect his social environment) than would a dull, lethargic child. We know that a person's behavior, whether hostile, friendly, depressed, or elated, affects other people and creates corresponding social environments. If a child's behavior is strongly genetically determined and draws certain types of responses from others, then genes indirectly create environments. If so, the inferred genetic influences would be as important in determining the child's behavior as the observable social influences in the child's environment.

The view that genetic endowment increases a person's chances of entering or creating particular types of social situations is called the **reciprocal gene-environment model** (Rende & Plomin, 1992). This model features the idea that genetic vulnerabilities can increase a person's exposure to the very situations that create problems for the person. For example, a person with a genetic tendency toward shyness and depression may be repelled by outgoing, optimistic romantic partners and may focus on potential mates who also are shy and depressed. This sets the scene for both the person and her partner to become depressed. In relation to antisocial behavior, those people who are genetically at risk because they have antisocial close relatives are the most likely to develop problems when placed in a disruptive and discordant environment (Rutter, Giller, & Hagell, 1998).

High heritabilities of such unlikely characteristics as being divorced appear to support the reciprocal gene-environment model. Divorce is shared by fraternal twins twice as often as by unrelated pairs of people, but is shared an amazing six times more often by identical twins than by unrelated individuals (McGue & Lykken, 1992). A problem with the view that divorce has high heritability is the difficulty in connecting genes with something as complicated as marriage and divorce. Do some people have such difficult personalities that divorce is inevitable, or do they tend to select partners who are detestable? Does being an identical twin place some unusual burden on the twins and their spouses? At this point, the causal path is not apparent, and everyone is free to speculate about what may be going on.

Perils of Behavioral Genetics Research

It is important to understand why it is so difficult to connect specific genes with specific psychological disorders. First, the complex and subtle contributions of many genes are much more difficult to trace than are those of a single gene. Another problem is that many psychological or mental disorders are difficult to diagnose, which makes them difficult to study genetically. For example, clinicians may disagree on whether a child has ADHD, conduct disorder, depression, or all three disorders. If the diagnosis is uncertain, there is little hope of locating a genetic problem since some of the children studied will actually have the disorder, while others will not. It's like trying to find the genes for blonde hair color when some of the people you erroneously identify as blondes are actually bleached brunettes. Having them in your study group only confuses the search.

In the case of June, learning disabilities could be her basic problem, but she could also be an insecure child with oppositional defiant disorder who refuses to pay any attention to her schoolwork and fails because of emotional and motivational problems. So a precise diagnosis is absolutely essential in the study of behavioral genetics, and many types of childhood mental disorder are difficult to assess and diagnose accurately (see Chapter 4 for a discussion of assessment).

In fact, as you can see, research in genetics is highly complicated, and many of the presumed causal paths cannot be directly observed. Present methods for assaying many physiological agents in the body are still imprecise, so we must often rely on studies of animals. Unfortunately, various species differences mean that animal studies do not apply perfectly to humans. Also, blood levels of many neurotransmitters and other substances do not invariably indicate behavioral problems in children, even if they do so with some accuracy in adults. For unknown reasons, individuals who have atypical levels of particular hormones or neurotransmitters may or may not eventually develop the disorder linked to their particular physical condition (Valenstein, 1998). There is no perfect correspondence between brain structure, genes, or biochemistry and behavior disorder. Instead, genetic endowment most often creates predispositions to develop certain disorders, given a particular set of biological and environmental conditions, and many different genes and circumstances must occur together to create a disorder.

Structure and Functions of the Brain

IN FOCUS 2 ▶ Describe the functions associated more extensively with the left and the right hemispheres of the cerebral cortex. When can one hemisphere compensate for damage to the other?

Everyday speech is rich with phrases that suggest that the brain controls behavior. Comments such as "It's all in your head" and "He should get his head examined" attest to the common belief that if there is something wrong with your behavior, it must be because there is something wrong with your brain. Scientists know that the brain-behavior link is not as simple as is commonly believed and, in fact, is one of the most complex phenomena they study. Modern neuro-

science is making unprecedented advances in revealing the operation of the nervous system, and especially the brain. To help you understand some of this new knowledge about the brain and behavior linkages, we must first explain some basics of the structure and activities of the nervous system. The central nervous system (CNS) consists of the brain and spinal cord and is connected to the peripheral nervous system (PNS), which consists of the somatic and the autonomic nervous systems. The brain is composed of billions of neurons (nerve cells) that are interconnected in complex ways. These neurons transmit information within the brain and throughout the body to control thoughts and actions. (The complexity and essentiality of the brain, plus its vulnerability, provide excellent reasons to wear protective sports helmets to avoid head injuries, no matter how much macho motorcyclists despise them.)

Neurotransmitters

There is a space between the spot where one neuron in a pathway terminates and the next one begins. To bridge the gap, chemical agents called **neurotransmitters** are released by the transmitting neuron and stimulate the receptors of the receiving neuron to transmit or inhibit the nerve impulse. This may sound like a simple process, but like many other physiological processes, it seems ever more complex as research advances. Each neuron is surrounded by many others, some of which connect with it functionally at junctions called **synapses.** Excitatory synapses affect the receiving neuron, making it more likely to respond, but inhibitory synapses act to decrease the activity of the receiving neuron. Whether a neuron will fire a signal to other neurons in its pathway depends in part on the accumulated strength of the excitatory versus the inhibitory synapses.

Let's take the neurotransmitter **dopamine** as an example. Originally, it seemed that excess dopamine might be responsible for schizophrenia, because antipsychotic drugs (which treated schizophrenia) were found to block dopamine receptors and lower dopamine activity. Thus, it seemed that overly active dopamine circuits could be responsible for schizophrenia. However, it was later discovered that some effective drug treatments for schizophrenia have little effect on dopamine receptors. So levels of dopamine do not seem to account for schizophrenia. Also, inter-

Table 2-1 Some Neurotransmitters and Their Presumed Actions	
Serotonin	Acts on many behaviors, particularly information processing and moods. Low activity levels in suicide, aggression, sexual excesses, impulsive overeating.
Gamma-aminobutyric acid (GABA)	Reduces anxiety, inhibits behaviors and emotions, reduces overall arousal, reduces emotional responses
Norepinephrine	May act generally to regulate or moderate behavioral tendencies. One circuit influences flight or fight reactions.
Dopamine	Activates other neurotransmitters to inhibit or facilitate emotions and behavior. Associated with exploratory, pleasure-seeking behavior. Associated with Parkinson's disease and possibly with schizophrenia.

connections of dopamine and **serotonin** (another neurotransmitter) circuits make the independent action of dopamine difficult to detect. To add complexity, there are five and possibly more different neuron receptor sites for dopamine, and each may respond differently to other neurotransmitters (Owens, Mulcahey, Stout, & Plotsky, 1997).

Some other neurotransmitters that are involved or probably involved in psychological disorders include norepinephrine and gamma-aminobutyric acid (GABA). These neurotransmitters and their presumed actions are described in Table 2-1. This table necessarily oversimplifies neurotransmitter activity, since many of these substances act on other neurotransmitters and on nervous system activity generally and their actions can be subtle and complex. Relatively little is known about them at this time, although they are under intense research scrutiny.

Links between Brain, Behavior, and Psychopathology

This section briefly reviews some of the basic anatomy and functioning of the brain, especially those aspects relating to psychological disturbances. Neuro-

science has made impressive advances in the past decades and has contributed important information about the role of the CNS in processes such as movement, speech, language comprehension, planning, and memory (Rapp, 2001). Less is known about the neural basis of most behavior disorders, although many theories have been offered. Later chapters will refer to brain structures, so the descriptions in this section will also be useful in understanding some specific disorders, especially anxiety, depression, autism, and learning disorders.

Figure 2-2 is a schematic drawing of the brain, showing portions of the hindbrain, midbrain, and forebrain. Many areas of the brain and peripheral nervous system are involved in behavior, whether normal or abnormal. As we explain these functions, it will also become clear that the linkages between what we experience, how we act, and how the central nervous system operates are so multiple and interactive that effects of nature and experience are difficult to isolate. The structure and functions of the brain are affected by what we experience, and, in turn, our behavior depends on brain activation.

Let's consider the large and prominent forebrain first. The **cerebral cortex,** which contains most of the neurons in the CNS, is a deeply wrinkled surface layer divided into obvious right and left hemispheres. The hemispheres are connected by nerve fibers, and each has some specialized functions. Popular psychology has greatly exaggerated the sex differences in hemispheric functioning and related hemispheric differences to alleged personality types. There is little research support for such claims. The left hemisphere is more responsible for speech and other cognitive processes, such as memory and reasoning, while the right hemisphere predominates in perception and creating images. However, some language functions, such as comprehending the positive or negative emotional quality of someone's speech and expressing emotional aspects of language are traced to activity in the *right* temporal area of the cerebral cortex and not the left hemisphere, which controls other language functions (Kandel, 2000). Thus, both right and left hemispheres are involved in speech and language. Usually, the two cerebral hemispheres coordinate smoothly with each other to produce normal, skilled behavior. Early in life, one hemisphere can assume some of the functions of a damaged opposite hemi-

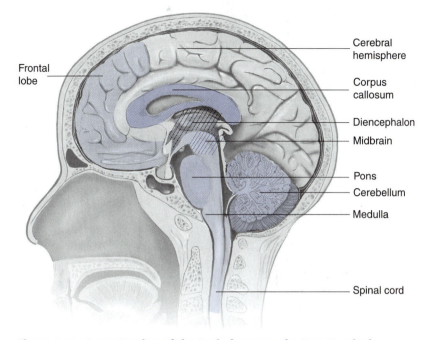

Figure 2-2   Cross-Section of the Brain between the Two Hemispheres, Showing the Main Parts of the Brain

sphere. For example, children younger than age 7 who have severe left cerebral hemisphere damage can still develop normal language, apparently through the functioning of the right cerebral hemisphere (Johnson, 2000). Different regions of the cortex appear to be involved in infants' language acquisition than in adults' language use, especially the extent and pattern of cortical lateralization (left or right hemisphere activity) related to expressive and receptive speech (Johnson, 2000).

The cerebral cortex has four lobes (frontal, parietal, temporal, and occipital), and each lobe has a different function. The forebrain also contains three deeper structures: the basal ganglia, the hippocampus, and the amygdaloid nuclei located in the amygdala. The amygdaloid nuclei are important to the study of abnormal behavior because they coordinate the functions underlying emotional states. Other brain areas important to psychological disorders include the diencephalon, which contains the thalamus and hypothalamus. The thalamus appears to process and transmit information from the rest of the CNS to the cerebral cortex, while the hypothalamus affects autonomic, en-

docrine, and gut functions. The hypothalamus and endocrine system form the **hypothalamic-pituitary-adrenalcortical axis (HYPAC);** see Figure 2-3. The hypothalamus affects the pituitary gland, which coordinates the endocrine system. If the pituitary gland stimulates the cortical portion of the adrenal glands (located on top of the kidneys), epinephrine is released to energize and support strenuous action. However, the adrenal cortex also produces a stress hormone called **cortisol,** which is elevated during stressful life events and in some cases of adult depression and anxiety.

The brain sites located below the cerebral cortex and closer to the rest of the body (the midbrain, cerebellum, pons, medulla oblongata, and spinal cord) are associated with the more automatic functions such as respiration, digestion, heart rate, movement, and balance.

How does this material on the nervous system relate to the case of June? Our brief summary of the genetic and neuroscience view of behavioral disturbances suggests that CNS dysfunctions may play a role in June's learning problems. However, it is difficult to determine whether her behavior and learning prob-

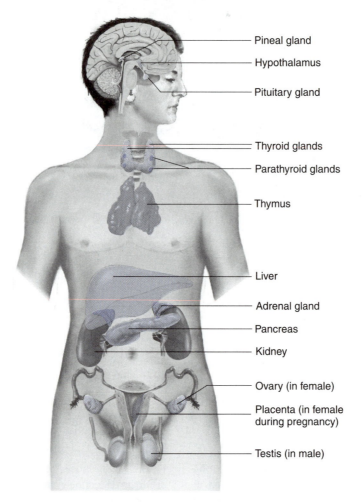

Figure 2-3 The HYPAC Axis and Locations of Some of the Major Endocrine Glands

lems come from a genetic predisposition, a neurotransmitter dysfunction, or some type of brain damage. We now turn to psychological theories to see what they can offer to help us understand June's behavior.

A PSYCHODYNAMIC EXPLANATION: FREUD'S PSYCHOANALYTIC THEORY

IN FOCUS 3 ▶ Identify the four main themes of Freud's theory of personality.

Many people would attribute June's learning problems and antisocial tendencies to her early relationships with her parents, particularly her mother. The common tendency to blame mothers for their children's adjustment problems may be attributable to the immense influence of one man, Sigmund Freud (1856–1939). Freud's theory of psychoanalysis has been the most powerful single influence on popular beliefs about the origins and nature of psychopathology. Formulated in the late 19th century, **psychoanalytic theory** (and many variants, all called psychodynamic theories) has long dominated in psychiatry, psychology, literature, and the arts, with forays into politics, sociology, and a host of other disciplines. Generations of authors and clinicians have been profoundly affected by Freud's dramatic explanation of

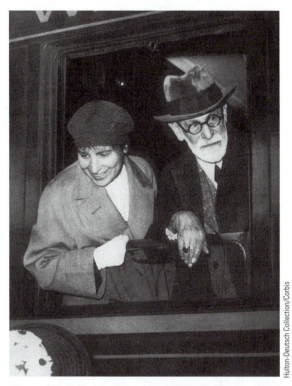

Sigmund Freud in later life, accompanied by his daughter, Anna Freud, who was also a prominent psychoanalyst.

is the first and most primitive component of personality. The id seeks immediate gratification of needs, regardless of consequences. "It [the id] is demanding, impulsive, irrational, asocial, selfish, and pleasure-loving. It is the spoiled child of personality" (Hall, 1954, p. 21). Clearly, it is impossible to get everything immediately, so the ego develops and operates more realistically. The ego operates on the reality principle, taking existing reality constraints into account. As the decision-making, executive branch of personality, the ego must deal with the id's demands, but must also serve a third, equally demanding system of the personality, the superego.

The superego represents the harsh moral code derived from what the child believes the strict, unforgiving parents want. The superego drives the person to try to meet unattainably high standards in controlling the sex and aggression instincts. Of course, that is impossible, so the superego punishes the ego with guilt even for merely thinking about satisfying the id's demands. There is no anatomical location for the id, ego, and superego in the brain or body. They are merely constructs meant to explain irrational and conflicted human behavior.

human development. Freud's theory is very rich in clinical observations and dramatic interpretations of behavior, but some of the main elements can be summarized as follows:

- People are irrational and seldom can act or think clearly.
- Even young children are naturally sexually jealous, aggressive, self-centered, and anxiety-ridden, although they are not conscious of these feelings.
- Our personalities are formed early in childhood and change little thereafter.
- Early hostile, competitive, and sexual attractions to parents must be confronted and worked through in order to achieve normality in adulthood.

The Structure of Personality

In Freud's view, personality is composed of three systems—the id, ego, and superego—which interact to produce both normal and abnormal behavior. The id

Stages of Psychosexual Personality Development

Freud believed that much of adult personality is formed during the first 5 years of life, when powerful, pleasant sensations are supposed to be focused on different parts of the body referred to as erogenous zones. These follow a developmental pattern in Freud's view, beginning with the oral area of the mouth and lips, which are stimulated during nursing and are a major source of gratification for the baby. Either too much gratification or too little can produce a fixation at the oral stage that is thought to result in lifelong character traits such as dependency and could lead to later oral dependence on cigarettes, alcohol, or drugs.

Next, in the anal stage, the area of the anus supposedly becomes the focus of pleasurable sensations. Toilet training occurs at this time and helps determine later personality traits such as overeagerness to please others by producing products such as art, writing, or other tangible creations. Frustration in the anal stage is supposed to produce a person who is compulsively neat and tidy, stingy, and unable to complete projects.

At around 4 or 5 years of age, the phallic stage begins, and the child's genital area becomes the primary focus for gratification. This is when the crucially important Oedipus complex is resolved. The child is supposed to become sexually attracted to the parent of the opposite sex, much as the ancient Greek mythical hero Oedipus did to his own mother. Freud paid most attention to sons, but also believed that daughters were sexually attracted to their fathers. In the Oedipus complex, the little boy feels sexual rivalry toward his father and becomes guilty and fears his father's retaliation by castration. To relieve his anxiety, the boy is presumed to repress his incestuous desire for his mother and his hostility toward his father by identifying with his father and trying to be as much like him as possible. In this way, the boy reduces anxiety, possesses the mother at least indirectly through his bond with his father, and forms a masculine sexual identity. Failure to resolve the Oedipal conflict presumably results in enduring psychological problems. Freud originally felt that girls never developed as satisfactory a moral sense as males because they do not experience and overcome a strong, complete Oedipus complex. The general principle is that even seemingly inconsequential events and minor adjustment difficulties during childhood are presumed to produce lifelong psychological problems.

Evaluation of Freud's Psychoanalytic Theory

Despite its implausibility, many internal inconsistencies, and lack of research support, Freud's theory remains perhaps the best known of all the psychological explanations of human conduct. Freud intellectually demolished the general beliefs that children lack sexual interests and adults behave rationally. He also contributed psychoanalysis, an intervention for psychologically disturbed people that guided psychiatric assessment and treatment for many decades. Many trained psychoanalysts and people who have been psychoanalyzed credit psychoanalysis with a profound understanding of their behavior and significantly improved functioning. These personal testimonials provide the major ongoing support of the psychodynamic approach. However, other theories inspired by psychoanalysis, such as object relations theory and attachment theory, have more research support and

continue to be important contributors to the field of child psychopathology (see later sections of this chapter and Chapter 15).

Yet Freud's work has been as savagely criticized as it has passionately defended. Well over a century after his work began, debate rages over the value and validity of his contribution (Crews, 1996; Macmillan, 1991). It is generally agreed that psychoanalytic theories are more self-contradictory, more complex, and less parsimonious (simple and straightforward) than competing models. Critics complain about the lack of rigorous research testing of psychoanalytic propositions. Crews (1996) termed Freud's theory "pseudoscience" because it lacks independent confirmation. In addition, the theory is too vague and inconsistent to be testable, relying instead on Freud's personal authority and on clinical experiences for support (Crews, 1996; Macmillan, 1991). There is also little empirical evidence for the effectiveness of psychoanalysis as a treatment, and the developmental basis of the theory is debatable, since it was built on the retrospective accounts of patients rather than on the study of children (Fonagy & Target, 2000). Critics complain that psychoanalytic theory is dated, because it contains gender, cultural, and ethnic biases and does not incorporate advances in the biological and social sciences (Frosh, 1997). Supporters draw largely on their personal conviction that Freud is right, based on their own psychoanalytic training and clinical work with troubled individuals.

Most writers no longer accept all of Freud's original theory, although many people have adapted it for their own purposes. The ego theorists, discussed next, regret the emphasis on sex and aggression in Freud's account of personality development. They suggest devoting greater attention to the more rational aspects of human nature and believe that personality development can continue into adulthood.

FREUD'S HERITAGE: EGO THEORY, ATTACHMENT THEORY, AND OBJECT RELATIONS THEORY

Erikson's Ego Theory

Unlike Freud, who focused on psychopathology, many theorists who were influenced by him stressed the more rational, less destructive components of personality. We

PEANUTS

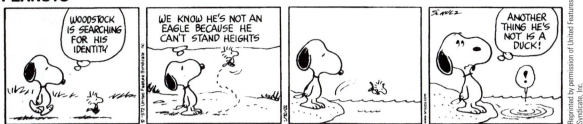

According to Erikson, identity crises can occur in early adolescence.

will consider one such theorist, Erik Erikson. Erikson wrote about the development of the healthy personality in the broader culture. Erikson's theme was **ego identity,** or the individual's healthy solution to a sequence of identity crises associated with each psychosocial stage of life. The person encounters a progression of eight major psychosocial crises, each of which must be mastered in order to achieve psychological health and ego identity and move on to the next maturational stage, until the highest level is achieved. Erikson's psychosocial stages are presented in Table 2-2.

Some of Erikson's stages derive from Freud's, while others are original and extend into maturity and old age. The stages are labeled in terms of opposites (e.g., industry v. inferiority), but Erikson believed that most people's adjustment lies somewhere between these extremes. For example, we all have some trust in others and some mistrust. Like Freud, Erikson believed that early childhood experiences with parents form personality. The mother's handling of the feeding situation could determine how trusting or wary the infant will be, both at the time and later. The crisis of autonomy v. shame and doubt surrounds toilet training and affects the child's growing sense of independence. Good experiences lead to self-control and high self-esteem, and bad ones produce problems such as compulsivity, stinginess, self-doubt, and hostility. The child faces another identity crisis in early adolescence (Erikson, 1968), when puberty and new role expectations can lead to confusion about who one is and should be. Successful resolution of this crisis produces a strong sense of individuality and self-confidence.

Erikson believed that the sequence and timing of the psychosocial stages are genetically determined, but

Table 2-2 Erikson's Psychosocial Stages		
Stage Name	**Age**	**Description**
Autonomy versus shame and doubt	Infant	The infant learns to trust or mistrust the mother and others.
Initiative versus guilt	Years 3–5	At the time of the toilet training, the child learns independence, self-control, and self-esteem or hostility, compulsivity, and low self-esteem.
Industry versus inferiority	Before puberty	At the resolution of the Oedipal conflict, the child develops initiative and competency or guilt and inability to function. The child realizes his abilities through work or sloth and inferiority.
Identity versus role diffusion	Adolescence	The adolescent's successful resolution of the identity crisis yields comfort and good adjustment or the opposite.
Intimacy versus isolation	Young adulthood	The young adult chooses between love and marriage or loneliness.
Generativity versus stagnation	Maturity	The adult chooses children and interests in others or selfish self-interest.
Integrity versus despair	Old age	The elderly person feels pride in her life or despair.

culture determines how the person resolves the identity crises. Unfortunately, Erikson's theory is scarcely more focused and scientifically verifiable than Freud's. Judged on this criterion, most of the psychodynamic theories fail, but attachment theory and object relations theory, which incorporate some psychodynamic features, have generated significantly more research support.

Attachment Theory

IN FOCUS 4 ▶ Explain how secure and insecure attachment develop, and describe the effect of each.

Attachment theory was originated by a British psychiatrist, John Bowlby (1969), who was struck by the importance of the infant-mother emotional bond in many species, including humans. Psychodynamic theories also consider such attachments between mother and infant to be among the most important events in early development. Attachment theory has become one of the most influential explanations of early social and emotional adjustment in humans. Developed in large part by the research and writing of Mary Ainsworth and her collaborators (Ainsworth, Blehar, Waters, & Wall, 1978), **attachment theory** is one of the few approaches that systematically analyze actual observations of mother-infant interaction to explain the emergence of normal and disturbed social behavior. According to attachment theory, attachment is focused on one person, ideally the mother, although secondary attachments to other people may develop. Many authorities believe that attachment is a lifelong process, and that how you function as a parent or a spouse depends in part on how good or bad your early attachment experience was when you were a baby. Normal social development throughout the formative years is based on the young infant's developing trust in a warm, sensitive caretaker called an **attachment figure** (this is the child's primary caregiver, usually the mother). People may form attachments to additional people throughout life, but the original attachment is the strongest and most influential. From experiences with the mother, the baby forms internal working models or mental representations of the mother's typical behavior toward him and his own behavior. In this way, the infant internalizes the mother's reactions as expectations of how

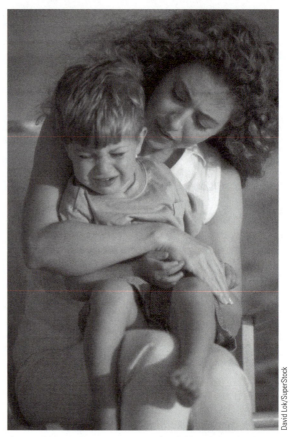

The positive or negative nature of a child's early relationship with his mother can affect his perceptions of her, himself, and other people throughout life.

others will behave, whether warm and sensitive, neutral, or distant and abusive. However, a person's mental model (understanding) of a relationship as an adult is not completely set in childhood, but is open to ongoing experiences with other people within meaningful relationships (Owens et al., 1995). This means that factors in addition to early attachments help determine the quality and meaning of adult relationships. Such formative factors include the child's growing cognitive capacity, changes in family structure and functioning, and conversations with parents that alter the child's understanding of events (Thompson, 2000).

A baby with a secure attachment feels safe in the caretaker's presence, and when the mother is near, the baby is free to roam and explore the environment (secure-base behavior) and freely express her feelings, learning a great deal in the process. Thus, a sensitive caregiver provides a source of affection, a safe haven during danger, and someone who can help the baby to minimize negative emotional states (Seifer & Schiller, 1995). In contrast, a child with an insensitive or rejecting parent and an insecure attachment behaves less adaptively when rejoining the mother after a brief separation. Some insecurely attached children appear to avoid their mothers when rejoining them, appearing to prefer solitary play, while others angrily reject their mothers' play overtures. Still others, probably the most disturbed, may appear dazed and unfocused, showing disorganized behavior. The children with disorganized attachment are the most likely to have mothers who are dysfunctional and preoccupied because they are seriously depressed, abusive, or addicted to drugs (Lyons-Ruth, Bronfman, & Parsons, 1999; Teti, Gelfand, Messinger, & Isabella, 1995).

Evaluation of Attachment Theory

The quality of the child's attachment to major caretakers may change over time, but more often it remains the same through the first few years of life. It is difficult to distinguish between effects of early attachment quality and the child's later relationships with parents, because parent-child relationship patterns most often persist over time. Child adjustment problems that are attributed to early attachment alone may in fact be due to the continuing poor quality of the parent-child relationship from birth throughout the preschool years (Lamb, Thompson, Gardner, & Charnov, 1985). It is reasonable to expect that both past and present experiences affect the child's adjustment. Research evidence suggests that the quality of early attachment influences a person's later relationships. But does a working model based on the primary attachment figure and self and formed early in life serve as the framework for later relationships (Owens et al., 1995)? Although quality of current attachment relates to a child's adjustment, there is insufficient evidence that early troubled attachment strongly predicts later psychopathology (Cicchetti, Toth, & Lynch, 1995). To summarize, the jury is still out on the question of whether later mental disorders can be traced directly to disturbed early attachments.

Object Relations and Interpersonal Theories

Elements of Freud's theory appearing in present-day **object relations theory** include the lasting importance of the emotional tone of early mother-child relations, identification with the parent(s), and the child's internalization of parents' attitudes and behavior toward the child. The term *object relations* refers not to physical objects, but to human social and emotional relations (Cashdan, 1988). Like attachment theory, object relations theory stresses the lasting influence of early relationships with important others, especially the mother. From this early emotional tie, the child forms stable, internalized beliefs about himself and other people.

Psychological problems arise if a mother is rejecting, preoccupied with her own concerns, or highly stressed and consequently insensitive to her child. The child comes to imitate and identify with the mother and other important caretakers, viewing herself as these people do (**introjection**). Like these caretakers, the child thinks of herself as dumb or bright, good or bad, reacting as though the person who was the original attachment object was still present (**internalization**). In this way, a child develops high or low self-esteem, which may endure throughout life. She reacts toward new people in a manner that draws the very same internalized reactions she expects. So people who view themselves as needy but rejected may be drawn to the particular types of partners who reject them. Expectations derived from early relationships with caretakers are exaggerated, persistent, and resistant to change.

Benjamin's Interpersonal Psychology

Lorna Benjamin (1974, 1993, 1995) presents a model of interpersonal functioning featuring interactive roles played by parents and children or by other pairs of emotionally involved people, such as spouses or psychotherapists and their clients. As shown in Figure 2-4, a mother who protects her child is more likely to have a child who is trusting and relying (complementary mother-child behaviors). A mother who is emancipating and grants her child independence will probably have a child who is assertive and separate. The major themes are that some patterns of behavior naturally elicit certain complementary behaviors in return and these interac-

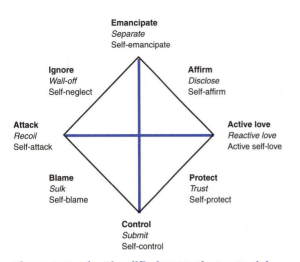

Figure 2-4   The Simplified SASB Cluster Model
The poles of the axes, starting at the right-hand side and moving clockwise, are Love, Enmeshment, Hostility, and Differentiation. Points between the poles consist of components of the nearest poles (see text for further explanation).

tion patterns can become stable and persistent, extending beyond the person's original interactions with the mother early in childhood. Thus, learning continues throughout the life cycle as the person develops new relationships. Attachment interactions that involve affiliation and warmth are considered necessary for positive interpersonal interactions and mental health. Those that involve hostility compose the disrupted attachment group and warn of adjustment problems to come.

Parent-child interaction patterns tend to become progressively more stable and predictable as children approach adolescence (Benjamin, 1974). The child's continuing goal is to maintain closeness with primary caregivers. In order to gain actual or psychological proximity to the parent or other caregiver, children develop and internalize specific ways of treating others and themselves. The physical presence of the parent is no longer necessary, since the child reacts to the parent's internalized presence. The attitudes and behaviors learned within early relationships with important others are internalized and re-experienced through identification, recapitulation, and introjection, processes described as follows:

- *Identification.* Through long experience with a caregiver, the child comes to act like the caregiver and display similar behaviors.

- *Recapitulation.* Over time, the particular behavior patterns of the caregiver come to reliably draw predictable responses from the child; for example, a mother's hostile belittling and blaming of her child are likely to produce a general pattern of hostile passive aggression in other relationships.

- *Introjection.* A person treats himself as he was treated by caregivers early in life. For example, a boy who was often criticized by his mother for expressing affection may come to criticize himself for expressions of affection, even when they are appropriate. According to Benjamin, copying of one's parents is an inevitable part of children's lives, and it is crucially important that what is copied is positive, healthy behavior.

Interpersonal theory has gained popularity because of its clinical usefulness in diagnosis and treatment and because of its growing research support. Nevertheless, it is extremely difficult to pinpoint the cause of interpersonal distress as mentally internalized expectations formed in the early years of life. Although Benjamin's model yields testable hypotheses, her theory has not yet been subjected to formal clinical trials. Nevertheless, many diagnosticians and therapists find this approach very powerful, insightful, and useful.

June's Case and Object Relations and Interpersonal Theories

In the case that opened this chapter, June's mother and father would be prime suspects in the development of at least some of June's problems, including her hostility toward her teacher, her growing resentment at her parents' nagging, and her stealing. June's mother probably tried to be a good parent, but her attitude toward her daughter might be described in object relations terms as controlling and blaming. Unfortunately, this parenting style is likely to draw hostile submission from June, possibly developing into active resentment as she enters her teens.

As always, there is an alternative explanation for the mother's negative reaction to her daughter. What if the mother's rejecting behavior followed rather than preceded June's problems? Perhaps the long-suffering mother finally lost patience with June's poor school performance and defeatist attitude and only then became controlling and blaming. Often only the retrospective reports of therapy clients attest to the aversive behavior of their parents, and no direct observations were made of the early parent-child interactions. In searching for a cause of their misery, troubled therapy clients are likely to exaggerate their parents' early ill treatment of them. Clinicians cannot verify that poor parenting was responsible for the child's later problems, and it is always possible that overburdened parents are inaccurately portrayed as villains. Memories are subject to a host of distortions. Note, though, that the same difficulty in reconstructing early parent-child relationships poses a problem for *any* theory that focuses on early socialization.

Developmental Psychopathology

Rather than competing with existing theories and facts, the developmental psychopathology perspective provides a broad, integrative framework within which the contributions of separate disciplines can be fully realized in the broader context of understanding individual development and functioning. (Cicchetti & Sroufe, 2000, p. 256)

Developmental psychopathology is an emerging theory of very broad scope that aims to understand the roots and development of child disturbances of many different types through the use of concepts derived from approaches ranging from neuroscience to behavioral and psychodynamic theories. Complexity is a key aspect of this theory, which holds that there are potentially many different paths to the development of a particular disorder and that more than one disorder can result from any particular risk factor. That is, some children become depressed because they are mistreated by their parents, while others have a strong genetic predisposition to depression and become depressed after their parents divorce each other, and still others are depressed because they were raised by depressed parents. Research reveals that some children respond to a risk such as having a severely depressed mother with depression, others become hostile and aggressive, and still others resist psychopathology and develop normally. The principles of equifinality (many possible causes for a particular outcome) and multifinality (many possible outcomes for a particular cause) are emphasized in this theory (and defined in Chapter 1). Developmental psy-

chopathology aims to uncover risk factors leading to children's problems, individual differences in vulnerability to risks, and individual responses to preventive and treatment interventions.

Developmental psychopathology aims for a comprehensive understanding of the origins, maintenance, and treatment of adaptation problems in *individual children* as they grow and develop. The approach seeks to understand the child by measuring the effects of all developmental influences including genetic, evolutionary, cognitive, emotional, biochemical, and social factors (Rutter & Sroufe, 2000). Most developmental theories concentrate on either environmental or biological-physiological factors, but developmental psychopathology aims to incorporate an understanding of both sets of interacting influences. The ultimate goal is accurate prediction of long-range outcomes from the study of early experiences and adjustment status. Developmental psychopathology seeks answers to questions such as these: How does infant insecure attachment affect the person's adjustment at later periods such as at preschool, elementary and high school, and adult periods? Does difficult infant temperament predict later adjustment under particular circumstances? Developmental psychopathologists advocate a wide-ranging, *interdisciplinary study* of the etiology and course of *individual patterns of behavior adaptation* for children with mental retardation, autism, externalizing or aggressive behavior, and hyperactivity (described in a series of volumes of the Rochester Symposium on Developmental Psychopathology and published by the University of Rochester Press). This approach rejects a rigid stage view of development but incorporates some concepts from the cognitive developmental theory of Piaget, developmental neurology, and physiology. It also draws on concepts from ethology (the evolutionary study of animal behavior in natural settings) and from attachment theory.

Developmental psychopathology emphasizes that we cannot understand the developing child or predict her future without understanding the many aspects of her physical and psychosocial functioning. This is an ideal since, of course, it is not possible to identify all the factors that could influence a child's behavior and development. The obvious drawback of this approach is that it is perhaps too ambitious. It is a great challenge to master even one of the major fields involved in understanding child psychopathology and nearly impossible to know and combine all of them.

June's Case and Developmental Psychopathology

A developmental psychopathologist would find it important to observe June in her usual home and school settings to gain clues as to the causes of her problems. A thorough medical and neurological exam would be conducted to identify possible physical problems and June's intelligence would be tested by standard intelligence tests, achievement tests, and special tasks based on Piaget's work to see whether she is functioning at a developmentally appropriate level. Other psychological tests and interviews would concentrate on June's social adjustment with her family, teachers, and other children. The goal of developmental psychopathology is to carry out as complete as possible a process of assessment and treatment, using a multifaceted and multidisciplinary approach.

CONDITIONING, LEARNING, AND COGNITIVE PSYCHOLOGY EXPLANATIONS

The following theories are distinctive because they do not consider experiences during infancy to be the dominant, crucial determinants of later personality characteristics and adjustment. Instead, these learning-based theories hold that our behavior is largely determined by our current social environment in combination with previous experiences. People are not doomed to become maladjusted because of negative childhood experiences, because behavior is at least somewhat malleable throughout life. Of the learning theories, Skinner's operant learning model places the greatest emphasis on the influence of current experiences on normal and abnormal behavior.

Skinner's Operant Learning Model

Harvard experimental psychologist B. F. Skinner (1953) used animal conditioning principles to explain human behavior. Of the two basic types of learning—operant and respondent conditioning—Skinner devoted most of his attention to operant conditioning, which involves behaviors that are voluntary and pur-

poseful. Examples of operant behaviors include actions such as walking, dancing, marching, and studying, as well as speaking, singing, helping, hitting, and a host of other intended acts. In contrast, respondent behaviors typically involve the more automatic physiological reflexes such as salivation, release of gastric juices, blood pressure, breathing, or heart beat. Some types of learning seem to include elements of both types of conditioning and are not easily categorized.

Positive Reinforcement

IN FOCUS 5 ▶ Describe operant behavior and tell how it can be increased and decreased. Give some examples of operant behavior.

Operant behavior alters or operates on the physical or social environment in some way and is cued by situations that precede it, called **discriminative stimuli,** and controlled by the events that follow it (reinforcers or punishment). Discriminative stimuli can consist of the presence or actions of others, such as an instruction to sit down, or physical cues such as the presence of toys, work, or a television set. These stimuli signal that certain behaviors can be reinforced. (See Figure 2-5.) Operant acts that produce **reinforcing consequences** are likely to be repeated in similar circumstances in the future. Any event that strengthens a preceding operant response or makes it more likely to recur is a **reinforcer,** no matter whether it appears neutral or unpleasant to other people. What a person responds to as a reinforcer may change from time to time, and what one person finds reinforcing might be ineffective or even distasteful to someone else. Even winning an Academy Award or a Nobel Prize might fail to act as a reinforcer for some people. It's completely subjective. Some generalized reinforcers such as money and praise are widely effective and are often used in interventions with children in classroom and treatment settings. However, even these stimuli aren't invariably reinforcing, since praise from the wrong people or delivered at the wrong time can be repugnant. Perversely, some children find adults' scolding to have reinforcing properties, simply because it is a form of attention. This means that scolding can and often does unintentionally increase the rate of children's misbehavior.

Operant behavior can be eliminated through **extinction,** in which the usual reinforcement is com-

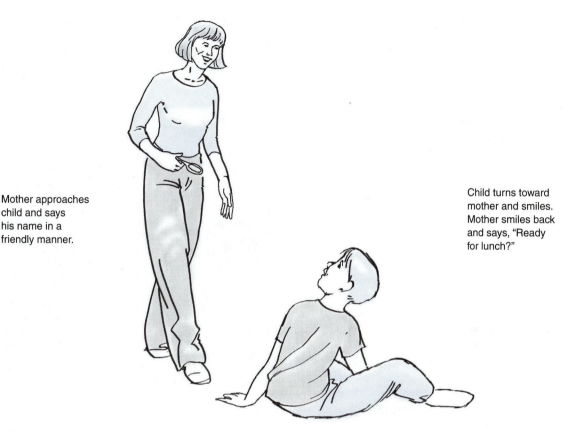

Mother approaches child and says his name in a friendly manner.

Child turns toward mother and smiles. Mother smiles back and says, "Ready for lunch?"

Figure 2-5   Skinner's Operant Conditioning Model
In operant learning, a parent's behavior, such as approaching the child in a friendly way, can serve as a discriminative stimulus, signaling the child to attend to the parent. Here, the child's operant behavior of turning toward the mother and replying is then reinforced by the mother's continued attention and announcement that it's time for lunch. What would happen if the child ignored the mother or defied her?

pletely withheld for a prolonged period. For example, parents may completely stop responding to their 2-year-old daughter when she refuses to go to sleep at bedtime despite reassurances and prolonged lullabies. Attempts at extinction may be unsuccessful if the behavior receives even occasional reinforcement (intermittent reinforcement), which is often the case. Deviant behavior that has been maintained by very occasional intermittent reinforcement may be highly resistant to extinction.

Punishment and Negative Reinforcement
Much human misery arises from punishment and negative reinforcement, two different procedures that are often confused. **Negative reinforcement** increases the rate of the behavior it follows exactly as positive reinforcement does. In negative reinforcement, the operant behavior is repeated because it removes an aversive stimulus. For example, yelling at a child to stop pulling the dog's ears will be reinforced if the child stops misbehaving. In contrast, **punishment** is the delivery of an aversive stimulus following some action, which reduces the future probability of that behavior. If the parent in our example abandons shouting and makes the child go to his room or slaps the child, the parent is using punishment.

Punishment can be cruel and often has unpredictable effects. The punished child does not learn what to do, but only what not to do or how to avoid detection while misbehaving. Skinner maintained that punishment is used much too freely and is often ineffective in deterring people from misbehaving. On the contrary, punishment creates resentment and invites retaliation.

Evaluation of Skinner's Model

Many of the behavior therapy procedures discussed in this book stem directly from Skinner's work. He aimed to improve human life in as many ways as possible, and he propounded one of the most focused, general, easily understood, and parsimonious explanations of behavior in humans and other species. Skinner proposed a limited number of well-defined, demonstrably powerful mechanisms to account for a wide range of abnormal and normal behavior across species. Critics such as linguist Noam Chomsky (1959) criticized Skinnerian theory as too simple and too much grounded in animal research to explain complex human activities such as language. Behavioral geneticists argue that much human behavior has a hereditary basis and is not simply learned. Applied behavior analysts, who use Skinner's principles, have made great strides in the treatment of persons with mental retardation, autistic and psychotic disorders, conduct disorders, antisocial personality disorder, and those with physical disabilities.

Bandura's Social Cognitive Theory

Skinner's psychology highlights the importance of environmental reactions such as other people's attention, approval, or disapproval in shaping and maintaining behavior. But can we break free of environmental forces and control our own lives? Albert Bandura's **social cognitive theory** (also called *social learning theory*) holds that humans' impressive mental abilities allow us to exert a significant amount of control over our own conduct regardless of powerful external influences. A person's *interpretation* of an event is the chief determinant of that person's reaction. For example, a student could view being called on to answer a question in class as a welcome opportunity to excel, a matter of little importance, or a trigger for an anxiety attack.

Mischel (1993) and Bandura stress the roles of both cognitive and social influences in human behavior. Cognitive social psychologists avoid ascribing general traits, such as hostile, dependent, or honest,

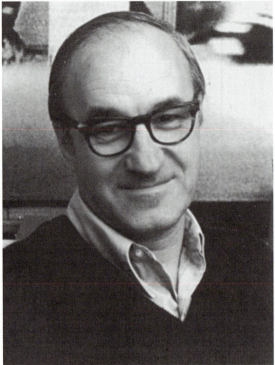

Courtesy of Dr. Albert Bandura

Albert Bandura changed psychology in the United States with his view that people initiate actions as well as being acted upon by their environment. He believes that one of the strongest determinants of behavior is a person's self-perception.

to people because trait concepts imply unrealistically high consistency and generality in responding in many different situations. People's behavior changes, depending on whom they are with, their current psychological and physical state, and whether they are relaxed, challenged, or stressed.

Bandura and Walters (1963) originally pointed out that humans are remarkably adept at **observational learning** (also called imitation, modeling, and vicarious learning). Their writing led to a vast amount of research illuminating the importance of modeling and imitation from earliest infancy to maturity. Many key skills are acquired though imitation alone. However, imitation is selective, and children imitate only some of the behavioral sequences they see in real life or the media. One important cause of faulty social learning is *exposure to socially deviant models,* for example, other children who behave highly aggressively or parents with mental disorders. In addition, other sources of children's abnormal behavior include:

- *Insufficient reinforcement,* which could lead to extinction of appropriate behaviors, as in a case where hostile or dangerously neglectful parents fail to reinforce a child's appropriate behavior.
- *Inappropriate reinforcement or reinforcement of undesirable behavior,* which can promote problem behavior. Delinquent gangs may differentially reinforce adolescents' cruel and violent acts, as shown by the remarks of a juvenile gang member about a murder in which he was involved: "If I would have got the knife, I would have stabbed him. That would have gave me more of a buildup. People would have respected me for what I've done and things like that. They would say, 'there goes a cold killer'" (Yablonsky, 1962, p. 8). This is a chilling example of the effects of social reinforcement of violence by a deviant group. Inappropriate reinforcement can also take the form of parental inconsistency. Parents can bewilder a child by violently punishing him for talking back to them on one occasion, ignoring him for the same behavior at other times, and then later praising him for sticking up for himself. In response, the child might come to behave erratically and perhaps violently because of his parents' inappropriate reinforcement and deviant modeling.
- *Faulty learning* of negative emotional states either directly or vicariously from observing another person. A child might develop a fear of doctors directly through being hurt and frightened while at the doctor's office or might be alarmed by observing a parent terrified at the thought of going to the doctor.
- *Fictional reinforcement contingencies* (Skinner's superstitious behavior) can exert great control over some people's behavior. Confused beliefs that household objects are dangerously contaminated by dirt can lead to compulsive cleaning and hand-washing rituals, and many other irrational beliefs may be acquired through the teachings of other people or may be self-generated. These fictional reinforcement contingencies can be more powerful than real ones.
- *Faulty self-reinforcement* can occur when people hold themselves to overly strict or overly lax stan-

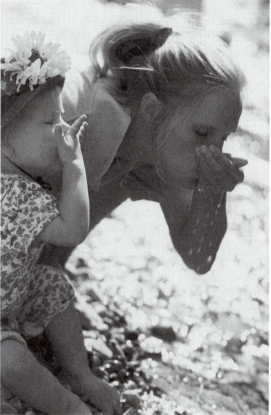

Humans are superb imitators, learning a wide variety of skills through simply observing others.

dards. Some people maintain such high standards for themselves that success is impossible and they eventually cease trying. Others are content with nearly anything they do, however minimal. Self-standards are learned from others through modeling and instruction from parents, teachers, or other influential people. Inappropriately demanding or highly permissive families and schools can instill unrealistic expectations and deviant self-reinforcement practices.

Self-Efficacy and Behavior

IN FOCUS 6 ▶ Define *self-efficacy,* and tell how high self-efficacy helps children solve problems.

Bandura's (1995, 1997) self-efficacy theory attempts to explain the mutual interacting influences of people's self-perceptions and their behavior. **Self-efficacy** is your belief in your own ability, a conviction that you can succeed at some type of task through skill, effort, and persistence. People high in self-efficacy are convinced of their own problem-solving effectiveness; those who are low in self-efficacy believe that they are doomed to fail. Self-efficacy convictions can prove self-fulfilling. People who have failed repeatedly in certain situations begin to believe they can never succeed at those types of tasks, so they don't try hard, fail, and come to avoid those types of tasks. Consider the student who is so terrified of failure and unconvinced of her own ability that she cannot think clearly while taking an achievement test and decides just to answer at random and leave as quickly as possible. With more self-confidence, she might pass the test. Lack of self-efficacy interferes with many types of skilled performance. Relevant self-efficacy beliefs act as shapers of children's career aspirations and progression into career paths (Bandura, Barbaranelli, Vittorio, & Pastorelli, 2001). Even with the necessary mathematical and spatial skills, a child who lacks confidence in her ability will not pursue a career in engineering.

Appropriate psychological treatment helps in several ways. A client's self-evaluation could be improved through positive self-talk, consisting of learning and practicing confident statements ("I'm smart." "I can do this.") in feared situations. Accomplishments are very important. Success at a series of tasks, beginning with the easiest and progressing gradually to more challenging ones further builds self-efficacy. Growing confidence leads to vigorous, persistent, and probably more successful attempts to cope with the problem. Success increases perceived self-effectiveness even further, creating a positive cycle of optimistic beliefs and effective behavior, as shown in Figure 2-6. Such success is the most potent and convincing source of increased self-confidence.

Other sources of information may also be helpful at times. Observing others succeed (vicarious success) can boost a child's self-confidence, but not as much as does experiencing actual success. People who have had problems tend to doubt their own skills until they have actually succeeded in performing a difficult task.

Instructional programs and psychotherapy rely on verbal persuasion, an even less convincing source of self-efficacy expectations than the preceding ones. You may have tried to convince a reluctant friend to engage in some feared activity or had others persuade you to try an activity that intimidates you. An even more formidable challenge is to try to convince a deeply depressed person to cheer up. It doesn't work very well. If only verbal persuasion and enthusiastic encouragement are used, improvement is unlikely.

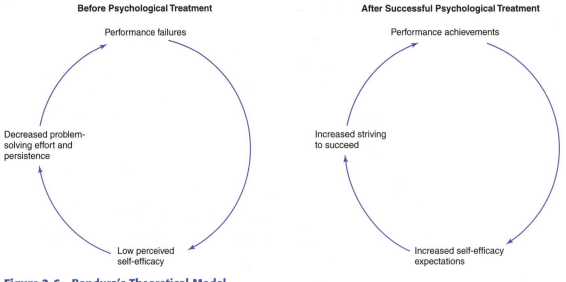

Before Psychological Treatment

Performance failures

Decreased problem-solving effort and persistence

Low perceived self-efficacy

After Successful Psychological Treatment

Performance achievements

Increased striving to succeed

Increased self-efficacy expectations

Figure 2-6   Bandura's Theoretical Model
SOURCE: From Benjamin (1996), p. 55. Reprinted with permission.

Back to the Beginning

Explaining June's Problems

You may have noticed some similarities in the different psychological theories of the origins of behavior problems. Many of these theories, particularly the psychodynamic ones, trace the origin of a problem to the child's very early experiences with parents, especially the mother. Mothers perhaps justifiably feel that they are blamed for their children's psychological difficulties, which may actually have other causes. However, these same theories describe the mothers themselves as victims of their personal history, of how they were treated by their own parents. That is, problems can be multigenerational, passed down from parent to child. June's mother could well have had a demanding, cold, and perfectionistic mother herself, and her childhood experiences may have determined how she is raising June. The developmental psychopathology approach stresses that all potential psychological, social, and biological influences must be carefully traced in order to understand and help individual children such as June.

Finally, the person's own emotional arousal can affect her expectations of success. The child who trembles at the thought of going to school may be less able to approach the school than a less shaky student. In observing our own emotional states, we reach conclusions about our own probable effectiveness. Anxiety reduction through relaxation training, tranquilizing drugs, or social support can bolster self-confidence and increase the chances of success.

Evaluation of Learning and Social Cognitive Approaches

Bandura's social cognitive theory has proved its usefulness in clinical practice, particularly in promoting children's academic skills, athletic performances, and health maintenance and in combating their fears, phobias, and anxiety (see Figure 2-6 and Chapters 7 and 15). Many research studies demonstrate the usefulness of social learning formulations. Although most of the supportive evidence comes from highly controlled laboratory studies rather than being confirmed by observations in everyday settings, the available evidence supports social cognitive theory. Mischel's longitudinal research on children's behavior patterns in a summer camp (see Shoda, Mischel, & Wright, 1994) is a case in point. Mischel's group found that individual children were not consistently aggressive or cooperative in all situations, but only in psychologically similar situations. Interactions with adult supervisors are psychologically different from those with peers, so children might behave consistently in one fashion with adults, but might react differently when with other children. For example, a boy named John was observed for a long time, and it was found that he behaved aggressively when criticized by adults but complied when threatened by other children. These different behaviors with adults and peers would be predicted by the social cognitive theory of personality, but not by psychodynamic theory, which would predict more behavioral consistency with different social groups. Bear in mind that complaints about incomplete validation of theories of psychopathology are common, and all of the theories we consider are difficult to validate.

June's Case as Viewed by Skinner and Bandura

Concerning June's behavior, as described in the chapter-opening case, the behavioral and social cognitive theories offer a somewhat different perspective from the psychodynamic theories. The behavioral approaches emphasize the here and now, while the psychodynamic theories emphasize the enduring effects of early childhood experiences, some of which are only imagined. Neither Skinner nor Bandura would say that June is encountering difficulties because she is suffering from a faulty early attachment or that she formed harmful internal working models of caretakers based on experiences during her childhood. Instead, Skinner would concentrate on the potentially reinforcing attention June receives when she complains or acts out and would improve her poor study habits through highly scripted training that featured repetition and reinforcement. Bandura might examine the type of behavioral models her parents and peers provide and offer her some less deviant, more desirable models, either in real life or on TV or videos. Social cognitive psychologists would also analyze her self-efficacy beliefs about her academic ability and her self-control and social skills. Success and reinforcement are essential features of both approaches. Both Skinner and Bandura stress the importance of teaching children the specific skills they need to succeed in life, such as how to do their schoolwork and how to get along with peers and adults.

SUMMARY

Biological explanations of abnormal behavior point to genetic, biochemical, disease, injury, or structural physical defects in combination with environmental circumstances. Known chromosomal abnormalities produce single or multiple-gene disorders. Behavioral genetics research has traced some types of mental retardation and progressive neurological disorders to genes. General mental ability appears heritable, as do some social behaviors, but virtually none of the recognized mental disorders have yet been specifically linked to genetic factors. Despite rapid advances in genetics research, previously unsuspected complexities plague the field: Researchers have discovered different genetic bases for the same psychiatric illness in different groups, apparent genetic contributions to behavior that influence an individual's social environment, lasting effects of experience on biochemical functioning, and low reliability in psychiatric diagnoses, particularly in children.

The original form of psychodynamic theory was Freud's psychoanalytic theory, which describes separate id, ego, and superego systems within the personality structure. Psychic energy for mental activity arises in the primitive, selfish id, while the more realistic ego balances id impulses and situational constraints and the harsh, perfectionistic superego demands to deter-

mine behavior. Personality development can be halted or impeded by overgratification or trauma at any early stage of personality development (oral, anal, or phallic) and is virtually completed during early childhood. Erikson's ego theory extends psychodynamic models to include social and cultural factors and views personality as continuing to develop into old age. Attachment theory stresses the lasting influence of very early secure, insecure, or disorganized attachment to the mother or other primary caregiver. Good caregiving leads to secure attachment, positive working models of attachment relationships, and healthy views of self and others. Benjamin's object relations theory emphasizes the enduring importance of relationships with mother or significant others in early childhood. The child forms an internalized representation of self and others that guides later self-evaluation and relationships with other people. Pairs interact in complementary fashion, often duplicating the roles of the person and the perceived, remembered mother.

The developmental psychopathology approach of Cicchetti, Rutter, and colleagues attempts to offer a comprehensive picture of development that includes all known physical and developmental psychological factors in the production of children's disturbances. This approach embraces the complexity of human development and states that a particular disorder can be produced by different causes in different children and that a particular causal factor can produce different types of disorders in different children.

Skinner's operant conditioning model and Bandura's social cognitive (or social learning) theory are both grounded in experimental research and reject the view that personality is determined early in childhood and changes little thereafter. Skinner stresses the continuous contribution of environmental events in determining behavior. Skinner's operant conditioning approach attributes normal and abnormal voluntary behavior to reinforcing and punishing events. Bandura's social cognitive approach acknowledges the importance of consequences, but also maintains that a degree of self-control is possible and that both self-efficacy beliefs and the probability of success determine a person's behavior. In the next chapter, we will show how well-designed research can provide some answers about potential causes and cures of children's abnormal behavior.

INFOTRAC COLLEGE EDITION

For more information, explore this resource at http://www.infotrac-college.com/Wadsworth. Enter the following search terms:

genetics
heredity
behavioral genetics
neurotransmitters
psychoanalytic theory
psychodynamic theories
attachment behavior in children
object relations
developmental psychopathology
cognitive psychology
operant learning
social cognitive theory

IN FOCUS ANSWERS

IN FOCUS 1 ▶ Identify four types of abnormality in normal gene replication that can cause physical or mental problems.

- A single defective gene
- Recessive genes
- Disarranged or excessively replicated gene sequences
- Incompletely divided chromosomes

IN FOCUS 2 ▶ Describe the functions associated more extensively with the left and the right hemispheres of the cerebral cortex. When can one hemisphere compensate for damage to the other?

- The left hemisphere is more responsible for speech, memory, and reasoning.

- The right hemisphere is more responsible for perception and for creation of mental images, and also for emotional aspects of speech.
- In younger children, the right hemisphere can compensate for a damaged left hemisphere in language acquisition.

IN FOCUS 3 ▶ Identify the four main themes of Freud's theory of personality.

- Irrationality of humans
- Unconscious aggression, sexual jealousy, anxiety
- Formation of personality in early childhood
- Need to recognize and overcome early irrational feelings about parents

IN FOCUS 4 ▶ Explain how secure and insecure attachment develop, and describe the effect of each.

- Secure attachment comes from having a warm, sensitive caregiver and promotes infants' social adjustment.
- Insecure attachment comes from an insensitive or rejecting caregiver and leads the child to expect problems with others in the future.

IN FOCUS 5 ▶ Describe operant behavior and tell how it can be increased and decreased. Give some examples of operant behavior.

- Operant behavior is voluntary and controlled by events that follow it such as reinforcing consequences.
- A child's remaining seated during class, doing schoolwork, answering questions, and hitting another child are all operant acts.

IN FOCUS 6 ▶ Define *self-efficacy,* and tell how high self-efficacy helps children solve problems.

- Self-efficacy is believing in your own competence, so you persevere in the face of difficulties.
- Children with low self-efficacy give up easily, so they often fail.

Research Methods Used to Study Child Behavior Disorders

In the Beginning

Jeremy Can't Read

Jeremy's first day at preschool had been very cool. It was fun to have all the other kids to play with, and even though his mother had seemed a little weird about him going to school, this was definitely an exciting place. He couldn't figure out why mom cried when she left him there, after all she had said about how neat school would be. After the first day, he agreed—it was neat.

That was a long time ago, way before Christmas. Now it wasn't so fun, and Jeremy didn't like school anymore. Everybody else learned faster it seemed, and that red-headed girl could spell and everything. Jeremy couldn't spell, and he didn't know the alphabet, and the book pages that most of the other kids read just had weird lines on them when he looked at them. Some of the kids made fun of him and called him a baby. Even though it wasn't as fun as it used to be, Jeremy's dad said it would get better. There were some things he was best at, like on the playground. It was like that crocodile man said in the movie, "No worries, mate."

But someone should probably be a little concerned. Research studies have clearly shown that early learning experiences are *very* important for young children, and the beneficial effects of positive early learning experiences seem to have a snowball effect. They lead to smoother academic growth and good experiences later on. There is enough research evidence that someone probably needs to be concerned about Jeremy and how his early school experience is going.

INTRODUCTION

As you read this book, you will encounter many references to research studies on various topics. The quality of these investigations varies greatly: Some provide reliable results, while others are less dependable, perhaps even misleading. This chapter introduces you to the fundamentals of research methods so that you can better evaluate research articles you read. After reading the chapter, you can expect to be able to answer a variety of questions such as these: Was an appropriate control group or condition used (or did improvement in speech occur because of therapy, maturation, or some other factor)? Was an appropriate dependent measure employed (or did the researcher observe behaviors unrelated to drug abuse or use unreliable measures)? Do

children grow out of phobias, or do phobias persist into adulthood? Are drugs or psychotherapy more successful in the treatment of schizophrenia during childhood? What are the most sensitive and accurate measures of children's emotions? Only well-planned and properly conducted research can answer the important questions parents ask professionals every day. Some of these questions are very practical (like "How do I get some more sleep when my kid won't go to bed?"), but they also have scientific relevance that many nonscientists may not see at first. We can guess at the answers to such questions, but children's lives are too important to base their treatment on such guesses. The best-quality research scrutiny is required.

Most children display both desirable and undesirable behaviors from time to time. It is often difficult to

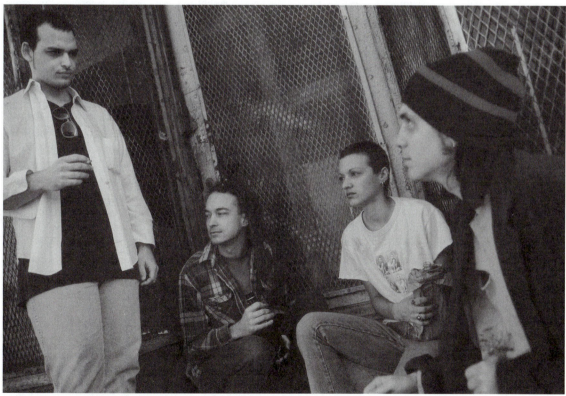

Casual observation will not produce reliable and systematic information because we may notice only certain individuals because of external characteristics, such as the young man in the stocking cap.

Lisette LeBon/SuperStock

determine which actions can be considered normal and which merit concern as deviating from the norm enough to require intervention. A child's behavior is often judged in terms of (1) a comparison to age-mates' behavior, (2) the intensity and persistence of any problem behavior, and (3) the degree to which behaviors are culturally appropriate. The fact that normalcy judgments rely heavily on comparing a child's behavior with that of a majority of peers raises the question of how we obtain information regarding behavioral norms and deviations from these norms.

In order to know how most people behave, we must have information that is gathered *systematically*. We cannot rely on casual observations alone, since such efforts are not systematic and will not produce reliable information that will be the same at different times with various observers. Informal observation, such as we might casually perform while shopping, is likely to be quite selective and inaccurate. We may notice only certain individuals (such as those who dress strangely) or certain behaviors that seem different or inappropriate. Such observation is highly unsystematic, and the resulting information will be incomplete. For more complete and accurate information, we must turn to a process that emphasizes its systematic acquisition—namely, research.

Like most terms, research has different meanings for different people. For our purposes, *research* will be broadly defined as a systematic method of inquiry, a systematic way of asking questions and obtaining information. This is a rather simple definition with the emphasis on the word *systematic,* or proceeding in a methodical, planned fashion. Certainly, there are many ways to obtain information. We constantly make decisions and take actions based on information. Often, our attention is focused mainly on the immediate decision needing attention or the action to be taken, and it can be highly focused (such as the driving need to buy *that* stereo equipment *today*). In research, the focus is on objective, systematic information gathering. The process may not produce the same immediate gratification as impulse buying, but it does tend to result in more rational decisions.

If research is planned and executed in a technically sound manner, the results should provide an objective answer to the initial question. Research processes that proceed in a methodical and systematic fashion may appear somewhat strange to the average person who is accustomed to making daily decisions in a more casual fashion. Research methods become even more perplexing when results appear to contradict widespread public opinion and are therefore counterintuitive or perhaps socially controversial. This was certainly the case with an article by Rind, Tromovitch, and Bauserman (1998) reporting a study on child sexual abuse, described in the Research Focus box. In fact, these researchers reached conclusions that created such a stir that some members of the U.S. Congress publicly ridiculed the specific methodology as "junk science," despite the fact that the article had been subjected to rigorous peer evaluation prior to publication. This shows how it may become fashionable in some quarters to question the value of research when results are politically sensitive. While such pursuits may be momentarily amusing or may serve a short-term political agenda, it is important to remember that many items and processes that make our daily life easier were once the results of some research that was perhaps thought silly at the time.

We are all consumers of research whether we are conscious of it or not. Scientific investigation has contributed immeasurably to the world around us. It influences the production of our food, clothing, medication, and modes of transportation, as well as the way we write term papers or go on diets, among many other products and procedures. Too frequently, we encounter poor-quality products that have allegedly been developed and evaluated with care. Consequently, we are skeptical when advertisements say that a product has been scientifically evaluated and is unsurpassed in quality. Having been misled in the past, we may become suspicious of scientific claims. However, with some knowledge of the characteristics of good research, we can make more informed choices as consumers.

This chapter attempts to make you a better informed consumer of research by increasing your ability to evaluate psychological and educational research studies. Both practitioners and parents are dependent on research of many types, for evaluating not only material products, but also educational and therapeutic or rehabilitation programs. For example, parents of a child with attention-deficit/hyperactivity disorder (ADHD) must make decisions regarding a treatment

Science, Politics, and Pedophilia

Rind, Tromovitch, and Bauserman (1998) published an article describing a meta-analysis of 59 previous studies that had examined child sexual abuse. As Rind and his colleagues pointed out, many people "... believe that child sexual abuse ... causes intense harm ... pervasively in the general population" (1998, p. 22). These researchers found that students who had experienced child sexual abuse were slightly less well adjusted than their peers, but concluded that they could not attribute this somewhat diminished psychological adjustment to the sexual abuse encounters. The authors' rationale for not drawing such a conclusion was sound to those trained in research methods but escaped the understanding of many without such background. Poorer psychological adjustment could not be attributed to child sexual abuse because it could not be separated out from another influence that confused the picture—that is, poor general family environment. Stated another way, the evidence did not make it clear whether the slightly poorer psychological adjustment was due to the child sexual abuse or to the influence of family environment variables such as marital conflict, having an addicted or criminal parent, or physical abuse.

Such a conclusion fits the general approach usually employed by scientists when analyzing evidence. How could it cause such a furor? The authors likely captured the reason why in the very last sentence of their abstract, which read "Basic beliefs about [child sexual abuse] in the general population were not supported" (Rind et al., 1998, p. 22). Added to this reason is the fact that issues pertaining to child sexual abuse are socially, and therefore politically, very sensitive. Sexual abuse of children runs counter to some fundamental beliefs that permeate our public persona and our religious and cultural heritage. Our social conscience is outraged by someone telling us that what we believe may not be true, and in this particular instance, the U.S. Congress (and some state legislative bodies) became the self-appointed voice of social conscience, decrying the review by Rind and his colleagues as "junk science." Resolutions were introduced and debated, and nationally syndicated media personalities demanded that the American Psychological Association repudiate the article.

All of this uproar highlights the very reasons why research and the scientific protocols involved in it are vitally important. In this case, science challenged a sacred cow, and the process resulted in arguments that were as public as they were heated and that put enormous political pressure on the researchers (Rind, Bauserman, & Tromovitch, 2000). Researchers using scientific methods go to great lengths to ensure objective collection and analysis of evidence on important questions and problems. The extent to which those steps are employed may make the process less understandable to lay persons. The article by Rind and his associates emphasizes how such a lack of understanding, combined with the extreme importance and sensitivity of some research questions, can lead to serious controversy.

NOTE: The title of this box was used by the journal *Psychological Science Agenda* in its September/October 1999 issue (Vol. 12, No. 5) in a commentary on the political turbulence about the article by Rind, Tromovitch, and Bauserman (1998). It captures the essence of this controversy and is used here thanks to the Science Directorate of the American Psychological Association.

program for their child. Likewise, teachers and other professionals must make decisions concerning educational or other treatment programs for children. The Research Focus box illustrates an investigation on the effects of a treatment program to help children with ADHD control their impulsive behavior (Posavac, Sheridan, & Posavac, 1999). For this study, researchers selected for treatment four boys diagnosed with ADHD because they frequently talked out, interrupting the class, and seldom raised their hands to be recognized appropriately. The boys were already participating in a program to improve their social skills. The experimental treatment involved providing a cueing procedure, a method for prompting them to focus their attention with the goal of getting them to raise their hand before speaking.

Table 3-1 Differences between Scientific Inquiry and Commonsense Reasoning

Area of Difference	Scientific Inquiry	Commonsense Reasoning
Use of theories and concepts	Studied systematically	Studied informally and unsystematically, if at all
Level of proof required	Very stringent and based on agreed-upon principles	Loose and variable
Control demanded	High degree	Little or none
Interest in relationships between phenomena	Systematic, constant study of relationships	Unsystematic, often only interested in phenomena of personal relevance
Types of explanations regarding phenomena	Couched in the observable, logical, empirically testable	Often extend beyond the empirically testable to metaphysical explanations

SCIENCE AND COMMON SENSE

There are many popular misconceptions and negative stereotypes regarding science and scientists. For example, some people think of scientists as unrealistic dreamers, space cadets, or arrogant "ivory-tower eggheads," incapable of relating to the "real" world. (We eggheads resent these labels.) This view implies that there is little relationship between science and common sense (a notion explicitly stated by some). Although there are some important differences between the two, it would be incorrect to conclude that science and common sense are totally unrelated.

Science is an extension of common sense that emphasizes systematic questioning. Generally speaking, common sense is characterized by a much less systematic approach to problems than that used by the scientific method. For example, common sense might dictate behaving in a traditional way, such as spanking unruly children ("spare the rod and spoil the child"). Someone using the scientific method would be more likely to investigate immediate and long-term behavioral effects of spanking compared to other methods of curbing disobedience. Table 3-1 summarizes some of the ways science and common sense differ.

RESEARCH QUESTIONS

IN FOCUS 1 ▶ What three types of research questions are typically addressed in psychology?

In general, research can be conceptualized as a process that begins with a question and progresses through a systematic series of steps aimed at obtaining an answer to that question. Knowing what type of research question is being investigated is very important to understanding a research study. Research questions in psychology generally fall into three basic categories: descriptive questions, questions regarding differences, and questions about relationships or correlations.

Descriptive research questions ask about the nature of a phenomenon. Such questions are aimed at describing a particular group or type of individual with regard to certain characteristics. For example, a descriptive research question might ask, "What behavioral patterns are typical of individuals with anorexia?" or "What is the average IQ of psychotic children?" Such questions are not simple to answer since they require samples of participants who are truly representative of the group of interest, such as autistic children or depressed ones, or of particular subgroups, such as autistic children with normal-range IQs or depressed adolescents.

Difference research questions ask, "Is there a difference?" Investigations addressing difference questions may compare groups (for example, "Is there a significant difference in academic performance between the group that received individual tutoring and the group that received structured group instruction?"), or they may compare a group's or an individual's behavior before and during treatment (as in the study described in the Research Focus box).

Relationship research questions ask to what degree two or more phenomena relate or vary together. These are often termed *correlational questions* (after the correlational statistical analyses used). A correla-

Research Focus

Getting Their Attention to Improve Treatment

This study investigated the effectiveness of a cueing procedure on the target behavior of hand raising in the context of a social skills training program for four boys with ADHD. In addition to observing hand raising, researchers also collected data on talking out, which was considered to be an important collateral behavior. All of the boys exhibited rather low rates of raising their hands and unacceptably high rates of talking out before the cueing procedure was implemented. As described by the authors, "The cueing procedure was aimed at increasing the frequency with which the participants raised their hand before speaking, to help them devote attention to and improve impulse regulation. In addition, we believed that reinforcing participants' hand-raising behavior may produce side effects on a related behavior (i.e., talking out of turn)" (Posavac, Sheridan, & Posavac, 1999, pp. 235–236).

This study used a reversal, or A-B-A-B, design: Participants' behavior was observed under untreated, or base-line, conditions first (A1), followed by an initial application of the treatment (B1), then a return to baseline (A2), and finally a reapplication of the treatment (B2). All of the participants demonstrated positive changes in raising their hands before talking. Figure 3-1 summarizes the data from Participant 2. These results show a relatively high rate of talking out and a low rate of hand raising during the baseline phase. With the implementation of treatment, hand raising increased substantially and talking out of turn reduced somewhat, returning nearly to pretreatment levels during the return to baseline. Behaviors during the final treatment phase indicated that hand raising and talking out nearly traded places from the beginning of the study, with hand raising showing a high rate of occurrence and talking out at a far lower rate than when the study began. The data suggest that cueing may be a useful element in an overall social skills treatment program, at least for promoting hand raising and reducing talking out of turn.

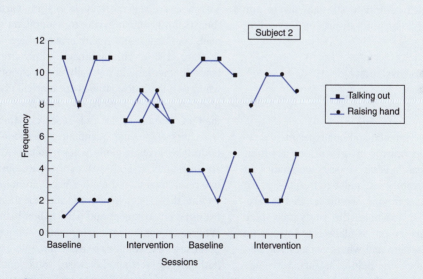

Figure 3-1   Direct Observational Data for Hand Raising and Talking Out (Target and Collateral Behaviors) for One Participant in a Study
SOURCE: Posavac, Sheridan, & Posavac (1999). Reprinted by permission of Sage Publications, Inc.

tional study might explore the relationship between annual family income and the frequency of mental health problems in children. Simply stated, the question might be "As family income varies, what tends to happen to the frequency of youngsters' mental health problems?" (To put it another way, "As income increases, does the frequency of child mental health problems tend to increase or decrease?")

RESEARCH PARADIGMS: DISTINCTIONS, DESCRIPTIONS, AND ILLUSTRATIONS

Scientists working in psychology and education often classify research into a variety of methodology categories, or paradigms. These paradigms have varied over the years in terms of their popularity in different disciplines. We will briefly examine certain differences between experimental and nonexperimental methods and between quantitative and qualitative approaches. Each is applicable in certain situations, and the selection of a particular method depends on the investigator's background, the question under investigation, and the setting in which a study is conducted. All of these methodologies contribute substantially to our understanding of child behavior disorders.

Methodology Distinctions

IN FOCUS 2 ▶ Discuss the differences between experimental and nonexperimental research methods.

In some ways, experimental and nonexperimental research methods are mirror images of one another. Experimental research often consists of studies in which the investigator manipulates the treatment given to a participant in an environment that is carefully controlled (for example, the study may take place in a lab where no one is allowed to intrude on the experimental setting and where noise, light, and temperature levels can be held constant). Investigators using nonexperimental research methods tend to observe, analyze, and describe phenomena as they exist naturally rather than manipulating treatments or conditions. Nonexperimental research does not typically impose as much control and may take place in a

more natural environment such as a classroom, a playground, or a home. Nonexperimental research may yield ideas to be tested in experimental research, or it may add richness and realism to experimental findings.

The bulk of research in psychology and education has historically used what most would term "quantitative" methodology. For the most part, this research has asked questions, developed hypotheses, manipulated experimental variables, and measured outcomes in a manner that allows results to be reduced to some numerical representation (such as, the number of correct responses or the number of tantrum outbursts). However, another approach to conducting research, known as "qualitative" methodology, has gained popularity in psychology and education during the past 15 to 20 years. Such methods have long been used in other disciplines, such as anthropology, sociology, and psychiatry.

The different terms suggest that one method (quantitative) collects data that are numbers, whereas the other (qualitative) collects some other type of data (e.g., case history description or a natural history of some behavioral problem in a child, a family, or a small set of cases). This is true, but it is not the only difference between the methods. Qualitative researchers are also more likely to study participants in their natural context, trying to understand the participants' perceptions of reality around them (Gall, Gall, & Borg, 1998). This approach emphasizes a reluctance to intervene in naturally occurring phenomena, whereas quantitative studies are more likely to manipulate experimental variables, situations, and other matters pertaining to the research question. Researchers employing quantitative methodology often undertake investigations whose points of departure are questions, hypotheses, or theories. Some qualitative researchers, on the other hand, are more likely to let the theories, hypotheses, and questions emerge from the environment and participants being studied. Whereas quantitative-experimental studies test hypotheses, case studies are more likely to generate hypotheses for testing. Likewise, some qualitative researchers are more likely to let definitions emerge as a study progresses, which would not be considered acceptable by most quantitative researchers, who first develop tests or observational procedures, assess their adequacy, and then make observations.

The growing popularity of qualitative research methodology in psychology and education has been prompted by a desire to learn more about the complexities of naturally occurring human behavior than has been possible with traditional quantitative approaches. The tension between controlled experimental and observational case methodology has generated heated debates heavily laced with stimulating intellectual (and even personal) attacks (Kopala & Suzuki, 1999; Wallen & Fraenkel, 2000). Perhaps only researchers could take this issue so seriously. It is important to remember that this transition period toward qualitative approaches is still ongoing. As we gain more experience, the "methodology wars" will diminish, and research methodology will eventually be strengthened by the addition of qualitative elements to the arsenal of quantitative tools, and vice versa (Gliner & Morgan, 2000). Table 3-2 summarizes the major differences between quantitative and qualitative research paradigms.

Both quantitative and qualitative research approaches have advantages and limitations. For example, one advantage of experimental over nonexperimental methods involves the extent of control. Experimental researchers exert more control and attempt to hold all influences constant except the treatment variable that is being manipulated. Because experimental research involves such high control, an investigator can be more confident in attributing his or her results to the treatment variable. If the only known difference between two groups of children is the treatment they receive, then posttreatment differences in their behavior can likely be attributed to the type of treatment received. But control has a limitation as well. Because they require a high degree of control, experimental studies are frequently conducted in a rather artificial environment. Results may be substantially altered by an artificial environment if the setting is so unusual that participants perform differently than they would normally. For example, children who have

Table 3-2 Major Differences between Quantitative and Qualitative Research

Quantitative Methods	Qualitative Methods
Preference for precise hypotheses stated at the outset	Preference for hypotheses that emerge as study develops
Preference for precise definitions stated at the outset	Preference for definitions made in context or as study progresses
Data reduced to numerical scores	Preference for narrative description
Much attention to assessing and improving reliability of scores obtained from instruments	Preference for assuming that reliability of inferences is adequate
Assessment of validity through variety of design procedures with reliance on statistical indices	Assessment of validity through cross-checking of sources of information (triangulation)
Preference for random techniques for obtaining meaningful samples	Preference for expert information (purposive) samples
Preference for precise descriptions of procedures	Preference for narrative/literary descriptions of procedures
Preference for design or statistical control of extraneous variables	Preference for logical analysis in controlling or accounting for extraneous variables (describing what else seems to be going on)
Preference for specific design control for procedural bias	Primary reliance on researcher to detect and minimize procedural bias
Preference for statistical summary of results	Preference for narrative summary of results
Preference for breaking down of complex phenomena into specific parts for analysis	Preference for holistic description of complex phenomena (describing the whole picture)
Willingness to manipulate aspects, situations, or conditions in studying complex phenomena	Unwillingness to tamper with naturally occurring phenomena

Source: Adapted from Fraenkel & Wallen (1996), p. 442. Reprinted by permission of McGraw-Hill Education.

Margaret Mead's Reporting of Samoan Sexual Behavior

Margaret Mead's research on the Samoan culture has long been a classic, widely known both within and beyond the disciplinary boundaries of cultural anthropology (Mead, 1928). One of the areas that received the most widespread interest in this research was Mead's reporting of Samoan sexual behavior. It was Mead's assertion that young Samoans made the best sexual adjustment in the world and that young females deferred marriage "through as many years of casual love-making as possible" (Freeman, 1983, p. 226). Based on her conversations with young Samoan women, it was Mead's conclusion that premarital sex was commonplace and a casual pastime. This perspective on Samoan culture became so prevalent that one author characterized it as "institutionalized premarital sexuality" (Honigmann, 1963, p. 273). As time passed, however, certain questions began to be raised regarding this aspect of Mead's report. In fact, what began to emerge as a characteristic Samoan behavior, rather than recreational sex, was "recreational lying," especially about sex (Freeman, 1989).

As other researchers probed this topic, evidence began to accumulate that perhaps Mead's questions to her informants about sexual behavior had produced responses that should not have been accepted at face value. Testimony in 1988 by one of Mead's actual participants indicated that the sexual questions touched on a taboo topic and embarrassed the young Samoan women. Their responses (indicating a common acceptance of premarital sex) were presented in what they intended to be a joking manner. However, unaware of the intent, Mead took the answers seriously, did not challenge the stories, and did not obtain corroboration from other sources. Such an error highlights dramatically the need for triangulation, or cross-checking of information through multiple sources, to provide confidence that data obtained in qualitative research are valid.

spent most of their time at home may be unusually active or frightened if they are brought to a laboratory or clinic (especially if they see unfamiliar adults in white lab coats who resemble doctors who might give injections). Such conditions might influence the participants' performance, causing them to behave or react uncharacteristically.

The fact that nonexperimental researchers use much less control than experimenters can be both an advantage and a limitation. On the positive side, many nonexperimental methods do not create artificial environments that substantially influence participants' responses. However, the relative absence of control is a limitation in that it can contribute to unreliable data. For example, the data obtained in a case study are likely to be influenced by the biases of the interviewer, especially if a structured protocol of questions is not used. Without the control imposed by a consistent set of questions, an interviewer may obtain information only in areas that he or she thinks are important. That is why researchers are careful to train interviewers

and examiners to a high standard. Nothing is so fundamental to high-quality research in psychology as the reliability of measurement (Oliver & Benet-Martinez, 2000).

Although there are researchers who conduct poor-quality research using either quantitative or qualitative methods, the standards for rigor in the use of quantitative methods are more widely accepted. Critical standards of rigor are not yet as widely evident for qualitative methodology in psychology and education, which increases the vulnerability of qualitative studies to accusations of poor-quality science. Errors or questionable results appear even in disciplines where qualitative methods have long been used, because of the reliance on informants as the fundamental source of data. The Research Focus box illustrates a case of such questions being raised about a classic study. No single strategy provides a perfect solution to all the challenges of collecting data. Scientists must select a method or set of methods and be fully cognizant of the strengths and limitations inherent in the chosen approach.

Nonexperimental/Qualitative Research

IN FOCUS 3 ▶ Describe how qualitative research methods generally differ from quantitative approaches.

If you are observing a 3rd-grade boy to see how he gets along with his classmates, you're informally engaging in nonexperimental research. Nonexperimental methods involve observation, analysis, and description of phenomena rather than the manipulation of treatment variables (as in experimentation). A variety of procedures may be viewed as nonexperimental. Some of these procedures are also considered qualitative methods, depending on the data collected. In this section, we examine certain nonexperimental and qualitative methods used in the study of child behavior disorders. Interested readers may wish to consult other sources for additional information on these approaches (e.g., Allen & Walker, 2000; Stebbins, 2001; Willig, 2001).

Observation

Observation is a data collection method that actually crosses a variety of methodological boundaries. It is used in both experimental and nonexperimental research and also in both qualitative and quantitative investigations. It is discussed in this section because manipulation of a treatment variable is not inherent in the observation process. Observation has been viewed by some as a distinct research method because it has traditionally been used by certain disciplines. However, for our purposes, it is best viewed as a data collection strategy that may be used in several research methods.

Observation techniques vary greatly depending on the type of investigation and the setting of a study. One variation involves the degree to which an observer participates in the activities of the group being studied. For example, qualitative researchers often use what is known as participant observation, wherein the individual collecting the data actually participates in the setting or activities being observed. Such a procedure is vastly different from an investigation in which a nonparticipant observer collects the data. Nonparticipant observers stay as inconspicuous as possible and do not become involved in the interactions under investigation.

Researchers in psychology have tended to use procedures in which the observer participates minimally or not at all and often is not even seen by those being observed (for example, observations are made through a one-way mirror or by means of audio or video recordings). Such procedures are employed not because researchers are unscrupulous snoopers but because they do not want participants' behavior to change as a result of being acutely aware of being observed. Teenagers and preteens may become agonizingly self-conscious about being observed, at least initially. By contrast, babies show no apprehension unless they are in the stranger-anxiety age range. Similarly, preschool and kindergarten children are delightful to observe because they adjust to nonintrusive observers' presence very rapidly, minimizing the influence on their behavior. Investigators must be very alert to the degree to which their participants are susceptible to being influenced by the presence of an observer in the context of the study. For circumstances in which participants are at risk regarding influence, the impact of known or evident observers on participants' behavior has been demonstrated frequently in the literature. Researchers using nonparticipant observation do so because they are concerned that participants will behave as naturally as possible (a factor of particular importance in some studies). Natural behavior is often achievable if participants become accustomed to the observer; however, many people may never behave completely naturally when they are aware of being observed.

Observation procedures may also vary in the amount of structure imposed by the researcher. Structure may be imposed on the environment or on the observer. For example, data may be recorded in an unstructured environment such as the setting in which the participants normally live or work. On the other end of this continuum, data may be collected in an environment that is very structured, even artificial and foreign to the participants (e.g., a contrived laboratory setting). Similarly, observer procedures may vary on a continuum of structure. Data may be recorded in an unstructured fashion (e.g., field notes recorded anecdotally without guidelines) or in a very structured and prescribed manner (e.g., on a standard checklist for counting frequency of disruptive behavior).

Case Studies

Case studies represent a second nonexperimental research method frequently used by qualitative re-

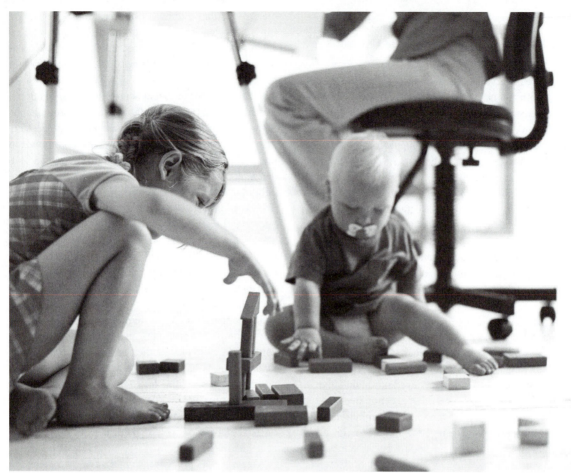

A qualitative research study might study these children in the natural environment of their home and family.

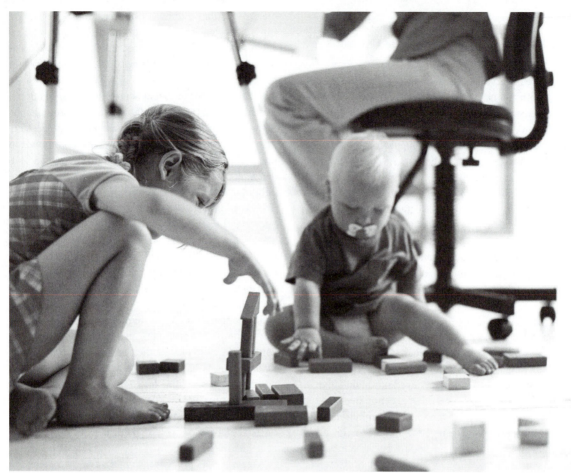
Jim Bastardo/Getty Images

searchers. A **case study** characteristically involves an in-depth examination of the behavior of an individual or a small social unit such as a family. Case studies in psychology are traditionally characterized by a lack of experimental controls (Kazdin, 1998). The researcher collects observations, perhaps in psychotherapy sessions, but does not introduce different types of treatment or record the client's reaction. The focus of a case study may vary depending on the nature of the research question. Usually the researcher attempts to determine all of the factors or influences that are important in a participant's development and current behavior. Data collected often include a developmental history, including physical, psychological, and social aspects of the person's development. The case study's purpose is to determine why an individual has reached his or her current status. An investigator describes the participant and attempts to reconstruct his or her past history and the nature and sources of any present problems.

For the most part, case studies address descriptive questions, to serve as a preliminary investigation, to verify a theory, or to understand and trace the history of a behavior disorder as it develops in a child. However, increasingly, researchers are reporting case studies that address difference questions about treatment. This is true of the case reported by Luiselli and Pine (1999), presented as Karen's Story.

Karen's Story

A Case Study on Stealing

Karen was a 10-year-old female who was diagnosed as having attention-deficit/hyperactivity disorder (ADHD) and, provisionally, obsessive compulsive disorder. At the age of 4.5 years, she was placed in the care of a foster family by the state's Department of Social Services subsequent to substantiated neglect and physical maltreatment at the hands of her biological parents. For several years, she experienced multiple foster family placements due to behavioral difficulties and adjustment problems. Eventually, she was adopted by her present parents when she was 8 years old. Karen was their only child.

Karen was described as a "highly distractible" child who was very active and frequently oppositional in response to adult requests. She seemed "hypervigilant" towards her surroundings, often dominated social interactions, and seemed to "constantly search for adult attention." Her interactions with peers were poor because she did not respond cooperatively and was disruptive in group contexts. At the time of referral, she had received medication trials of methylphenidate, nortriptyline, and sertraline, none of which were associated with meaningful behavioral improvement. Karen's academic abilities were at a 2nd-grade level.

Stealing behavior was identified by school personnel several months after Karen's enrollment in a public elementary school. Typically, stolen items included food (e.g., candy, cookies) or personal possessions (e.g., pencil, pad of paper) that were taken from students and adults. Karen's parents reported that stealing also was a problem at home and in the community, but they were able to control its occurrence by removing temptation (e.g., keeping particular objects under "lock and key") and providing close supervision (e.g., keeping Karen in sight when shopping in stores). . . .

Karen attended a public elementary school located in a suburban community. She participated in a self-contained, resource room classroom with nine other students who had learning and behavior challenges. . . . For portions of the day, she also experienced instruction with grade-level peers within a 3rd-grade classroom. In this context, she received individualized support from either the resource room teacher or the instructional assistant.. . . .

Baseline data were recorded for 7 weeks under conditions that were operative preceding the study. There were several procedures in effect at this time that had been introduced by staff in an attempt to manage stealing behav-

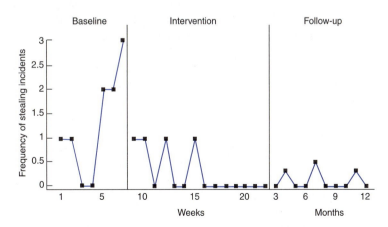

Figure 3-2 A Quantitative Case Study of a Difference Question Treatment Intervention

Source: Luiselli & Pine (1999). Used by permission of Elsevier Science.

ior.... Before an intervention plan was implemented, several types of functional assessment were performed. The [researcher] reviewed baseline data that had been collected, looking specifically at any antecedent or consequence events that appeared to be associated consistently with stealing incidents....

As a result of hypothesis formation, intervention was based on removing sources of attention for stealing. The plan included several components, each of which represented the elimination of preintervention (baseline) procedures that were judged to be reinforcing (Luiselli & Pine, 1999, pp. 231–239).

Figure 3-2 summarizes the data on stealing incidents during baseline, intervention, and follow-up phases.

Case studies are valuable for the depth, complexity, and quantity of information typically obtained (Powell, Calkins, Quealy-Berge, & Bardos, 1999; Sigafoos & Littlewood, 1999). They also have a characteristic limitation, however. Case studies usually describe one or, at most, a few participants, such as members of a family, and the information may not apply to other individuals or situations that differ from those studied. That is, the information may not be generalizable. Another limitation of the case study approach is the possible bias of the investigator or of informants such as the child or family members. In many cases, there are no objective records of the child's past interactions. Information must come from the individual or perhaps from interested third parties such as parents or other relatives. Such data may be biased because informants are aware of the existing problem and consequently interpret earlier events differently than they would without such knowledge (e.g., viewing previous normal play incidents as abnormal because the child has now been labeled as emotionally disturbed). Data inaccuracy may also arise from informants' faulty memories. Individuals providing information may selectively remember certain types of incidents, recall only more recent events, or confuse one child's reactions with those of another child. Case study data may also be biased by the investigator's or therapist's interpretations. Information for a case study comes from the individual or other informants and is necessarily filtered through the investigator before it is recorded. Such data are quite vulnerable to the biases and expectations of an investigator, who may enter data into the record in a manner that is incomplete or inaccurate to some degree. It should also be noted that case study methodology is viewed as being limited because it does not adhere totally to certain elements of the qualitative paradigm. For example, questions under investigation may sometimes be at least partially determined before the data collection begins. While this would suit experimental and quantitative researchers just fine (actually, they would want the question to be completely specified), some qualitative researchers see such predetermination of the questions disquieting and prefer to have the questions emerge as the investigation progresses.

Experimental/Quantitative Research

As noted earlier, experimental research is characterized by manipulation of the treatment or condition under study. The factor under study, manipulated by an experimenter, is known as the **independent variable** (also called the *experimental variable*). If, for example, we were interested in determining the effectiveness of a new treatment for childhood autism, our independent variable might be "type of treatment." We might be comparing a new treatment with one that had been used previously and contrasting the effects of these different treatments on autistic behavior. As researchers manipulate a treatment, they must have some way of measuring its effect. For example, we might count the number of times per hour that a child exhibits what is considered "autistic behavior" (which must be defined operationally, perhaps as particular hand or body movements, lack of interest in other people, unusual speech content, etc.). The measure or means by which researchers determine a treatment's effect is known as the **dependent variable.** So they manipulate an independent variable (e.g., treatment type) to observe its effects on the dependent variable (e.g., counting the frequency with which a particular behavior occurs under different treatment types). Such an investigation is an example of an experimental study that collects quantitative data.

Quasi-Experimental Designs

An experimental/quantitative study might be conducted by sampling a population of autistic children and then randomly assigning half of the sample to one group and the other half to a second group. Because of random assignment of the children to the groups, the groups would be very similar in their behavior and other characteristics until after the two treatments were applied. There are, however, situations in which a researcher cannot manipulate the independent variable. This might be the case if we were interested in comparing the performance of children with mental retardation and their peers of normal intelligence on some task. In this example, the focus of study would be on performance differences between the two populations, and our independent variable might be labeled "participant classification" (those having retardation versus those who do not). We could not actually manipulate the independent variable, since the intelligence differences were preexisting and impossible to alter. Investigations such as this, in which participants cannot be randomly assigned to groups, are known as **quasi-experimental designs,** while those in which an independent variable is literally manipulated are viewed as "true" experiments (or simply, experiments).

Quasi-experimental studies have particular limitations that do not arise in true experiments. We just used the example of comparing participants of normal intelligence with those having mental retardation on some task performance. As we design such a study, our aim is to control or hold constant everything except the independent variable. There are, however, other influences that cannot be readily controlled. Each participant has a history of having mental retardation or being of normal intelligence. That history carries with it a myriad of experiences that cannot be precisely assessed or controlled. For example, the participants who do not have mental retardation are likely to be healthier and more self-confident than those who are diagnosed with mental retardation. Thus, if we obtain results that suggest differences, we must be cautious about how the findings are interpreted. Although we would like to attribute differences to the independent variable (in this case, mental retardation), some of the experiential factors (e.g., general health status, social rejection, or vitality) might also differentially affect the participants' performance. Lack of control is a continuing problem with quasi-experimental

studies, one that researchers must constantly address. Although it does not preclude the use of such studies in psychology and other behavioral sciences, it does require that researchers proceed with caution. There are many areas of great interest to psychologists that can only be investigated using quasi-experimental designs, and such investigations have provided enormous amounts of useful information over the years.

Longitudinal and Cross-Sectional Designs

IN FOCUS 4 ▶ What are two experimental research designs commonly used to study human development?

As Chapter 1 noted, human development is one of the fundamental themes of this book. Development is fundamental to the study of child behavior disorders, as it is in so many different areas of psychology and related fields. We are continually interested in and puzzled by how children (and all humans, for that matter) change as they grow older and how advancing age interacts with behavior and ability. The study of child behavior disorders is often undertaken within a developmental framework. That is, a researcher may be interested in how a particular disorder develops or in the developmental course of children's behavioral problems. Two basic approaches have been commonly employed in such research: longitudinal designs and cross-sectional designs. **Longitudinal designs** select a sample of participants, test or observe them, and follow these same participants for an extended period of time, repeating the assessment intermittently. For example, a researcher may be interested in observing the development of social skills in youngsters with mental retardation as they progress from age 3 to age 15. **Cross-sectional designs,** on the other hand, simultaneously sample different groups of participants at several age levels (e.g., 3 to 5, 6 to 8, 9 to 11, and 12 to 15) and compare the dependent variable (e.g., social skills scores or self-esteem) across the age groups. With both longitudinal and cross-sectional studies, researchers attempt to draw conclusions regarding the developmental trajectory of the dependent variable being measured. Time or age serves as the independent variable in both strategies. These approaches cannot readily be categorized as experiments (illustrating that most classification schemes are somewhat arbitrary). Longitudinal studies typically do not involve manipulation of an independent variable, but only repeated observations or

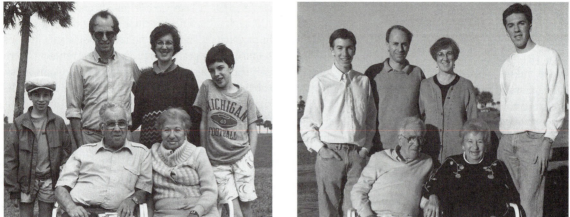

Longitudinal research collects data on the same individuals or families over an extended period of time.

measurements over time. Cross-sectional investigations seem to fit the quasi-experimental mold, because pre-existing differences (e.g., in age) are present at the time of assessment.

Longitudinal and cross-sectional designs also have certain advantages and limitations that must be considered in developmental studies. As noted previously, longitudinal investigations measure the same participants repeatedly, usually over an extended period. This permits observation of change in the same individuals as they develop, which is a distinct strength of the longitudinal approach with regard to developmental interpretations. A potential problem with this approach is that participants' development may be altered by the repeated assessments as they become more "test-wise" or that events such as war or economic depressions may affect their development (which would mean that researchers would not be evaluating development *only*). Thus, it is important to assess the performance of other comparison groups as well as the group of particular interest, so that all groups receive the same repeated testing. Another limitation often encountered in longitudinal studies is participant attrition. As an investigation proceeds over an extended period of time, it is not uncommon for a certain portion of the participants to be lost because they move away, refuse to continue, or die. The researchers may not actually have the *same* group of participants at the conclusion of their study. Thus, data collected toward the end of a study may be differ-

ent from data collected earlier because of the particular characteristics of the lost participants rather than because of an actual developmental trend. Moreover, in really lengthy longitudinal studies, the measures originally used may become outdated and fail to address matters of contemporary concern. Finally, such studies are often prohibitively expensive, and so most longitudinal studies are now limited to no longer than 4–5 years.

Cross-sectional studies are more convenient to conduct than longitudinal investigations, since participants from several age levels are sampled and typically assessed once, at about the same time. This approach circumvents the difficulties of participant attrition and the possible effects of repeated testing. However, cross-sectional developmental studies have other problems. One of the most serious limitations is inherent in the cross-sectional approach—the fact that different cohorts or groups are being compared. There is a strong tendency to interpret differences between groups as representing developmental trends, similar to the way longitudinal conclusions are drawn. Such inferences must be viewed with great caution since differences may be caused by factors that are not a result of development. In some cases, the age range from the youngest to oldest groups is so great that sociocultural or historical changes have been substantial (e.g., groups were born in such different times that social mores regarding child rearing have changed, or prevailing teaching practices or permissiveness levels have changed). For example, people's behavior differed before and after the appearance of television, AIDS, computers, synthetic drugs, and so on. Consequently, differences between groups could be due to development, sociocultural variations, or a combination of the two. Developmental interpretations from cross-sectional studies must be made with great care, although such designs can contribute to research methodology in psychology if employed prudently.

Time-Series Designs

IN FOCUS 5 ▶ Explain how time-series designs investigate the effects of an intervention with children.

The examples of experimental research described so far have involved investigations in which groups of participants are studied. Traditionally, such studies have been conducted with no fewer than ten participants in each group (and often many more). Yet another type of experiment that characteristically does not compare groups of this size is the time-series design. **Time-series designs** involve investigations in which an independent variable is manipulated across two or more phases (e.g., applied, then withdrawn, and then reapplied, or applied at different times to different participants) and the dependent variable is monitored at each phase. Data collected are often graphed as in Figure 3-3 to visually summarize any changes across the different experimental phases.

Figure 3-3 represents a *reversal time-series design* because the sequence of experimental phases runs from baseline to treatment, reverses to baseline, and, finally, returns to a second treatment phase. A variety of specific design configurations are used in time-series research (Drew, Hardman, & Hart, 1996; Richards, Taylor, Ramasamy, & Richards, 1998).

Time-series studies are often used to assess the effect of treatment on the behavior of a small number of participants or even a single participant. If treatment manipulation reliably changes behavior, then researchers can conclude that the treatment is effective. Time-series designs have provided researchers with a powerful tool for investigating the effects of treatment in applied settings where limited numbers of children with similar problems are available for study, something that is not always possible in large group studies. Figure 3-4 illustrates data from such an experiment, in which four children were treated for noncompliance with bedtime. The graph shows that three of the four children improved substantially, reducing the total number of minutes out of bed per evening. The fourth child (Victoria) did not improve as much, and in fact, she seemed to be worse at follow-up.

Time-series designs are particularly well suited for situations in which there is a scientific purpose and an immediate clinical need at the same time (Morgan & Morgan, 2001). With disorders that strike less than 1 child in 1000, it may not be feasible to find a group of children with a problem in order to investigate its na-

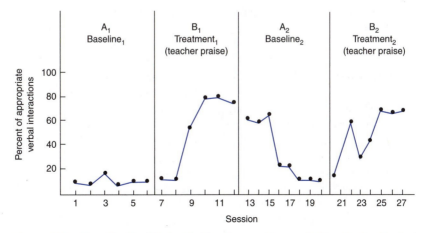

Figure 3-3   Hypothetical Data Display from a Reversal Time-Series Design

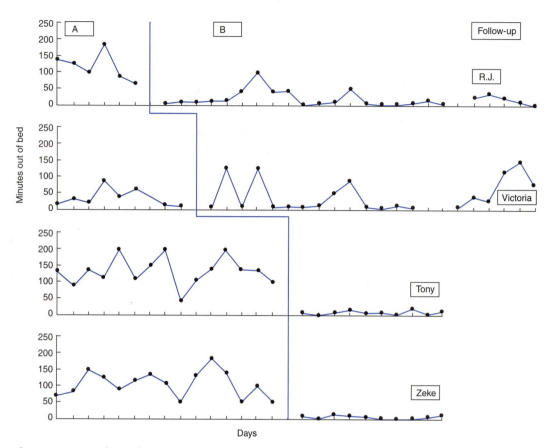

Figure 3-4   Total Number of Minutes Out of Bed per Evening for Four Children
Source: Robinson & Sheridan (2000). Reprinted by permission of The Haworth Press, Inc.

ture. Additionally, if the time is taken to gather an experimental group, it may mean neglecting a clinical responsibility for the *individual child.* Time-series designs provide a means by which clinicians can treat individuals and at the same time systematically collect scientifically sound information regarding the effectiveness of a treatment.

Time-series designs have an advantage over group experiments because *many more measurements* are collected on the same individuals over some period of time. Group experiments often involve only one test or measurement after treatment has been applied, although sometimes there are two or three repeated assessments. Even in longitudinal studies, far fewer measurements are obtained than is typical in time-series investigations. In time-series studies, many observa-

tions are made (perhaps several daily) under both untreated and treated conditions. In fact, because of the ongoing data collected over time from participant(s), these are occasionally termed *continuous measurement studies.* This continuity represents an important strength since one can actually observe the process of change as well as determine the end product.

On the other side of the coin, time-series studies have been criticized because of the small number of participants that are studied (often only one). The concern here involves the generalizability of data obtained for only one or a few individuals. Can one 3rd-grade boy with a conduct disorder tell us how children with conduct disorders will generally respond to a particular treatment? Additionally, the types of participants frequently studied in time-series research are often quite atypical—they really need treatment because their problems are severe. How do we know that the results would be similar if other, more typical people were tested? Basically we do not—unless several replications of the same investigation with different participants show very similar results. For example, a particular medication may have disastrous side effects in only 1 in 10,000 patients. Testing only a few children may fail to reveal such a rare but potentially lethal reaction.

Group Experiments

IN FOCUS 6 ▶ How do group experimental studies differ from time-series studies?

Group experimental studies represent a mirror image of time-series designs in terms of strengths and limitations. More participants are included in a group experiment, so the concern about generalization is lessened. Researchers are more likely to obtain a representative sample of behavior from 30 or 60 participants than from 1 or 3. However, one limitation arising from group experiments, as they are frequently executed, relates to the small number of measurements that are obtained. If, for example, an experiment is conducted on highly similar groups, different treatments are applied, and participants are then tested, we have only one sample of behavior—that provided by the test after experimental treatments have been administered. Any posttest differences observed could have been produced by existing pretreatment differences. It is certainly possible that this one assessment involves atypical performance and the researcher is not aware of it. This concern is somewhat offset by the fact that many participants are usually tested. It is unlikely that all individuals (or even a substantial number) would be behaving in an extremely atypical fashion unless all had some contagious disease or all were subjected to some stress such as an earthquake or fire.

Various types of designs are used for group experiments. For example, two configurations of experimental designs are those that involve comparisons of several groups and those where a pretest-posttest comparison is performed on the same group (repeated measures design). In this context, a separate group design refers to investigations in which a different group receives each of several experimental conditions (i.e.,

Group A receives one treatment and is compared with Group B, which receives a second treatment). This is distinguished from a pretest-posttest study in which the same participants are being assessed twice. The point of interest is the magnitude of change from pretest to posttest. Figure 3-5 diagrams two simple group experiments: one involving comparisons of three groups and another illustrating a pretest-posttest configuration in which the same group is tested before and after treatment is applied. Both of these studies involve one experimental variable. It is labeled "Method of Treatment" in Figure 3-5a and "Learning Stage" in Figure 3-5b. Group experiments may include two or more experimental variables (such studies are also termed *multifactor designs*). Many variations of multifactor designs are used to study child behavior disorders. Discussions are found in sources that focus on research methods (e.g., Kazdin, 1998; Maxwell & Delaney, 2000).

There are strong designs and weak ones, procedures that produce reliable results and others that might prove misleading. The particular advantages and limitations of specific experimental designs could more than fill this book. Interested readers should consult any of the various available sources on research design (Drew et al., 2000; Gay & Airasian, 2000; Wallen & Fraenkel, 2000). The limitations of experimental research cannot be discounted as inconsequential or viewed as insurmountable difficulties. Experimentation remains one of our most powerful tools in the search for causes and treatments of behavior disorders. Its limitations can be circumvented to a substantial degree if a researcher carries out careful and thorough planning prior to execution of an experiment.

Table 3-3 summarizes advantages and limitations of different research strategies.

Meta-Analysis

One aspect of the scientific method that is difficult for nonscientists to understand relates to the slow and incremental nature by which single studies contribute to the overall knowledge base. It may seem simple enough to ask a research question: "Does medication help children with ADHD?" But answers to such a question are often slow to come, and scientists working on the question often seem frustratingly detail-oriented. Impatient research consumers, especially

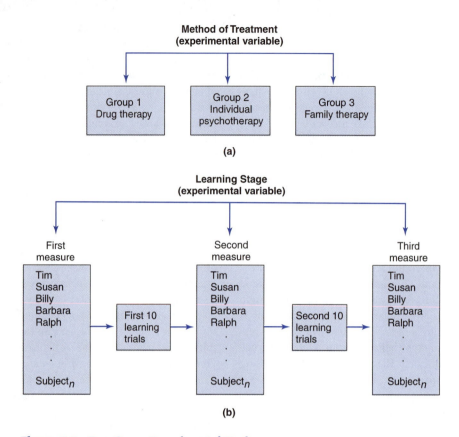

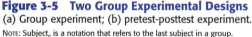

Figure 3-5 Two Group Experimental Designs
(a) Group experiment; (b) pretest-posttest experiment.
NOTE: Subject$_n$ is a notation that refers to the last subject in a group.

parents, may feel they want a simple answer (yes or no) to an apparently simple question. Researchers, on the other hand, do not see the question as simple since there are many subquestions or related issues that require attention (e.g., the child's age, type of ADHD, chemical tolerances, allergies, types of behavior or performance needing attention, and many others). Scientists' approach is to painstakingly address each aspect of the question, one at a time, allowing information to accumulate until they can ultimately answer the larger question—in this case, whether or not medication helps children with ADHD. Such an incremental accumulation of research evidence may involve many individual studies on children; it may take several years of work by multiple investigators in different locations and with different children.

One research procedure that facilitates the analysis and interpretation of multiple results from different studies is **meta-analysis**. This procedure allows a researcher to statistically analyze and synthesize the findings of many previous empirical studies on a given topic in an attempt to discern a consensus or uncover similar findings. This was the technique used in the study by Rind and colleagues (1998) presented in the Research Focus box on page 51. Meta-analysis involves statistical combining and therefore draws conclusions based on the actual data of the previous studies. A meta-analysis indicates whether there is a statistically significant effect based on all the studies combined and how powerful it is. The power evaluation is important, since a treatment effect can be statistically significant but so weak that the treatment is not

Table 3-3 Advantages and Limitations of Various Research Strategies

Strategy	Advantages	Limitations
Observation	Permits precise behavioral descriptions of participants' behavior and of changes caused by intervention.	Data may be inaccurate if observer is biased or unreliable if observer is not trained or if target behaviors are defined ambiguously.
Interview	Data may be rich and informative because interviewer can probe and interrogate further when answers are unclear or incomplete.	Data may be biased or inaccurate because of interviewer bias and interaction between respondent and interviewer.
Questionnaire	Economical means of obtaining data from a large, geographically dispersed sample if distributed by mail.	Data obtained may be limited by format of questionnaire or biased by low response rate.
Case study	Considerable depth and breadth of information on a given patient's problems.	Data may be biased or inaccurate if informant is biased or does not remember accurately or if investigator holds a strong bias.
Quasi-experimental	Permits the study of populations that are different prior to the investigation.	Difficult to control for pre-existing differences other than the independent variable.
Experimental (generally)	Exercises considerable control to minimize effects of extraneous factors.	Amount of control exercised may create artificial environment and alter participants' behavior.
Longitudinal	Permits observation of participants' development over an extended period of time.	Repeated assessment may alter participants' performance; attrition of sample may be substantial over the extended time period.
Cross-sectional	Much more convenient to execute than longitudinal studies.	Group differences may make developmental inferences difficult or incorrect.
Time-series	Many measurements on same participant permit observation of change process as treatment is manipulated.	Often criticized for using small number of participants, which may limit generalizability of results.
Group experimental	Use of many participants promotes greater confidence in generalizability of results.	Taking few measurements on participants does not permit observation of change process.

worth using. Also, methodologically stronger studies can be given more weight than weaker studies in calculating the overall effect.

Far from being junk science, meta-analysis can give a clearer picture of group differences and treatment effects than any single study. (Sorry, U.S. Congress, but you were wrong.) This approach has some clear advantages over drawing logical inferences about some overall trend by reading and interpreting many specific results, which was the approach used by many authors for hundreds of years. Conceptually, meta-analysis is an important research tool because it gives researchers the ability to look at many investigations on a topic, with an intent to synthesize the data into an integrated picture of the overall results (Fuller & Hester, 1999; Kavale & Forness, 2000).

FUNDAMENTALS OF RESEARCH DESIGN

Previous sections have alluded to the process of designing or planning an investigation, an essential step in research. No investigation that is designed poorly or planned in a haphazard fashion can generate results that are very reliable or useful. Regardless of which approach is being employed, the importance of this crucial step cannot be overemphasized.

The purpose of this section is to provide background regarding the fundamentals of research design. You will see how the process of designing high-quality experiments involves a highly systematic way of thinking about what factors influence the outcome, and you will appreciate how important it is to impose control on the research setting. The focus here on experimental investigation is not meant to discount the value of non-experimental and qualitative research in studying child behavior disorders. Space limitations preclude a more complete examination of all research methods.

The Concept of Control

IN FOCUS 7 ▶ What is the concept of control, and why is it important in experimental research?

The concept of control in experimental research warrants specific attention here because it is so central to a well-designed experiment. Many different factors can influence children's behavior, including their intelligence, language skills, motivation, and relationship with the examiner. The object of experimentation is to identify those factors that actually do affect a child's task performance and to eliminate the other factors. In experimental research, **control** involves *eliminating the systematic influence of all variables except the one being studied*. For example, perhaps we want to compare the effectiveness of two treatment programs and we have decided to conduct a group experiment. One group will receive treatment A, whereas the second will receive treatment B (the independent variable is thus type of treatment). The concept of control dictates that all factors must be equivalent for both groups except the independent variable (treatment). That is, the groups must be equivalent with regard to any factors that may influence the results (e.g., age, sex, problem severity). Procedures must also be similar for the two groups, except for any procedural details that are actually part of the treatment. Unless other factors are held constant, or controlled, we will not be able to attribute any differences to the effect of the treatments. For example, we might not be able to infer that participants in group A performed better than those in group B because they received individualized instruction (treatment A) if they also had more time to complete the task than group B did. The concept of control is basic to experimental design—a notion we will encounter repeatedly.

Common Design Mistakes

Classic textbook examples are seldom found outside the environment in which they were contrived—in classroom lectures and textbooks. This is the case for research designs just as for other subjects of study. The standard designs often must be altered to answer a particular research question or to suit a specific set of circumstances. In many cases, situations are encountered during the research study that may threaten the soundness of the investigation and require design or procedural changes. For example, the more disturbed, resistant families may drop out of therapy, raters may become unreliable, or a school may withdraw from a study. Some problems such as these can be prevented by careful planning. This section examines some common design mistakes.

Internal and External Validity

IN FOCUS 8 ▶ Distinguish between internal and external validity.

Validity is a term used in many different contexts and is misused perhaps as often as it is properly employed. With respect to experimental research, two types of validity—internal and external—represent crucial concepts and major criteria by which investigations are evaluated. These forms of validity have been important to experimental research methodology for many years and continue to be central (Babbie, 2001; Schloss & Smith, 1999). **Internal validity** refers to the technical soundness of an investigation in terms of control—that is, how well designed is the study? Experiments that are internally valid are those that have controlled all systematic influences except the one under investigation (i.e., the experimental variable). **External validity,** on the other hand, refers to an experiment's generalizability—that is, how well can its results be generalized to other participants, settings, and treatments?

Both internal and external validity are important, although they may be incompatible in certain circumstances. In some situations, the achievement of adequate internal validity requires conducting an investigation in a controlled or contrived laboratory setting. For example, one might best assess the social perception of juvenile delinquents in a laboratory, but at the risk that the participants will behave uncharacteristically in that setting. To the extent that a research study creates an artificial environment and influences participants' performance, the generalizability of results may be reduced. The reverse may also be true, in that studies may be representative but poorly controlled. Research is a process of constant compromise aimed at achieving an appropriate balance between internal and external validity. Particularly in the early stages of a research program, internal validity may be the primary concern; later, as the fundamental knowledge base grows, more attention may be given to external validity and the issue of to whom the results will apply. In all cases, however, care must be taken not to sacrifice internal validity to a point that the value of any knowledge gained is diminished. Without a satisfactory level of internal validity, confidence about the accuracy of the information is seriously reduced. That is, internal validity is necessary for researchers to be confident that children will ultimately benefit from research results.

A number of factors can threaten the internal validity of an investigation, and total elimination of all possible threats is often impossible. Nearly every study could be strengthened in some fashion. From a practical standpoint, a researcher's task is to eliminate or minimize the influence of as many internal validity problems as possible. Those that cannot be eliminated in a particular study must be accounted for as the results are interpreted.

Internal validity pertains very specifically to the important concept of control mentioned previously. Without control of confounding extraneous influences, a researcher will not be able to attribute results to the experimental variable. For example, suppose we are investigating the effects of a new treatment for obesity. Certainly, if differences are evident, we want to be able to say that this treatment probably generated the participants' weight loss. This would not be possible if, say, some other treatment for obesity, such as fasting or drinking a low-calorie concoction was also used by the overweight participants and thus became a rival explanation for the results. Similarly, we would not be able to determine the effects of our treatment if the scales were adjusted (changed or recalibrated) between two measurements of the participants' weight. In either case, observed weight differences may be caused by our treatment *or* by the other factors, and we could not say, with confidence, what caused the changes.

We have mentioned only a few threats to internal validity. Interested readers, particularly those who must complete an undergraduate or graduate thesis project, should consult sources that more completely examine these topics (e.g., Drew et al., 1996).

Related to internal validity concerns are the influences of placebo effects. **Placebo effects** are changes in participants' behavior or performance that occur simply because they are in an experiment and not because of the impact of a particular treatment or intervention. Placebo effects can make it difficult to attribute changes in participants to treatment. Such a situation is a concern in some drug research (Dienstfrey, 2000; Price, 2000), in which some control participants may show powerful, clinically relevant body changes after taking a placebo treatment (no actual medication). Placebo effects present a substantial challenge to researchers studying child behavior disorders since they are likely to be present in some form and to some degree in nearly all therapeutic interventions. Additionally, placebos may sometimes be quite potent, actually altering disorders that are quite severe (Kazdin, 1998) through a beneficial impact on participants' expectations and behavior.

As stated earlier, external validity refers to the generalizability of results, which can also be threatened by a number of factors. The basic notion of external validity is that the experimental results must be applicable to participants, materials, and settings other than those used in the particular experiment. Such generalizability may not be attainable if there are substantial differences between the participants, materials, or setting of the experiment and those in the world outside the experiment. For example, if the sample of participants is substantially different from the population at large (or the population to which the researcher wishes to generalize), then the results will likely *not* be generalizable. This is a problem when only a few people from a target group, such as mothers of autistic children, volunteer to participate in a study. The volunteers may be more highly educated and their children less seriously disturbed than the others in the target group. Similarly, the environment in which a study is conducted, such as a brightly lit, sparsely furnished, sterile laboratory equipped with one-way viewing windows, may be too unusual or different from the participants' routine environment. If this is the case, participants may behave differently than usual, and the results would not likely generalize to their behavior in their homes, schools, and neighborhoods.

The examination of threats to internal and external validity highlights the importance of thorough planning prior to the execution of a study. Effective planning requires training, foresight, and meticulous attention to detail. Often more time is spent in planning than in actually conducting an investigation. Without such initial efforts, an investigation may provide inaccurate information that is of little or no value in the treatment of behavior disorders in children.

Avoiding Design Pitfalls

Researchers have several methods of avoiding the threats to validity described above. Being sure to choose the appropriate experimental design is a key first step, since some designs are particularly vulnerable to certain problems. Procedures employed during the actual execution of a study can also be very important in minimizing threats to internal and external validity. Techniques for selecting participants and assigning them to groups or treatments are powerful procedural tools for strengthening internal and external validity of investigations.

Behavioral researchers seldom study an entire population. In most cases, it is necessary to select a sample of individuals from a given population to serve as participants. This immediately increases the importance of carefully defining and describing the participant population. Unless this is accomplished, an investigator does not know which individuals are potential participants and to what population the results can generalize. Population definition is of crucial importance as a foundation of external validity and for selection of an appropriate sample. Many sampling procedures are available, and choosing the most appropriate one depends on the specific nature of an investigation. Space restrictions preclude a detailed examination of all sampling techniques that may be employed. Once again, interested readers may wish to consult a source that gives more attention to details of sampling (e.g., Babbie, 2001; Drew et al., 1996).

One of the most generally used methods of selecting participants is known as **random sampling.** This procedure, like sampling in general, is aimed at obtaining a sample of participants that will be representative of the population under study. To accomplish this goal, researchers use a selection process in which each individual in the population has *an equal chance* of being chosen to participate in a study. Since each person has an equal chance of selection, it is assumed that the characteristics of the participant sample will represent those of the entire population. Certainly, this is an assumption, and random sampling does not totally ensure a representative sample, particularly if small groups are being studied. (If a very small number of participants are sampled from a large population, it is unlikely that all or most of the population characteristics are represented in that sample.) However, random sampling procedures do decrease the probability that some systematic bias is operating in the selection process. Even if the resulting sample is found to be unrepresentative in some important way, statistical corrections can be used to control for the differences. The most simple and effective technique for selecting a random sample involves using a random number table (available in most statistics texts) and assigning participants to groups according to whether each successive random digit is odd (Group 1) or even (Group 2); there are also variations of this procedure.

We have repeatedly stressed the importance of group equivalence on the characteristics other than the experimental variables (remember, control is essential to internal validity). The basic tool a researcher can use to accomplish group equivalence is participant assignment. In addition to random assignment, researchers can use **experimental matching.** Experimental matching basically involves procedures by which a researcher forces group equivalence in terms of some characteristic(s) thought to be important for the particular study being conducted. For example, if chronological age (CA) is thought to be important, groups might be formed by matching children on this characteristic. This is often accomplished by replacing participants or switching group assignments for pairs of participants until the average CA is the same for the treatment and control groups.

Random assignment procedures (usually accomplished using random number tables) have become favored over experimental matching. In fact, some researchers believe that matching should be employed only as a last resort, if ever. There are many reasons for favoring random assignment over experimental matching. Perhaps the most compelling relates to the identification of the characteristics on which equivalence is desired. Experimental matching requires a clear knowledge of those factors on which control is to be exercised. Using this procedure essentially requires a declaration that "these are the important factors and others are not." Selectively placing participants (i.e., switching, replacing) raises a substantial possibility that the groups will be made different on some factors in addition to those being matched. The major strength of random assignment is that, because of the nature of the process, there is little reason to expect any *systematic* differences between the groups. Thus, the researcher is probably forming equivalent groups on those factors that are known to be important and those that are as yet unidentified as being important for control (a nice touch and good insurance for the durability of internal validity).

ETHICAL ISSUES IN CONDUCTING RESEARCH

IN FOCUS 9 ▶ Why are ethics vitally important in psychological research on children, and how is the physical and psychological welfare of participants protected?

Ethical issues are vitally important in psychology because the field centrally involves people working with other people and controlling aspects of their lives. When children's behavior is given a diagnostic label and they are treated, ethical problems may arise. Educational, medical, and mental health professionals are the caretakers, the treatment specialists, and generally the professionally authorized arm of society for addressing children's problems. As such, they must be especially concerned about fairness and avoidance of harm to children. Researchers must not take unfair advantage of their responsible positions. They must act ethically, or they may be punished by their professional societies or state licensing offices.

One of the major ethical concerns in behavioral research relates to harming participants. Individuals must not be harmed by serving as participants in any study. Obviously, harm includes physical injury, but the notion of harm also extends to such effects as psychological stress, social embarrassment, and many others. Avoidance of harm is a difficult and complex consideration. Ordinary living is not stress-free. A researcher must judge how much added stress would prove harmful. If pushed to its conceptual limits and interpreted in an extremely literal manner, this consideration would significantly detract from the ability to conduct psychological research (or perhaps eliminate it). Of course, there is *some* stress for participants par-

ticipating in most investigations, and it is not feasible to take a position that there must be absolutely no psychological infringement. It is necessary for researchers to balance carefully the avoidance of harm and the potential risk for harm as they undertake each study. For this reason, independent review boards (e.g., human participants committees, institutional review boards, or IRBs) operate in most agencies to examine research proposals and attempt to protect participants' rights. The questions involved are complex, and there are no simple answers. One must turn to professional guidelines and colleagues for guidance (e.g., Bersoff, 1999; Jones, 2001).

Ethical concerns hold a place of particular importance in psychological and other behavioral research because of the nature of the undertaking. To investigate patterns of normal and abnormal behavior, psychologists do invade, look into, and explore the lives of others. They do this not for personal curiosity or advantage, but in order to find causes of problems and more effective treatments. Because psychological research involves people's lives, great care must be taken to ensure fairness to those being studied. A researcher's task is not limited to the design and execution of a technically sound investigation. Constant vigilance must be maintained regarding ethical issues as they pertain to research procedures and related professional activities, especially in the area of child behavior disorders. Consequently, each national professional society requires members to abide by written codes of ethics.

Institutional review boards or human participants committees oversee research ethics, as do federal offices, school district research participation committees, and other bodies. The typical child research project is scrutinized by at least three such bodies in order to protect the welfare of participating children and their families. In addition, public agencies and research sponsors require that researchers obtain informed, written consent from participants or their parents. For children, parental consent is required, and the children themselves must consent if they are able to do so. Participants are also informed that they may withdraw from the study at any time without penalty.

Concern for research ethics is not new, although it has gained prominence in recent years. In addition to establishing ethical codes of conduct for their members, some professional organizations (e.g., the Amer-

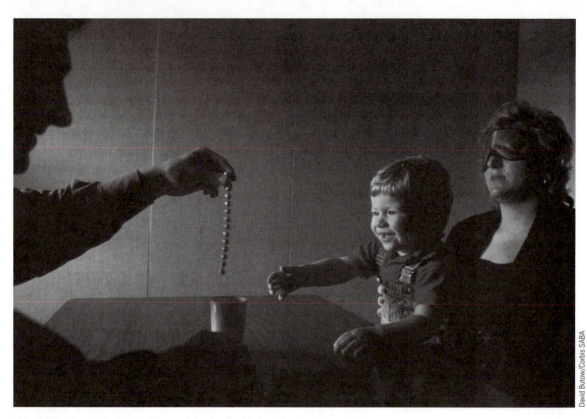

This child must not be harmed by participating in this learning experiment.

ican Psychological Association) have made a practice of investigating allegations and expelling individuals from membership for breaches of ethical conduct. Additionally, federal agencies funding research activities typically have regulations regarding appropriate and ethical treatment of participants. Entire books have been written on research ethics, and as we shall see, the issues can be complex ones.

Probably the most conspicuous concern in research ethics relates to the protection of the physical and psychological welfare of participants (Brandon, 2000; Sales & Folkman, 2000). This concern has been sharpened by two major influences: periodic though rare cases of flagrant abuse of research participants' rights, and a generally heightened societal sensitivity regarding individual rights. Of particular concern in psychological research is obtaining participants' fully informed consent to participate in a research project.

Consent may be viewed simply as the means by which participants openly declare whether or not they wish to participate in a research investigation. On further inspection, this apparently simple process involves a number of complexities. To be valid, consent must include three elements: capacity, information, and voluntariness. All three elements must be present for consent to be meaningful; the researcher must also be aware that consent is not permanent. It may be withdrawn at any time. That is, participants must be allowed to discontinue their participation whenever they wish to do so and without penalty of any type, psychological or material.

Capacity refers to a person's ability and legal authority to consent to participate in a research project. Although a 12-year-old boy who is a juvenile delinquent may have the ability to decide whether to agree to participate in a study, he does not have the legal authority to do so since he is considered a minor. His parent or legal guardian must grant consent for him to participate, but he must also agree that he wants to do so. This issue is even more sensitive and difficult when people with psychosis or mental retardation or very young children are studied. Because they lack capacity to determine whether they should participate, their caretakers and the investigators must take special pains to protect them from exploitation. At the same time, caretakers must bear in mind that progress in treatment can come about only through procedurally sound research. Thus, participation in research studies is in the public interest and may be advantageous for participants who receive a thorough assessment, a new intervention, or monetary compensation.

The second element of consent is information. *Information,* in this context, refers to the information given to the research participants. Generally speaking, the researcher is responsible for the information provided to the participants. It is his or her responsibility to assure that the information is designed to be fully understood and that it *is* understood (Drew et al., 1996). The investigator must carry the burden of satisfying these responsibilities, and IRBs will carefully review the protocols to make sure this has been done. The need to provide complete information causes a particular problem in that examination of the consent information may sometimes alert participants to what the research hypothesis is, which may make them act unnaturally.

Voluntariness, the third element of consent, is, once again, more complex than it may appear on the surface. Clearly, the notion of voluntariness suggests that participants in a study must agree to participate of their own free will. This requirement also places a great deal of responsibility on researchers studying child behavior disorders. Certainly, there should not be any constraint or coercion, either explicit or implicit. In some cases, even a reward for participation may be coercive, as might be the case with destitute families.

Researchers studying child behavior disorders must be particularly cautious regarding ethical practices. In many cases, it is difficult to meet the requirements of the three elements of consent (Drew & Hardman, 2000; Drew et al., 1996). First, researchers must obtain consent from a child's parents, guardian, or other agent who is legally responsible and authorized to act on the child's behalf. Even then, a researcher must be confident that the consenter's interests are not at odds with what may be the best

interests of the child, which is not always the case (Drew & Hardman, 2000). For example, a nervous or autocratic parent might desire an inappropriately quiet and timid child. In nearly all cases, researchers are ethically bound to obtain consent from the child as well, despite the fact that there is no legal requirement to do so. Ethical appropriateness concerning consent often goes far beyond what is legally necessary, as illustrated by the material presented in Table 3-4.

Another ethical issue in psychological research (related to harm in some senses) involves the degree to which researchers invade participants' privacy. Privacy has been long treasured in Western society. When researchers collect and analyze information (data) on participants, they are invading those people's privacy to some degree. Although total privacy does not exist, each of us has some concept of the degree to which we want to share certain matters with others outside our close circle of family and friends, and the form in which that sharing is acceptable. As with avoidance of harm, respect for participants' privacy must be carefully balanced with the need to conduct research that will help solve people's problems. It is clearly an invasion of privacy to secretly tap someone's telephone, but is it also an invasion to observe people in a public place such as a supermarket or a schoolyard? Once again, there are no simple answers. The best that one can do is to be sensitive and remain vigilant to procedures that may unduly or unnecessarily invade privacy.

Deception is another issue that frequently surfaces in examining research ethics. *Deception* is any misrepresentation of information regarding the purpose, nature, or consequences of a research study. Such a misrepresentation may occur because of either omitting information or giving false information. Either, if serious and potentially harmful to participants, is unethical. It would seem that the solution to this problem is to simply avoid deception. However, like so many other issues, matters aren't quite that simple. Deception in one form or another is rather widespread in psychological research. In some cases, researchers do not fully inform participants about the purpose of the study, such as by withholding details about the treatment. Sometimes informed consent forms are written at a higher reading level than is appropriate for the participants being investigated, which raises serious questions regarding the effectiveness of the participants'

Table 3-4 Problems with Consent in Research with Behavior Disordered Children

Consent Element	Guideline	Problem	Potential Solution
Capacity	Participants must be mentally and psychologically able to give consent and also of legal age to give consent.	Children with behavior disorders are not typically old enough to give legal consent. In many cases, they are also unable to give consent by virtue of mental or psychological limitations.	Consent must be obtained from the legal guardian of the child who has the authority to make decisions for the child. The child should also give consent, despite the fact that it is not legally required in most cases.
Information	Participants and legal guardians must be fully informed regarding purposes and procedures of the study. The information must be understood.	Participants with behavior disorders may have difficulty understanding the information, regardless of how well it is communicated.	Researchers must be certain that the legal guardians understand the information and make every attempt possible to make the children understand.
Voluntariness	Participants and guardians must give consent of their own free will, without explicit or implicit coercion of any type. They must be aware that they can withdraw consent at any time.	Participants and guardians may feel some degree of coercion simply because the researcher may represent a power figure for them. Similarly, children may feel coerced if their guardian(s) consent(s).	Researchers must be very sensitive to any evidence of reluctance to consent of desire to discontinue participation. This is true for both participants and guardians.

NOTE: Additionally, participants and guardians have the right to confidentiality concerning the information obtained by a researcher, as well as the right to non-harmful treatment, knowledge of results, and full compensation for the time spent participating.

consent. Issues of deception remain controversial and of intense interest to researchers (e.g., Crook & Dean, 1999; Karlawish, Hougham, Stocking, & Sachs, 1999; Loftus, 1999). There are a number of reasons why this is so. Certain psychological research cannot be conducted at all or would be extremely difficult with totally nondeceptive procedures. There are circumstances when having full information might change participants' behavior or performance. For example, if we were studying the amount of influence friends have on opinions concerning drug use, complete information about the purpose of the investigation might alter participants' susceptibility to such influence. Additionally, there are situations where the focus or method of a particular study actually requires deception. These types of studies necessarily involve deception—so are they unethical? There is no simple answer. Deception must be considered in relation to the risk of harm and may require discussions with experienced colleagues, school personnel, and ethics boards.

Children and adolescents are generally more "at risk," or more vulnerable to being taken advantage of

by thoughtless or uninformed investigators, than are adults. Beyond this fact, the nature of many of the problems studied in the field of child behavior disorders further complicates ethical considerations. Research on child behavior disorders thus presents a considerable challenge—improving the knowledge base for more effective treatment while simultaneously providing the necessary protection for a vulnerable group. Is it ethical to single out a child with learning disabilities or a seizure disorder for study and observation, even treatment in a classroom, and thus draw more attention to her disorder? When is it justified to try a new, unresearched treatment on a child? Is it ethical to prescribe a drug that has only been used with adults to treat a 6-year-old with bed-wetting problems? How accurate must an assessment technique or diagnostic test prove to be before it should be used routinely? Is it ever better to choose treatments based on clinical experience rather than on controlled research tests? If a researcher discovers a promising treatment, can it ethically be withheld from control participants in order to study its effects? Both design

Back to the Beginning

Jeremy Begins to Read

Jeremy basically liked school in the 5th grade, although it had not always been that way. He remembered when he first went to preschool, he had been all excited, but then it had gotten a little rocky at times. While all the other kids seemed to be reading and spelling, the pages didn't tell him anything. All he saw was just a bunch of lines and marks. Then his mom and dad had taken him to a doctor who talked to him and made him do some tests. And after that he had help from a young woman who went over the lines again and again, until they began to make some sense.

Jeremy is a fortunate boy. His parents realized that he was having some difficulty early in his preschool experience. Without making a big deal about it, they took him to a psychologist for some diagnostic work, despite the fact that Jeremy was still a little young for most of the tests that assess the types of difficulties he *seemed* to be showing. Although it was too early to determine

definitively whether Jeremy had a learning disability, it wasn't too early to try to make his preschool experience more positive, and that was important to his parents.

Jeremy spent only a few months with the psychology graduate student on some structured tutoring, but it helped immensely. He was soon beginning to say his alphabet and even starting to read. The reading wasn't an easy thing for him, but he was getting better, and it felt really good to be able to do it like the other kids even if he wasn't the best at it. Although there are likely to be further challenges for Jeremy in school, the early intervention and the low-key approach used by his parents were likely quite important. Without labeling him as having a disability, they were able to provide some specialized individual instruction aimed at helping him learn the initial skills needed for letter and word recognition and then taking the next step to beginning reading skills.

---

considerations and ethical questions affect the answers to such questions in all research settings (Arhar, Holly, & Kasten, 2001).

SUMMARY

Research is a major source of objective information regarding the nature of child behavior disorders, their causes, prevention, and treatment. Because information produced from research is systematically and objectively collected, it tends to be more accurate and reliable than information obtained by casual observation or from commonsense reasoning. Research procedures are much more systematic and the requirements of evidence are much more stringent than those used in more informal information seeking. Therefore, some knowledge of research principles is important for those who are consumers of research and are attempting to make decisions about identification (or diagnosis) and treatment of children with behavior disorders.

Psychological research may be classified into several general types, including experimental, nonexperimental, quantitative, and qualitative. These categories are not mutually exclusive and, in fact, overlap in some research strategies. Nonexperimental research tends to be descriptive, whereas experimental research often examines causal relationships through manipulation of participants' behavior. Qualitative research tends to use data expressed in nonnumerical forms (e.g., words) and studies participants in their natural environment. Quantitative research analyzes data in the form of numbers and is more likely to manipulate naturally occurring events in order to achieve control. Each approach is appropriate for some research questions and settings, and each has certain advantages and limitations that must be considered. Within each general approach are a variety of specific designs or methods that may be used depending on the circumstances of the particular study being planned.

The planning of an investigation is crucial to the soundness of the methodology and the reliability of the results. Many procedural matters must receive attention in selecting an appropriate research design. The design must minimize threats to the study's validity. When an experimental study has high internal validity, the results can be attributed to the experimental variable (e.g., the type of treatment used) rather than some other influence. With high external validity, research findings from the sample studied can be generalized to the larger population from which the research participants were drawn. These types of validity are essential for research to be dependable and meaningful.

In addition to being concerned about validity, a researcher must take precautions to avoid ethical violations in the process of conducting a study. Behavioral scientists face some particularly difficult ethical issues when studying child behavior disorders since children (and their caretakers) may lack the capacity to make informed judgments about the advisability of participating in research projects. In all cases, children as well as adults must be allowed to terminate their research participation at any time they choose.

We now take the opportunity to terminate this chapter. Students who have found these concepts intriguing may well become the researchers of tomorrow. Those who have found it uninteresting or unintelligible may find graduate work requiring research and statistics to be a real trial. There are more important and valid tests of one's career interests, of course, but most graduate research programs in clinical and counseling psychology, nursing, and medicine involve training in research theory and practice. Practitioners must be knowledgeable consumers of research in order to keep pace with new developments.

INFOTRAC COLLEGE EDITION

For more information, explore this resource at http://www.infotrac-college.com/Wadsworth. Enter the following search terms.

deceptive research
experimental control
experimental design
data analysis
qualitative research
quantitative research
statistical tests
ethics and research

IN FOCUS ANSWERS

IN FOCUS 1 ▶ What three types of research questions are typically addressed in psychology?

- Descriptive questions concern the characteristics of a particular group or type of individual.
- Difference questions compare different groups or they may compare a single group's or an individual's behavior before and after treatment.
- Relationship questions (or correlational questions) ask to what degree two or more phenomena relate or vary together.

IN FOCUS 2 ▶ Discuss the differences between experimental and nonexperimental research methods.

- In experimental research, the investigator manipulates the treatment a participant experiences in an environment that is carefully controlled.
- Nonexperimental research methods tend to emphasize observing, analyzing, and describing phenomena as they exist naturally, rather than manipulating treatments or conditions. Nonexperimental research does not typically involve as much control as in experimental research.

IN FOCUS 3 ▶ Describe how qualitative research methods generally differ from quantitative approaches.

- Qualitative research collects data often by observing participants in their natural context. With participant observation, the individual collecting the data actually participates in the setting or activities being observed. Alternatively, the observer participates minimally or not at all and may not even be seen by those being observed (for example, observations made through a one-way mirror or by means of audio or video recordings).
- For the most part, quantitative research asks questions, develops hypotheses, manipulates experimental variables, and measures outcomes in a manner that can be reduced to some numerical data.

IN FOCUS 4 ▶ What are two experimental research designs commonly used to study human development?

- Longitudinal designs select a sample of participants, test or observe them, and follow these same participants for an extended period of time, repeating the assessment intermittently.
- Cross-sectional designs, on the other hand, simultaneously sample different groups of participants who are at several age levels (e.g., 3 to 5, 6 to 8, 9 to 11, and 12 to 15) and compare the dependent variable (e.g., social skills or self-esteem) across the age groups.

IN FOCUS 5 ▶ Explain how time-series designs investigate the effects of an intervention with children.

- Time-series experiments involve investigations in which an independent variable is manipulated across two or more phases (e.g., applied, then withdrawn, then reapplied, or applied at different times to different participants), and the dependent variable is monitored.
- Time-series studies are often used to assess the effect of treatment on the behavior of a small number of participants or even a single individual participant. If treatment manipulation reliably changes the behavior of the participant(s), then the researcher can conclude that the treatment is effective.

IN FOCUS 6 ▶ How do group experimental studies differ from time-series studies?

- More participants are included in a group experiment, so generalization of the results is enhanced. Researchers are more likely to obtain a representative sample of behavior from 30 or 60 participants than from one or three.
- Group experiments tend to take fewer measurements than time-series experiments, often using only one, two, or three assessments.

IN FOCUS 7 ▶ What is the concept of control, and why is it important in experimental research?

- The concept of control involves eliminating the systematic influence of all variables except the one being studied. Thus, all factors are equivalent for both groups except the independent variable (treatment).

- Control is important so that the research can attribute any differences between the groups to the treatment and not to other factors that might be influential.

IN FOCUS 8 ▶ Distinguish between internal and external validity.

- Internal validity concerns the technical soundness of an investigation in terms of control—that is, how well designed is this study? Experiments that are internally valid are those that have controlled all systematic influences except the one under investigation (i.e., the experimental variable).
- External validity, on the other hand, relates to generalizability—that is, how well results can be generalized to other participants, settings, and treatments.

IN FOCUS 9 ▶ Why are ethics vitally important in psychological research on children, and how is the physical and psychological welfare of participants protected?

- One of the major concerns in psychological research is that no harm be done to participants. Individuals must not be harmed by serving as participants in any study. Many participants in psychological research are vulnerable in that they are young or have emotional or mental limitations that make them susceptible to being taken advantage of.
- Independent review boards (e.g., human participants committee or institutional review boards, or IRBs) operate in most agencies to examine research proposals and attempt to protect participants' rights. The typical child research project is scrutinized by at least three such bodies in order to protect the welfare of participating children and their families.
- Public agencies and other research sponsors require that researchers obtain informed, written consent from participants and/or their parents. For children, parental consent is required, and the children themselves must consent if they are able to do so.
- Participants are also informed that they may withdraw from a study at any time without penalty.

4 Assessment and Classification of Child Behavior Disorders

WILLIAM R. JENSON   CLIFFORD J. DREW   DANIEL OLYMPIA

In the Beginning

"What's Wrong?" "He'll Grow Out of It."

"He's just growing up. He'll grow out of it and catch up." Margie and Jeff had said these words to each other thousands of times. But it gnawed at them. Thinking about it, Margie would get a pain in her stomach and feel a bit sick. Jeff would become preoccupied, not hearing his coworkers' comments. Brian was the first-born child of Margie and Jeff. They were so proud when he was born, big eyes that just looked right through you. At first Margie thought he was a really good baby because he didn't cry or fuss like other children she had seen. He seemed shy and always wanted to be close to her. As he got a little older, he did not talk around other people. He would talk to Margie at home, but he didn't pronounce words very well and seemed to have difficulty making sentences. And when adults other than Margie did hear him, they couldn't understand what he said. Sometimes he seemed to be in his own world, not responding to his parents' questions unless they made him look at them. The family doctor seemed baffled, and said to wait. He would grow out of it— "catch up," the doctor said. Anyway, the doctor was not concerned because Brian seemed healthy and did not have any obvious physical problems.

But then things changed after one holiday when all the families got together and there were wall-to-wall children. Comparisons were natural, and Brian was now 5. He refused to talk, gestured for what he wanted, and seemed anxious around the relatives. Margie's more experienced sister who had three children said something might be wrong. "Things should be checked out," she said, noting that Margie had held Brian back from preschool because she didn't think him ready.

What does "checked out" mean? It means entering the world of testing, assessment, and classification—a world few parents are aware of or ready for. What is a test? Would classification and a label follow? What would be the effects of the assessment and classification procedures, and would they help? Or simply result in the stigma of a label?

INTRODUCTION

What does it take to accurately assess and classify a child like Brian? Are complicated psychological tests and classification systems needed? Or can parents and teachers easily and accurately identify children with psychological and developmental difficulties? Obviously not, in the case of Margie and Jeff with Brian's perplexing behavior. What are the advantages and limitations of psychological assessment and classification?

In this chapter, we will discuss several assessment and classification methods that are used to make decisions concerning children's behavior problems like Brian's. We will review specific assessment techniques such as psychological testing, structured interviewing, behavioral observation, and functional behavior assessment. We will also survey the most commonly used systems for classifying and labeling children. But, most important, we will discuss criteria for judging the adequacy of assessment and classification procedures.

ASSESSMENT AND CLASSIFICATION: ALIKE BUT DIFFERENT

Assessment and classification can be as controversial as religion, politics, or the newest approaches to treatment. It is difficult to get a consensus on these subjects from a majority of professionals. In the field of child development, **assessment** means the process of collecting information regarding the psychological, medical, and academic achievement status and performance of a child. The assessment is conducted through observation of behavior and testing of performance and status using instruments or other protocols that result in reliable information about the child. **Classification** involves categorizing the child into a grouping based on diagnostic analysis of the assessment information. Such classifications, at best, provide guidance for interventions and delivery of educational, medical, and psychological services. In their less useful forms, classifications result in groupings for administration of programs, but clinicians need to gather more detailed information to guide interventions.

First, precise *measurement* is stressed in most definitions of assessment. Second, comprehensive *information* gathering is essential to good assessment prac-

Table 4-1 Collection Procedures Used in Assessment	
Tests	Standardized intelligence and achievement tests
	Projective personality tests
	Objective personality tests
	Criterion-referenced tests
Observations	Objective behavior observations by an independent observer
	Self-recording
	Behavior ratings by teachers or parents
Interviews	Behavioral interviews
	Social histories
	Child psychiatric interviews

tices. Assessment methods used to gather information vary from systematic procedures (such as structured behavioral observation) to relatively unstructured procedures (such as informal interviews). Table 4-1 lists various types of procedures used to collect information. However, good assessment should go beyond merely collecting information; it involves making decisions about classification, diagnosis, placement, treatment, and research for children (Anastasi & Urbina, 1997; Merrell, 1999; Sattler, 2001).

Classification systems, however, are different from most assessment methods. They rely almost entirely on interviews to gather basic information about a child and then use prescribed guidelines to reach a decision and assign a label. The process is somewhat like ordering from a menu. If so many of the child's characteristics or behaviors are found in one list of the classification system and so many in another list, then a child may be diagnosed with a disability. Table 4-2 gives some of the classification systems most commonly used with children.

Although most classification systems use interviews to collect information, many also use some type of assessment information to help generate a diagnosis. For example, psychological measures such as IQ tests are used to help in the classification and diagnosis of mental retardation or a learning disability. Similarly, federal special education legislation mandates that the classification of a student with disabilities be based on measures that are designed specifically to assess the disabilities validly [Individuals with Disabilities Act (IDEA), 1997]. Some classification sys-

Table 4-2 Commonly Used Classification Systems
Diagnostic and Statistical Manual of Mental Disorders, 4th Edition—Text Revision (DSM-IV-TR) of the American Psychiatric Association
International Classification of Diseases (ICD-10) of the World Health Organization
Categorical Educational Classification derived from the Individuals with Disabilities Education Act, 1997 (IDEA)
Categorical Classification derived from the Rehabilitation Act of 1973 (Section 504) and the Americans with Disabilities Act (ADA)
Functional Behavior Assessment and Classification

tems use several types of related assessment measures (i.e., behavior checklists, academic testing, and observations) and several informants (i.e., teachers, parents, and the child) to rule out other disorders and arrive at a diagnosis. Others, such as functional assessment and classification, use interviews, observations, and probing of the child's behavior to understand what may be controlling the behavior in the child's environment.

Assessment information is generally used along with a classification system in arriving at a diagnosis for a child. In the chapter-opening example, Brian and his parents will be given several psychological assessment measures, and Brian will be observed. The data will be reported to a professional who has interviewed Margie and Jeff and examined Brian. This professional will then use an accepted classification system to arrive at a diagnosis and label. Hopefully, this will help Margie and Jeff answer the questions "What does my child have?" (i.e., the diagnostic label) and "What's wrong?" (i.e., the specific problem areas identified by the psychological assessment data).

The next sections deal with psychological assessment, specific assessment methods, and standards for evaluating their adequacy. Later, the chapter will deal similarly with classification systems commonly used with children.

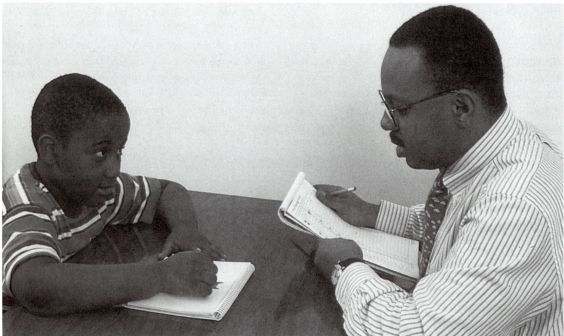

Laura Dwight/PhotoEdit

Because assessment information substantially affects the appropriateness of the decisions made concerning a child, assessment often includes individually administered tests.

PSYCHOLOGICAL ASSESSMENT

First, in psychological assessment, measurements are taken and information is gathered. Second, based on the information, decisions are made regarding classification, placement, treatment, and evaluation of a child. The information-gathering phase of assessment substantially affects the appropriateness of the decisions made concerning the child (Gronlund, 1998). If the information is erroneous or inadequate, the quality of the decisions will be affected. It is critical to understand how to judge the quality of assessment information. To help judge assessment procedures, the American Psychological Association (APA) has developed joint standards for educational and psychological testing (APA, 1999). These standards cover test development, measuring error, fairness in using tests, and responsible use of test information.

Standards for Assessment

IN FOCUS 1 ▶ Identify the sources of systematic and random error.

Any type of assessment method is subject to error. In a sense, all assessment data includes a "true score" and an "error score" (Sattler, 2001). No method is perfect. For instance, if we are trying to measure the motor activity of children in a classroom and several of the children are ill, then our activity measurements will probably be lower than if all the children were in good health. In a sense, the information gathered by an assessment method is only an approximation of the real phenomenon that is being measured because error is always present. In our example, the random event that some children were sick would result in an underestimate of the true motor activity of the group. This type of chance error is known as **random error**. Another type of error that also affects assessment is **systematic error**. With systematic error, the assessment procedure or the person using it is *always* off to a certain degree. For our example study of motor activity, a systematic error in measurement might occur because the pedometer (a device that measures motor activity) is malfunctioning and always records too low a measurement. Both random and systematic errors are important because they are at the root of problems with assessment reliability and validity. Using assessment measures that have poor reliability and validity can lead to serious consequences in selecting psychological treatments (Gronlund, 1998).

Reliability

The **reliability** of an assessment procedure is an indication of the consistency of the procedure (Anastasi & Urbina, 1997; Sattler 2001). For example, if a measure is repeatedly taken, it would be considered reliable if the same or similar scores are yielded each time. As mentioned earlier, we can assume that the information given by an assessment tool contains the true score (Sattler, 2001). However, on each administration of the assessment procedure, random error is present and affects the true score. If the assessment procedure is unreliable, then large amounts of random error will be present, causing the scores to vary greatly. If only a small amount of random error is present, then the scores will be similar and cluster around the true score. For example, if an intelligence test is repeatedly given to a child who has a true IQ score of 100 and the test results are 50, 107, 36, and 129, the test is unreliable. However, if the test scores are 105, 99, 103, and 101 (which are close to the true score of 100), the test is reliable.

Factors that reduce the degree of consistency of information and result in significant random error include:

- Ambiguous assessment procedures that leave a great deal of interpretation up to the evaluator
- Poorly trained evaluators who are not familiar with the assessment procedures
- Widely varying behavior of the children being evaluated (as in our example of motor activity and ill children)
- Growth and development, which cause differences in children's ability and behavior (common when significant periods of time elapse between assessments)
- Varying assessment conditions (such as a noisy or distracting environment)

If the information that is gathered by an assessment procedure is not reliable, then a child is at risk. If the procedure has poor reliability, then it becomes difficult to use it to judge treatment effectiveness. Is the difference between the measures taken before and after treatment a function of the treatment's true effectiveness or an artifact of random error? Similarly, interrater reliability is important in identifying behaviorally disordered children. If one observer judges a child's behavior to be problematic and another judges it to be normal, then the disagreement may result in the child's not getting help.

Validity

Although reliability is a measure of random error, it is not a measure of systematic error, which also affects assessment information. Validity is a much better measure of systematic error. **Validity** is a reality check on the meaning of an assessment procedure or how accurately it measures what it is supposed to measure (Anastasi & Urbina, 1997; Sattler, 2001). For instance, if a new test purports to diagnose children's behavior disorders accurately, we might compare the results of the new test on several children with the diagnostic judgment of a group of experienced clinical psychologists. If the test's results closely match the results from the psychologists, we could assume that the test has good validity. However, if the results are not similar, we would question the test's validity. Several other types of validity are associated with how well an assessment method measures what it was designed to measure. Different types of reliability and validity are listed in Table 4-3.

Utility

Assessment information is only valuable if it is useful in making decisions concerning a child's placement and treatment. Without these decisions, the assessment process is only half accomplished. Yet, many children are expensively assessed with little thought about treatment. This link from the assessment process to the decision process is called *utility*, and it is often overlooked. The **utility** of an assessment procedure is the extent to which the assessment information that is gathered is used to make practical, cost-effective, and correct decisions to help the child (Drew & Hardman, 2000; Gronlund, 2000).

No practitioner, teacher, or parent wants to use an assessment technique that can lead to incorrect decisions. However, many assessment techniques result in dubious decisions if they are used incorrectly or with the wrong population. The cost of an incorrect

---

Table 4-3 Types of Reliability and Validity

Test-retest reliability: This type of reliability is assessed by administering an assessment instrument and then readministering the same instrument after a certain time interval (e.g., 30 days). The similarity of the two scores indicates the level of test-retest reliability.

Alternate form reliability: When an assessment measure has two equivalent forms (e.g., Form A and Form B) and both are administered, the similarity of the two scores from the two measures is the measure of reliability.

Internal consistency reliability: This type of reliability is calculated when an assessment measure is split in half and administered. The division creates two alternative forms of the same test. The similarity in the two scores from the two halves of the test yields the reliability score.

Inter-rater reliability: When two raters or observers simultaneously use an assessment measure (e.g., behavioral observation), the similarity between their scores indicates the level of reliability.

Face validity: This type of validity refers to what a test seems to measure intuitively, what the test appears to assess based on visual examination. Face validity does not mean that the test actually measures that property.

Content validity: This type of validity refers to whether the items in the assessment instrument or protocol actually contain or represent items found in the content area that it is designed to measure.

Concurrent validity: This type of validity is measured when a new assessment measure is given at the same time (concurrently) as a well-accepted measure. The similarity between the new measure and the criterion measure is an indication of validity.

Predictive validity: With this type of validity, the correlation between the assessment measure score and some future outcome it predicts is an indication of validity.

Construct validity: This type of validity indicates how well an assessment procedure score represents some theoretical construct such as a trait, ability, or characteristic.

---

decision also varies with the type of behavior disorder. For example, making a wrong decision and not identifying for treatment a child with autism may later have dramatic implications for the child because of the delay. When a condition truly exists but is missed, the error is called a **false negative**. In the opposite type of situation, an assessment technique can incorrectly identify a child as having a behavior disorder. This error is called a **false positive**, meaning that the assessment process has positively identified a problem when one does not exist. False negatives waste valuable time that could have been used for early intervention. False positives may be quite problematic if the label attached is stigmatizing to the child.

In the case of Brian, his parents may be in a quandary. How much will the testing and assessment cost? Will insurance pay? But, most important, what if they wait and he gets worse and early opportunities for treatment are lost? However, like all concerned parents, they do not want their child assessed inappropriately and saddled with an incorrect diagnosis and label. Brian's parents can take heart. Recent evidence has shown that well-administered psychological tests and assessment procedures have validity comparable to the standard medical tests ordered by the family doctor (Meyer et al., 2001).

Psychological Tests

IN FOCUS 2 ▶ List the characteristics of a standardized measure.

Generally, when people think of assessment, they think of psychological tests. However, psychological testing is a procedure by which a specific instrument yields a specific score (e.g., an IQ score). In contrast, psychological assessment is a more general process in which a variety of test scores, referral information, and additional data are collected to be used to answer referral questions about placement, treatment, or research (Meyer et al., 2001; Sattler, 2001).

In general, a **psychological test** is an objective and standardized measure of a sample of behavior (Anastasi & Urbina, 1997). An important aspect of this definition is the term **standardized measure**, which indicates that explicitly defined procedures are to be employed in administering the test. Intelligence tests, developmental tests, academic achievement tests, and personality tests for children are standardized so that comparisons can be made between each child taking

the test and a large group of children on whom the test was first developed. Holding the testing conditions constant generally means that:

1. The same items or test questions are given in the same order to all subjects.
2. The same test instructions are given to all subjects in an identical fashion.
3. All subjects have the same amount of time to finish the test.
4. The testing environment is held relatively constant and free from noise and distraction for all subjects.

If these conditions are met, then the results obtained from the standardization group define what is normal for other children, and these results are commonly referred to as testing norms (see Research Focus box). The distribution of test scores generally fall along a bell-shaped normal curve, with the average score in the middle of the curve and the two tails or ends representing extreme scores. The simplicity of the normal curve concept has led to considerable controversy when it is used to relate intelligence and class structure, as in the book *The Bell Curve* (Frisby, 1995; Hernstein & Murray, 1994).

To make valid comparisons, children included in the standardization group should generally resemble those who will be tested later. The group should reflect the characteristics of the population of children with whom the test will be used routinely. For example, the standardization group should be of the appropriate age, developmental level, ethnic background, socioeconomic level, and geographical distribution (Anastasi & Urbina, 1997).

What Psychological Tests Measure

The definition of a psychological test includes the idea that a person's behavior is sampled. This definition emphasizes the fact that some type of behavior, whether it is academic performance, intellectual ability, or abnormal behavior, is directly sampled or observed in a specific situation. Once the sample has been collected or the observation has been made, comparisons to standardized norms can be carried out to determine the child's abilities and/or deficiencies.

Alternative views to this sample-situation approach propose that psychological tests measure *traits* (this view is described but not advocated by Mischel, 1993). The trait view holds that test scores are signs of under-

Research Focus

The Normal Curve and Assessment

The *normal curve* is a mathematical concept that allows meaningful comparisons of different assessment scores. An example of the normal, or bell-shaped, curve is given in Figure 4-1. Actually, this curve is a representation of many scores; some are high, some are low, but most of them are average. The *average* or *mean* score is represented on the curve by the X. The hump at the average indicates that most scores are average or near-average. As we get to the extreme scores (at the ends of the curve), the curve gets flatter, indicating that there are fewer scores in these ranges. The SDs on the curve are *standard deviation markers*. A standard deviation is a statistical measure of variability. It is also an indicator of the percentage of scores that fall within the standard deviation markers. For example, approximately 68% of all scores are within 1 standard deviation above and 1 standard deviation below the mean. Also, standard deviations can be measured from the ends of the curve. For example, 97.7% of all the scores fall on or below the +2 SD mark on the curve.

The normal curve is important for assessment because it allows us to make meaningful judgments about how av-erage or different a particular score might be. If a score is average, we know that approximately 50% of all the other scores are above and 50% are below the average score. In a sense, the average score is right in the middle of the distribution. Also, if a score is +2 SD from the mean, it is in the range that many psychological tests and checklists describe as "clinically different." For instance, if a score on the hyperactivity factor of the Achenbach Child Behavior Profile is +2 SD from the mean, then the score is considered clinically significant. This is because 98% of all the other children in the standardization group fell on or below this mark. Only 2% (a very small number) of the children in this group were above the +2 SD mark. These were the very hyperactive children.

There are also several different types of standard scores that are used in assessment. A T score has a mean of 50 and a standard deviation of 10. A Z score has a mean of 0 and a standard deviation of 1. These scores are important because such tests as the Personality Inventory for Children (PIC) and the Achenbach Child Behavior Profile use T-scores in measuring a child's performance on the normal curve.

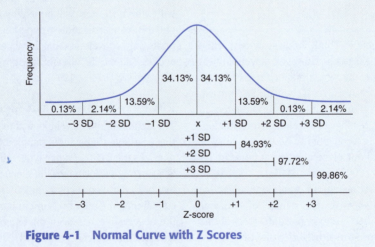

Figure 4-1   Normal Curve with Z Scores

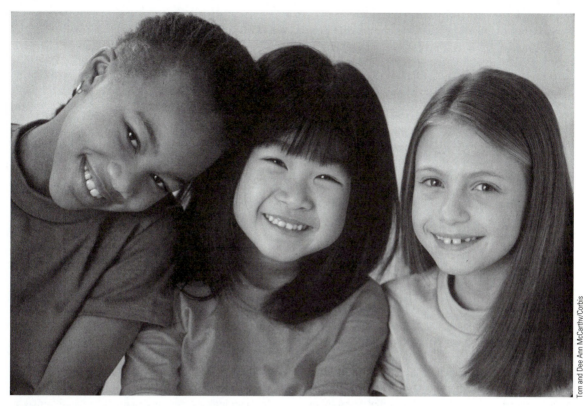

Children's ethnic and socioeconomic diversity creates significant challenges for assessment.

lying traits that govern behavior. These traits are assumed to be stable across time and situations. In a sense, a trait is a shorthand method of describing a child's personality and behavior. For example, a child might be labeled lazy, outgoing (extroversion), shy (introversion), or dependent. For assessment purposes, it is good to recognize the existence of traits but observe and record several samples of the behavior.

Intelligence Tests

IN FOCUS 3 ▶ Identify the abilities assessed with standardized intelligence tests.

When "psychological test" is mentioned, many individuals think of intelligence tests with their various tasks, questions, and puzzles. These tests were originally designed as a series of complex problems to screen children for academic readiness. The original 1905 version of Alfred Binet's test was developed by administering the problems to normal children as well as children and adults with mental retardation. What made Binet's work unique was the development of norms so that comparisons could be made between children with and without disabilities (Sattler, 2001).

Shortly after Binet's original work, L. M. Terman helped refine and standardize the test on American children in 1916. Terman and others developed the concept of the IQ, or intelligence quotient, for use in comparing the relative intelligence of children at different ages. To calculate an IQ, a child's mental age (as determined by how well he does on the test) is divided by his chronological age and multiplied by 100 (IQ = MA/CA × 100). For example, if a child scores at the 76 month level (mental age) on the test and is 8 years old (chronological age is thus 96 months), his IQ is 80 = 76/96 × 100. The average child has a mental age approximately equal to his chronological age, and so has an IQ of approximately 100 (i.e., IQ 100 = 96 months MA/96 months CA × 100).

Table 4-4 Examples of Children's Intelligence Tests

Wechsler Intelligence Scale for Children-III (WISC-III): This is one of the best intelligence tests for children and adolescents (6–16 years). It contains both a verbal and a nonverbal performance component and yields a Verbal IQ, a Performance IQ, and a Full Scale IQ. Excellent reliability and validity characteristics.

Wechsler Preschool and Primary Scale of Intelligence–Revised (WPPSI-R): This test is similar to the WISC-III except that it is used with younger children (3–7). It also yields a Verbal IQ, a Performance IQ, and a Full Scale IQ. Excellent reliability and validity characteristics.

Stanford-Binet Intelligence Test–Fourth Edition (SB-4th): This test is an outgrowth of Binet's early work with intelligence. It has been revised several times with the newest revision done in 1986. It yields a global measure of intelligence and can be used with children aged 2–12. Excellent reliability and validity.

Leiter International Performance Scale (LIPS): This is a nonverbal intelligence test that is useful for individuals who cannot talk. The test is a series of puzzles based on small blocks. The test can be used with 2-year-old children up to adults. This test has been criticized because the norms are outdated and the standardization is inadequate. This test should be used with children only when other verbally based intelligence tests cannot be used.

Kaufman Assessment Battery for Children (K-ABC): This intelligence test is designed for children aged 2–12. It assesses two types of intellectual processing: simultaneous processing and successive processing. This test has excellent reliability and validity characteristics, but more research is needed to determine if it adds any useful information that the WISC-III or Stanford-Binet misses.

Since Binet's intelligence test was first devised, many types of intelligence tests for children have been developed (see Table 4-4). One of the most frequently used children's intelligence tests is the Wechsler Intelligence Scale for Children—Revised (WISC-III-R). A basic advantage of the WISC-III-R is that it combines both verbal subscales and performance, or motor, subscales in assessing a child's intellectual ability (see Table 4-5). The WISC-III-R thus yields an overall intelligence score, plus separate verbal and performance IQ scores, which can be useful in assessing children who are more proficient in one area than the other.

Both the Stanford-Binet Fourth Edition and the WISC-III-R are popular intelligence tests for children, and both have good reliability. However, there is a great deal of controversy over the construct validity of intelligence tests. That is, exactly what is intelligence?

Binet (Binet & Simon, 1905) considered intelligence to be a set of abilities that include comprehension, reasoning, judgment, and the ability to adapt. Wechsler (1958) similarly defined intelligence to be a set of abilities that include the capacity "to act purposefully, to think rationally, and to deal effectively with the environment." Frequently, intelligence has been described as the *g factor*, or general ability factor, which has its origins in Frances Galton's (1869) pioneering work in measuring individual sensory and motor differences. Spearman (1927) refined the concept of the g factor to mean basic mental energy, with

complex mental tasks containing the greatest amount of "g."

However, there may be a problem in assuming that intelligence is an entity existing within a child. All of the above definitions and the concept of the g factor rely on an indirect measure of intelligence obtained by sampling selected behaviors under controlled conditions. In essence, intelligence is inferred from behaviors sampled under strict environmental stimulus conditions. Intelligence tests primarily sample and measure (1) *verbal ability*, which is associated with general information and language acquired at home, and a general factor of (2) *perceptual and performance ability* associated with reasoning, problem solving, and comprehension. Other factors that may be measured by intelligence tests include the ability to attend to a task, numerical reasoning, recall, and memory. Since all of these abilities are particularly important in school settings, intelligence tests are good at predicting success in schools (Aiken 1997; Anastasi & Urbina, 1997; Rourke, 1997; Van den Broek, Golden, Loonstraa, Ghinglia, & Goldstein, 1998).

Beyond simple two-factor models of intelligence, theorists have also proposed multiple-factor explanations of intelligence. Robert Sternberg (1997) has proposed a triarchic theory of intelligence, which includes a metacomponent of intelligence that is involved in planning, monitoring, and evaluating performance, a performance component that consists of

Table 4-5 Descriptions of the WISC-III Subtests

Subtest	Description
Picture completion	A set of colorful pictures of common objects and scenes, each of which is missing an important part which the child identifies.
Information	A series of orally presented questions that tap the child's knowledge about common events, objects, places, and people.
Coding	A series of simple shapes (Coding A) or numbers (Coding B), each paired with a simple symbol. The child draws the symbol in its corresponding shape (Coding A) or under its corresponding number (Coding B), according to a key. Coding A and B are included on a single perforated sheet in the Record Form.
Similarities	A series of orally presented pairs of words for which the child explains the similarity of the common objects or concepts they represent.
Picture arrangement	A set of colorful pictures, presented in mixed-up order, which the child rearranges into a logical story sequence.
Arithmetic	A series of arithmetic problems which the child solves mentally and responds to orally.
Block design	A set of modeled or printed two-dimensional geometric patterns that the child replicates using two-color cubes.
Vocabulary	A series of orally presented words that the child orally defines.
Object assembly	A set of puzzles of common objects, each presented in a standardized configuration, which the child assembles to form a meaningful whole.
Comprehension	A series of orally presented questions that require the child's solving of everyday problems or understanding of social rules and concepts.
Symbol search	A series of paired groups of symbols, each pair consisting of a target group and a search group. The child scans the two groups and indicates whether or not a target symbol appears in the search group. Both levels of the subtest are included in a single response booklet.
Digit span	A series of orally presented number sequences that the child repeats verbatim for Digits Forward and in reverse order for Digits Backward.
Mazes	A set of increasingly difficult mazes, printed in a response booklet, which the child solves with a pencil.

Source: Wechsler (1991).

strategies used in the execution of a task, and a knowledge acquisition component used to acquire information in learning new tasks. Howard Gardner (Gardner, 1998; Gardner, Kornhaber, & Wake, 1996) has expanded the notion of intelligence to include ten basic components, ranging from spatial intelligence to higher-order spiritual and existential intelligence (see Figure 4-2).

Possibly the greatest controversy surrounding the use of intelligence tests centers on their use with children from diverse cultures (Brems, 1998), especially children who use English as their second language in their homes. Language differences present a particularly challenging issue for psychological assessment, since they open enormous opportunities for errors and test bias (Battle, 1997; Lamison-White, 1997; Perez, 1997). The inappropriate use of intelligence tests has led to overidentification and mislabeling of minority children as having disabilities (a false positive error). Errors like this are testing artifacts, emerging from an assessment that reveals cultural background rather than psychological status (Drew & Hardman, 2000; Hopkins, 1998; Saccuzzo & Johnson, 1995). Such errors resulted in a federal court ruling in *Larry P. v. Riles* (1974, 1984), restricting the use of intelligence tests in California for assessing minority and culturally diverse children. The situation has improved as test manufacturers have expanded the standardization norms of their tests to include more diverse populations and specific guidelines have been developed for assessing minority children (American Psychological Association, 1990; Sattler, 2001). Issues regarding cultural bias and unfairness in psychological assessment are far from resolved, however, and continued efforts

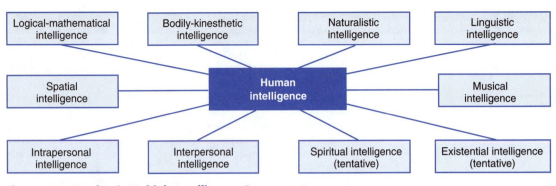

Figure 4-2   Gardner's Multiple Intelligence Components

SOURCE: Gardner (1983, 1998).

are essential to provide more appropriate and fair evaluations for children from ethnically and culturally diverse backgrounds (Drew & Hardman, 2000; Mayfield & Reynolds, 1997; Paolo, Ryan, Ward, & Hilmer, 1997).

Projective Tests

IN FOCUS 4 ▶ Explain why projective tests are better viewed as clinical tools than as psychological tests.

Projective tests are some of the most popular assessment procedures used with children (Watkins, Campbell, Nieberding, & Hallmark, 1995; Wilson & Reschly, 1996). In a recent survey of clinical psychologists, approximately 80% indicated that they used projective tests at least occasionally in their practices (Watkins et al., 1995). Only recently have these tests been supplanted by more objective behavior rating scales (Kamphaus, Petoskey, & Rowe, 2000).

Projective tests have been called "a clinician's delight and a statistician's nightmare" (Lilienfeld, Wood, & Garb, 2001). This is because most popular projective tests are not based on rigorous standardization procedures but instead are based on a psychoanalytic assumption that a child is driven by underlying psychological forces such as sexual and aggressive urges (Anastasi & Urbina, 1997; Knoff, Batsche, & Carlyon, 1993). These urges emerge early in a child's development and are affected by family interactions. For some children, these underlying forces can be so disturbing that they are blocked from consciousness by repression and denial. To attempt to reveal the unconscious urges, projective tests employ ambiguous or open-ended stimuli onto which the child has to project

meaning and structure, thereby revealing unconscious conflicts. Pathological traits and underlying emotional forces are supposedly revealed by deviant responses to the ambiguous projective stimuli.

Projective techniques offer some interesting assessment options and can be categorized into five basic groups (Silverstein, 2001; Westen, Feit, & Zittel, 1999):

1. *Association techniques.* A child is asked to tell what he sees in a set of materials (such as inkblots) or to give the first word which comes into his mind after the therapist says a word (word association).
2. *Construction techniques.* A child is asked to create a product such as a story after she has seen some test materials (e.g., in the Thematic Apperception Test, the child makes up a story to accompany a set of pictures).
3. *Completion techniques.* A child is asked to complete a statement or brief story (sentence completion test).
4. *Choice of ordering technique.* A child is asked to rank a set of materials in order of preference (e.g., to indicate which of a set of picture activities would be most enjoyable).
5. *Expressive techniques.* A child is asked to create a product of his own choice (e.g., sculpting in sand or finger painting).

Most frequently used with children are the association and construction techniques—for example, the Rorschach Inkblot Test and the Thematic Apperception Test (e.g., Ackerman, Hillsenroth, Clemence, Weatherill, & Fowler, 2001; Milne & Greenway, 2001). The Rorschach Inkblot Test (see Figure 4-3) was first

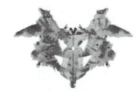

Figure 4-3   An Inkblot Used in the Rorschach Test

SOURCE: Rorschach (1948). Reprinted by permission.

developed in Germany for use primarily with adults, but it has also been widely used with children. The test consists of ten cards with symmetrical inkblots; half are black and white and half are colored. The cards are shown to the child one at a time in a set order, and the child is asked what each inkblot represents (free association stage). Later, more detailed information is gathered by asking the child to justify her responses and to describe them in more detail (inquiry stage). There are several ways to score and interpret Rorschach responses (Hunsley & DiGiulio, 2001); one is shown in Table 4-6.

The Thematic Apperception Test (TAT) is second only to the Rorschach in both clinical usage and published studies (Teglasi, 2001). The TAT is a constructive projective technique in which 20–30 cards (such as the one depicted in Figure 4-4) are shown to a child; each card consists of a drawing or fantasy scene. As each card is shown to a child, he is asked to make up a story about the picture. The child's stories are tape-recorded or transcribed. After a sufficient

number of cards have been shown (the number may vary from clinician to clinician), the results are interpreted. The interpretation generally includes major elements of the story, such as the choice of a hero, the needs and qualities of the hero, the basic themes of the story, the emotional tone, and the general outcome of the story. In clinical practice, there is no universally accepted method for scoring the TAT.

A technique similar to the TAT is the Children's Apperception Test, or the CAT. This technique is used with younger children (aged 3 to 10) and is based on pictures of animals instead of adults (Faust & Ehrich, 2001). The pictures depict scenes that are designed to elicit responses on sibling rivalry, attitudes toward parents, aggression, feeding problems, toileting behavior, acceptance, and loneliness. It is assumed that young children relate more easily to animals than to adults.

One of the most popular projective techniques for use with children is called Draw a Person or Human Figure Drawing (Fu, 1999; Wilson & Reschly, 1996). With this test, a child is asked to draw a human figure and through the drawing reveals emotional difficulties. Figure 4-5 shows an example from a 9-year-old boy who was having emotional difficulties with anger, poor school achievement, and hostility toward his father. It is assumed that the picture is a representation of the child's father, who was authoritarian and punitive. The basic appeal of drawing human figures is that drawing is generally a nonthreatening and enjoyable task for a child. From this test, inferences have

Table 4-6 Interpretation of Data from the Rorschach Test for Children and Adults

Response to Cards	Interpretation
Blood content followed by evasion	Hostile impulses defended against by avoidance, resentful passive compliance, or withdrawal
Color naming, cool colors	Depressive trend which is defended against
Color denial and avoidance	Withdrawal tendency
Body mutilation	Fantasies or fears
Smoke	Children with average or above average intelligence; apprehension, depression, social maladjustment
Gums and teeth	Aggressive response to frustrated dependency needs; more common in adolescents and children; resentfulness
Completely unmodified, unqualified terse responses	Children; organics; people in trouble with the law; persons resistant to social pressure

SOURCE: Gilbert (1978). Copyright © 1975 by Van Nostrand Reinhold.

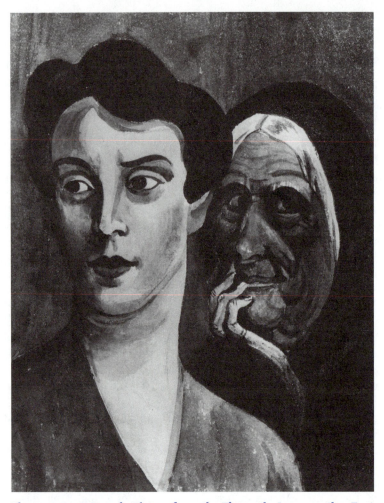

Figure 4-4 A Sample Picture from the Thematic Apperception Test

Source: Murray (1943). Reprinted by permission of the publishers from Henry A. Murray, *Thematic Apperception Test*, Plate 12F. Cambridge, MA: Harvard University Press, copyright © 1943 by the President and Fellows of Harvard College, © 1971 by Henry A. Murray.

been drawn concerning emotional problems, indicators of intelligence, and predictions of academic achievement (Bardos, 1993; Holtzman, 1993; Naglieri, 1993).

Although projective techniques have been extremely popular, their usefulness with children with behavior disorders has been repeatedly criticized. Since by definition (projective hypothesis) the stimuli associated with these tests have to be ambiguous, their reliability is generally low. Even the validity of the projective hypothesis itself has been criticized

(Anastasi & Urbina, 1997). Anastasi and Urbina (1997) regard projective techniques as "clinical tools" and not psychological tests because they do not measure up to acceptable psychometric standards of basic reliability and validity. Similarly, research reviews of projective techniques and their use with children having behavior disorders have questioned their reliability, validity, and utility (e.g., Lilienfeld et al., 2001). Some researchers have noted that projective tests "rarely add much to information that can be obtained in other, more practical ways such as by conducting interviews

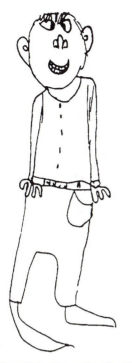

Figure 4-5   Koppitz's Example of a Human Figure Drawing

Source: Koppitz (1968).

or administering objective personality tests" (Lilienfeld et al., 2001, p. 87).

Personality Inventories and Behavior Rating Scales

IN FOCUS 5 ▶ Summarize the advantages and limitations of personality inventories and behavior checklists.

Personality inventories and behavior rating scales are similar in that they identify traits or consistent behavior patterns in children. Personality inventories generally ask a parent to respond "Yes" or "No" on whether a child exhibits a certain behavior or characteristic. Some of the most familiar personality tests are the California Psychological Inventory, the Minnesota Multiphasic Personality Inventory (MMPI-II), and the Jessness Personality Inventory. For children, the Personality Inventory for Children—Revised (PIC-R) and the Personality Inventory for Youth (PIY) are two of

the most familiar instruments (Lachar & Gruber, 1994; Negy, Lachar, Gruber, & Garza, 2001; Saunders, Hall, Casey, & Strang, 2000).

When behavior checklists or rating scales are used, raters who are familiar with a child are asked to score the child's behavior along several predetermined dimensions. An adult (parent, teacher, or ward attendant) is asked to rate a child's behavior in comparison to a standard or to the behaviors of other children. For example, the Child Behavior Checklist (Achenbach, 1991) shown in Figure 4-6 requires a parent to rate items as 2 = "very true," 1 = "somewhat true," or 0 = "not true" of their child's behavior in the past 6 months. This checklist identifies many problematic behaviors and is used for screening. Generally, behaviors in such checklists are grouped into *broad-spectrum factors*, such as internalizing behaviors (problems directed inward toward the self) and externalizing behaviors \problems directed toward others and the environment). The broad-spectrum factors are then further subdivided into *narrow-band factors*, such as aggression, hyperactivity, depression, and social withdrawal.

Figure 4-7 gives an example of a profile sheet from the Child Behavior Checklist (Achenbach, 1991; 1992), which shows the broad-spectrum and narrow-spectrum factors. A parent fills out the checklist in Figure 4-6, and then the scores are transposed onto the profile sheet. In this example, both the father (dashed line) and the mother (solid line) rated the child's behavior with their individual scores of 0, 1, or 2 for each item listed at the bottom of the profile sheet (i.e., "Argues" rated as a 1 by the father and a 2 by the mother under "Aggressive Behavior"). The profile sheet also allows a normative comparison to a standardization group. For example, 98% of the standardization population had scores that fell on or below the line at T-70 (note the higher dashed line across the profile). The T-70 scores, which are two standard deviations from the mean (T-50), are considered to mark the level of clinical significance for most of the factors. In this particular case, the mother rated the child's "Aggressive Behavior" as significant (T-76), while the father rated it as nonsignificant (T-65), indicating disagreement between the parents about the severity of the child's aggressive problems.

Personality inventories and behavior checklists have many qualities in common. They are generally

CHILD BEHAVIOR CHECKLIST

Below is a list of items that describe children and youth. For each item that describes your child now or within the past 6 months, please circle the 2 if the item is very true or often true of your child. Circle the 1 if the item is somewhat or sometimes true of your child. If the item is not true of your child, circle the 0. Please answer all items as well as you can, even if some do not seem to apply to your child.

0 = Not True (as far as you know)   1 = Somewhat or Sometimes True   2 = Very True or Often True

0 1 2 1. Acts too young for his/her age	0 1 2 31. Fears he/she might think or do something bad
0 1 2 2. Allergy (describe): _____	0 1 2 32. Feels he/she has to be perfect
	0 1 2 33. Feels or complains that no one loves him/her
0 1 2 3. Argues a lot	0 1 2 34. Feels others are out to get him/her
0 1 2 4. Asthma	0 1 2 35. Feels worthless or inferior
0 1 2 5. Behaves like opposite sex	0 1 2 36. Gets hurt a lot, accident-prone
0 1 2 6. Bowel movements outside toilet	0 1 2 37. Gets in many fights
0 1 2 7. Bragging, boasting	0 1 2 38 Gets teased a lot
0 1 2 8. Can't concentrate, can't pay attention for long	0 1 2 39. Hangs around with others who get in trouble
0 1 2 9. Can't get his/her mind off certain thoughts; obsessions (describe): _____	0 1 2 40. Hears sounds or voices that aren't there (describe): _____
	0 1 2 41. Impulsive or acts without thinking
0 1 2 10. Can't sit still, restless, or hyperactive	0 1 2 42. Would rather be alone than with others
0 1 2 11. Clings to adults or too dependent	0 1 2 43. Lying or cheating
0 1 2 12. Complains of loneliness	0 1 2 44. Bites fingernails
0 1 2 13. Confused or seems to be in a fog	0 1 2 45. Nervous, highstrung, or tense
0 1 2 14. Cries a lot	0 1 2 46. Nervous movements or twitching (describe): _____
0 1 2 15. Cruel to animals	
0 1 2 16. Cruelty, bullying, or meanness to others	0 1 2 47. Nightmares
0 1 2 17. Day-dreams or gets lost in his/her thoughts	0 1 2 48. Not liked by other kids
0 1 2 18. Deliberately harms self or attempts suicide	0 1 2 49. Constipated, doesn't move bowels
0 1 2 19. Demands a lot of attention	0 1 2 50. Too fearful or anxious
0 1 2 20. Destroys his/her own things	0 1 2 51. Feels dizzy
0 1 2 21. Destroys things belonging to his/her family or others	0 1 2 52. Feels too guilty
	0 1 2 53. Overeating
0 1 2 22. Disobedient at home	0 1 2 54. Overtired
0 1 2 23. Disobedient at school	0 1 2 55. Overweight
0 1 2 24. Doesn't eat well	56. Physical problems without known medical cause:
0 1 2 25. Doesn't get along with other kids	0 1 2 a. Aches or pains (*not* headaches)
0 1 2 26. Doesn't seem to feel guilty after misbehaving	0 1 2 b. Headaches
0 1 2 27. Easily jealous	0 1 2 c. Nausea, feels sick
0 1 2 28. Eats or drinks things that are not food—*don't* include sweets (describe): _____	0 1 2 d. Problems with eyes (describe): _____
	0 1 2 e. Rashes or other skin problems
0 1 2 29. Fears certain animals, situations, or places, other than school (describe): _____	0 1 2 f. Stomachaches or cramps
	0 1 2 g. Vomiting, throwing up
	0
	1
0 1 2 30. Fears going to school	2 h. Other (describe):

Figure 4-6 Sample Items from the CBCL

SOURCE: Achenbach (1991), p. 11.

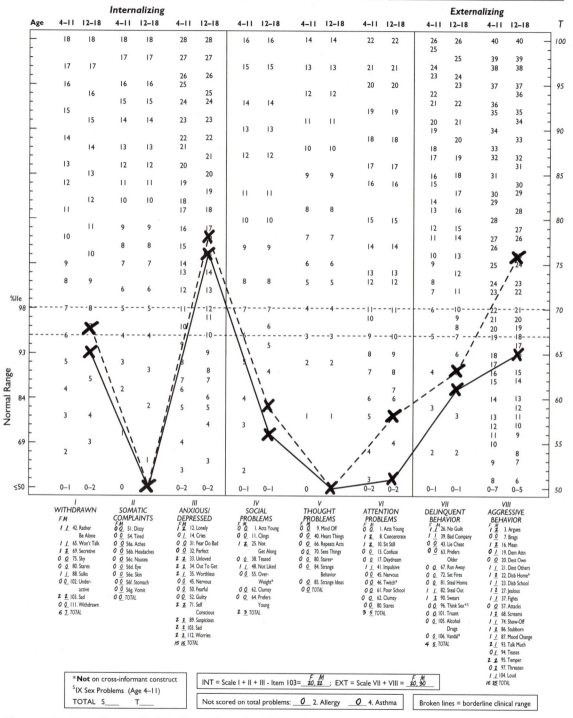

Figure 4-7 Sample of a Profile Sheet from the CBCL

Source: Achenbach (1991), p. 169.

derived statistically through factor analysis and are well standardized with normative groups for comparison. Both types of instruments also require a knowledgable rater to judge the presence of a specific behavior or personality characteristic. However, these instruments also have differences. Personality inventories tend to identify broad traits that together help describe a whole personality (i.e., delinquency) with dysfunctional characteristics (i.e., noncompliance). Behavior checklists are more behavior-based and tend to identify broad-band characteristics (i.e., externalizing) that can be broken into specific problematic behavior patterns (i.e., aggression). The popularity of behavior checklists or rating scales in the assessment of children has increased dramatically in the past decade (Kamphaus et al., 2000; Mash & Terdal, 1998). However, like intelligence tests, behavior checklists are prone to cultural problems (Reid, 1995). What is behaviorally acceptable in a minority culture may differ from what is behaviorally acceptable in the majority culture on which the behavior checklist was standardized. Many of the newer behavior checklists and other assessment instruments have included minority children of diverse cultures in their normative standardization groups, as well as modifying their protocols for

both administration and interpretation (Connors, 1997; Hopkins, 1998; Janda, 1998).

Behavioral Observation and Self-Recording

IN FOCUS 6 ▶ Give some advantages and limitations of behavioral observation.

Behavioral observation is the most direct form of assessment based on a sampling method. A basic assumption of behavioral assessment is that public events, rather than private or assumed underlying traits, are the important target for measurement. With behavioral observation, a sample of behavior is taken in the child's natural environment or a clinic setting that is relevant for the child (Haynes, 2001; Mash & Terdal, 1997). Behavioral observation has been used to assess "bullying" behaviors (Atlas & Pepler, 1998), social competence and conflict resolution skills in children with conduct disorders (Webster-Stratton & Lindsay, 2000), autistic behavior in structured play settings (Klinger & Renner, 2000), and medication effects on behavior of children with attention deficit disorder (Ardoin & Martens, 2000).

Gathering information in the natural environment in which the child's problem behavior occurs may be

---

Table 4-7 Methods for Collecting Observational Data

Frequency recording: Has also been called *tallying* or *event recording*. With this method, an observer simply counts the number of times a behavior occurs within a predetermined amount of time (for example, the number of head bangs in a 10-minute period). A restriction of the frequency method is that it should be used with discrete behaviors—that is, behaviors that have a clear onset or offset, such as head bangs. Behaviors that do not have a clear start or ending, such as conversation between two people, are difficult to measure with the frequency method. The types of behaviors with which the frequency method has been used include eye contact, self-stimulation, and self-injurious behavior.

Interval recording: The most popular method of recording behavior, because it can be used with both discrete and nondiscrete behaviors. With interval recording, a block of time is divided into small equal units. For example, a 10-minute period of observation time may be broken into ten 1-minute intervals of time. If the target behavior occurs during a 1-minute interval, it is scored. Generally, only one behavior is scored per interval even if more than one behavior occurs. This type of system does not depend on the starting or stopping of a behavior. The only requirement is that the behavior must be scored if it occurs during the 1-minute interval. The types of target behaviors that interval recording has been used with include play activity, aggressive behaviors, and eating and drinking.

Duration recording: This method must also be used with discrete behaviors that have a clear onset and offset. The duration of a behavior is generally timed from the onset to the offset of the behavior. This type of method is useful when the amount of time a subject engages in a behavior is important. Duration methods have been used to assess time spent doing homework, watching television, engaging in an exercise program, and thumbsucking.

Latency recording: With this method, the amount of time from some stimulus to the start of a behavior is timed. Again, this requires a discrete response with a clear onset. The latency method is useful when the lapse in time from a stimulus to the starting of a behavior is important. For example, latency recording has been used to measure how long it takes a child to start to comply after a request has been given by an adult.

more informative in that events that precede the behavior (antecedents), the behavior itself, and events that follow the behavior (consequences) can be directly observed and measured. This type of observation leads to a functional behavior assessment that reveals under what conditions and why a behavior occurs. It is a popular and increasingly utilized method of assessment and classification that will be discussed in more depth later in this chapter (Ellingson et al., 2000; Olympia, Heathfield, Jenson, & Clark, 2002).

There are several methods for collecting observational data (see Table 4-7), each of which has advantages and disadvantages depending on the type of behavior being observed. Each of these methods, however, requires the precise definition of **target behaviors**, which leaves little guesswork or interpretation to the observer. For example, an adequate definition of in-seat behavior for a hyperactive child may read: "The child must be sitting in the chair with both feet on the floor, both buttocks touching the seat, with hands on the desk." Target behaviors are generally defined in terms of: (1) the duration of time involved in responding, (2) the intensity or amplitude of the response, or (3) the topography of the response. Target behaviors can also be classed as discrete responses with a clear beginning and ending, such as biting or

hitting, or nondiscrete responses without a clear beginning or ending, such as a long conversation between two people.

A set of explicitly defined target behaviors designed for observation in one environmental setting, such as a classroom, playground, or home, is called an **observation code**. An observation code has the advantage of describing several different behaviors that can occur in one setting, giving a global picture of the child's behavior in that setting. This global picture is somewhat like a photograph. If the camera's settings (the observation code) are incorrectly adjusted or the camera (the observation system) is improperly used, then the picture will be inaccurate and fuzzy. A good example of an observation code that is used with an interval data collection system is given in Table 4-8. This code includes 29 behaviors that are used to describe the interactions between a child and his family. These behaviors range from positive behaviors such as "approval" and "play" to very negative behaviors such as "humiliate" and "destructiveness."

Although behavioral observation may be one of the most accurate methods of collecting data on problematic behaviors, it also has several drawbacks (Mash & Terdal, 1997). It is expensive and time-consuming in both the collection of the data and the training of observers. Observers have to be trained to a high degree of accuracy to ensure reliability. However, there is a tendency for observers to "drift" over time and thus require periodic retraining. There is also the problem of reactivity. Simply placing an observer in the child's naturalistic environment can cause the child to change her behavior in the presence of this stranger. The less obtrusive the observer, the less the reactive change in the child's behavior. Despite these problems, behavioral observation remains the "gold standard" for much of the research and treatment that is currently done with children. Major advances have been made in using hand-held computers for collecting observation data, which facilitates cost-effectiveness and reliability of the data (Oswald, Rhode, & Jenson, 2001; Sanders, 2001).

However, behavioral observation does not necessarily require trained independent observers. A child can be taught to collect data on herself, which saves money and training time and provides useful clinical and research assessment data (Cone, 1999; Foster, Laverty-Finch, Gizzo, & Osantowski, 1999; Korotitsch

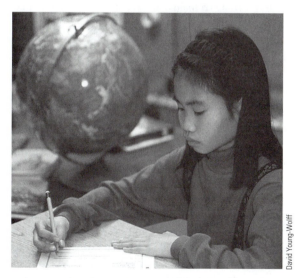

To be scored as showing in-seat behavior, the child must be sitting in her chair, not slouching, and have both feet on the floor and her hands on the desk.

David Young-Wolff

Table 4-8 Behavioral Observation Code Used with Families

Code	Behavior	Code	Behavior
AP	Approval	NE	Negativism
AT	Attention	NO	Normative (routine behavior which fits no other code)
CM	Command		
CN	Command negative	NR	No response
CO	Compliance	PL	Play
CR	Cry	PN	Physical negative
DI	Disapproval	PP	Physical positive
DP	Dependency	RC	Receive (when a person receives an object from another person and shows no response)
DS	Destructiveness		
HR	High rate (occurring at a high frequency and over time so that the behavior is aversive)	SS	Self-stimulation (a child bounces, rocks body, or sucks thumb)
HU	Humiliate	TA	Talk
IG	Ignore	TE	Tease
IN	Indulgence (doing something helpful for another individual who is capable of doing it for himself without being asked)	TH	Touch
		WH	Whine
LA	Laugh	WK	Work
NC	Noncompliance	YE	Yell

SOURCE: Reid (1978), p. 38. Reprinted by permission of the author and the publisher.

& Nelson-Gray, 1999; Shapiro & Cole, 1999). This self-collection of data has been called self-recording, self-monitoring, and self-observation, and it provides an added benefit: Simply recording data on oneself often therapeutically changes the observed behavior. In a sense, the person reacts to collecting data on a target behavior, which produces behavior change (Shapiro & Cole, 1999). Self-recording has been used to increase social skills and reduce disruptive behavior in children with autism (e.g., Akande, 1998; Koegel, Koegel, Hurley, & Frea, 1992). It has also been used extensively to improve on-task behavior and academic performance of students with attention deficit disorder, learning disabilities, and brain injury (Clare, Jenson, Kehle, & Bray, 2000; Davies & Witte, 2000; Lam, Cole, Shapiro, & Bambara, 1994; Selznick & Savage, 2000).

The observed behavior changes are assumed to be due to reactivity, which frequently increases appropriate behaviors and decreases inappropriate behaviors. However, these effects are generally temporary unless they are specifically rewarded. In a sense, the child gets used to the data-collecting process, and as the novelty wears off, the old behaviors tend to return. However,

the temporary treatment effects of self-recording can be made more permanent by combining them with reward and self-management contingencies (Clare et al., 2000). Self-recording remains an important technique that bridges the gap between assessment and treatment (Cone, 1999; Shapiro & Cole, 1999).

Interviewing

Interviewing has been called one of the basic "four pillars of assessment" (Sattler, 2001) and the "cornerstone of assessment" (Hechtman, 2000). Interviewing a child and his or her parents is generally used to start an assessment process that may involve other evaluation techniques. In a sense, the initial information gathered in this interview helps the clinician decide which other assessment techniques should be used. Other widely used types of interviews include a social history (a history of a child's social development), an intake interview (a method used to decide whether an agency's facilities meets a child's needs), a child psychiatric interview (a health and psychiatric history), a diagnostic interview, and many more.

There are several reasons why interviewing is such a popular assessment technique (McConaughy, 2000). First, interviewing generally utilizes open-ended questions, which allow a child or parent to explain or elaborate on answers instead of being forced to choose an alternative from a predetermined list. They can put the information in their own words (Sattler, 2001). Second, interviewing helps to establish a relationship between the clinician and the child, which facilitates the assessment process. Unlike formal psychological testing in which the interaction between the evaluator and child is kept to a minimum, interviewing involves a less structured exchange of information. Interviewing both child and parent(s) together (conjoint interview) can give the clinician a picture of the family's interactions. Interviewing can also utilize creative methods to help elicit information from children who may be scared or have limited verbal abilities for answering complex clinical questions. For example, the Berkeley Puppet Interview for children uses two hand puppets of dogs (Iggy and Ziggy) to solicit clinical information through the question "How about you?" (Ablow et al., 1999). Similarly, the Dominic-R uses pictures to help illustrate each of the interviewer's questions about an emotion or problem behavior that a child might not understand from the words alone (Valla, Bergeron, & Smolla, 2000).

One of the most frequently used interviewing techniques in hospitals and mental health facilities is the child psychiatric interview. The more traditional psychiatric interview consisted of a mental status exam and a basic content section. The mental status exam is a detailed description of the child's behavior and appearance during a prescribed time period dedicated to psychiatric interviewing. The basic content section includes the child's direct answers to the psychiatrist's questions, which helped establish a formal diagnosis and treatment recommendations. Although the psychiatric interview has a long history of use, its format is frequently informal and unstructured, which can lead to interviewer bias and error. It has been re-

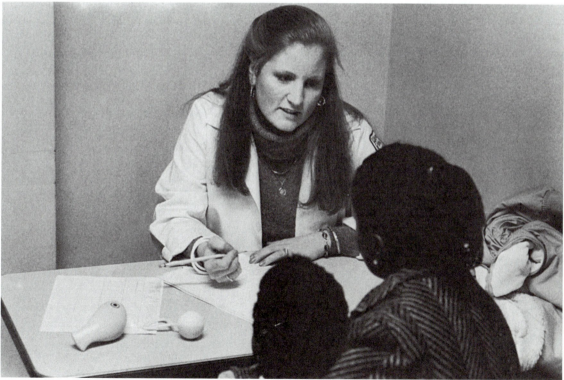

David Witbeck

Interviewing is a popular assessment procedure used with children and their parents. It allows a clinician to obtain a range of information, including a developmental history.

placed in much research and clinical practice by more highly structured interviews. Several structured diagnostic interviews have been developed and are used primarily to diagnose and classify children with a high degree of rigor (McConaughy, 2000). They contain a series of questions which parallel the major childhood disorders listed in the *Diagnostic and Statistical Manual of Mental Disorders* (DSM). These interviews include the Diagnostic Interview Schedule for Children (DISC-IV) (Shaffer, Fisher, Lucas, Dulcan, & Schwab-Stone, 2000), the Child and Adolescent Psychiatric Assessment (CAPA) (Angold & Costello, 2000), and Children's Interview for Psychiatric Syndromes (ChIPS) (Weller, Weller, Fristad, Rooney, & Schecter, 2000).

CLASSIFICATION SYSTEMS

The diagnostic process involves assigning behaviors to alternative groupings within a classification system. A diagnostician may identify a mental disorder by matching the child's observable behavioral characteristics with the operational definitions included in a diagnostic classification system. The operational definitions are the descriptive rules that allow the sorting of behaviors into groups or classification categories. Diagnosing a behavior disorder is the process of using an accepted classification system and a set of operational definitions to identify a child's atypical behavioral characteristics. In clinical practice, this process allows a clinician to assign a child's behavior to a particular subcategory of the classification system. The matching and assigning of behavior to a subcategory not only result in a label or diagnosis for the child's behavior disorder but also reveal its prognostic outcome and possible treatment options.

It is important to note that a *child* is not diagnosed by the classification process; only the child's *disorder* is diagnosed. It is particularly inappropriate to classify children in terms of disorders because, even more than adults, children can be expected to change over time. It is a mistake to believe that any child conforms exactly to the behavioral description of a diagnostic category. Each child is unique, and exceptions are the rule in the classification of children's psychological disorders.

Characteristics and Functions of Behavior Classification Systems

Like assessment techniques, classification systems have error built into them. They are only models of children's behavior and are subject to the psychometric properties of reliability and validity. Good classification systems share several features. A good system can be used with high reliability (consistency) by different diagnosticians. It includes a managable number of behavior disorders, and it describes, as closely and as concisely as possible, how these disorders are manifested. A classification system should be utilized by clinicians and researchers for its practical information and not as a mere mechanism to secure treatment and research funds. In addition, since the nature of psychopathology changes with age, classification systems for use with children should be flexible enough to address issues of growth and development.

The scope and coverage of any classification system are important characteristics. The *scope* of a classification system refers to the breadth of its coverage, the system's ability to cover either a broad or a narrow spectrum of clinical conditions. If a system has 100% (extremely broad) coverage, it has a category for every possible problem presented by patients. If a system has only 10% coverage (narrow coverage), it can classify only 10% of the cases presented by patients and leaves the rest unclassified. Excessively broad coverage results in what are known as "wastebasket" or "catchall" categories. These are broadly defined categories that are designed for idiosyncratic or exceptional cases that do not really fit any other category. The phrase "not otherwise specified (NOS)" means that the behaviors do not specifically fit the established classification criteria but may come close. For example, "adjustment disorder not otherwise specified" in the *Diagnostic and Statistical Manual of Mental Disorders* (American Psychiatric Association, 2000), or the DSM-IV-TR, is commonly used for troubled individuals when other diagnoses do not apply. Overly narrow coverage can also create problems. With narrow coverage, a system's reliability can be quite high, because the operational definitions of the categories are very specific and limiting. The system's validity can also be quite high, but only for a few conditions. If too many conditions remain unclassified because the system is not appropriately flexible, then clinicians and researchers will not use the system.

Mental disorders are classified so that children with those problems can be treated, often by placing them in a treatment program or facility. It is a little surprising to realize that the most frequently used classification system in the United States is an educational classification based on the federal special education law mandating free and appropriate education services for students with disabilities (IDEA 97). Special education services are available for students only after they have been appropriately classified as meeting the criteria for an accepted disability under the law, such as emotional disturbance or autism. Classification systems are also used for research, for making outcome or prognostic predictions, and for helping understand the causes of many childhood disorders. The DSM-IV-TR is well-accepted for these purposes.

Psychiatric Classification

IN FOCUS 7 ▶ Describe the DSM-IV-TR classification system for mental disorders and explain how it could be improved.

The DSM-IV-TR is perhaps the most widely known classification system used in the mental health field today. Although successful, the DSM-IV-TR classification scheme has also been criticized (Beutler & Malik, 2002; Follette, 1996). Some of this criticism has focused on the shortcomings concerning the basic psychometric characteristics of reliability, validity, and utility (e.g., Reeb, 2000). Other criticism has been leveled at its handling of difficult conditions such as pervasive developmental disorders and childhood schizophrenia (Nathan & Lagenbucher, 1999; Szatmari, 2000), where the behavioral symptoms for different cases can run a spectrum of intensity from mild to severe. There can also be problems when the diagnostic criteria of the DSM are used with very young children (Nicholls, Chater, & Lask, 2000; Pavuluri & Luk, 1998). Poor inter-rater reliability can result when one informant is a parent and the other is a teacher (Mitsis, McKay, Schulz, Newcorn, & Halperin, 2000). Other problems with validity can occur when the system is used with diverse cultures that hold different values and acceptability standards for behaviors (Canino, Canino, & Arroyo, 1998; Drew & Hardman, 2000).

There are other psychiatric classification systems such as the *International Classification of Diseases*

(ICD-10) developed by the World Health Organization (WHO, 1992). But in the United States, the DSM has been the standard for mental health workers, who rarely use other systems.

Functional Behavior Assessment and Classification

One alternative to the DSM has been a functional assessment and classification of behaviors (Hayes et al., 2001; Wulfert, Greenway, & Dougher, 1996). Functional behavior assessment procedures are not new to psychology; they have their roots in early applied behavior analysis. In 1953, B. F. Skinner described the cause-and-effect relationship between behavior-controlling stimulus events and the consequences that followed the behavior. With functional behavior assessment and classification, there is less emphasis on labeling and categorizing and more emphasis on how a behavior is functionally controlled in the environment.

Environmental control over a behavior is accomplished using antecedents (stimuli that come just before a behavior) and consequences (positive reinforcement, negative reinforcement, and punishing stimuli that follow the behavior). Antecedents can be specific people, a special time when the behavior is likely to occur, or events that precede and set the occasion for the problematic behaviors. Consequences can be special sensory feelings that follow a behavior or positive reinforcements such as peer attention or avoiding compliance with a command from a parent. In this system, there is great care to define the behavior of interest objectively and make a careful analysis of environmental events. It has been called the ABC (A = antecedent, B = behavior, and C = consequences) system.

Functional behavior assessment and classification can involve interviewing (O'Neill et al., 1997; Reavis, Jenson, Morgan, Likens, & Althouse, 1998) (see Table 4-9). In this type of interview, specific information is collected on possible antecedents and consequences as well as on the rate of the behavior, when it last occurred, and previous modification attempts. Other aspects of functional assessment and classification are direct observation and recording of the behavior in the ABC format and sometimes a review of past clinical or educational records.

Table 4-9 Initial Caretaker Interview

These are basic questions to ask caretakers concerning the child's problem behavior:

1. *Specific description*
   "Can you tell me what (child's name)'s problem seems to be?" (If caretaker responds in generalities such as, "He is always grouchy," or that the child is rebellious, uncooperative, or overly shy, ask him to describe the behavior more explicitly.)
   "What, exactly, does (he or she) do when (he or she) is acting this way? What kinds of things will (he or she) say?"

2. *Last incident*
   "Could you tell me just what happened the last time you saw (the child) acting like this? What did you do?"

3. *Rate*
   "How often does this behavior occur? About how many times a day (or hour or week) does it occur?"

4. *Changes in rate*
   "Would you say this behavior is starting to happen more often, less often, or staying about the same?"

5. *Setting*
   "In what situations does it occur? At home? At school? In public places or when (the child) is alone?" (If in public places) "Who is usually with him? How do they respond?"
   "At what times of day does this happen?"
   "What else is (the child) likely to be doing at the time?"

6. *Antecedents*
   "What usually has happened right before (he or she) does this? Does anything in particular seem to start this behavior?"

7. *Consequent events*
   "What usually happens right afterwards?"

8. *Modification attempts*
   "What things have you tried to stop (him or her) from behaving this way?"
   "How long did you try that?"
   "How well did it work?"
   "Have you ever tried anything else?"

SOURCE: Gelfand & Hartmann (1984), pp. 230–232. Reprinted by permission.

A more thorough and sophisticated form of this classification system is functional behavior analysis. With this system, information is not collected passively through interviews, observations, or review of records. Instead, the child is probed under experimental conditions with specific antecedents and consequences, and the reactions are recorded. This type of analysis has been used extensively with self-injurious and very aggressive behaviors to isolate the specific controlling environmental variables and then try to modify them (Iwata, Dorsey, Slifer, Bauman, & Richman, 1994; McComas, Hoch, & Mace, 2000).

The importance of functional behavior assessment and classification has been highlighted by some in the field of clinical treatment who recommend that these procedures always be used before any intervention is implemented (O'Neill et al., 1997). Also, federal edu-cational legislation for children with disabilities [Re-authorization of the Individuals with Disabilities Act (IDEA, 1997)] requires a functional behavior assessment in certain situations (Drasgrow & Yell, 2001). Thus, functional behavior assessment and classification has become one of the most important classification/assessment approaches in the past decade.

SUMMARY

Assessment and classification are the gateways to treatment and the foundation of research on childhood behavior disorders. Both of these processes involve structured information gathering that leads to a decision on intervention. However, both assessment and classification methods are only models of a child's

Back to the Beginning

"It Wasn't What We Thought."

In the absence of information, Margie and Jeff had imagined a lot of things. Despite their repeated assertions to each other that Brian would grow out of it, they knew something was amiss and believed they needed help. Margie had imagined a brain tumor that prevented Brian from developing language—and in the worst moments, late at night, she imagined that Brian's condition worsened and he died in pain. Many times, in the absence of information, we imagine matters to be much worse than they are.

Margie and Jeff finally no longer accepted their family physician's claim that Brian was developing normally just slowly. This was difficult because the doc was like a trusted member of the family. But Margie talked with one of her friends who had experience with having children evaluated. This gave her some courage and also some information on where to turn. She really hadn't paid attention to her sister and now wished she hadn't been so negative about that advice (but her sister was so pushy!).

Margie made an appointment with a staff member of the preschool she hadn't sent Brian to. She now knew what information she needed, how to contact a reputable and qualified school psychologist to request a screening assessment—she had written it down since it involved terminology she was not familiar with (but she would soon understand these and many other terms related to assessments and Brian's functioning).

The school psychologist did some extensive interviews and testing and made Margie quite comfortable with a referral to some other clinicians. Testing, interviewing Margie and Jeff, and observing Brian resulted in some findings: The behavior rating scales and observations showed him to be an internalizing child who is clinically anxious, especially in social situations. Further testing revealed no language, developmental, or intellectual problems. What was most revealing was the functional behavior assessment of Brian. It showed that he would talk only when alone around his mother (an antecedent), whispered sometimes with his mother present in social situations, and clearly showed a fear reaction when she left. It was also revealed that in kindergarten he could gesture for what he wanted and the teacher and other children catered to his needs (positive consequences). The diagnostic conclusion was that Brian's condition is selective mutism and separation anxiety from his mother. He is scheduled for a new type of treatment, self-modeling, which has been shown in the research to be promisingly effective in reducing anxiety and getting children suffering from selective mutism to talk in social situations.

This was a story about Brian, but it was also a story about his parents. Because of his age, they had to be the ones to realize that help was needed, that evaluation was needed, and that they weren't making headway by simply talking to each other (although talking with each other was very important, the content of the talks just needed to move from "He'll grow out of it" to something more proactive).

---

behavior and have inherent error. This error can be random error involving reliability problems or systematic error involving validity problems. No assessment or classification system is 100% accurate.

The leading types of assessment and classification methods reviewed in this chapter are structured interviewing, behavioral observation, standardized testing, and behavior rating scales. Less optimal are the popular but nonstandardized projective techniques. For classification of childhood behavior disorders, the *Diagnostic and Statistical Manual of Mental Disorders* (DSM-IV-TR) is the system most frequently used by mental health professionals. Educational classification used in qualifying children for special education services is the most often used classification system in the United States. Over the past decade the advent of functional behavior assessment and classification has set a new standard for pretreatment assessment and has furthered understanding of how the environment functionally controls behavior.

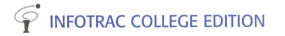

INFOTRAC COLLEGE EDITION

For more information, explore this resource at http://www.infotrac-college.com/Wadsworth. Enter the following search terms:

> intelligence tests
> projective tests
> psychological tests of children
> assessment
> diagnosis
> personality tests
> clinical interviews
> diagnostic and statistical manual

IN FOCUS ANSWERS

IN FOCUS 1 ▶ Identify the sources of systematic and random error.

- Systematic error stems from some constant source, such as a poorly trained observer who always overestimates aggression.
- Random error happens by chance and is unpredictable, leading to poor reliability.

IN FOCUS 2 ▶ List the characteristics of a standardized measure.

- Explicitly defined test administration procedures are used.
- The test questions are always given in the same order.
- The same test instructions are always used.
- Everyone is given the same amount of time to complete the test.
- A similar, distraction-free test room is used every time the test is given.

IN FOCUS 3 ▶ Identify the abilities assessed with standardized intelligence tests.

- Verbal ability
- Perceptual and nonverbal performance abilities

IN FOCUS 4 ▶ Explain why projective tests are better viewed as clinical tools than as psychological tests.

- They are not acceptably reliable or valid.
- Consequently, they are of little value for diagnostic purposes.

IN FOCUS 5 ▶ Summarize the advantages and limitations of personality inventories and behavior checklists.

- They are empirically derived, based on children's actual behavior problems.
- They are standardized and permit comparison of a child with normative groups.
- Like other tests, they may be inappropriate for use with children from minority cultures.

IN FOCUS 6 ▶ Give some advantages and limitations of behavioral observation.

- Observations show the child's behavior in a natural setting.
- Observational data can be used in a functional behavior assessment of what is supporting the child's problem behavior.
- The method requires hours of expensive observer training and observation and coding time.
- Children can react to being observed.

IN FOCUS 7 ▶ Describe the DSM-IV-TR classification system for mental disorders and explain how it could be improved.

- The DSM was developed by the American Psychiatric Association and is the classification system most often used in the United States.
- Some aspects of the DSM are low in reliability, validity, and utility.
- The DSM is of questionable value with very young children and children from minority cultures.

Drugs and Social Issues

5

In the Beginning

How Many Kids Use Drugs?

When my class on child and adolescent psychopathology was studying illicit substance use, I (Donna Gelfand) presented a statistic on drug use among American high school students: 54% of the students in a recent national survey said they had used some illicit (illegal) drug before finishing high school [National Institute on Drug Abuse (NIDA), 2001]. A couple of my students looked surprised, so I asked them if this number seemed high. Quite the opposite! They said that every single one of the students in the high schools they came from, in two different states, had probably used recreational drugs. My students said that popular drugs such as home-grown marijuana, animal tranquilizers, and meth (methamphetamine, an easily manufactured, powerful but cheap stimulant) are within the reach of nearly every student in most high schools. If so, illicit drug use today is more common than drinking alcohol was during Prohibition in the 1920s.

The information from my students was chilling. Even if their estimates of usage rates are much too high, illicit drugs have reached all corners of our country, affecting students of all socioeconomic levels and a wide range of ages. Most youngsters escape serious consequences, but they still face risks of criminal prosecution and school and family conflict about their drug use. If they use the more dangerous illicit drugs in large quantities, they face serious drug-related health effects, dependence or addiction, accidental poisoning, suicide risk, and even death from overdose or the wrong combination of drugs. The individual and social toll in loss of education, earning power, consumption of goods and services, demands on service agencies, and interrupted lives is beyond calculation. Young people's illicit substance use is not new, but the sheer extent of usage now far surpasses that at any time in the past.

INTRODUCTION

IN FOCUS 1 ▶ Distinguish among substance use, substance abuse, and substance dependence.

In this chapter, we examine problems associated with young people's use of drugs. In communities throughout the United States, children encounter drugs such as home-grown or imported marijuana, meth from local illicit labs, cocaine, inhalants used to produce intoxication (e.g., paint thinner or fuel), and prescription medications or animal tranquilizers. Our concern focuses on problematic use patterns that lead to serious interference with daily functioning, drug dependence (also called addiction), and substantial health risks from unknowingly consuming adulterated or unexpectedly pure and powerful street drugs, which can result in overdose. Addicts must get large amounts of money for maintaining a drug habit, which drives them into criminal activity and drug-related problems with the law.

The distinction between *substance use* (which may be a one-time or casual experience) and **substance abuse** (which is heavier and more frequent use, with adverse effects) is based on the degree of hazard and impairment in functioning caused by taking the substance. According to the DSM criteria (Table 5-1), the effects must be substantial in order for use to qualify as substance abuse. Even more serious is **substance dependence** (see Table 5-2). Not all drugs of abuse produce dependence, but those that do produce a nearly irresistible pattern of repeated self-administration that can result in tolerance, withdrawal, and compulsive usage (American Psychiatric Association, 2000). People who become dependent on a substance report strong cravings for it as well as tolerance, or the need for escalating amounts in order to become intoxicated. There are wide differences among substances and users regarding the severity and timing of dependence. Withdrawal symptoms can be minor or absent for some substances, such as marijuana, but sedatives, alcohol, and opiates (heroin, codeine, and morphine) can produce very uncomfortable, even deadly withdrawal syndromes. An unhealthy, compulsive pattern of usage can be diagnosed as substance dependence even in the absence of tolerance, withdrawal, or both.

This chapter presents research-based information on why so many young people use illegal drugs, the characteristics of the users, and their adjustment prob-

Table 5-1 DSM-IV-TR Criteria for Substance Abuse

A. A maladaptive pattern of substance use leading to clinically significant impairment or distress, as manifested by one (or more) of the following, occurring within a 12-month period:

(1) recurrent substance use resulting in a failure to fulfill major role obligations at work, school, or home (e.g., repeated absences or poor work performance related to substance use; substance-related absences, suspensions, or expulsions from school; neglect of children or household)

(2) recurrent substance use in situations in which it is physically hazardous (e.g., driving an automobile or operating a machine when impaired by substance use)

(3) recurrent substance-related legal problems (e.g., arrests for substance-related disorderly conduct)

(4) continued substance use despite having persistent or recurrent social or interpersonal problems caused or exacerbated by the effects of the substance (e.g., arguments with spouse about consequences of intoxication, physical fights)

B. The symptoms have never met the criteria for Substance Dependence for this class of substance.

SOURCE: American Psychiatric Association (2000). Reprinted with permission from the *Diagnostic and Statistical Manual of Mental Disorders*, 4th ed., Text Revision. © 2000 American Psychiatric Association.

lems. It emphasizes the many contributors to substance abuse, especially chronological age, which relates to this book's developmental theme. Drug use is closely tied to the young adolescent's development of autonomy and longing to be grown-up and independent from parents. Another developmental basis for drug use is the growing power of peers during adolescence. Adolescents may pose as sophisticated drug users and actively encourage their peers to try drugs. Such peer influences are strongest when parents spend little time with their children and are distant and rejecting (Dishion, 1990; Roth & Brooks-Gunn, 2000). Modeling and imitation entice children to use drugs when the drug-taking models are parents or older siblings, admired peers, or media personalities. The social context in which many young people grow up— their families, schools, and communities—includes heavy drug and substance use and is thus a contributor to the nation's drug problem.

Table 5-2 DSM-IV-TR Criteria for Substance Dependence (Abridged)

A maladaptive pattern of substance use, leading to clinically significant impairment or distress, as manifested by three (or more) of the following, occurring at any time in the same 12-month period:

(1) tolerance, as defined by either of the following:

    (a) a need for markedly increased amounts of the substance to achieve intoxication or the desired effect

    (b) markedly diminished effect with continued use of the same amount of the substance

(2) withdrawal, as manifested by either of the following:

    (a) the characteristic withdrawal syndrome for the substance (refer to Criteria A and B of the criteria sets for Withdrawal from the specific substances)

    (b) the same (or closely related) substance is taken to relieve or avoid withdrawal symptoms

(3) the substance is often taken in larger amounts or over a longer period than was intended

(4) there is a persistent desire or unsuccessful efforts to cut down or control substance use

(5) a great deal of time is spent in activities necessary to obtain the substance (e.g., visiting multiple doctors or driving long distances), use the substance (e.g., chain-smoking), or recover from its effects

(6) important social, occupational, or recreational activities are given up or reduced because of substance use

(7) the substance use is continued despite knowledge of having a persistent or recurrent physical or psychological problem that is likely to have been caused or exacerbated by the substance (e.g., current cocaine use despite recognition of cocaine-induced depression, or continued drinking despite recognition that an ulcer was made worse by alcohol consumption)

SOURCE: American Psychiatric Association (2000). Reprinted with permission from the *Diagnostic and Statistical Manual of Mental Disorders*, 4th ed., Text Revision. © 2000 American Psychiatric Association.

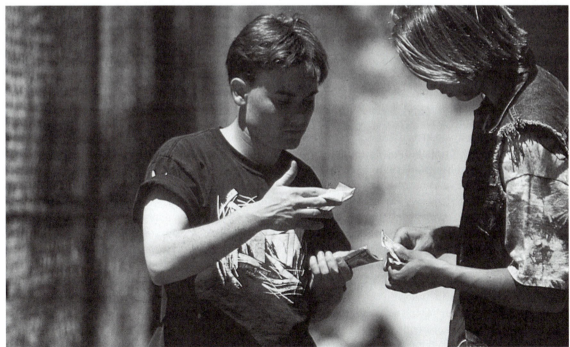

Robert Bruce Ayres

Students can purchase drugs at school or in their neighborhoods, often from other kids. Are stricter drug laws and harsher penalties needed, or should drug use be decriminalized?

The research theme of this book appears in this chapter at many points. Research studies provided vital information on which young people use drugs and why. Research revealed that many early drug prevention programs did not work, in part because they were devised by adults without the participation of young people or knowledge about their psychology. Research provided clues about how to construct more effective prevention and treatment programs and tested their effectiveness. It turns out that adult and adolescent drug abusers require different types of prevention and treatment programs, another example of the need to gear interventions to the recipients' level of development.

Because so many types of psychoactive substances are misused, this chapter's coverage must be selective. Discussion is limited to young people's use of several of the more frequently abused substances, including alcohol, tobacco, marijuana, Ecstasy, and several misused prescription drugs. The chapter concludes with a discussion of the various types of prevention and treatment programs available for young people. Although much work remains to be done to prevent and treat illicit substance use, there has been encouraging progress.

WHAT ENCOURAGES SUBSTANCE USE?

Psychological and Physical Drug Effects

The most obvious attraction of illicit substances is their powerful and compelling biochemical and psychological effects. Archeological evidence of alcoholic brews in containers in ancient ruins and shipwrecks throughout the world suggests that for eons people have used psychoactive substances to become inebriated or to get relief from pain. The lure of intoxication continues to be a strong motivator for drug use to this day. These drug effects clearly relate to this book's theme that behavior has biological roots.

There is an interaction between the attraction to intoxication and a youngster's living situation. The more stressful, negative, and apparently hopeless the adolescent's life, the more likely he is to use substances that make him feel good, provide a sensation of power, and offer escape from worries. Accepted and

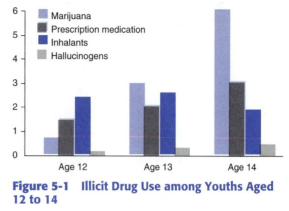

Figure 5-1   Illicit Drug Use among Youths Aged 12 to 14

Source: Leshner (2001).

successful adolescents are less likely to become heavy drug users than are their peers who have fewer advantages and more troubles, although there are exceptions to this rule. Unhappy teens may shun drugs, while popular and successful ones sometimes become drug dependent. One positive note is that, as a group, high school students are somewhat cautious about the drugs they use. They say they are most attracted to substances that seem safer and are more affordable, such as marijuana (see Figure 5-1), and tend to avoid the more dangerous types of drugs that are clearly addictive, are sometimes adulterated with cheaper, more toxic fillers, and can prove lethal (Ballie, 2001b).

Acting Like Grown-ups

"Drugs are for cool grown-ups, not for babies." That is what millions of preteens and adolescents believe, and it tempts them to become smokers, drinkers, and drug users at an early age. The lure of adult status and the power and independence it confers is immense. So even very young children try to look and act older, like the people they admire and would like to be. Children are strongly motivated to imitate powerful, high-status role models, such as the ones they see at concerts and sports events and daily on TV programs and videos (Bandura, 1969). When the people they admire openly use illicit drugs, kids are almost irresistibly attracted to the drug scene. This tendency for youngsters to equate drug use with maturity leads some social scientists to view alcohol, cigarette, and illicit drug use as a transitional fact of life for many children entering adolescence (Jessor & Jessor, 1977).

Employment and Teen Drug Use

Some of the adult roles that society approves for adolescents are not necessarily healthy. Most adults believe that exposure to the world of work is good for teenagers and teaches them good job skills and responsibility. However, the quality of the job and the number of hours the teenager works make a huge difference. Good jobs that teach valuable skills for future employment, offer close adult supervision, and perform community services may benefit young people. Bad jobs may require too much of their time, produce overload that induces chronic fatigue and interferes with school achievement, expose them to health hazards and accident dangers, and disrupt social relationships (Roth & Brooks-Gunn, 2000). About half of U.S. teenagers are employed part time, a higher proportion working longer hours than in other developed countries (Children's Defense Fund, 2000). Despite adults' high expectations for the beneficial effects of employment, adolescents who work more than 15–20 hours per week (and many do) are in danger of becoming cynical about the world of work and alienated from school and their parents. They are also more likely to use alcohol and drugs than their peers who are not in the labor market (Barling, Rogers, & Kelloway, 1995; Steinberg, Fegley, & Dornbusch, 1993).

Coworkers are important socialization agents, and their influence is not always good. Teenagers who take jobs in food preparation and food service work side by side with fellow employees who admit to moderately high levels of illicit drug use and heavy alcohol use, according to an analysis conducted by the Substance Abuse and Mental Health Services Administration (cited in Smith, 2001). (See Table 5-3.) Is it likely that the habits of their coworkers have no effect on younger workers? Teenagers employed in retail sales are just as likely to encounter drug users working beside them, and those who land the higher-paying jobs in construction, moving and transportation, or manual labor are especially likely to associate with heavy drinkers and drug users. Adolescents employed in blue-collar jobs are also more likely to be of lower socioeconomic status and at greater risk for substance abuse than middle-class, achievement-oriented youngsters, more of whom work at office jobs that teach them skills useful in their future careers. Clearly, drug use risks are not confined to homes, schools, and neighborhoods but extend to the workplace as well.

Table 5-3 Percentage of Full-Time Workers, Ages 18–49, Reporting Current Illicit Drug Use and Heavy Alcohol Use, by Occupation

	Current Illicit Drug Use	Heavy Alcohol Use
Total	7.6	8.4
Executive, administrative and managerial	5.5	6.5
Professional specialty	5.1	4.3
Technicians and related support	5.5	6.2
Sales	11.4	8.3
Administrative support	5.9	3.5
Protective service	3.2	6.3
Food preparation, waitstaff and bartenders	11.2	12.2
Other service	5.6	5.1
Precision production and repair	7.9	13.1
Construction	15.6	17.6
Extractive and precision production	8.6	12.9
Machine operators and inspectors	10.5	13.5
Transportation and material moving	5.3	13.1
Handlers, helpers and laborers	10.6	15.7

SOURCE: "An Analysis of Worker Drug Use and Workplace Policies and Programs," Office of Applied Studies, Substance Abuse and Mental Health Services Administration, U.S. Department of Health and Human Services, July 1997.

Predicting Drug Use

Researchers have searched long and fruitlessly for a way to predict which individuals will become drug users. This search is unlikely to be completely successful because so many different types of youngsters try so many different types of drugs and substances. Although no single personality type marks potential users, some personal characteristics often accompany drug use. Risk-takers who crave excitement, are rebellious, avoid school, and feel unaccepted are more likely to be users (Epstein, Griffin, & Botvin, 2001). And antisocial, externalizing behavior beginning in early childhood is a risk factor for teenage substance use (Dishion, French, & Patterson, 1995). In fact, adolescents treated for substance abuse often also have another diagnosable mental disorder, especially conduct disorder (Foxhall, 2001; Grella, Hser, Joshi, & Rounds-Bryant, 2001). Adolescents with a co-occurring psychological disorder are more likely than those without such a disorder to relapse, or resume illicit substance use following treatment. A combination of early drug use, conduct disorder, and encounters with the law greatly increases an adolescent's odds of continuing a pattern of substance abuse into adulthood (Gilvarry, 2000).

Being One of the Gang

IN FOCUS 2 ▶ Describe how friends, celebrities, and family members can lead youngsters to use drugs.

Adolescents tend to share the illicit substance use patterns of their friends, whether they are users or abstainers (Kilpatrick et al., 2000; Wills, Sandy, Yaeger, & Shinar, 2001). A preponderance of users in a school or community makes it difficult for teens to abstain because they have many deviant companions and few who avoid drugs. When a neighborhood is dominated by delinquent, antisocial youths, the usual controls exerted through adult monitoring and informal rules break down and delinquency escalates (Roth & Brooks-Gunn, 2000; Sampson & Morenoff, 1997). Associating with a deviant peer group provides one of the strongest incentives to use drugs (Weinberg, Rahdert, Colliver, & Glantz, 1998), especially if a teen's parents are neglecting or rejecting (Dishion, 1990). Parents warn their children against associating with known drug users and dealers, but are often powerless to influence their children's choice of friends.

Immigrant parents who speak little English and are unfamiliar with the new culture feel particularly helpless to protect their children from bad influences (Portes & Rumbaut, 2001). On many issues regarding customs, manners, and proper behavior, these parents must defer to their more knowledgeable children, who are more fluent in English and know more about American culture than their parents do. Also, the parents often lose their children's respect because, as recent immigrants, they must take poor-paying menial jobs and are on the bottom rung of society. Formerly high-achieving, obedient young people such as Khae, the son of Laotian Hmong refugees described in the Family Focus box, may turn defiant and join a local gang. Many children of immigrant parents are at risk for drug use and gang involvement because their families exist at the margins of a rich society.

Drug Use by Entertainers and Athletes

It is not uncommon for entertainment and sports stars to get into trouble because of their illicit drug use. No doubt you can name several well-publicized cases in the recent news. Young people know that the rich and famous use illicit drugs, and they yearn to be like them. They want to be in the spotlight, sport tattoos, gang-inspired clothing, body piercing, and gold and diamond jewelry, and ride in limousines. This glamorization of a life-style based on drugs undoubtedly affects young people and motivates them to obtain drugs.

Family Problems

Parents must assume some of the responsibility for their children's drug use. Although most people believe that having a healthy family protects children from drugs, the exact nature of the association between the family and children's drug use is not immediately obvious. We consider the family context in some detail because parent-child relationships are critically important to children's decisions to use drugs as well as to the treatment of drug abuse. There are many ways in which families directly or inadvertently encourage children to use drugs.

Drug Use by Other Family Members

It is common for children to watch their parents using dangerous substances and illegal drugs (National In-

Family Focus

Khae, Son of Pao Yang, American

The San Diego home of Mr. Pao Yang and his family was in disarray . . . because they were packing to move to Fresno. As refugees, both Mr. Pao and his wife Zer Vue receive federally supported assistance. Pao Yang complements this with some odd jobs, but his options are limited as he speaks little English. The interview was conducted in Hmong. Before starting, the interviewer asked for his 18-year-old son, Khae, who had not yet completed the project's follow-up schedule. Pao responded that his son had just stepped out of the house, but they could begin the interview. Ten minutes into it, the porch screen door slammed, and Khae stepped in. He wore no shirt and had shaved his head.

The father called, "Khae, come here; you have some questionnaire to fill up." The young man replied, "No, I don't care for it or anybody." He went to his bedroom, slamming the door after him. Fifteen minutes later he was out; he was now confronted by his mother who politely asked him to cooperate. Khae answered, "No, all of this is shit." He left the home, again slamming the front door. In Hmong, the mother reported, "It was not like this before. He was obedient, well-behaved, went to school every day.

Two years ago, he joined the Mesa Kings [a local gang] and last year he quit school. He does what he likes, does what he pleases. If you try talking to him, he yells louder and leaves."

Pao added, "We cannot control him; once I hit him and he pulled a gun on me. He knows English better than us—thinks that he knows everything. If he continues this way, he'll never finish high school; he'll be killed first." By the end of the conversation, it became clear that Khae was the reason why the family was moving to Fresno. There is a larger, more concentrated Hmong population there, and the family had several relatives living in the city. The parents hoped to put him back to school and garner the help of the extended family and clan to keep him away from gangs. Zer, the wife, accompanied the interviewer to the door. "I want to apologize for the bad attitude of my son," she said. "It would not have been like this back home; it is this country that is so hard to understand."

SOURCE: Portes & Rumbaut (2001), p. 93, from *Legacies: The Story of the Immigrant Second Generation*, 2001. Used by permission of the University of California Press.

---

stitute on Drug Abuse, 1996; Smith, 2001). In a recent national survey, one half of the children had at least one parent who reported smoking cigarettes in the past month. Fourteen percent of the children lived with a parent who reported past-year use of illegal drugs, 6% had a parent who needed treatment for illicit drug abuse, and 8%, or 6 million kids, lived with a parent who was dependent on alcohol (is an alcoholic). Parents' alcoholism is associated with their children's use of alcohol and illicit substances in adolescence and early adulthood, particularly if the children had early conduct problems and exhibited other externalizing behaviors (Chassin, Pitts, DeLucia, & Todd, 1999). Any type of adjustment difficulty in the preschool years appears to increase future drug use. Boys who were anxious and inhibited at age 3 (internalizing problems) as well as those with behavioral undercontrol (externalizing problems) had more alco-

hol problems when they became young adults (Caspi, Moffitt, Newman, & Silva, 1996).

In sum, parents model the very drug abuse they warn their children against, and children are more likely to follow their parents' actual examples than their admonitions to abstain. Further, the substandard parenting that accompanies alcoholism and drug abuse and addiction can cause children to reject and avoid their parents.

No One Is Watching the Kids: Poor Monitoring and Supervision

Darrell felt his parents kept him under surveillance 24 hours a day, and he hated it. The other kids at his high school didn't have to report in after school, eat dinner with their families, and then spend a couple of hours on homework every school night, so why should he? Darrell's situation reflects a dilemma of many American families. Peers put tremendous pressure on their friends to go out and do things rather than stay home completing homework. Parents want to make sure their children are keeping up with their schoolwork and are protected from bad peer influences, and so they want to know where their kids are and what they are doing. Adolescents are at a developmental period when they naturally want freedom and autonomy. These competing interests generate a tremendous amount of parent-teen conflict. Yet the statistics suggest that the parents have a case.

Columbia University's National Center on Addiction and Substance Abuse found that the more regularly children and parents ate dinner together, the less likely children were to smoke, drink, or use drugs (Hewlett, 2001). There is no guarantee that the family that eats together abstains together, since other factors may account for the correlation between eating to-gether and abstinence. Traditional values, including abstinence, may be typical of families that eat together, and it may be that general family life-style accounts for children's remaining drug-free. Other factors, too, could be responsible, such as better relationships between parents and children, higher socioeconomic status, or better parent and child mental health. However, impressed by this research, the U.S. Senate unanimously passed a resolution in June 2001 declaring a "National Eat Dinner with Your Children Day."

Dinnertime may be one of the only times during a day that busy parents and children can enjoy being together for any extended period. Changes in the American family, such as increases in the number of parents working more than 40 hours a week, in maternal employment, and in mother-headed households, have decreased the amount of time children spend with their parents, particularly in the after-school hours

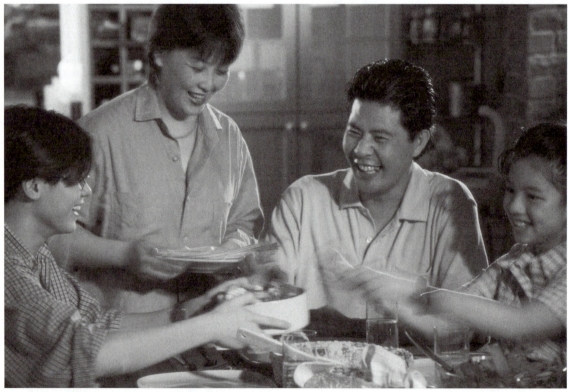

Nasi Sakura/SuperStock

When a family eats dinner together regularly, the children are less likely to use drugs.

(Hofferth & Sandberg, 1998). Most violent juvenile crime (and probably drug and substance use) occurs during these same hours, from 3 to 8 p.m. (Sickmund, Snyder, & Poe-Yamagata, 1997). Youngsters who do not regularly eat dinner at home with parent(s) have very high rates of smoking, drinking, marijuana use, fighting, and early initiation of sexual activity, with accompanying early parenthood (Council of Economic Advisors, 2000). It appears that undersocialized peers take over from parents during times when parents are occupied elsewhere. So Darrell is lucky that his parents show such concern about where he is and what he is doing. Although he currently sees them as overconcerned, he may later come to appreciate their tight supervision and treat his children the same way when he becomes a parent.

When parents and adolescents get together, do they talk about avoiding drugs and alcohol? Apparently not, because most children surveyed say they don't remember having a conversation with their parents on these subjects. On the other hand, most parents claim they have spoken to their kids about not using drugs (Ballie, 2001a). Perhaps the parents did broach the subject, but the comment was so brief and general that the children didn't notice it. Drugs, like sex education, may be a topic parents know they should discuss with their kids but often avoid because they don't know what to say.

Rejection and Harsh Punishment

Simple lack of supervision can lead to substance abuse, but harshness and rejection by parents can be even worse. Anything that alienates young people and sends them into the company of other rebellious teens is likely to promote substance use. The same child and family characteristics that encourage substance use also increase children's risks for developing externalizing disorders such as conduct disorder, delinquency, oppositional defiant disorder, and attention-deficit/hyperactivity disorder (ADHD). It is not clear whether drug use and externalizing behavior are caused by rejection, abuse, and family problems or by general social conditions. Whatever the causes, there is a regrettable tendency for poor parenting practices, child drug use, and children's antisocial behavior patterns to occur together, with a devastating effect on the children (White, Loeber, Stouthamer-Loeber, & Farrington, 1999).

Parents under Stress

Family risk factors such as conflict between parents and children, parental substance use, and negative life events (e.g., a parent's serious mental or physical illness or loss of job) increase children's risk of substance use (Wills et al., 2001). Children's risk for substance use is further increased if they have a high activity level and a negative, emotional temperament. A child with negative emotionality tends to be irritable and easily becomes upset. In contrast, children are at less risk for substance abuse if they are task-oriented (can focus on performing tasks) and have a positive outlook (Wills et al., 2001). It seems that children and adolescents who have more vulnerable, negative temperaments and are less easily controlled by caretakers are more likely to turn to drugs under adverse family situations.

Disadvantaged Neighborhoods: Poverty and Prejudice

What often strikes observers about the most impoverished neighborhoods is a paradox: How is it that people who live there manage to obtain large amounts of alcohol, cigarettes, and illicit drugs? Sick alcoholics, junkies, and crack addicts feeding their addictions are seen on the streets in the most desperate parts of cities. Even people who cannot always afford to eat are driven to obtain mind-altering and addictive substances to take their minds off their other problems or feed their addictions for a while. And many of these people are disabled, mentally ill, new immigrants, or minorities forced to live at the edges of society, their hope ebbing that they will ever do better. They form a familiar part of many very poor children's lives and a warning to them: "You could become like us."

Despite this obvious evidence of the consequences of drug use, children are more likely to turn to illicit substances if they live in disadvantaged neighborhoods and suffer from high levels of stress, as many in such surroundings do. Delinquency and drug abuse rates are highest in neighborhoods with high rates of poverty, unemployment, resident turnover, and single-parent families and a changing cultural mix (Brody et al., 2001). Children living in these chaotic conditions rightfully feel anxious and depressed about their unhealthy situations. For their own safety, children must be wary in areas with high crime levels, where they are often victimized and gunfights are common occurrences.

Good and Bad Schools

Schools in these neglected areas are among the worst in the nation and are grossly underfinanced, badly maintained, and overwhelmed by large numbers of extremely needy students. So the children either attend or avoid attending overburdened and inadequate schools, where too little learning goes on to give them basic skills and prepare them for employment. Under these grim circumstances, many young people turn to gangs and use illicit substances for excitement or self-medication. Crime becomes their most likely source of money.

Fortunately, some public schools in poverty areas defy the odds and achieve excellence, with much higher than expected achievement levels and graduation rates. Although attending a poorly functioning school seems to increase children's antisocial and delinquent behavior, a good school environment can help protect students from these adjustment hazards (Rutter, 2000). Like good families, good schools are led by capable, caring adults and have teachers and administrators who provide models of healthy behavior.

Teachers' substance use affects their students. When faculty members are prohibited from smoking within view of students, adolescent students have lower smoking rates (Perry, Kelder, & Komro, 1993). Students also profit from the emotional support of a favorite teacher who serves as a role model and confidante (Werner & Smith, 1992). Good teachers care intensely about their students' progress, have high standards for students' work, and administer fair and consistent discipline (Gottfredson, Gottfredson, & Hybel, 1993). Disadvantaged young participants in a large national health study were less likely to use drugs and alcohol if they reported strong emotional attachments to their teachers. They were also less likely to attempt suicide, act violently, or become sexually active at an early age (Resnick et al., 1997). Positive relationships with teachers seem to have a greater influence on adolescents' drug use and other risky behavior than do such school characteristics as class size, attendance, dropout rate, and amount of teacher training (Roth & Brooks-Gunn, 2000). However, it is immensely challenging for a teacher to stay optimistic and build good relationships with individual children while working in a poorly functioning school serving highly disadvantaged children in a neglected, dangerous neighborhood. Cynicism and burnout are ever present dangers for teachers in such schools.

Segregation, Crime, and Drug Abuse

Fortunately, communities are beginning to learn how to overcome the strict segregation along the lines of income level, ethnicity, and race that divides cities and consigns poor children to the worst lives. Diversity in the socioeconomic composition of the student body is important, since grossly underfunded schools that serve only poor students cannot keep good teachers and have students who fail and drop out early. Communities that are segregated by income and race typically have completely separate and highly unequal school systems, with excellent schools in the higher-income areas and shockingly bad ones in low-income neighborhoods.

As the Family Focus box describes, some communities have decided to reduce inequality in opportunity by integrating students of all socioeconomic levels in their schools. Income-based school integration has improved school atmosphere and performance, offering better academic opportunities for impoverished children regardless of race or ethnicity (Walker, 2001). When a school and a community are united in their determination to help children of all backgrounds to succeed academically, the school can counteract some of the many bad effects of poverty on children's academic development, future employment, and upward mobility.

Sometimes the best solution is to move a family from a dangerous, dilapidated, and poorly served neighborhood into a better one. The Yonkers Project moved families from such locations to middle-class neighborhoods. An evaluation of this program found that teens who remained in impoverished neighborhoods were more likely to develop problem drinking and marijuana use than were those who moved to better surroundings (Briggs, 1997). Other urban family removal projects have reported similar beneficial effects. Compared with youths who remained in public housing in Baltimore, those who moved into higher-income areas had lower crime rates and fewer drug, truancy, runaway, and weapons offenses (Ludwig, Duncan, & Hirschfield, 1998).

In general, substance abuse is just one of a constellation of problems—including school failure, antisocial

What Happens When Rich and Poor Kids Attend School Together

With poor and minority children's academic achievement and school graduation rates at a dismally low level, it seemed like a good idea to try to give them an education as good as that given to kids from wealthier families. Children from all areas were bused to superior magnet schools. Unfortunately, busing involved using race in student assignments, which the courts declared unconstitutional. The result of this judicial decision was to consign most poor and minority students to the worst schools and the poorest outlooks. Resegregation of the schools proceeded rapidly in the late 20th century, especially in the South. African American and Hispanic American students became among the most highly isolated, educationally deprived groups in the nation, except for Indians living on remote reservations (Portes & Rumbaut, 2001).

Some communities reacted in an innovative way, because they wanted to retain their diverse student enrollments. When schools are segregated by race, they are almost invariably also segregated by family income, with whites being much more advantaged. Why not integrate schools by family income rather than race, which would also provide educational advantages for impoverished white students? Communities across the United States are considering socioeconomic desegregation in their schools, including districts in North Carolina (a leader in this movement), Wisconsin, California, Connecticut, Florida, Kentucky, Massachusetts, and Washington. The process faces many difficulties, including ensuring that rich and poor children do receive equally good programs even within the same schools. Also, "white flight" by white, middle-class parents might undermine the economically integrated public schools whether or not they are succeeding.

The alternative to integration is to have greater and greater isolation of the poor from middle-class society. Across the nation, gated communities are going up because better-off people fear the resentful poor. Since all must live together in the same country, integration may be a more realistic alternative than further segregation. Many people will watch the experimental mixing of wealthy and poor public school students with great interest.

Sources: Kahlenberg (2001); Walker (2001)

---

behavior, and criminal activity—that flourish in pockets of poverty. The fight against drug abuse must address this larger social issue of creating healthy communities if we are to make any substantial progress in eliminating a variety of social ills.

> *Drug, alcohol, and tobacco abuse is the cause of more deaths, illnesses, and disabilities than any other preventable health condition, and seriously undermines America's family life, economy, and public safety. (Martin, 2001, p. 10)*

Cumulative Risk Model

People find drugs appealing for a range of reasons, and there is no single risk factor leading to drug use. The **cumulative risk model** says that drug use, like other adverse developmental outcomes, is better predicted by the number of personal and environmental risks in a child's life than by any one specific vulnerability factor (Carta et al., 2001; Sameroff, Seifer, Barocas, Zax, & Greenspan, 1987). In sum, while many individual factors can increase children's vulnerability to drugs, the addition of factors further increases the likelihood of substance abuse. Finally, some individual factors that appear to increase risk, such as prenatal exposure to illicit drugs, may not themselves add much to a child's future vulnerability to illicit drugs. Instead, prenatal exposure to illicit drugs may co-occur with other harmful influences, such as the parents' limited schooling, extreme poverty, and inadequate diet or the mother's use of other harmful substances such as alcohol or nicotine (Carta et al., 2001). Thus, a child's illicit substance use is likely to develop in a context of multiple risks, making it difficult or impossible to identify a single major risk factor.

SOME FREQUENTLY USED SUBSTANCES

IN FOCUS 3 ▶ Identify the possible effects on the fetus if a pregnant woman drinks, smokes, or takes some form of cocaine.

Alcohol, Cigarettes, and Marijuana

A major problem with alcohol, cigarettes, and marijuana is that their immediate effects are enjoyable, but their regular usage can lead to serious consequences. Cigarettes contain nicotine, which often leads to dependence, and continued smoking greatly increases the individual's risks for cancer, cardiovascular disease, and other major health problems. Alcohol intoxication causes or contributes to traffic accidents and violence, and marijuana, especially in its highly refined forms, can also induce intoxication. In addition, juveniles can get into trouble with the law for using any of these three substances. Yet recent surveys show that over one-third (35%) of high school seniors smoked in the past month, and 23% said they smoked every day (NIDA, 2001). Despite the widespread concern about the grave dangers of smoking, adolescents continue to take it up in huge numbers.

Alcohol

What are the historical trends in alcohol consumption among high school students? Alcohol use has always been high, and it is growing among very young women. Several decades ago, in the 1960s, only 7% of 10- to 14-year-old girls were beginning to use alcohol, but now nearly one-third, or 31%, of girls that young have begun to drink. Any unhealthy practice that increases by more than fourfold over a period of 40 years and can produce serious physical illness demands the nation's immediate attention.

Both smoking and drinking are particularly alarming in girls and young women because of their potential effects on their children. Heavy drinking during pregnancy can produce lasting effects, such as fetal alcohol syndrome, which affects both physical and cognitive development. Symptoms of **fetal alcohol syndrome** include physical abnormalities of the face, marked by widely spaced eyes with short eyelid openings, a small head, suggesting that the brain is not fully developed, thin upper lip, and small, upturned nose,

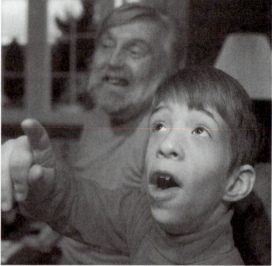

A child with fetal alcohol syndrome shows distinctive facial features (small head, widely spaced eyes, prominent groove from nose to top lip) and may also have mental retardation.

along with other anatomical defects. These children often suffer from mental retardation, poor motor coordination, and deficits of memory, attention, and language, and they have adjustment problems of many types. Other children have a related disorder, **fetal alcohol effects**, in which only some of these abnormalities appear, probably because their mothers drank less than the women whose children developed fetal alcohol syndrome. Scientists have not established a safe level of drinking during pregnancy, and pregnant women are advised to refrain from drinking alcohol.

Cigarettes and Marijuana

The 12% of expectant mothers who smoke regularly (Ebrahim, Floyd, Merritt, Decoufle, & Holtzman, 2000) expose their babies to the risk of **low birth weight**, which can be associated with slow learning throughout childhood. In addition, the risk of miscarriage, prematurity, impaired heart rate and breathing abnormalities while asleep, infant death, and childhood cancer also increase if the mother smokes (Franco, Chabanski, Szliwowski, Dramaix, & Kahn, 2000; Walker, Rosenberg, & Balaban-Gil, 1999). And the more cigarettes she smokes, the greater the risk to her fetus.

Marijuana is the favorite illicit drug of young adolescents, far outpacing illegally obtained prescription medications and other types of drugs (Leshner, 2001). Younger teens are attracted to inexpensive and easily obtained mind-altering substances. Since the hemp plant, the source of marijuana, is easily grown, families and children can become their own suppliers of very inexpensive, low-grade marijuana. This form is generally less dangerous than street marijuana, which tends to be much more potent and can produce dependency if consumed in large doses over an extended period of time. Some youngsters limit their experimentation to marijuana, while others move on to stimulants, tranquilizers, and narcotics.

The Alluring Stimulants

The stimulants are the illicit drugs of choice for many adults and adolescents. This large group of drugs includes some that are legal and commonly available, such as coffee, chocolate, and some soft drinks, all of which contain caffeine. Other stimulants are the nicotine in cigarettes and smokeless tobacco products and the amphetamines found in some diet drugs, nasal decongestants, prescription drugs to treat ADHD, and both over-the-counter and prescription drugs to increase alertness and combat sleep. Cocaine in any form is a powerful and highly addictive stimulant.

Amphetamines

Various amphetamines have long attracted users of both sexes, many cultures, and various ages. Young women in particular find methamphetamine (meth) enticing because it is inexpensive, greatly increases their energy, and suppresses their appetite, resulting in weight loss. A single dose, which can be snorted, smoked, injected, or swallowed, produces what users describe as a thrilling high, stimulates the senses, increases feelings of self-esteem, and greatly increases activity over many hours (see the case study of a meth mom). These are the pleasant, mostly subjective effects that appear when someone first uses meth. However, the honeymoon does not last, and the list of later negative physiological and psychological effects caused by amphetamine intoxication and dependence is long and frightening.

Amphetamines in large quantities increase the activity of the neurotransmitters norepinephrine and dopamine to excessive levels in the central nervous system, which causes hallucinations and delusions. All of the stimulants can have major, very dangerous negative effects, including panic, agitation, and paranoid delusions, which can impel the user to strike out irrationally at other people. Users crave the intoxicating feelings of euphoria and high energy derived from consuming lower doses of stimulants, but many soon find themselves with a drug habit that is no longer fun and is escalating beyond their control. When they develop dependency, they require more and more meth to get high and their lives center on the drug, causing them to ignore all responsibilities. Sleep deprivation combined with the effects of the drug can produce dangerous paranoia. Parents who become dependent on meth neglect family, friends, and work, eventually becoming unable to function and unemployable. (See the Family Focus box.) Drug-dependent parents become so negligent that they endanger their children, who must be taken away from them for the children's protection.

An amphetamine called MDMA (methylenedioxymethamphetamine), or Ecstasy, is popular among some college students. Like other amphetamines, it is extremely addictive. Ecstasy is often referred to as a "club drug" because it is widely used at night clubs and dance clubs, in combination with alcohol and other drugs such as Ritalin. Young people who take Ecstasy and dance and drink for hours at a time can overdose and experience overheating and dehydration (which can be fatal), panic attacks, and fainting. As Ecstasy became increasingly popular, its bad effects became obvious. Some users attending nightclubs and rave parties collapsed and required emergency medical treatment. Alarmed communities attempted to close the clubs as a public health measure. Predictably, the party crowd just went someplace else but did not stop using Ecstasy.

Bad Companions: Cocaine, Crack Cocaine, and Heroin

Cocaine's effects on the brain are similar to those of amphetamines. Dopamine accumulates in the synaptic space between neurons and continues stimulating the receiving neuron, creating an intensely pleasurable "high." Once thought to produce euphoria without being addictive, cocaine is now recognized as producing dependence after a prolonged period of use. Crack, a crystallized form of cocaine that is smoked, is

Meth Moms—A Contradiction in Terms

Life becomes a nightmare for anyone with an addiction to a stimulant, but especially so when a mother of young children is dependent on methamphetamine. Women find meth appealing at first because it is an appetite suppressant that allows them to lose weight, while feeling so positive and energetic that they look for extra things to do around the house in the many hours when they cannot sleep at night. However, they aren't thinking clearly, and their activities have a compulsive, irrational tone: Some do things like sort everyone's clothing by color, size, and label; others start on senseless redecorating projects that are never completed or try to paint the house by themselves. Imagine how appealing this drug must be to busy young mothers who never have enough time and energy to do everything they'd like.

The adverse effects of stimulants are very bad indeed, and often bring addicts into trouble with their spouse and family and employer, as they become ever less dependable. Addicts also risk encounters with the law if they turn to drug dealing or other illegal activities to support their habit. Staying awake for days at a time brings on wild paranoid hallucinations and delusions. These are not happy dreams.

Convinced that some innocent person is a monster or evil enemy, the meth addict may attack that individual with fists or a weapon. Such behavior endangers children directly as possible victims of the violence and indirectly through the loss of trust and of the safe base that children need from their parents.

A 26-year-old mother had this to say about trying to take care of her 3-year-old son while she was in the grip of meth:

> There were a lot of times I'd put a movie on [for my son] and say, "God, just watch the movie and let me get high." I had all these little rationalizations, justifications, addict rules—you can't use it if he's in the room. But if he's in the bathtub, I can run in the other room and get high. (From "Speed Trap," by J. Santini and A. Estes, *Salt Lake Tribune*, Sunday, Sept. 2, 2001, p. A-1. Reprinted with permission.)

Many recovering meth addicts are fighting to regain custody of the children they neglected while on the drug. It is not easy for them to convince child welfare workers and the courts that they are once again responsible, loving, and consistent parents.

---

a popular drug of abuse among disadvantaged youth in urban areas but is rejected by many middle-class adolescents as being too dangerous (Foxhall, 2001; Grella et al., 2001).

A pregnant woman's use of cocaine, particularly if she smokes crack and is dependent on it, affects her newborn adversely—at least temporarily. The baby is born irritable and addicted to cocaine and often has a low birth weight, with decreased head circumference, and other problems. However, babies born to cocaine-addicted mothers show no obvious cognitive or motor skills delays at birth or in the first months of life (Gold, 1997). Because of public outcries that cocaine addiction is a form of child abuse, some 200 low-income, mostly African American mothers have been prosecuted for endangering their babies by using cocaine while pregnant (Paltrow, Cohen, & Carey, 2000). But are these babies in fact harmed in any

major, permanent way? Recent medical studies fail to support this view (Frank, Augustyn, Grant Knight, Pell, & Zuckerman, 2001; Hurt, Betancourt, Brodsky, & Giannetti, 2001). The babies of crack users do suffer developmental problems, but not because of the unique contribution of cocaine (Chavkin, 2001). The desperately poor mothers who take cocaine during pregnancy often smoke, drink heavily, take other illicit drugs, eat a poor diet, and fail to get adequate prenatal medical care, all of which adversely affect their children. Combined with poor parenting practices, these influences can have a devastating effect on children's development. This is not to say that fetal exposure to a powerful drug such as cocaine is harmless, but the effects have been found to be much less distinctive, severe, and lasting than was originally widely believed.

Use of opiates, particularly heroin, dwindled with the increased availability of other types of drugs, but heroin is returning in a potent drug mixture in combination with cocaine. Partly because the fashion industry publicized "heroin chic," a gaunt and haunted appearance of some high-fashion models, this drug combination has gained popularity and is taking its toll of young people. In addition to producing addiction and overdose problems, this injected drug puts users at risk for HIV infection and AIDS.

Prescription Drugs Gone Wrong: Ritalin and OxyContin

IN FOCUS 4 ▶ Describe the illicit use of Ritalin and OxyContin and the direct and indirect effects of these prescription drugs on children.

> *Data from the National Household Survey on Drug Abuse show that 12- to 14-year-olds reported prescription medications as one of two primary drugs used. (Leshner, 2001)*

With the explosive growth of the pharmaceutical industry and the development of medications for a growing number of illnesses has come misuse of many prescription drugs. Especially popular are the amphetamines, such as Ritalin and Dexedrine, and the opioid pain relievers, notably OxyContin. Other frequently misused prescription drugs are the central nervous system depressants used to treat anxiety and sleep disorders; these include the barbiturates and benzodiazepines such as the best-sellers Valium and Xanax (Botsford, 2001). Abuse of these drugs can be physically hazardous, and some create tolerance and dependence syndrome. Young people try these drugs because they are readily available from fellow students or from relatives for whom they are prescribed. Two prescription medications that are popular as illicit drugs of abuse are Ritalin and OxyContin.

Ritalin

Stimulants are always in demand as drugs of abuse. The stimulant Ritalin is one of the most widely misused prescription drugs for children. Attention-deficit/hyperactivity disorder (ADHD) is a very common childhood disorder for which Ritalin is often prescribed, since it is usually effective in reducing symptoms and has relatively few and mild unwanted effects. Children give or sell their prescribed Ritalin to other youngsters, and family members may secretly

use or distribute the child's Ritalin. An obvious and overdue reform measure is to place much tighter restrictions on the prescription and sale of stimulants. It should become obvious to pharmacists and prescribing physicians when a child seems to be consuming much more of a stimulant than was ordered. If parents prescription-shop from one physician and pharmacist to another, accumulating the medication, it is difficult to detect misuse under the current system. Tighter controls may be cumbersome and unpopular with drug manufacturers and many parents, but they may be essential to protect the health of young people.

OxyContin

People who have not yet heard of OxyContin will probably do so soon, because this very powerful and effective painkiller used in cases of severe and chronic pain has become a favorite drug of abuse in communities throughout the United States. The active ingredient in OxyContin is an extremely addictive and potentially lethal substance called oxycodone, which is also present in less concentrated form in other painkillers such as Tylox and Percodan. OxyContin is often prescribed to older people with serious illnesses but is sold by some of them to provide extra income, is simply taken from them by their ostensible caregivers, or is stolen from pharmacies. OxyContin is usually administered as a time-release pill, but it can be crushed and injected or snorted by abusers to produce a quicker reaction. Taken either alone or in combination with other substances, OxyContin has been linked with a number of overdose deaths (Meier, 2001; National Clearinghouse for Alcohol and Drug Information, 2001). An ideal public health system would mandate changes in drug manufacture to reduce the possibility of dangerous misuse, particularly by young people.

PROGRESS IN PREVENTION

IN FOCUS 5 ▶ Identify the types of programs that have proven to be least and most successful in preventing drug abuse.

Admittedly, the U.S. war on drugs is not going well, despite ever tougher criminal penalties, mandatory prison sentences, international enforcement programs, and drug czars appointed at the federal, state, and local levels. Social scientists have taken up the challenge to reduce the number of youths who become victimized by the use of illicit substances. Initial studies indicate that professional knowledge of child psychology is necessary in order to devise a successful program, because straightforward, commonsense approaches rarely work. Nevertheless, simple educational programs such as the popular Drug Abuse Resistance Education (DARE) program are offered in most high schools in the United States. DARE presents police officers who warn students about the dire physical and social effects of drug abuse. Officers welcome this role as a relief from burdensome and dangerous duties, and parents, teachers, and principals like the program, but popularity of a prevention program does not ensure its success. Thus far, there is no credible research evidence that the DARE program or

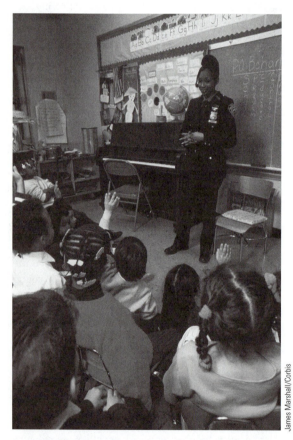

James Marshall/Corbis

Some popular prevention programs featuring authority figures such as police officers may have little impact on children's illicit drug use.

others like it deter students from substance abuse (Smith, 2001). However, the national DARE program received a $13.7 million grant from the Robert Wood Johnson Foundation to devise a new curriculum that might prove more effective. The new version is less dependent on speeches by adults and involves students more actively in discussion of topics of interest to them. In general, programs designed to involve young people and meet their needs are more successful than one-way, adult-dominated efforts.

The Drug Free Schools and Communities Act of 1986 provided support for elementary and secondary classroom programs to prevent alcohol, tobacco, and illicit drug use, but the programs had only mixed success. Many of these funded programs, like DARE, emphasized drug-related information but neglected students' needs and interests. More successful have been ambitious multicomponent community-wide prevention programs involving the youth, parents, schools, and local governments (Smith, 2001). These programs look beyond the individual vulnerabilities of children to analyze the many aspects of their lives that might lead to drug abuse (such as those discussed earlier in this chapter as risk factors). Children with special needs, such as those living in poverty or with alcoholic, criminal, or mentally ill parents, receive targeted interventions tailored for their personal situations. In many instances, families are recruited to help children learn and practice skills to help them avoid drugs.

Family involvement may be key to a successful prevention program with young adolescents. In a community-wide prevention program in Iowa (Spoth, Redmond, & Shin, 2001), researchers provided volunteer families with brief **family skills-training interventions** that promote bonding of 6th graders to their parents and others who provide positive models through greater child involvement in family activities, planning, and rule setting. Children are also trained to resist antisocial influences, and their parents learn skills to support this. Behavioral training for parents focuses on how to provide increased rewards for children when they conform to family rules and expectations as well as appropriate consequences for violations. As compared with children of control families who received drug prevention reading material alone, the children of families who received the skills-training intervention were significantly slower to begin substance use and had current lower use rates. This outcome is promising, but the drug problem is not yet solved. It is essential to develop some means of deterring young people from destructive drug use and abuse, because our nation has made little or no progress in reducing the availability of illegal drugs and harmful substances to children.

TREATMENTS FOR YOUNG DRUG AND SUBSTANCE ABUSERS

IN FOCUS 6 ▶ Discuss why family therapy is particularly effective in treating drug abuse and dependence.

For many young people, prevention efforts have failed, and treatment for drug and substance abuse is necessary. Nearly 60% of these adolescents are in trouble with the law, and more than 60% have some diagnosable mental disorder, mostly conduct disorder, but also depression and ADHD (Hser et al., 2001). These co-occurring conditions indicate that the adolescents treated in community-based programs are typically seriously disturbed and require treatment beyond help through drug withdrawal.

Most interventions for juvenile drug abusers are expensive. The adolescents' drug use must be closely monitored through frequent urine testing, since many have learned to lie about taking drugs. Some must be hospitalized for drug withdrawal because they are addicted, others enter drug-free residential or wilderness survival programs, and still others participate in family and group therapy. Which of these alternatives is the most successful and cost-effective? A group of over 1,000 adolescents between the ages of 11 and 18 were treated in various outpatient, residential, or short-term inpatient programs in several cities throughout the United States. The different treatments, which were all conducted by mental health professionals, produced encouraging results. In the year following treatment, the teenagers who received any type of treatment felt less disturbed and reported better school performance, and their heavy drinking, use of marijuana, and criminal activities dropped substantially. Although their use of other illicit drugs was also significantly decreased, they did not totally abstain from drugs and so may be in danger of further drug abuse in the future (Hser et al., 2001). Most treatments were brief, but teens who remained in treatment longer had the best outcomes.

Since many different treatments seem to have an overall positive effect on adolescents, it is natural to ask which treatment modality is best for which teens. Some interventions are based on educational principles, and others are inspired by the personal experiences of ex-addicts, while still others draw on psychological theory and research. The various types of treatments for drug abuse include:

- *Short hospital inpatient programs* lasting 4 to 6 weeks and offering comprehensive counseling, group therapy, medication, family therapy, school programs, and recreation. These very expensive programs include both medical and psychological treatment, and most are private rather than public.
- *Outpatient programs* led by mental health professionals, focusing on various types of individual counseling, family therapy, or both. These are scheduled for one or two sessions per week and may last as long as 6 months.
- *Therapeutic community residential programs*, which are highly regimented and lengthy with high dropout rates. These programs are largely staffed by former substance abusers and have very strict rules governing most aspects of residents' lives. Individuals who do not abide by the rules (such as many conduct-disordered teens) are excluded.
- *Life skills-training programs* such as Outward Bound take youths camping in primitive wilderness settings for an intensive 3- or 4-week group experience usually consisting of a survival trek. The theory is that when removed from their familiar, unhealthy surroundings and fellow drug abusers, teenagers learn survival skills through dependence on themselves and fellow campers. Their newfound maturity is presumed to allow them to return to their homes better able to resist bad companions and drugs. These outdoor programs are privately operated, very expensive, and largely unregulated. Their value as drug abuse treatments remains to be demonstrated.

Research may have identified a preferred treatment for teen drug abuse. *Outpatient family-based therapy* is one of the best established and most effective interventions for adolescent drug abusers (Ozechowski & Liddle, 2000). Treatment evaluation research shows that outpatient family-based therapy is effective in curbing the behavior problems that accom-

Back to the Beginning

Inadequate Drug Control Programs

The students in my class on child and adolescent psychopathology have never known a time when kids did not casually use illicit drugs of many different types. They believe that for most youngsters in most regions of the country taking drugs is the norm and that it is rare to find abstinent communities with large numbers of abstinent teenagers. At the same time, some of my students liked the educational abstinence training programs used in high school, such as DARE, and believe they may be effective—with teens other than themselves. Although schools officially discourage illicit drug and substance use, my students point out that schools are the major drug marketplace for young users. Similarly, parents who use drugs and/or alcohol sternly prohibit their youngsters from following their example. My students criticize such inconsistency and see it as leading to more drug use. As one student said, "The double standard is all too apparent to the child." Another student commented, "Scare tactics in schools have proved ineffective."

In general, the undergraduates in my classes are unimpressed by current prevention programs. They say after-school programs are helpful in giving teens something to do, but this is not enough. My students would like to see a genuine and unified prevention effort among federal and local government, communications and entertainment media, churches and agencies, schools and families. The psychology students I teach believe that our society is obligated to reduce the temptation to use psychoactive substances, greatly limit their availability, and treat abuse and addiction promptly and effectively for all young people who need it, regardless of family wealth and circumstances.

---

pany adolescent drug abuse as well as in reducing the abuse (American Academy of Child and Adolescent Psychiatry, 1997; Spoth, Redmond, & Shin, 2001). Family therapies of various types appear to be effective in reducing adolescents' drug abuse, most for at least a year after treatment ends (Ozechowski & Liddle, 2000). This is the best outcome achieved by any psychotherapy intervention with drug abusers to date.

Types of family therapies include *family systems therapy*, which focuses on parent, sibling, and extended family interactions that relate to the adolescent's drug abuse. Family functioning is seen as integral to the development and maintenance of the adolescent's problem behavior, and the family, rather than the child alone, is the focus of treatment. Family members are taught to recognize disruptive, counterproductive interaction patterns and to replace them with positive reactions. Many family therapy models also integrate principles and techniques of behavioral therapy, such as completing behavioral homework assignments, re-

hearsing desirable behaviors, and charting progress, with praise and privileges for meeting the goals. In behavioral therapy, a parent typically attends treatment sessions to help the teenager meet the goals and to reinforce desirable behavior, such as learning to shun tempting situations and spend more time in drug-free activities. Azrin's behavioral therapy is effective in helping teens quit using drugs, remain drug-free following treatment, and improve at school and home (Azrin et al., 1996). The whole social system, including the school, peers, neighborhood, community, and culture, may also be considered in the therapy (Liddle, 1995). In *multidimensional family therapy*, the teen's behavior is changed in multiple ways in different settings. Individual and family sessions are held in a clinic, home, or school, with family members at the family court, or in other relevant community locations. The teenager is helped to develop decision-making, negotiating, and social problem-solving skills. At the same time, sessions with parents and other key family members help them become aware of the impact their parenting and interacting style has on the child. This approach also has resulted in decreased drug use and improved family interactions (Diamond & Liddle, 1996). *Multisystemic therapy* is a related approach in which young drug abusers and their parents are treated intensively in their homes, schools, and neighborhoods. This approach also significantly reduced drug use at the follow-up evaluation 6 months after treatment (Henggeler, Pickrel, Brondino, & Crouch, 1996).

Treatments like the approaches described here tend to be more successful when teens' use of substances is limited rather than extensive, meaning that the earliest possible treatment works best. The treatment effects are also improved when parents and peers provide support for abstinence (Williams, Chang, & Addiction Centre Adolescent Research Group, 2000). Unfortunately, these benign conditions are not often found in the troubled lives of adolescents who require formal treatment for drug abuse. New and more effective programs are badly needed for the young people whose families and friends can provide no help in overcoming their serious drug problems.

SUMMARY

Drug use among young Americans continues unabated, although the popularity of particular substances changes from time to time and new drugs emerge. Youngsters use illicit drugs for various reasons: They try to appear worldly and sophisticated, desperately want to be accepted by the drug-using ingroup, and identify with the many drug users among media stars and famous athletes or, closer to home, among their own parents, older siblings, and friends. Living in neighborhoods ravaged by poverty and attending schools where drug use is rampant encourage children's experimentation with forbidden substances and their later heavy use of drugs, tobacco, and alcohol. In addition, having negligent, rejecting, and harsh parents alienates children and drives them into the drug culture. Adolescents who rely heavily on illicit drugs and substances risk truancy, school failure, dropout, conduct disorders and delinquency.

Some, but not all, illicit drugs produce dependency, in which the user typically must take increasing amounts of the drug to produce the same effect and experiences an unpleasant or physically dangerous withdrawal syndrome. Use of some common substances such as tobacco and alcohol can lead to dependency, as can heavy use of marijuana. The addictive stimulants are especially appealing to young people, and they are readily available as potent drugs in the various forms of cocaine and illegally diverted prescription drugs such as Ritalin and OxyContin. Club drugs such as Ecstasy have become a part of rave parties, in combination with alcohol and other drugs, and can produce dangerous dehydration and overheating during prolonged dancing. Opiates, particularly heroin, continue to be used by some young adults in combination with cocaine, but high school students know about the bad effects and most confine their drug use to marijuana and milder forms of stimulants.

Drug abuse prevention programs are often simplistic and based on common beliefs rather than research. The Just Say No and DARE programs featuring police officers giving warnings about drug use are popular with the public but ineffective as preventive measures. The multiple roots of youthful substance use are better addressed in more multifaceted prevention programs. Effective programs include several of the following features: Family interventions with preteens (an especially effective tactic), after-school programs to keep youth busy and supervised during high-risk times, skill-building interventions that teach effective methods of resisting peer pressure, coping with stress, and building social skills.

Treatment programs for juvenile drug abusers include wilderness survival outings, therapeutic community residential treatments, brief hospitalization, and therapy, especially family therapy, for youngsters living at home. Many drug abuse treatments for young people are of questionable effectiveness, and some are intuitively appealing but expensive and ineffective. Family therapy provides less costly, more powerful treatment that is supported by evaluative research and recommended by professional societies. Family therapy may be effective because it draws the family together and counteracts many of the causes of illicit substance use in children, such as poor family communication, parental harshness and rejection, and parental modeling of illicit substance use.

INFOTRAC COLLEGE EDITION

For more information, explore this resource at http://www.infotrac-college.com/Wadsworth. Enter the following search terms:

substance abuse
drug abuse prevention
drug abuse treatment
smoking
alcoholism in adolescents
drug addiction
drug dependence

IN FOCUS ANSWERS

IN FOCUS 1 ▶ Distinguish among substance use, substance abuse, and substance dependence.

- Substance use is a single or casual drug experience, neither serious or repeated.
- Substance abuse is heavy or frequent substance use with dangerous or impairing effects.
- Substance dependence is repeated use often resulting in tolerance, withdrawal, and compulsive drug taking.

IN FOCUS 2 ▶ Describe how friends, celebrities, and family members can lead youngsters to use drugs.

- Deviant peers model and advocate drug use.
- Celebrities make drug use appear glamorous.
- Family members may use drugs themselves; parents may fail to supervise their children, reject them, or punish them harshly.
- Family stress can increase risks for children with negative temperaments.

IN FOCUS 3 ▶ Identify the possible effects on the fetus if a pregnant woman drinks, smokes, or takes some form of cocaine.

- Drinking can produce fetal alcohol syndrome.
- Smoking is associated with low birth weight and other physical problems.
- Cocaine use is associated with low birth weight, decreased head size, irritability, and addiction.

IN FOCUS 4 ▶ Describe the illicit use of Ritalin and Oxy-Contin and the direct and indirect effects of these prescription drugs on children.

- Ritalin, a stimulant, is used by children to get high and is dangerous in high doses.
- OxyContin is dangerous because it is an opioid that can be addictive and lethal in high doses and in combination with other illicit drugs.

IN FOCUS 5 ▶ Identify the types of programs that have proven to be least and most successful in preventing drug abuse.

- Least successful are simple educational programs using police officers to warn students about the perils of drug abuse.
- Most successful have been family skills-training interventions.

IN FOCUS 6 ▶ Discuss why family therapy is particularly effective in treating drug abuse and dependence.

- The family therapy approach recognizes that the problem isn't the child's alone but arises from dysfunctional family interactions.
- The family therapy approach allows family members to help in implementing the treatment.
- Family members learn new, healthier ways to interact so that stress is reduced and the child is less motivated to use drugs.

Abuse, Neglect, and Children's Rights

In the Beginning

Abuse and Neglect—All Too Common

Tony was only 5, but he knew enough to be afraid when his parents screamed at each other even longer and louder than usual one night. They had been sitting in front of the TV, drinking and doing drugs for hours. They were running out of everything, but neither one wanted to go out for more. And neither remembered to feed the kids. Their quarreling continued; next would come the sickening thud of someone getting hit. Tony pulled the covers over his head and tried not to whimper, because that would make them notice him. He still had bruises from the last beating. It was always dangerous for a child to be noticed in this house.

Newspapers and TV news programs regularly present stories like Tony's—of shocking cruelty to children. Other reports of severe neglect and abuse of children include the following:

- A preschool boy was found very emaciated and much too small for his age. His father explained that he fed the boy only lettuce in an attempt to keep him spiritually and physically pure. The mother shared her husband's bizarre beliefs, and so did not feed her son either. The boy was taken into custody and soon thrived with proper feeding and medical care. How far can parents go in the name of religious beliefs?

- An air-conditioning repairman was babysitting his 2-year-old son and decided to give him a bath. He put poisonous Freon solution in the boy's bath water in order to make bubbles. The little boy died, and the father was charged with killing him. Why did he do it?

- A mother left her 6-month-old baby in the care of her boyfriend when she went to work. She returned to find the baby severely injured and barely clinging to life. The child later died of multiple injuries, including skull fractures and brain injuries consistent with severe shaking and beating. The boyfriend claimed the baby had fallen down the stairs, but his story was not believed and he was convicted of killing the baby. What was the mother's responsibility?

- When neighbors called the police to report suspicious activities in a certain apartment, the officers found a prostitution business. Marcie's stepfather was forcing her to act as a prostitute at the age of 14. Her mom claimed she didn't know anything about it, and Marcie, shamed and afraid, had no one to turn to for help. How could this tragedy be avoided?

INTRODUCTION

It is hard to imagine how anyone could hurt defenseless children in such ways, and it is important to answer the question "Why?" in order to prevent this type of harm and exploitation. Although some topics discussed in this chapter are very upsetting, there is no avoiding them, especially by the child victims. As you read this chapter, try to maintain some emotional distance from the material, just as a physician or child protective services professional must do when dealing with actual cases of child maltreatment. Unfortunately, we must inquire about the worst circumstances children endure in order to stem the tide of child maltreatment. Furthering this book's theme that research protects children, this chapter presents current research-based knowledge about neglect and physical and sexual abuse of children. The stress here is on *research-based*, since there is a desperate need for solid facts on which to base prevention and child protection efforts.

Young children's injuries and deaths from trauma were long attributed to accidents or the causes were listed as unexplained until John Caffey (1946), a radiologist, published a medical paper describing the association between chronic subdural hematoma (bleeding inside the head) from head injuries and multiple fractures of infants' arms and legs. The clear implication was that someone was intentionally injuring these babies. Today, physicians are alert to signs of physical abuse and have developed refined techniques to detect the difference between accidental and intentional injuries.

Long overlooked, the maltreatment of children has become a major national concern, a serious problem that affects the physical and mental development of thousands of children each year. In this chapter, we review how maltreatment affects children, what psychological treatments are available, and what might be done to reduce cruelty to children. We also examine children's moral and legal rights to humane treatment and why children's rights are sometimes restricted. The impact of reduced public spending on children's welfare is also considered, as is the increased burden on charitable and religious organizations to provide needed child welfare and protective services formerly administered by the government. Government funding and charitable spending to improve children's education and mental and physical health constitute a humane policy and an enlightened investment in the future.

Child maltreatment is unlikely to diminish spontaneously if nothing is done. Rates of child abuse and neglect are high, despite the best efforts of the schools, health care providers, social services agencies, and religious institutions. Children cannot help themselves, but must depend on adults to do it. Mandatory reporting laws in the United States and other countries require health professionals, teachers, and child care workers to report suspected cases of child abuse. Although laws vary from state to state, the main aim is to protect children. People who suspect that a child is being abused are legally protected against retaliation, so they can safely inform child protection authorities (see Table 6-1 for reporting tips).

Most adults recognize young children's vulnerability and do all they can to protect children from harm, but some people are neglectful or abusive—either out of ignorance or because they were mistreated and have personality problems. The ignorant abusers simply do not understand young children's limitations.

Table 6-1 Tips about Reporting Suspected Child Abuse

1. *Who can report child neglect or abuse?* You can. When you suspect or know that a child is being abused and is in danger, you are morally obligated to take action. You are legally obligated to inform authorities about suspected child abuse if you are a teacher or health care provider. Most states also require social workers, day care staff, police, and judges to report child abuse, and some states require *everyone* to report.

2. *To report, use a 24-hour child abuse and neglect helpline.* Helpline numbers are usually listed in the front section of the telephone book. These calls are confidential. You can also report suspected abuse to the police or call 911 if someone is being physically attacked.

3. *Can I get into trouble for making a child abuse report that is dismissed?* Not unless you are doing it out of personal malice against the alleged perpetrator. Many states protect the informant even then. All states provide legal immunity for mandatory reporters (teachers, health care providers, and others).

SOURCE: Hempelman (2000).

Family Focus

Alcohol and Abuse

For 6-year-old Shawna, perhaps even more terrifying than being hit herself was watching her father beat her mother during his violent, alcoholic rages. Alex, her father, was a frequently unemployed construction worker who spent his days drinking. Irascible, paranoid, and assaultive when drunk, Alex took his rage and frustration out on his wife, Toni, their two little boys, and Shawna. Following a bout of heavy drinking, Alex would lash out at his wife for imaginary offenses, punch her in the face and stomach with his fist, drag her by the hair, and throw her out of the house, locking the door behind her. When she tried to take the children and escape, Alex would follow them, insist on their return, and loudly threaten to "kill the bitch." He recently hit Shawna, cutting her lip, which required stitches, and blackening her eye when she failed to get him more beer because the refrigerator was empty.

Once a bright, inquisitive child, Shawna has become extremely shy and insecure, avoiding eye contact with people, mumbling rather than speaking clearly, and staying to herself. She has no friends, suffers from terrifying nightmares, and shows little interest in or affection for family members. Her teacher says that Shawna doesn't seem to pay attention or concentrate on her schoolwork, but spends much of her time sitting quietly by herself and staring vacantly out the window. Shawna's family is being investigated by the state child protective services agency for possible child abuse, but there are so many cases to investigate and so few staff available that much time may pass before the family can be helped. The mother has been counseled about the availability of a community shelter for abused women and children, but she insists that Alex is a good husband and father except for his drinking. Once again, Alex has vowed that he loves Toni and promises to reform.

The prognosis for this family, including Shawna, depends on the control of the father's alcoholism and rage and on the family's and society's ability to protect the mother and children from physical and psychological harm. Too often, a parent's alcoholism or drug abuse go untreated and the spouse is too helpless to leave the relationship, so the abuse and its evil effects on the family continue for many years. Adequate prevention programs are needed, ones that feature parenting skills, skills for independent living for single parents, anger management training, effective alcohol and drug abuse treatments, and better law enforcement to protect battered spouses and children.

They were never taught how to care for children, and they do not realize that children are less mentally and physically capable than adults. These inadequate adults don't know that children cannot provide their own food and shelter and are incapable of caring for themselves. Other adults are so angry and self-centered that they become enraged when young children inconvenience them in any way. They feel outraged that little children are unable to understand and follow their complex commands, cry loudly for hours, or wet and soil themselves. The boyfriend who apparently shook and beat the baby is a clear example: Not only was he ignorant of the infant's needs and how to meet them, but he was probably also resentful that he had to stay and take care of the baby rather than doing something more enjoyable. The stepfather who sexually exploited his stepdaughter saw her as a sexually mature woman, although she was only 14 and still emotionally and legally a child. He was ignorant of her psychological development status, may have had an antisocial personality, and did not care what he did to her. In many instances, abuse stems from both ignorance of development and some diagnosable mental disorder or criminal history.

In this chapter, we see how maltreatment may injure a child's emotional stability, make the child mistrustful of adults, lower school performance, distort sexual functioning, and sometimes impair later adjustment and parenting performance. Reviews of the best available social science research studies provide clues for understanding why adults attack children and how their cruelty hurts children and affects their development. This book's theme that research protects children is reflected in the importance of the task of protecting children from maltreatment.

TYPES OF MALTREATMENT

IN FOCUS 1 ▶ Describe the various types of child abuse.

Children can be harmed through lack of appropriate care, attacks of some type, or both forms of maltreatment. Child neglect occurs when caretakers persistently fail to feed, clothe, or clean children or to provide normal health care. The Family Focus box on page 125 describes a tragic case of combined child abuse and neglect, like those that frequently appear in the files of child protection agencies. **Physical abuse** occurs when caretakers attack and injure a child, sometimes inflicting serious, even fatal, wounds. Physical abuse is often accompanied by **emotional abuse** (or psychological abuse), in which the perpetrator endangers the child's psychological welfare by attacking the child's self-esteem, self-confidence, and well-being. Although emotional abuse has not been precisely defined, it is usually understood to consist of verbal assault, confinement, and exploitation or punitiveness toward the child (Hamerman & Ludwig, 2000). The stepfather's sexual exploitation of young Marcie involved emotional abuse as well as criminal behavior. Emotional or psychological abuse necessarily occurs in cases of physical abuse but can also occur independently. Because it is not precisely defined and is seldom studied, emotional abuse is probably greatly underreported (Hamerman & Ludwig, 2000).

PREVALENCE OF MISTREATMENT

The amount of damage to children is heartbreaking. Homicide is one of the five leading causes of child mortality in the United States, and child abuse and neglect cause many additional fatalities. A national study found that nearly 1 million U.S. children (903,000) were harmed in a single year, which amounts to 12.9 children per 1,000 [U.S. Department of Health and Human Services (DHHS), 2000]. Neglect was the most frequent form of mistreatment, accounting for more than half of the child victims (53.5%). In comparison, emotional abuse and medical neglect (failure to provide necessary medical care) are less prevalent, possibly because they are more difficult to detect and define than obvious neglect and physical damage (see Table 6-2).

Each year in the United States, nearly 5 children per 1,000 (22.7% of maltreated children) are reported to be physically abused and more than 2 per 1,000 are sexually abused (DHHS, 2000). Many of the children suffered from more than one type of maltreatment (Ryan, Kilmer, Cauce, Watanabe, & Hoyt, 2000). Infants and toddlers have the highest maltreatment rate, 14.8 children per 1,000, which is considerably more than the overall rate of 12.9 per 1,000 for children of all ages. The most frequent types of abuse differ somewhat for boys and girls. Many more boys suffer physical abuse and become homicide victims, and many

---

Table 6-2 Definitions of Neglect and Abuse

Physical neglect: Refusal of or delay in seeking health care for a child, abandonment of a child, expulsion of a child from the home, or not allowing a runaway child to return home. Inadequate supervision. (Extreme poverty is not an acceptable excuse for failure to care for a child.)

Educational neglect: Chronic failure to obey state laws regarding compulsory school attendance; permitting a child's chronic truancy, failure to enroll a child of mandatory school age in school, or inattention to a child's special education needs.

Emotional neglect: Refusal of or failure to provide needed psychological or emotional care; can include spouse abuse in the child's presence, exposing the child to violence, or permitting the child to use drugs or alcohol. (Usually occurs together with physical or educational neglect.)

Physical abuse: Cruel treatment that goes beyond customary or justifiable corporal punishment and threatens the physical health and may threaten the mental health of a child. Includes a serious attack on a child with or without a weapon; the attack can cause major injuries or death.

Child sexual abuse: Any type of age-inappropriate sexual exploitation of a child. Sexual acts may include exhibitionism, exposing a child to pornography or using a child to produce pornography, genital fondling, or sexual relations with a child.

---

more girls than boys are sexually abused, particularly among low-income white families. It is shocking to realize that almost 1 child in 100 is so badly treated as to meet the criteria for physical neglect, and nearly 1 child in 200 is physically abused. A hopeful note is that the overall rate of maltreatment is decreasing slightly, although it remains unacceptably high.

DEFINING PHYSICAL ABUSE

People sometimes disagree about exactly which actions should be considered abusive to children. College students express strong and sometimes diametrically opposed opinions about physical punishment: Some totally disapprove of physically punishing children, including spanking, and consider that to be physical abuse, while others equally vigorously defend spanking as the best way to teach children proper discipline. Usually some male students offer personal testimonies that strict discipline, including spanking, kept them away from drugs and bad company when they were kids and they see no other way this could have been accomplished. Others, most often female students, are horrified by these stories and say that using physical discipline on children just teaches them that you are a bully on a power trip, willing to overpower a child to get your own way.

This type of principled disagreement makes it difficult to classify many disciplinary practices as clearly appropriate or abusive. In any case, many children are spanked. In one large survey, 94% of parents said they occasionally use mild physical forms of punishment with their 3- and 4-year-olds (Straus & Stewart, 1999). Furthermore, although some psychologists have found that physical punishment increases children's misbehavior, others have reported beneficial results of mild spanking when used as a backup after nonphysical methods have failed (Larzelere, 2000). (Mild spanking consists of no more than two open-handed slaps on the young child's buttocks.)

Research shows that mild physical punishment can be effective when used with restraint and according to a plan or family rule. Physical punishment should *not* be used under the following circumstances:

- To punish children of inappropriate ages, namely, those younger than 2, who cannot understand why they are being punished, or those older than 6, for

whom methods such as reasoning and loss of privileges are preferred
- To punish a child impulsively, when parents are angry, feel they are "losing it," or want to show the child "who is boss"
- To punish a child overly severely, as when beating the child produces bleeding, bruising, or other physical damage, an object is used to increase the pain, or the child is beaten frequently for minor infractions

Exactly where is the line between acceptable corporal discipline and physical abuse? Nearly all parents admit to slapping or spanking their children at some time, but they also abhor child abuse, so clear distinctions between physical abuse and legitimate physical punishment are needed. In extreme instances, it is easy to decide. Physical abuse clearly goes beyond minor physical reprimands, such as slapping, pushing, or spanking a child, and consists of seriously assaulting the child and causing physical injury. Attacks that are illegal against adults are also illegal against children. Physical abuse of children has included attacks with a weapon such as a knife or firearm, beatings with an electrical cord or belt buckle, knocking the child to the ground and repeatedly kicking him, and choking, seriously biting, scalding, or otherwise seriously injuring the child. Such attacks are abusive and illegal, regardless of whether the adult claims to have acted out of concern for the child's spiritual, social, or educational welfare. Abuse has always been with us, but children have not always been protected by laws, as revealed in Mary Ellen's Story.

THE ROOTS OF CHILD ABUSE

There are various sources of child abuse; some of them lie in traditional social and cultural practices, others in unhealthy family relationships, and yet others in the ignorance, cruelty, or mental disturbance of the perpetrator.

Cultural Differences Regarding Corporal Punishment

Among the social factors influencing abuse rates are cultural practices and religious beliefs that can either promote or inhibit the use of physical force with

First We Protected the Animals, Then the Children

In 1875, it was safer to be an animal than a little girl. The Society to Prevent Cruelty to Animals (SPCA) had already been organized by citizens who were concerned about public acts of cruelty toward animals, such as vicious beatings of dying horses who could no longer pull heavily loaded carts. But there was no such society to protect children from battering and abuse. In that year, the case of a 9-year-old girl named Mary Ellen came to light. Mary Ellen was legally the indentured servant to Francis and Mary Connolly and possibly the daughter of Mary's ex-husband. She was whipped every day, stabbed with scissors, and tied to a bed. She was painfully thin and had visible scissor wounds on her legs and cheek. A church worker, Etta Wheeler, learned about her plight from neighbors and reported the situation to the police. She discovered there was no law against cruelty to children and no legal means to help rescue the girl, although there were laws preventing people from doing the same things to animals. The SPCA successfully brought court action to have Mary Ellen removed from the abusive home, arguing that the child was a member of the animal kingdom and animals had the protection of the law. Mrs. Connolly served a year in prison, and Mary Ellen went to a new home. Later, the New York Society for the Prevention of Cruelty to Children was formed, and laws were passed forbidding child maltreatment.

And despite vigorous attempts to stop child abuse, it still goes on over 100 years later. In January 2001, a relative discovered that two little boys, Clarence, aged 7, and Ernest, aged 8, had sustained terrible stabbing and slashing wounds to their faces, and she took them to a hospital immediately. Their mother had a history of prostitution, drug addiction, and domestic violence with various partners, and she had been sent to prison for stabbing their father 18 times. In the indictment against her, the mother was accused of assaulting the boys with a knife, a metal pipe, and the sharp heel of a high-heeled shoe. This terrible case illustrates how much more must be done to protect children.

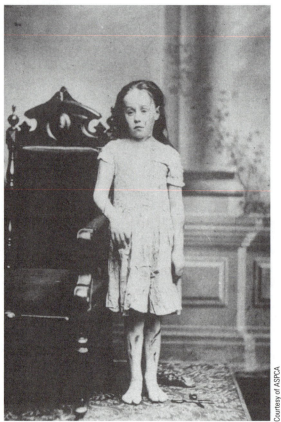

Mary Ellen, at the time of her rescue by the SPCA.

Courtesy of ASPCA

SOURCES: *New York Times*, April 10, 1874; Bernstein (2001, February 2).

children. Some scholars argue that corporal punishment of children should be prohibited as a means to prevent physical abuse (Straus, 2000). Indeed, England is in conflict with its trading partners in the European Union over a British legislative act that permits the physical punishment of children. This legislation violates the U.N. Convention on the Rights of the Child. The British Government has been required by the European Court to amend the law permitting parents to use physical punishment (Lansdown, 2000). The nations of the European Union view physical punishment as ethically and morally unacceptable. In contrast, in the United States, certain extremely conservative religious groups and some cultural groups, such as African Americans, are outspoken supporters of corporal punishment of children. Although there are wide individual differences of opinion among them, African Americans use spanking more frequently and with more positive effects than do other groups (Deater-Deckard & Dodge, 1997; Gunnoe & Mariner, 1997). Many African Americans see spanking as a desirable practice when used by responsible, concerned parents to teach their children proper behavior. In contrast, more European Americans see spanking negatively, as signifying parental rejection of the child (Deater-Deckard, Dodge, Bates, & Pettit, 1996). Their cultural traditions may make African-American parents and children more likely to accept spanking as a reasonable and appropriate form of discipline. When spanking is customary, children may resent it less and learn more from it than when it is culturally unacceptable. How spanking is viewed within a culture may be as important in its effects on children as the spanking itself.

Family Factors Associated with Maltreatment

IN FOCUS 2 ▶ Summarize the family factors that are associated with child maltreatment.

Many people are deeply shocked to learn of the full extent of neglect and violence toward children by their own parents. In the United States, one or both parents account for 87.1% of the officially reported cases of maltreatment of children (DHHS, 2000). We wonder how parents can so pitilessly neglect or attack their own children. Contrary to popular belief, abuse

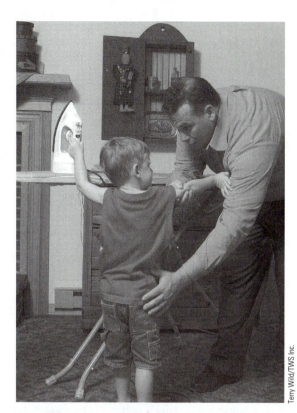

Will a swat on the backside teach a child to avoid a hot iron? Children punished by spanking may comply immediately but not learn a long-term lesson.

does not usually stem from parental mental illness, and only rarely do abusing parents have diagnosable mental disorders (Oliver, 1993). However, many abusers do have difficult lives and face significant problems, such as domestic violence, a childhood history of abuse, desertion, burdensome child care responsibilities, unemployment, and poverty. None of these risk factors necessarily produces child abuse by itself, but each one raises the likelihood of abuse and other psychological and criminal problems.

Sometimes abuse stems from an unwilling caretaker's resentment about having to bear the burden of tending a child. Caring for young children is a 24-hour-a-day job with no pay, no vacations, and little time for relaxation or recreation. A prized and welcome opportunity for some, parenting can be demanding, exhausting, expensive, and isolating for inexperienced or self-centered caretakers. Child abusers often resent children's demands on them and complain of unbearable stress from being a parent. In one Scottish study of nearly 1,500 cases of abuse and neglect, the strongest predictor of child physical abuse was unemployment of the man of the house (Gillham et al., 1998). Abuse can arise from a man's anger and frustration over being fired, financial strain due to unemployment, resentment at having to act the feminine role of babysitter while the mother is at work, lack of child management skills, and feelings being tied to the house by tedious child care duties. Add to this the temptation for a jobless father to pass the time drinking and using illicit drugs and it is easy to see why unemployed men can become dangerous. Unemployed mothers can suffer from similar frustrations, with similar resulting potential for abuse.

Parents' limited education, resources, and opportunities may also be associated with child maltreatment. Lower-income, less well-educated people are more likely to be identified as child abusers than are middle-class parents, but it is unclear whether they actually are more abusive or are under closer surveillance by welfare case workers, police officers, and public health home visitors. Wealthier parents who abuse their children are less likely to be reported to authorities, and they may be better able to deny their abusive acts and avoid detection. Certainly, most people are responsible parents, regardless of their wealth or educational background and whether or not they are currently employed.

A family's social isolation may breed abuse. Abusing families frequently have few social contacts and lack friends. In part, they may avoid being seen by others because their abusive practices are something they want to hide, but another reason is their lack of social skills. Moreover, stressful transitions such as the parents' separation or divorce, job loss, financial problems, or a move to a new neighborhood can lead to loss of friends and decreased contacts with family and former neighbors. Added to the stress of a transition like a move is the loss of emotional support, advice, and help from friends and relatives. Often there is no one in the new neighborhood to act as a moderating factor, the voice of reason and restraint, on the stressed parent's discipline of the child. When the parents and children begin to irritate each other, the parent may "lose it" and become violent. Children are best protected from deviant peers and abusive parents in neighborhoods that have a high level of collective socialization, which is the residents' tendency to monitor and supervise all the children in the area and not only their own kids (Brody et al., 2001).

Curiously enough, a family's characteristic interaction style can predispose members to physical conflicts and abuse. Certain families have abnormally high levels of both activity and irritability—arguing, fighting, and physical roughness—and they engage in more child abuse than do calmer, more controlled families. Family activity level differences can stem from genetics, environmental factors, or both. Impatience, hyperactivity, and a tendency to strike out at others make a dangerous combination. Although they also share good moments, such battling parents are unusually hostile and irritable toward each other and toward their children. Parents' coercive and explosive behavior usually extends to their treatment of their children; however, abusive parents tend to treat certain victimized children the worst (Garfinkel, McLanahan, Meyer, & Selzer, 1998; Lamb, 1997).

Does having been abused as a child lead people to become abusive with their own children? Many people are convinced this is true and unavoidable. Some over-zealous case workers have refused to place children with foster or adoptive parents who were abused as children, believing they would be unfit parents. This belief is very probably wrong and is undoubtedly exaggerated. It is much more accurate to say that the experience of being abused as a child is just one of many factors that might heighten the risk of using abusive physical punishment. Research indicates that children whose mothers experienced physical abuse as children and are exposed to domestic violence in their homes are at greater risk of being abused (Bowen, 2000; Fleming, Mullen, & Bammer, 1997), which would seem to point to the experience of being abused as causing mothers to become abusers themselves. The problem is that we cannot separate the adverse effects of poverty, extreme stress, poor parenting skills, and social isolation from the effects of having been abused as a child. All are closely linked, and each factor alone *weakly* predicts child abuse (Peterson & Brown, 1994), but not strongly enough to allow detection of potential abusers. The experience of childhood abuse does not invariably produce abuse of others (Golden, 2000), just as having an abuse-free childhood does not always prevent parents from abusing their children.

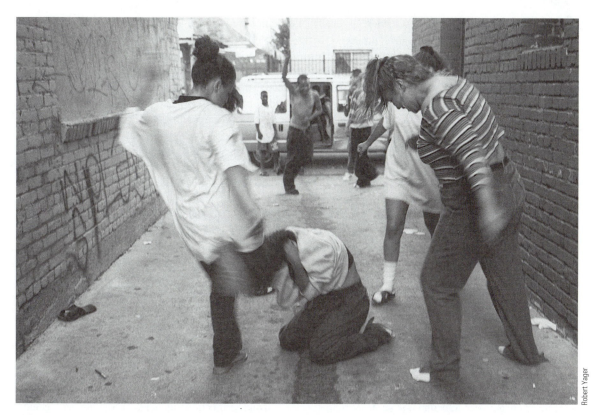

Children are more often victims of violence than are adults, and often at the hands of other children. Through being victimized, many learn to attack others and have never become adequately socialized.

Most people believe that parents are the ones who most often physically attack children, but in fact siblings and other children are many times more likely to physically attack children than are their parents (Finkelhor & Dziuba-Leatherman, 1994). Ironically, attacks by siblings are the most prevalent type of physical assault on young children. There are several reasons why some youngsters physically abuse their sisters and brothers: First, children in a family spend a great deal of time with each other and are often unsupervised by adults. Because many children have not yet learned to share and cooperate, their disputes often end in physical force. Second, the older children within a family may be forced to serve as unwilling babysitters for long periods of time while their parents are out of the house at work or elsewhere, and they can become bullies who enjoy dominating their younger, weaker siblings. An older child or teenager

who is forced to care for younger siblings instead of being out with friends may turn on the siblings, both psychologically and physically.

Characteristics of Victimized Children

Children are not all equally vulnerable to physical abuse. High-risk children may have physical or behavioral characteristics that annoy caretakers and encourage victimization. Infants may have a difficult temperament, be socially unresponsive and difficult to soothe, and have a piercing, high-pitched cry. Other victimized children may have a chronic physical illness or disability or be physically unattractive. Sadly, the weak are especially endangered; children may also be a higher risk for abuse if they are developmentally delayed or below average in intelligence. Moreover, chronic, frequent misbehavior and hyperactivity by a child can lead parents to abusive behavior. Ironically, abusive parents are often inadequate, unsuccessful disciplinarians, whose ineptitude inadvertently creates the very type of defiant behavior by the child that irritates them the most (Larzelere, 2000). The mother who tries to control her misbehaving child by negative tactics is doomed to fail. Loudly screaming "no" and hitting the child without explaining how to behave appropriately and never acknowledging good behavior will create a confused, resentful, and defiant child. Punitive and rejecting parenting promotes antisocial child behavior; mothers who rely heavily on physical punishment thus tend to have defiant and impulsive children. This sets the stage for possible child abuse.

Although we know that certain types of children are at higher risk for abuse, we do not know whether the distinguishing child characteristics preceded and caused the abuse, were caused by the abuse, or stemmed from some other factor. Some children are at greater risk for abuse than are other children mainly because their physical appearance or behavior irritates, inconveniences, or displeases their parents. Even then, other factors must be at work to precipitate the abuse, such as a baby's prematurity, low birth weight, or chronic ear infections or an early mother-baby separation. However, these factors alone are not sufficient to produce abuse, and most difficult babies and unattractive children are loved and cared for tenderly by their parents. It is likely that several factors—including child characteristics, family factors, and social beliefs and customs—dynamically interact to result in child maltreatment. Because there are many different causes and effects of child abuse, it would be misguided to seek a single cause or outcome.

CHILD SEXUAL ABUSE

Only recently have Americans begun to realize the full extent of sexual abuse of children in this country. Each year, child sexual abuse victims constitute nearly 12% of all children who are maltreated. In 1998, 104,000 substantiated cases of child sexual abuse were identified by state child protection agencies (DHHS, 2000). (Substantiated cases are those that have some officially accepted confirmation of the validity of the complaint.) As might be expected, the es-

timated prevalence of child sexual abuse depends largely on how sexual abuse is defined and on whether all reported cases (termed indicated cases) or only the substantiated cases are included. Efforts to study, treat, and prevent child sexual abuse are impeded by the absence of a clear definition of child sexual abuse (Haugaard, 2000), and so reported rates vary greatly. Very high prevalence rates come from national surveys of random samples of adults who were asked whether they were sexually abused as children. Between 2.1 and 6.3 persons per 1,000 reported being sexually abused before they reached the age of 18. Moreover, national surveys of teenagers have yielded astounding lifetime prevalence rates of up to 118 rapes per 1,000 teens (Finkelhor & Dziuba-Leatherman, 1994). Most of these occurrences were never reported at the time, and some may be erroneous or exaggerated. Until the past several years, official estimates of sexual abuse prevalence increased, in part because of growing public vigilance and because of laws to protect people who reported possible cases. Recently, there has been a welcome leveling off or slight decrease in reported and confirmed sexual abuse cases (DHHS, 2000).

Child protection agencies, hospitals and clinics, and law enforcement agencies have always been aware of child sexual abuse, but few outside of these organizations had any idea of how many children are sexually exploited. Family members or neighbors who suspect that such abuse is taking place fail to report it, and child victims are afraid or unable to complain about their abusers. Because many sexually abused children are very young, they may not realize what is going on, or if they know it is wrong, they fear they will not be believed if they try to report it. To make matters worse, there is often a huge power discrepancy between the abuser and the child. It is not easy for a child to say no to any adult or to report what happened to anyone else, even to a parent. Since children are easily intimidated, much sexual abuse goes undetected and unpunished.

Defining Sexual Abuse

In general, **sexual abuse** consists of the age-inappropriate sexual exploitation of a child for the perpetrator's pleasure or benefit. The abuse can be direct, as in sexual contact of any type, or indirect, as in exhibitionism or exposure of a child to pornography. The legal system assumes that any form of sexual abuse is harmful to the child in some way. Certain types of sexual abuse are obvious, but others are more subtle and difficult to identify. For example, an adult's having sex with a child who is well below the legal age of consent clearly constitutes sexual abuse, but what about the teenager who is just a few weeks or months below the age of consent? Is fondling a clothed child equivalent to rape of a very young child, and will it have equally bad effects?

Different people hold strongly opposed views on the definition and effects of child sexual abuse. A national debate is raging about whether all types of sexual involvement with children constitute abuse and are equally destructive to the children. Some people hold a strong faith-based or morality-based conviction that all adult-child sexual interactions of any type are criminally depraved and permanently harmful to the children. Moderates share this repugnance of adults' sexual involvement with children, but see it as having a range of effects. Moderates are more likely to rely on research evidence and call for empirical investigations to assess the harm to the children of various types of experiences and to determine appropriate treatment. This chapter attempts to present the fairest view of the best possible research on a very sensitive subject. Much national debate and many crucial research studies are underway, so the information presented here must be considered provisional, as a work in progress.

There is much public concern about possible abuse at child care centers. Physical abuse is the most frequent type of problem and takes the form of overdiscipline, inadvertently supported when parents give their permission for their child to be physically punished if necessary (Schumacher & Carlson, 1999). Sexual abuse often occurs with physical abuse, and the combination of the two is particularly likely to cause psychological problems in the children.

Cases of child care workers, church workers, and private citizens being accused of bizarre and outrageous sexual attacks on children have received widespread publicity in the 1980s (e.g., the McMartin day care case in California and the Little Rascals day care case in North Carolina). These criminal cases have led to the conviction and imprisonment of some defendants, some successful appeals, and some acquittals. Successful countersuits by defendants have made accusers cautious and have discouraged charges based on the testimony of very young children. There is growing national skepticism about the more dramatic charges against child care workers, accusations of slaughtering giraffes and other exotic animals, conducting nude rituals in vast underground tunnel systems, and other highly emotionally charged accusations from preschool children.

While publicity about sexual abuse of children has increased public vigilance, there are some unintended bad effects as well. People whose jobs require them to associate with children in a close teaching, supervisory, or voluntary role are afraid of being falsely accused of child sexual abuse. Men in particular may avoid working with or caring for children out of fear of arousing suspicion about their motives. Activities such as bathing, toileting, and diapering infants and young children may be risky, and schools and child care centers have instituted restrictive rules about the procedures to be followed. Even fathers may be suspected and accused, sometimes mistakenly, as the Family Focus box describes. Clear and reasonable standards of care must be developed in order to protect vulnerable children from abuse and appropriately shield their caretakers and teachers from groundless and damaging accusations.

Sexual Abuse Victims and Perpetrators

Victims of sexual abuse tend to be young. According to adult victims' recollections, nearly two-thirds (64%) were abused when they were younger than 12 or 13 years of age (Holmes & Slap, 1998). New York state records showed that nearly 40% of the official sexual abuse cases involved children younger than 7 years (Doris, 1993). Perpetrators may target vulnerable younger children in order to protect themselves from detection and punishment. They may take advantage of their position as a relative, mother's boyfriend, babysitter, or other child care worker. Younger children lack the language, cognitive skills, and self-confidence to report the abuse, and if they do attempt to seek help, their complaints may not be understood or believed by adults. Younger children are also less likely

Family Focus

When Adult Daughters Falsely Accuse Their Fathers of Past Sexual Abuse

Imagine you are a 68-year-old grandfather of four and father of an adult son and daughter. Your life is stable; you have been married for over 30 years, and, although your marriage is not ideal, you are content. You have worked hard as sales manager in a men's clothing store and plan to retire in the next couple of years. Then you get a phone call from your daughter's psychotherapist asking you to come to a joint therapy session with your wife and daughter. The topic is your daughter's recovered memory of the many times you had sex with her beginning when she was 10. You say there must be some mistake, such things never happened, you would never think of doing such a thing, but your daughter insists that suddenly, through her psychotherapy, she remembered what you did to her and that is why she developed depression and an eating disorder. You pretty much left the child raising to your wife and never knew your daughter very well, but how could she say this? Why would she do it?

There is a huge, continuing controversy about what some people call recovered memories and critics call false memories of early sexual abuse. Harold Lief and Janet Fetkewicz (1999) interviewed seven falsely accused fathers, whose daughters initially accused them but later retracted their claims and said they became convinced that their memories of being abused by their fathers were false. Most of the women had recovered the memories of their alleged abuse in therapy sessions, usually following a direct suggestion by their therapist. Their complaints were dramatic and difficult to believe. Some claimed they witnessed satanic rituals, violence, and sexual abuse and were abused; others said they had watched cannibalism, sodomy, and pornography. Each woman later said these charges were not true.

The daughters' accusations of sexual abuse had serious consequences for their families. One father had a stroke, another had a heart attack soon after being accused and blamed it on the stress caused by the accusation. However, the most common reaction was continually wondering "Why me?" The fathers reported feeling numb, devastated, frustrated that no one would believe them, fearful, angry, and in some cases emotionally detached from their situation. The men came to doubt their own memories and wondered whether they had actually committed the abuse without being able to remember it. Or perhaps, they thought, their daughters were abused, but by some other person. Among the more functional reactions were seeking consultation with a therapist, joining local support groups, and seeking scientific information from the False Memory Syndrome Foundation (3401 Market Street, Suite 130, Philadelphia, PA 19104) or mental health professional societies (American Medical Association, 1994; American Psychiatric Association, 1993; American Psychological Association, 1994; Canadian Psychiatric Association, 1996).

Since such a small group of families was studied, these findings must be considered tentative. However, the results of false accusations of sexual abuse seem potentially very harmful to all involved. The daughters and their therapists became thoroughly convinced that the abuse actually happened, and even some of the innocent fathers and their wives were unsure of what they might have done. Not surprisingly, the accused men's marriages suffered. Baffled wives were forced to choose between believing their husbands or their daughters. Surprisingly, few of the long-time couples divorced, and many said they grew closer as a result of their daughters' accusations. However, scars remained, and the men felt undermined in their roles in the family.

to understand what is happening to them and less able to provide a coherent description of the experience. They are particularly likely to give erroneous information if they are asked direct, focused questions about an encounter that occurred half a year or more ago

(Lamb, Sternberg, & Esplin, 2000). The limited mental ability and credibility of preschool informants present major social and legal issues about their own and others' protection and require special assessment procedures (discussed later).

The mother's competence to protect and instruct her children may be especially important in preventing their sexual and physical abuse. The majority of victims of sexual abuse are girls. According to national crime statistics, girls are eight times more likely to be raped than are boys (Finkelhor & Dziuba-Leatherman, 1994). Women report twice as many incidents of all types of childhood sexual abuse as do men (Ceci & Bruck, 1993). Girls who lack a mother's protection and guidance are more likely to fall prey to sexual abuse outside the home, especially if they were also previously physically abused and are socially isolated from friends and neighbors (Fleming et al., 1997). Sexual abuse victims of both sexes are more likely than most children to lack social support, have experienced the death of their mother, have a mentally ill mother, or have previously been physically abused (Fleming et al., 1997). The lack of a competent mother's protection endangers children of both sexes, but particularly girls.

Because many fewer boys than girls have been legally identified as sexually abused, less is known about these boys' characteristics and the circumstances of their abuse. However, a review of studies over a 12-year period (Holmes & Slap, 1998) revealed that victimized boys were often young (under 13 years of age), of lower socioeconomic status, non-white, and not living with their fathers. The father may act to prevent abuse for boys just as the mother does for girls. The perpetrators were mostly known to the boys, but unrelated to them. The sexually abused boys reported adjustment difficulties including psychological distress, substance abuse, and sexually related problems. There is reason to suspect that sexual abuse of boys is grossly underreported, particularly among more economically advantaged groups, because boys are expected to be able to protect themselves from being molested or raped and are reluctant to admit that they didn't. Consequently, the prevalence rates for boys may be much higher than the statistics indicate.

We now turn to the methods used by clinicians and the justice system to assess whether abuse has occurred. Accurate assessment is crucial to the detection of abuse and to appropriate treatment, as well as the prosecution of sexual offenders. Because this is an individually and socially important issue, it deserves special attention.

ASSESSMENT OF CHILD ABUSE

In many cases, child abuse leaves physical evidence. As mentioned previously, professionals and the public became aware of the extent of child maltreatment when physicians began to publish findings that many children who were believed to be accident victims were actually injured intentionally (Coury, 2000). Although there are still many cases in which health professionals are uncertain of the cause of a child's injuries, identification of the physical and psychological evidence of abuse has advanced. In one long-term study, almost 20% of children hospitalized with head injuries were identified by medical teams as probably physically abused, and in more than half of those cases, family members could not provide a convincing explanation for the child's injuries (Reece & Sege, 2000). Further, the 13% mortality rate in those cases was higher than for accidental head injuries and many other serious diseases such as meningitis. A similarly high mortality rate was reported in a larger national survey, with child abuse producing 10% of child hospitalizations for trauma (DiScala, Sege, Li, & Reece, 2000). Physical abuse can and does kill many young children each year.

How to accurately assess sexual abuse of children is a hotly debated issue in the field of child mental health and jurisprudence. With society's sudden realization that sexual abuse of children is a serious community problem came insistent demands for immediate steps to protect children, stop the abuse, and punish perpetrators harshly. All of these measures require accurate assessment of sexual abuse, which presents a difficult diagnostic problem for several reasons:

- Sexual abuse is concealed and often occurs within the home or some other private setting.
- Usually only the abuser and the child know about it with certainty.
- There is a power disparity between perpetrators and victims. Abusers are usually older than their victims and more physically and socially powerful. They may be parents or other blood relatives (in which case, sexual abuse constitutes incest), stepparents or stepsiblings, caretakers, youth workers, babysitters, or friends or acquaintances of the family. Less frequently, they are the dangerous strangers that parents so often warn their children about.

Candid Camera on Suspected Child Abusers

Much child abuse is difficult to detect and prevent because the victims are very young, often just babies, and there is no way to observe the behavior of the suspected abusers in their own homes. When they know they are under surveillance, abusive parents display only their best behavior, appearing to be affectionate and loving to their children. But in private, they can behave in shockingly abusive ways.

A British team of researchers and pediatric care staff members took a dramatic action to detect abusive parents. With the permission of British child welfare authorities, they installed hidden video cameras in the hospital rooms of children who had injuries consistent with physical abuse. During a period of nearly 10 years, cameras at two hospitals filmed 39 children between the ages of 2 months and 4 years together with their parents. In 33 of the 39 cases, the cameras recorded one or both parents attacking the child. Of course, all of this occurred while the parents believed they were alone and unobserved. The observers

would have intervened to prevent serious harm to the babies.

One father, who later admitted to the earlier manslaughter of a stepson, was spotted pinching his 6-week-old baby's hand, tweaking his ear repeatedly, flicking the sleeping baby's eyelids, placing his hand over the boy's mouth, digging his nail into the baby's palm repeatedly, and trying to suffocate him by placing his hand over his nose and mouth. This father was committed to a mental institution, while other parents were arrested and eventually lost custody of their children. Many had serious personality disorders, and some had drug abuse histories, which would help to account for their bizarre and cruel behavior. The researchers advocate installing concealed cameras in treatment centers to catch child abusers in the act.

SOURCE: Southall, Plunkett, Banks, Falkov, & Samuels (1997).

- Abusers' parental or supervisory responsibility over their victims discourages others' suspicions about their abusive actions and confuses their young victims. The youngsters may interpret sexual approaches by adults they know well as being appropriate and condoned by other adults.

Thus, assessment of childhood sexual abuse and other physical abuse is impeded by the covert nature of the act (see the Research Focus box above), the lack of witnesses, and some abusers' positions of authority as parents, educators, coaches, caretakers, or others.

Interviewing Children

It is difficult to obtain accurate, reliable information from young children about suspected abuse. Very few standardized tests or interviews are available, so clinicians often rely on informal interviews and play observations. Unfortunately, in most instances, these interview and observation techniques either have unknown accuracy or have been studied and found to be suscep-

tible to examiner bias. That is, unless great care is taken, the assessment results could reflect the examiner's initial expectations about whether or not abuse occurred. The most frequently used assessment device for sexual abuse is the anatomically correct doll, which, unlike children's usual dolls, has detailed genitalia (see the Research Focus box on page 137). This type of doll is used to allow young children, who may not be able to express themselves in words, to show the examiner what the perpetrator did to them. At the beginning of the interview, the clinician might use an anatomical doll to provide the child with an opportunity to discuss sexual issues ("Does this doll look like a girl or a boy?"). Also, the child can be asked to name the parts of the doll to reveal greater than usual knowledge of sexuality and sexual anatomy, which is presumed to come from the sexual abuse experience. Anatomical dolls have been used to aid children's recall of events and to allow children to demonstrate what happened (Boat & Everson, 1993). It is this last use that is the most controversial. Critics claim that examiners grossly influence the child's statements.

Testing for Abuse Using Anatomically Correct Dolls in Child Interviews

People differ in their opinions regarding the appropriateness of using anatomically detailed dolls in interviews with children who may have been sexually abused. In general, social workers, juvenile justice workers, and prosecutors are more likely to favor using the dolls, while opponents of their use include many research psychologists, defense attorneys, and civil libertarians, who favor strict adherence to defendants' legal rights. Both sides vigorously argue their positions, and both are strongly committed to justice and the protection of children.

Reasons to Use the Dolls

- Doll play is the natural language of children, putting them at ease. Anatomically correct dolls reveal whether the child has age-inappropriate knowledge of sexual terms and practices.
- Children with limited verbal expression skills can point to parts of the doll to show how they were sexually abused. The child's shame and embarrassment in recounting the crime can be reduced through use of dolls.
- The dolls prompt children's memories of abuse, serving as a trigger for the child's memory about traumatic experiences.
- Sexually abused children may play with the dolls in a distinctive manner, so doll play serves as a diagnostic test of sexual victimization. Children may use the dolls to show anger or fear toward the perpetrator or their own fear or arousal.

Reasons Not to Use the Dolls

- Examiners lacking education and training in child development or clinical service provision are using anatomically correct dolls in interviews and reaching unjustified conclusions about child sexual abuse.

- Even if trained in child interviewing, some clinicians are overzealous in attempting to protect the children. They insist that children use the dolls to "show how he hurt you" and do not question the guilt of the accused perpetrator.
- The dolls excite children and may confuse them. Research shows that it is not unusual for children who have never been abused to enact abuse themes in play with anatomically correct dolls. The unusual appearance of the dolls is sufficient to stimulate children to play out sexual encounters.
- In cases of suspected child sexual abuse, children are subjected to repeated interviews using the dolls over a period of time, in which different interviewers insistently suggest that the children were abused by certain people. This scenario is particularly likely to lead to children's accusations against the alleged perpetrators, according to research by Ceci and Bruck (1995).
- There are no standard doll play procedures and no child age and sex norms indicating which play features are normal and which indicate probable abuse.

Recommendations

Although anatomically correct dolls are widely used in questioning children about suspected sexual abuse, a growing body of research evidence dictates caution. Children must be protected. However, examiners must be sophisticated about children's cognitive development and suggestibility and must have relevant training in the proper use of the dolls in child interviews. Examiners and prosecutors must maintain professional objectivity despite heightened family, community, and media indignation about alleged sexual abuse. A number of highly publicized court cases in recent years have resulted in either hung juries or verdicts of innocence, and the cases were seen as having been tainted by questionably obtained children's evidence.

In reply, clinicians who use the dolls assert that children are unable to report their experiences in adult-style interviews, and so the dolls are necessary to help the children make accurate statements. For example, Boat and Everson (1993) advocate the use of anatomical dolls to focus the interview, assess the child's knowledge of sexuality, stimulate memories of sexual experiences, and enable the child to show what happened. However, simple observation of the child's behavior with the doll does not, by itself, prove abuse.

Some defenders of the diagnostic use of anatomical dolls believe that children never lie when asked about their abuse experiences, and thus their testimony must be trusted. A more moderate version of this claim is that children are suggestible, but not about events that involve their own bodies and experiences. The consensus from research on children's memories contradicts even this more moderate view. In fact, children's accuracy varies widely, and they may be especially inaccurate about personal bodily experiences such as genital examinations administered during medical examinations. Young girls who received genital exams incorrectly demonstrated on anatomical dolls that the doctor had inserted fingers into their anal or genital cavities, which did not occur. An amazing 75% of the girls who did *not* receive genital exams demonstrated with the dolls how the doctor supposedly had touched their genitals or buttocks (Bruck, Ceci, Francoeur, & Barr, 1995). If these results apply to the assessment of sexual abuse in interviews employing anatomical dolls, there is serious question about the validity of such interviews.

As an example of what *not* to do, consider the following suggestive, accusatory child interview techniques used in actual cases of alleged sexual abuse (Ceci & Bruck, 1995). These tactics are highly controversial because they may lead a child to give the answers the interviewer expects rather than what the child actually thinks and remembers:

- Children are interviewed repeatedly, many times under emotionally charged circumstances, often with their parents, who are accusing a defendant of molesting the children.
- Bribes and threats are used to lead the children's testimony. The interviewer calls them "smart" for agreeing and "dumb" if they disagree.

- Children are told that other children have already told about the abuse. The other children are pointed to as models for imitation.
- The interviewer asks the children about events of several years ago, when they were preschool age or younger and unlikely to form clear memories.
- The interviewer may name a doll after the defendant and scold the doll for abusing the child: "You are naughty for hurting Allison."
- The interviewer may simply appear more enthusiastic, approving, and supportive when the child says something that confirms the interviewer's expectations. These behavior patterns may suffice to lead children to tell the interviewer what he or she apparently wants to hear.
- The interviewer refuses to allow the interview to be audiotaped or videotaped. Note that many of these tactics would be unethical or even illegal if used with adult witnesses. Legal and administrative steps have been taken in many states to prevent examiners and prosecutors from putting words into children's mouths.

Much more research is needed to answer the important question of how young children can be credible witnesses in sexual abuse cases. We need high standards for examiner training and age-appropriate, standardized tests, interviews, and child behavior observation checklists.

Standards for Accurate Testing

IN FOCUS 3 ▶ What steps can be taken to improve the accuracy of children's reports of sexual or physical abuse?

Adequate psychological testing of children must take into account their cognitive and social immaturity, characteristics that make them poor informants. Even if accurate, their accounts of happenings tend to be extremely brief and unelaborated, especially those from children younger than 4 years. For example, when asked where he went with his father, a young boy might simply say "to the zoo" or "to McDonald's," without any further description. Much questioning and prompting might be required in order to obtain a fuller description. Unfortunately, pointed or suggestive questioning itself might alter the account given by a child, especially one under the age of 4 (Lamb et al., 2000). General questions and supportive comments are much more likely to elicit accurate accounts, even from very young children. Yet, even well-trained interviewers rely heavily on direct, suggestive questions ("Was he wearing a white T-shirt?" "Did he touch you here?"), which are likely to yield misleading results (Lamb et al., 2000).

Adults are much more powerful than children in all ways, so children are frequently nervous or even frightened at being questioned by adults. Unfamiliar adult interviewers can be especially threatening to children if they are businesslike, formally dressed, work in an imposing office building, are associated with the law (perhaps as police officers or child protection agency employees), and are obviously important people. Even most adults are intimidated to some degree if questioned by someone in authority. Child protection agency and police interviewers and prosecutors are dedicated to defending children, so they are eager to help punish adults who prey on children. In their zeal, some dedicated officials may underestimate their own power to influence children's claims about what happened to them. In the interests of accuracy and fairness, it is vitally important to obtain the child's own story without influencing it in any way.

A growing body of psychological research indicates that several steps can be taken to improve the accuracy of children's reports of incidents involving possible abuse:

1. Professionals trained to interview children are necessary. Relevant interviewer training is an essential ingredient. Interviewers require special formal training in interviewing and observing children who may have been abused, so the clinicians will be appropriately sensitive but objective and fair to all parties in the case. A number of forensic psychology, psychiatry, and social work programs offer graduate training in this area, and in-service workshops are offered by professional associations and public agencies. Child sexual abuse investigators require special, advanced training, professional credentials, and expertise in assessing children of the alleged victim's age.
2. Developmentally appropriate tests are needed, but this goal is difficult to achieve in the case of sexual abuse. Effects of sexual abuse are difficult to detect on tests, since they are highly diverse. Clinicians employ widely used symptom checklists and questionnaires such as those described in Chapter 3.

3. Age-appropriate, open-ended questions must be used. Research evidence suggests that reports are the most accurate and complete if the children are first invited to tell their own stories about the incident, free of any direct, possibly suggestive questions.
4. The timing of the interview is important. Reports need to be obtained as soon as possible after the incident, since children are more likely to offer inaccurate or incomplete reports when questioned months later (Lamb et al., 2000). Research has shown that children can be reliable informants if they are interviewed in an age-appropriate fashion as soon as possible after the alleged incident (Lamb, Sternberg, Orbach, Hershkowitz, & Esplin, 1999).
5. Multiple informants and information sources are necessary. At present, the best course seems to be to obtain information about the abused child from as many informants as possible (the child, parents, siblings, teacher, and others) using several different assessment techniques (interviews, psychological tests, observations) in diverse settings (Haugaard, 2000; O'Donohue & Elliott, 1991). This approach is expensive and time-consuming, but necessary, since there may be severe consequences to the child or to the accused abuser if the child's information is wrong.

NEGLECT

IN FOCUS 4 ▶ Describe the different forms of neglect.

Physical neglect includes refusal of or delay in seeking health care, abandonment, expulsion from home or not allowing a runaway to return home, and inadequate supervision. Educational neglect includes permission of chronic truancy, failure to enroll a child of mandatory school age, and inattention to a special educational need. Emotional neglect includes such actions as chronic or extreme spouse abuse in the child's presence, permission of drug or alcohol use by the child, and refusal of or failure to provide needed psychological care. (DHHS, 1989, p. 6)

You may be surprised that the official definition of neglect sounds like a common everyday experience in many children's lives. A very low-income mother who cannot afford child care while she is at work may leave her young children alone, waiting for hours for food. Parents who cannot deal with defiant and hostile teenagers sometimes lock them out for a time, or they find it impossible to take a firm stand on their persistent truancy from school. Impoverished, uneducated, physically or mentally ill, or highly stressed parents find it difficult to provide responsible care and supervision of their children. And many parents are unwilling or unable to prevent their teenage children from joining rebellious groups or criminal gangs and using alcohol and illicit drugs. However, it is possible to tell the difference between neglect and lapses in good parenting. Many parental disciplinary actions are designed to teach some lesson about good behavior or are temporary expressions of anger, after which more normal relations are restored. For actions to qualify as **neglect**, the parents must leave the child without adequate food, shelter, health care, or protection for a significant amount of time and endanger the child's health.

The most common pattern of maltreatment is child neglect by a mother (DHHS, 2000). Neglect is different from abuse. An abuser must be active in some way in order to mistreat a child, while neglect is more passive; it is an act of omission or failing to meet the child's basic physical, emotional, or educational needs. In **physical neglect**, the caretaker may fail to provide food essential to the child's nourishment and normal growth, may leave the child unsupervised for extended time periods, may not clothe the child appropriately for the weather (may send the child to school without shoes or a sweater in freezing weather), or may leave the child's serious illnesses untreated. The case of the father whose unconventional religious beliefs led him to feed his baby son only lettuce to keep him pure is an extreme example of physical neglect. The little boy was malnourished and in danger of dying from this deficient diet.

Emotional neglect is somewhat more difficult to identify than physical neglect, but it occurs when the child's psychological needs are obviously not served, as when the child is not protected from frightening scenes of marital violence, substance abuse, or criminal activity, which might be terrifying or encourage antisocial conduct. Physical abuse or neglect is almost always accompanied by emotional neglect, but emotional neglect can occur alone in children whose physical needs are being met, but whose psychological needs are not. Psychological abuse and medical neglect currently account for 6% or fewer of the cases of maltreatment each year (DHHS, 2000).

Educational neglect is defined by state laws concerning mandatory school attendance. Caretakers are considered to be educationally neglectful if they (1) defy school attendance laws and fail to send their children to school, (2) do not provide state-approved home education if their children are not attending school, or (3) encourage or condone truancy.

Characteristics of Neglectful Families

Some types of parents are statistically more likely to neglect their children than others. This does not mean that all parents who fit this profile are or will become neglectful; only that neglect is more frequent in families with certain characteristics. Risk factors for child neglect include very low family income, parents with little formal education, and large families. If larger families are also low-income, their rate of neglect is nearly double that for families with three or fewer children (Paget, Philp, Abramczvk, 1993). However, families who have many children because of their religious convictions, such as members of the Church of Jesus Christ of Latter-Day Saints (Mormons) and Catholics, typically are not at heightened risk for child neglect. More neglect is found in deteriorating neighborhoods with low-income, single-family dwellings, many vacant houses, and high family mobility (Zuravin, 1989). (However, as previously mentioned, cases of neglect are more likely to be detected in such neighborhoods.) Neglectful mothers of infants are likely to appear consistently less sensitive and responsive to their children and more withdrawn and uninvolved with them than most mothers (Crittenden, 1988). However, these behavioral patterns are also characteristics of depressed and highly stressed mothers, so, by themselves, they do not necessarily indicate neglect. The youngest children are most at risk, and the highest victimization rates are for children between birth and 3 years, with neglect rates declining steadily afterward (DHHS, 2000). Older children are better able to care for themselves and each other if their parents are unable to do so. Fatalities stemming from neglect are most likely to occur for boys younger than 3, who have two or three siblings and live in a single-parent household headed by their mother (Margolin, 1990). These families are very stressed because of poverty and inadequate resources, and the mothers often lack both the knowledge and the means to care for their children adequately.

EFFECTS OF MALTREATMENT

IN FOCUS 5 ▶ How does maltreatment affect young children's mental health and academic achievement?

Children are capable of great physical and psychological recovery, yet many suffer immediate and long-term consequences of maltreatment of various types. The effects depend to some extent on the type, severity, and frequency of the abuse, but also on the child's age, relationship to the perpetrator, and circumstances. Although it is customary to discuss the effects of abuse and neglect separately, we consider them together because they so often co-occur. The sad truth is that many children suffer from multiple types of maltreatment. For example, in one recent study of mistreated children from low-income urban families, 77.8% of the children actually suffered two or more types of abuse and neglect (Shonk & Cicchetti, 2001). This is a matter of great concern, because children who have been both physically and sexually abused are the most disturbed and at greatest risk for future victimization (Ryan et al., 2000).

Effects on Infants and Young Children

Infants and young children who have been neglected or abused early in life tend to have attachment problems, especially of a disorganized and disoriented nature (Lyons-Ruth, Melnick, & Bronfman, in press). In contrast to normal, securely attached babies, insecurely attached infants do not greet their mothers happily when reunited with them, but avoid or resist them. As the discussion in Chapter 2 on attachment theory stated, the most disturbed type of attachment is the disorganized/disoriented type. These children may appear alternately dazed, depressed, or highly active in an almost random fashion. Their erratic, inconsistent behavior when rejoining their mothers suggests future adjustment problems. These disorganized

attachment patterns may be handed down from one generation to the next, when caregivers display frightened, frightening, or other contradictory or atypical parenting behaviors.

Young maltreated children may also show delays in cognitive development. Girls are more likely than boys to become withdrawn and wary, and children of both sexes can become aggressive and noncompliant.

Preschool and kindergarten children who have been sexually abused tend to develop internalizing problems, including fear and depressed mood, and are especially likely to display strong anxiety (Trickett & McBride-Chang, 1995). Young sexually abused children also may exhibit inappropriate sexual behavior, such as excessive or public masturbation, or may make socially inappropriate overt sexual advances to others.

Moreover, more than 50% of sexually abused children of different ages meet some or all of the diagnostic criteria for **posttraumatic stress disorder (PTSD)**, a constellation of symptoms that can follow serious injury, threatened death, or a comparably devastating psychological experience (Saywitz, Mannarino, Berliner, & Cohen, 2000). As described in Chapter 7, PTSD symptoms include persistent re-experiencing of the traumatic event or avoiding of things associated with the event, either anxiety or numbing of responsiveness, and possible amnesia for an important aspect of the event. Children may become disorganized and distracted and may experience irritability, headaches, stomachaches, and sleep problems, which are easily confused with other mental and physical conditions.

Effects during Middle Childhood

Many physically abused elementary school children have low self-esteem and high rates of adjustment problems of all types, including rejection by their peers. Neglected children in particular have low school grades, academic deficiencies (especially in reading), and low tested intelligence, possibly because neglectful parents fail to provide them with cognitive stimulation in the form of talking and reading aloud to them. However, a recent study showed that all maltreated children (not just neglected ones) tend to show academic achievement problems, probably mainly because of their lower academic engagement, as measured by self-initiated, regulated, and persistent attempts to

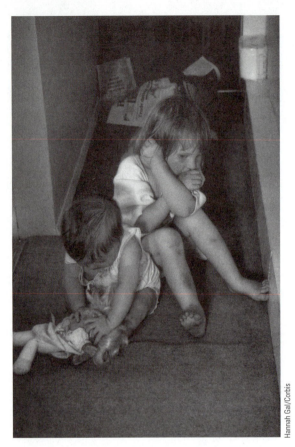

Physically abused children live in fear and pain. Detection and prevention of child maltreatment have improved, but too many children still suffer.

Hannah Gal/Corbis

master the subject matter (Shonk & Cicchetti, 2001). The troubled, maltreated children require more inducements to do their schoolwork and are less internally motivated to learn than other children their age. Sexually abused and otherwise maltreated elementary school girls may withdraw and become socially isolated, and a small number may become aggressive and angry. Maltreated boys have more academic achievement problems and adjustment problems of both internalizing and externalizing types than maltreated girls do (Shonk & Cicchetti, 2001).

Maltreated Adolescents

Adolescents who are maltreated experience both internalizing and externalizing problems and have poor peer relations. Some sexually abused adolescent girls

develop antisocial, delinquent behavior and become sexually active when still quite young (Trickett & McBride-Chang, 1995). Long-term adjustment problems include greater risk of substance abuse, binge eating, physical symptoms, depression, and self-injurious and suicidal behavior (Brown, Cohen, Johnson, & Smailes, 1999; Polusny & Follette, 1995). As a group, adolescents who have been abused and neglected in various ways show disturbances of many types, low self-esteem, low social competence, and poor school and peer adjustment. The neglected group has the lowest academic achievement (Eckenrode, Laird, & Doris, 1993).

It is impossible to say without qualification that one type of maltreatment is any more dangerous to children's adjustment than any other. Rather, effects of maltreatment vary in severity, and maltreatment is often associated with difficulties in social, emotional, and cognitive development. Contrary to popular public opinion, physical abuse seems to affect children as negatively as sexual abuse (Stevenson, 1999). Victimization rarely occurs in untroubled families, so most of these abused and neglected youngsters also bear the burden of parental marital conflict, family social isolation, economic and interpersonal stress, illness in the family, or other problems. Researchers have concluded that much of the increased risk of later depression and suicide among abused young people is accounted for by their adverse family environment and relationships with their parents (Brown et al., 1999). Sometimes victimized children require professional care of many types, not only immediately after the maltreatment, but also long afterward (Saywitz et al., 2000).

PREVENTION OF MALTREATMENT

IN FOCUS 6 ▶ What societal changes might help protect children from becoming victims of violence?

Prevention of Physical Abuse

The attitudes that tolerate and ignore violence in the society as a whole also tolerate the violence acted out in individual communities and homes throughout the country. (Osofsky & Fenichel, 1994, p. 40)

Violence toward children is part of a national and global climate that tolerates and even encourages violence as a solution to human problems. People fear being attacked, which makes them become more aggressive, which leads others to retaliate. Violent acts and fear of becoming a victim fuel each other, raising the level and intensity of assaults. Children are brought into the climate of violence. When many people possess weapons, children will find those weapons and shoot each other or be shot, either accidentally or in anger. TV shows and movies are highly and increasingly violent, offering the insistent message that violence is everywhere and that it works. For most people, this is merely entertaining, but for some young people media violence has tragic results. Youngsters may copy violent media and real-life models and improvise violent solutions to interpersonal conflicts (Bandura, 1969). Juvenile gangs rule the streets in many neighborhoods, juvenile detention facilities, and even some public schools. Violent attacks are provoked by use of alcohol and illicit drugs or disputes about drug sales. Many parents feel unprotected from assault at home and work and helpless to protect their children. Terrorist acts escalate the everyday violence level. Guns are commonly found in homes and schools, even elementary schools, and, in response, the schools themselves begin to resemble correctional facilities, with weapons detection systems, windowless walls, and tight police surveillance. More and more of our national resources are being poured into military preparedness, law enforcement, and prisons, yet people do not feel safer. Is this situation inevitable, or can something be done? Several reforms should be considered.

Protect Children from Weapons

The Study Group on Violence of the National Center for Clinical Infant Programs (Osofsky & Fenichel, 1994) examined the roots of violence against children. The study group concluded that there should be a national agenda to combat our society's apparent complacency about and tolerance of growing violence. They noted that Canada is a much less violent society. One difference between the two countries is the easier access to firearms in the United States. When nearly everyone of every age has ready access to a gun, shootings are inevitable. In addition to homicides, guns increase the rate of accidents and suicides. Too many children accidentally shoot and kill someone, often another child, using a loaded gun that was not secured. The availability of weapons and widespread incitement to use them against others result in the ac-

cidental and intentional deaths of many U.S. children. Present efforts to provide trigger locks on firearms, other mechanical protective devices, and gun safety classes and to pass laws requiring guns to be secured in locked cabinets are all essential measures. But are these efforts sufficient? Should gun possession and use be further restricted? It's a matter of opinion (hopefully, opinion based on objective facts), but few Americans believe that people should be barred from gun ownership.

I (Donna Gelfand) grew up in the tall timber in rural Oregon, where guns were a fact of life. Every family had at least one gun. Fathers taught their boys and girls how to shoot, clean, and store a rifle, and most of us at least did some target practice, if not actual hunting. No one in our neighborhood fired guns recklessly, except some who did when they got drunk at the dance hall on Saturday nights, and no kids were there. (Road signs were also an endangered species, although there was surprisingly little vandalism other than shooting signs.)

Why did it seem so much safer then? Our families provided some protection. Most of our parents gave us good training and kept weapons safely stowed away. We were also protected by the very nature of our society then. There were some bullies and a few outcasts, but there were no violent gangs. Kids could get alcohol, but there were no illicit drugs, no well-armed marijuana farmers, drug dealers, or the highly violent entertainment media that kids must deal with today. All the kids traded Spiderman, Batman, and Superwoman and Superman comics, but they were pretty tame compared with what kids see on TV and computer games today. And even though we lived in a lumber camp in a very poor part of the state, we did not have to be afraid that we would be attacked by anyone with a gun or bomb.

It is sad that times have changed, even where I grew up. Drug dealers and marijuana farms moved in near my sister's place in the woods of Oregon. Sometimes you can hear gunfire at night and it does not feel so safe there anymore.

Improve Parenting Skills

Children are more likely to suffer injury or abuse if their parents are emotionally disturbed, were abused as children, are risk-taking, substance-abusing, young, and single, hold unrealistic expectations of their children, and have poor parenting skills (Peterson & Brown, 1994). Thus, child protection programs have targeted mothers with these types of problems, and many of these programs have proved effective in preventing abuse and neglect by first-time, at-risk mothers (Eckenrode et al., 2001; MacMillan, 2000). One program (Olds et al., 1997) successfully reduced the rate of child abuse in a group of high-risk families through nurses' home visits to teach improved parenting practices and help parents form supportive social networks. During pregnancy and the child's first 2 years of life, mothers also received free transportation to prenatal and well-child health appointments. Abuse and neglect rates were 19% in comparable families studied, but only 4% in the families who participated in the prevention program. This study indicates that home visits and well-baby medical services can reduce the incidence of child abuse. One of the ways in which the nurse home-visiting program reduced the likelihood of later child maltreatment by parents was through reduction of problem behaviors when the children were preschoolers (Eckenrode et al., 2001). Children who are defiant, oppositional, and aggressive are likely to provoke abuse, and reducing these types of problem behaviors helps protect the children from attacks by annoyed parents. Physical abuse during the preschool period is particularly likely to lead to children's aggression and antisocial behavior (Manly, Kim, Rogosch, & Cicchetti, 2001).

Provide Self-Control Training for Older Children

Other abuse prevention services can focus on teaching the potential child victims skills that help them avoid physical abuse. Abused children tend to be difficult, hyperactive, distractible, and provocative, for example, disobeying and engaging in "back talk" to caregivers (Peterson & Brown, 1994). These children's chances of goading their parents into physically abusing them might be reduced if the children learned self-control techniques (described in Chapter 14). If children were taught to avoid talking back and other provocative behavior and to avoid negative interactions at high-risk times, they could escape much abusive treatment. Programs should also include other self-control techniques, including relaxation skills, positive self-directed talk, and problem-solving techniques stressing nonconfrontive tactics for resolving disputes.

Improve State and Private Social Services

Some states are providing social services that might help prevent child neglect and abuse. Since abuse can have many different causes, many different prevention measures must be used. Hawaii's Healthy Start Program offers families of newborns a wide array of services designed to promote physical and mental health, educate parents, and reduce their stress (Osofsky & Fenichel, 1994). Prevention services, emotional support, family crisis resolution strategies, and mental health services are provided to at-risk families in the belief that this is a good investment. It is much cheaper in terms of state tax revenues to prevent conflict and maltreatment of children than it is to incarcerate them later, after they have become criminals. In addition, in most of the nation's major cities, university-affiliated projects coordinate law enforcement agencies and human services to intervene in cases in which a child witnesses or is the victim of a violent crime.

Prevention of Neglect

A number of effective parent training programs have been developed to teach neglectful mothers to care for their youngsters. Cognitive behavior therapy techniques that have been shown to be effective include training in self-observation, self-reinforcement for good performance, and problem-solving strategies. Mothers with mental retardation have been taught to provide adequate diets for their children; abusive and neglectful mothers were successfully prompted to remove hazardous conditions in the home; and parents were helped to improve their children's personal hygiene through the application of behavioral treatments (Lutzker, 1990). This research suggests that child neglect may stem largely from mothers' deficits in relevant parenting skills or motivation, both of which can be effectively treated (Paget et al., 1993). A limitation of the behavioral approach is that, as yet, only small numbers of cases have been intensively treated and observed. Because so many neglectful families need help, a less labor-intensive, less costly intervention approach is needed, such as a parenting course in the schools for current and future child caretakers.

Neglected children have many psychological and educational needs. They are the most likely of the maltreated children to perform poorly on intelligence tests and on schoolwork, suggesting that they would profit from special education services. In addition, they may need social skills training to enable them to make and keep friends. Younger neglected children need a parent or surrogate to provide them with verbal stimulation, emotional responsiveness, warmth, and security. Parent training is the most effective intervention for neglected infants, toddlers, and preschoolers. These various treatment alternatives are presented in more detail in Chapter 15.

Prevention of Sexual Abuse

Many elementary schools offer child sexual abuse programs that focus primarily on warding off attacks by strangers. In reality, the vast majority of sexual abuse incidents involve adults who are known to the child. However, potential sexual abuse by relatives, friends, and acquaintances is a sensitive subject, so school-based programs continue to address the more remote possibility of abuse by strangers. As a group, the school-based child sexual abuse prevention programs are successful in teaching children some of the facts about such abuse and how to avoid dangerous situations (Davis & Gidycz, 2000). The more successful programs feature four or more sessions and actively involve children in demonstrations and skill rehearsal. However, the programs' effectiveness in reducing actual sexual abuse in everyday life remains to be demonstrated. This is a research area greatly in need of public attention and support, since it is possible that ineffective but popular programs give a false impression of protecting children.

TREATMENT OF ABUSED CHILDREN

There is hope for abused children: If the maltreatment is not severe, most sexually and physically abused children improve over time, whether or not they receive professional treatment. This resiliency is fortunate, particularly because so few children who need effective treatment will receive it. Factors that are important in an abused child's recovery are the family's cohesion and adaptability and the intensity of the parents' reactions to the abuse. Children's recovery is faster when their parents remain strong, calm, and supportive, rather than becoming distraught and accusatory (Cohen & Mannarino, 1998). Children who believe they have greater control over what happens to them (an internal locus of control) also tend to recover more quickly than those who feel helpless (Cohen & Mannarino, 2000).

Certain abusive or neglectful parents are considered treatment-resistant. These parents are typically young, have a long history of violent behavior, antisocial personality disorder, or substance abuse, and are socially isolated and living in poverty. Under these circumstances, the child must be protected through termination of parental rights and placement of the child permanently in foster care (Gelles, 2000).

When professional treatment is needed, several types of educational and therapeutic programs are available.

Psychoeducational Programs

Some children display no discernable psychological harm from being abused. Nevertheless, child protection workers and mental health experts advise monitoring these children for possible delayed reactions. For example, psychoeducational training and periodic follow-up assessments are advised for sexual abuse victims who show little or no disturbance over their experiences. It does not appear necessary to offer psychotherapy to these children immediately, but it is important to realize that they may show signs of disturbance up to a year or more later, when they will require more extensive mental health services. In psychoeducational interventions, the child and nonabusing parent are offered an opportunity to discuss the occurrence with a case worker, who gives them realistic advice and reassurance and tells them how to protect the child from further abuse. Parental involvement is very important to support and guide the child through the recovery process.

Foster Home Placement

Children whose family members have severely abused or neglected them may be placed in foster homes in order to protect them. Such removals from the family are avoided except when the maltreatment is sufficiently severe or persistent as to endanger the child's physical safety or threaten the child's life. Child welfare and protection services in many states focus on the preservation of families and have kept families together even when there was evidence of further severe physical abuse of the child. News stories of small children being fatally assaulted by family members in Connecticut and New York (Stoesz & Karger, 1996) led to heightened official alertness to possible murderous attacks on children and quicker placement of endangered children in foster care (McLarin, 1995).

But does the foster home system adequately protect these children? Unfortunately, foster care itself can also endanger children, who may stay in the system for years and are sent from home to home with little regard for their wishes or feelings. One New York boy was placed in 37 different homes during a 2-month period, while another lived with 17 families in less than a month (Stoesz & Karger, 1996). It is difficult to see how such treatment would help a child, unless the child's life was in danger. The seriously inadequate and underfunded child welfare system simply fails to protect too many children.

Psychotherapy

Many sexually abused children receive psychotherapy to help them deal with their experiences. Research indicates that cognitive-behavioral therapy (CBT) is consistently more effective in treating physical or sexual abuse than the other forms of treatment to which it is compared (Berliner & Kolko, 2000; Cohen & Mannarino, 1998; Deblinger, Lippman, & Steer, 1996). Such therapy may help children and teenagers who have experienced sexual abuse and suffer from anxiety, depression, and possibly posttraumatic stress disorder (PTSD, which is discussed previously in this chapter and in Chapter 7). In cognitive-behavioral therapy, the therapist gently induces the child to remember the trauma under close guidance so that the fear can be re-experienced in less severe form and then modified (Foa & Riggs, 1995). Over several sessions, the child repeatedly listens to and rehearses information that is incompatible with the fear (e.g., that the threat is now absent and the child is strong and can handle it). Evaluations of the effectiveness of the cognitive-behavioral therapy have yielded encouraging results when a child shows clear evidence of feeling anxiety, panic, or depression (Foa & Riggs, 1995). Less is known about how to treat sexual victimization that does not involve trauma and extreme fear and anxiety, but the involvement of the parents is usually important. Also, psychotherapy has been less effective with children who react to the abuse with anger and aggressiveness or sexualized behavior (Saywitz et al., 2000).

It is regrettable and somewhat surprising that we are only now beginning to obtain research-based evidence concerning effective therapy for sexual abuse victims, since such treatments have long been needed. Some of Freud's earliest patients complained about this type of victimization, yet well over a century later, many children still lack understanding and adequate care.

CHILDREN'S MORAL AND LEGAL RIGHTS

The topics of neglect and abuse raise questions about children's moral and legal rights, which sometimes conflict with the rights of their parents. Children's rights and status are changing. This section considers new developments in the field of child law and definitions of children's legal and human rights as they relate to child maltreatment. Issues of child custody and professional treatment are considered in other chapters. Some basic legal questions will be considered here. For example, are children considered *persons*, just as adults are, or are they the *property* of their parents and subject to their parents' wishes? What happens when parents and children disagree on whether the children have problems and, if so, what type? In fact, when children and their parents at a mental health clinic were asked to list the child's problems, 63% of the pairs did not agree on even a single problem (Yeh & Weisz, 2001). It seems unlikely that the children were truly willing to enter treatment, since many did not agree with their parents that they had major psychological problems. Are children's rights and prerogatives much more restricted than those of adults, and should this be the case? These searching questions address core beliefs about the capacities of

What Would It Mean to Have Equal Rights for Children?

Some believe children should be entitled to all of the rights adults enjoy in law and in custom. This view contrasts sharply with the prevalent law and opinion that children should be protected at all costs, even when it deprives them of their liberty. For example, children's custody may be awarded to the parent they dislike; a hated parent may have visitation rights; children may be unwillingly removed from the home of legally defined "unfit" parents or caretakers; they are legally compelled to attend school; and their lives may be otherwise controlled for their ultimate welfare.

In Cohen's (1985) view, one should treat people equally unless and until there is a justification for unequal treatment. This implies that the burden of proof is on those who would treat adults and children differently. That children lack adult mental capacities cannot be taken for granted, but must be scientifically demonstrated. In fact, it is sometimes difficult to distinguish between the mental abilities of adults and children. For example, both adults and children can be misled. Millions of adults can be enticed into buying harmful products or supporting unscrupulous politicians through clever advertising programs.

People of all ages can act impulsively or irrationally and contrary to their own long-term interests. After all, it is the adults, and not the children, who go to war. Both children and adults suffer from distortions in memory as well as in reasoning. And because individual children develop their full reasoning capacities at different ages (and some older people may lose their mental acuity), it is unfair to maintain that 21 years or some other arbitrarily selected age represents the age of reason.

Even proponents of equal legal rights for children recognize age differences in capacity, however, and would not choose to extend all liberties to inexperienced and cognitively limited preschoolers. Children may require educational and financial advisors to help them make wise decisions, but then so do most adults. With such assistance, children would not harm themselves nor be harmed by others; they could choose whom to live with, seek the type of medical treatment they prefer, and manage their own financial affairs with the assistance of objective adult counselors. Perhaps it would be good if adults had to provide good reasons for the requirements they set for children under their care.

children and the nature of childhood. The quest for answers opens many different areas of study, including law, ethics, social science, education, and government, illustrating the interdisciplinary nature of the field of childhood psychopathology. (See the Research Focus box.)

It is important to distinguish between legal rights and human (or moral) rights. **Legal rights** are guaranteed by the U.S. Constitution or by statute or state laws and are enforced by the police and the courts. **Human rights** are more broadly and less precisely defined and pertain to the conditions necessary for children to become healthy, well-adjusted, competent, and productive citizens. Many people believe that children have a right to be loved (a human right), and that they are harmed by parents who do not want or love them. Yet

no legal right to loving care exists in law, although children's physical health and safety are protected.

A Bill of Rights for the World's Children

Many of the world's nations attempt to guard children's welfare by agreeing to certain standards and attempting to persuade other nations to share these standards. Reflecting this concern, the United Nations General Assembly held a convention on the rights of the child, and in 1989 adopted a declaration that children are persons who are entitled to both protection and respect. After 20 nations (not including the United States) ratified the document, this treaty went into force (Limber & Flekkov, 1995; Wilcox & Naimark, 1991). Parents' rights groups in the United States oppose the U.N. declaration as depriving parents of their traditional power to determine rules for the family. That is, they believe any announcement of the independent rights of children will undermine the family. The treaty states that certain rights should apply to all children:

1. The best interests of the *child*, not of parents, teachers, or others, should be the most important consideration in legislation to protect children.
2. All children should have adequate prenatal and post-natal care, nutrition and housing, free, compulsory primary education, and recreation opportunities.
3. Children should be protected from economic exploitation as laborers, and their government should financially assist parents who cannot provide an adequate standard of living for their children.
4. Children have a right to live. Children under the age of 15 should not be recruited into armed conflict, and they should be protected from illegal narcotic and psychotropic drugs, and physical abuse.
5. Children should be raised in an atmosphere of affection and emotional security. Ideally, they should live with their parents, but if separated from their parents, they should receive society's protection.
6. Children should be spared all forms of cruelty, neglect, and exploitation for commercial gain. They should be among the first to receive relief in times of natural disaster, famine, or war.
7. To ensure peaceful relations among the peoples of the world, children should be protected from discrimination and prejudice, whether racial, religious, political, or any other type.

Some Nobel Peace Prize laureates have recently added their own statement about the protection of children. Nelson Mandela, Mother Teresa, Henry Kissinger, and Aung San Suu Kyi, along with many other distinguished individuals and groups, issued a joint statement to the heads of state of all member countries of the General Assembly of the United Nations, entitled "For the Children of the World." They said, in part, "Today, in every single country throughout the world, there are many children silently suffering the effects and consequences of violence. This violence takes many different forms: between children on streets, at school, in family life and in the community. There is physical violence, psychological violence, socioeconomic violence, environmental violence and po-

litical violence. Many children—too many—live in a 'culture of violence.'" The Nobel Peace Prize laureates go on to propose that nonviolence be taught at every level in all societies during the Decade for a Culture of Nonviolence (2001–2011) in order to reduce violence against children and all humanity. (See http://209.238.73.41/eng/index.htm for information on the Decade for a Culture of Nonviolence.) Protecting children is a challenging task in a world in which millions of children are suffering, even in economically advantaged nations. Any day's news stories typically describe violent encounters involving children and demonstrate just how far we are from achieving these humane goals.

Increases in rights have been associated with increases in the degree to which children are considered to be persons. (Hart, 1991, p. 55)

Children's Legal Rights

This section reviews some legal rights of children, many of which have been only recently enacted into law. Three fundamental principles guide legal and ethical codes affecting children; they are autonomy, beneficence, and justice (Levine, Anderson, Ferretti, & Steinberg, 1993).

1. The principle of *autonomy* refers to the ability to make personal decisions based on an adequate understanding of the circumstances. Previously, children were regarded as their parents' property and were almost completely subjected to their parents' decisions, however ill-advised or cruel. Today, children and adolescents are granted greater autonomy from parents.
2. The principle of *beneficence* advocates protecting children by preventing or reducing harm, working to benefit them, and not intentionally harming them.
3. The principle of *justice* asserts that children and adults should have equal rights, and juveniles' rights should be limited only by their still-maturing judgment and intelligence. Children should be treated justly so that they will not be goaded into alienation and rebellion (Levine et al., 1993).

Although children have some legal rights as persons, they also require special protection, first because they are more vulnerable than adults. They are

Back to the Beginning

Prevention Is the Key

What have we learned about child maltreatment that sheds light on the situations of the abused children described at the beginning of this chapter?

First, children are often abused in many ways, so it is important to examine them for more than one type of cruelty. Tony, the little boy lying in bed listening to his parents drinking, taking drugs, and hitting each other, was physically abused (indicated by his serious bruises) and also emotionally abused by witnessing the violence and substance abuse of his parents. There was a hint that he was also neglected, since neither parent remembered to feed the children; alcohol and drugs probably took most of their attention and money. The teenager who was forced into prostitution by her stepfather suffered several forms of abuse, including the repeated sexual abuse, the physical and psychological threat from her stepfather, and the terrible neglect from her mother, who could hardly have ignored what was going on.

Children are at greater risk of abuse from their parents or caretakers than from a stranger. That was true of Tony and the other children described at the start of the chapter. If a nonabusing parent does not choose to protect them or is powerless to intervene, then a violent or psychotic spouse, stepparent, or boyfriend is free to abuse them.

Neglect and abuse have many causes, including lack of education, poverty, unemployment, chaotic households, dangerous neighborhoods, substance abuse, extreme or bizarre religious and moral beliefs, mental disorders, and selfish concern for one's own gratification coupled with callous disregard for children. The cases presented at the chapter's beginning illustrated a number of these conditions. Tony's parents were engaged in drug use and domestic violence and also had little thought for their children. The man who was starving his son to cleanse him mentally was in the grip of a delusion that his son was some special, holy being who would not be harmed by such a lim-

ited diet. It isn't clear why the father put the fatal Freon in his little boy's bathwater; he claimed to be ignorant of its toxic effects, despite his training as a refrigeration technician. It is possible that he resented having to be a babysitter or that he was of limited intelligence or education and so didn't realize he could kill his son by making bubble bath with Freon. The boyfriend who bashed in the baby's skull clearly resented having to tend him, may also have had very little education, may have felt diminished because he was unemployed, and may have had other risk factors in his background. The girl forced into prostitution was cruelly victimized by both parents, who used her as a source of income and ignored her pain.

How should the perpetrators and victims be handled? If the police and child protection agencies become involved, they get emergency medical treatment for the physically abused child, put the child into protective custody and perhaps foster care, assess the evidence, and seek indictment of the alleged perpetrator. In the most extreme and dangerous circumstances, the child is placed in foster care and may or may not be returned to the parents depending on all of the evidence. In less serious cases, the child is returned to the parents, who are kept under regular surveillance for an extended time period. They may also be required to enroll in parenting classes, and perhaps anger management, addiction treatment, and family therapy. The outlook is not a rosy one for maltreated children. Sometimes a relative can provide good care for the child, but too often the child enters an inadequate foster care system. Treatment is available for only some of the children, and cognitive behavior therapy has been demonstrated to be helpful. The best alternative would be prevention of maltreatment, but that effort is just beginning. Any reduction in the level of violence in homes and communities would probably reduce some of the violence to children.

prohibited from harmful activities such as smoking, drinking alcohol, using drugs, and engaging in dangerous and taxing work that might endanger their health. Children cannot make informed decisions about important matters because they are relatively uninformed and unable to foresee the long-range consequences of their decisions. Law and custom hold that the family is the best and most appropriate source of socialization and protection of the child. The child is legally prohibited from leaving the family and from defying the parents' wishes so that family strength, cohesion, and discipline can be maintained (Teitelbaum & Ellis, 1978).

Many decisions pit the child's personal liberty and considerations of due process against the authority of parents and the state (Cohen, 1985; Koocher & Keith-Spiegel, 1990). In the process, parental rights may be limited. For this reason, conservative religious and political groups that view firm parental control as vital sometimes advocate new restrictions on children's rights. For example, although adults have the moral and legal right not to be punished with spanking or beating, conservative opinion strongly upholds parents' and sometimes also teachers' rights to spank disobedient children. (Recall that there are national and cultural differences in the acceptability of physical punishment of children.) Further, although the U.S. Supreme Court ruled in *Riggins v. Nevada* (1992) that under certain conditions adult defendants could not be forced to take antipsychotic medications, it is questionable whether similar protection would extend to children (Winick, 1997). However, there is a growing national consensus that children's legal rights should be safeguarded and possibly expanded if their welfare is endangered.

SUMMARY

Public approval of corporal punishment may unintentionally encourage physical abuse, especially in highly stressed families. Physical abuse is assaulting a child and inflicting physical damage. This clearly goes beyond ordinary corporal punishment. Sexual abuse involves the child in age-inappropriate sexual activity, either as a passive witness or a participant. Neglect is the most frequent form of abuse and typically involves very young children whose parents are unskilled, im-

poverished, and unmotivated to care for them. Physical neglect deprives a child of essential food, clothing, health care, or shelter. Emotional neglect is poorly defined, but includes parents' failure to protect their children from harmful situations such as substance use and domestic violence. Educational neglect occurs when parents fail to see that their child attends school regularly and gets an education.

The child's well-being is the primary concern in all cases of maltreatment. Typically, the child protection agency or court removes the child from the home or other unsafe situation, either temporarily or permanently. There are many reports of psychological disturbance stemming from child victimization, although it is often unclear whether most of the problem comes from poverty, ignorance, crime, and stress or from the maltreatment itself. Whatever the cause, cruelty to children is immoral, illegal, and harmful to them and to society and must be prevented.

International child protection groups suggest that children have moral or human rights to health, safety, freedom (including freedom of expression and belief), and education. Children's legal rights are much more limited, and their medical and mental health treatment, including institutionalization, are determined by their parents, if the parents are not abusive or neglectful. Children's liberty is restricted because they are presumed to lack mature judgment and are more vulnerable to harm than are adults. Restrictions on children are also imposed in order to maintain family strength and avoid parent-child conflict.

INFOTRAC COLLEGE EDITION

For more information, explore this resource at http://www.infotrac-college.com/Wadsworth. Enter the following search terms:

child abuse
child neglect
child sexual abuse
families and violence
prevention of abuse
posttraumatic stress disorder in children
child therapy
children's rights

IN FOCUS ANSWERS

IN FOCUS 1 ▶ Describe the various types of child abuse.

- Physical abuse consists of seriously assaulting a child and causing physical injury.
- Emotional or psychological abuse consists of serious, prolonged attacks on a child's self-esteem, self-confidence, and happiness.
- Sexual abuse is age-inappropriate sexual exploitation of a child for the perpetrator's pleasure or benefit.

IN FOCUS 2 ▶ Summarize the family factors that are associated with child maltreatment.

- Caretaker resentment of the demands and drudgery of tending children
- Poorly educated, impoverished parents
- Socially isolated parents
- Highly active, easily irritated family members
- Having been abused as a child in a disadvantaged family

IN FOCUS 3 ▶ What steps can be taken to improve the accuracy of children's reports of sexual or physical abuse?

- Use specially trained examiners who are qualified to assess children of the particular chronological age.
- Ask open-ended, nonleading questions
- Use reliable and valid tests standardized for use with children.

- Interview the child as soon as possible after the event.
- Obtain information from many sources, not just the child.

IN FOCUS 4 ▶ Describe the different forms of neglect.

- Physical neglect involves failing to provide food, clothing, shelter, or appropriate health care.
- Emotional neglect is failing to provide a child with a sense of safety by exposing her to domestic violence, substance abuse, or other criminal activity.
- Educational neglect is failing to send a child to school or tolerating chronic truancy so that the child does not receive a proper education.

IN FOCUS 5 ▶ How does maltreatment affect young children's mental health and academic achievement?

- Maltreated children have more attachment problems, especially the disorganized/disoriented type.
- They exhibit delays in cognitive development.
- They exhibit aggression and withdrawal, particularly girls.
- They exhibit symptoms of posttraumatic stress disorder in many cases.

IN FOCUS 6 ▶ What societal changes might help protect children from becoming victims of violence?

- Reducing children's exposure to weapons
- Improving parents' caregiving skills
- Helping older children avoid provoking attacks by giving them self-control training
- Improving state protective services for children

7 Anxiety, Posttraumatic Stress, and Obsessive-Compulsive Disorders

In the Beginning
The Aftermath of Kidnapping

This is the shocking story about the abduction of a group of elementary school children as they were traveling in their school bus. The children were held hostage for days inside the bus, buried in a landfill to avoid detection. This was the notorious Chowchilla, California schoolbus kidnapping, the effects of which haunted the children and their families long afterward. Here is the recollection of a 12-year-old girl who was threatened and held captive in the buried bus in the dark, together with several of her friends. Months later, she still suffered from posttraumatic stress disorder, as she describes here:

> I don't like to turn off the lights. I'm afraid someone would come in and shoot and rob us. When I wake up I turn on the light. . . . At night in Bakersfield (where she was staying with her brother) it feels like someone broke in. Nothing is there. I hear footsteps again. I keep going to check . . . I check where the sound is coming from . . . I'm very frightened of the kitchen because no one's there at all. I completely avoid it. At home I kept feeling someone was looking in and watching me. I kept the light on. I was afraid they'd come in and kill us all or take us away again. (Terr, 1981, p. 18.)

This child shows an extreme reaction to an extreme situation. In this chapter, we review children's fears and anxieties of many different types, ranging from reactions to traumatic events, such as that of this girl, to anxiety and fear that have no easily detected source. This chapter deals with incapacitating anxiety disorders and specific phobias that meet DSM diagnostic criteria and are very seldom adaptive.

INTRODUCTION

No child, no matter how privileged, is completely free from fear and anxiety. It is not surprising that anxiety disorders are among the most common psychological problems of childhood. Approximately 10% of all children will develop some type of anxiety disorder during their lifetime (Mitka, 2000). Stress and anxiety come from life challenges, and people differ in their threshold for experiencing stress and in their tolerance for resisting the debilitating effects of prolonged stress. Some children have a very low threshhold for stress and respond to simple changes in daily routine as stressful, while others adapt to new routines without any trouble. Tolerance for stress also depends on situational factors, such as illness, divorce, or death in the family, losing friends through moving to a new neighborhood, or even losing parents' attention as the result of the birth of a baby sister or brother.

Some vulnerable children respond to stress with anxiety, depression, physical complaints, or other maladaptive behavior patterns. We can call these *anxious children*. Kendall (1993, p. 239) offers a good description of them: "Anxious children . . . seem preoccupied with concerns about evaluations by self and others and the likelihood of severe negative consequences. They

seem to misperceive characteristically the demands of the environment and routinely add stress to a variety of situations." These anxious children may develop general or global anxiety, obsessive-compulsive symptoms, a specific phobia, or a combination of several of these problems. One feature of the anxiety disorders is that several types of these disorders frequently co-occur. It is not uncommon for a youngster with a specific phobia to also develop social phobia or school phobia. Children who suffer from obsessive-compulsive disorder may also experience school refusal. In addition, the most frequent combination is anxiety disorder in association with depression. As this chapter reveals, young children's severe and persistent anxiety symptoms should not be simply dismissed as a harmless phase, since they may last for months or years.

DEFINING FEAR AND ANXIETY

Compared to the obvious antisocial behavior of children with externalizing behavior problems, the problems of anxious children are much less obvious to others. The children may appear withdrawn and unhappy and may avoid certain situations, but close observation is required to detect the extent of their emotional distress. It is even more difficult to assess the particular type of distress they feel. Anxieties and fears are very similar in that both are distressing emotional states. However, there are differences between fear and anxiety. **Fear** is a strong emotional alarm reaction to real or perceived (even imagined) danger that is happening at the present and motivates escape or avoidance. When a person is afraid, the sympathetic branch of the autonomic nervous system surges into action to facilitate running away or attacking (this is called the *flight or fight reaction*). **Panic** is a sudden, overwhelming state of extreme fear or terror. In contrast, **anxiety** is more persistent and is marked by concern about bad things that might happen in the future, for example, dread about having the house burn down or of doing something wrong in public and having everyone think you are a fool. While everyday worry is likely to be adaptive and to trigger problem-solving efforts, anxiety is by definition less constructive, especially in its extreme form.

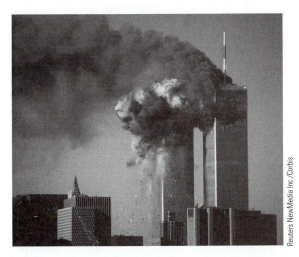

Reuters NewMedia Inc./Corbis

Children cannot be completely protected from witnessing or experiencing terrorist attacks and natural disasters. Psychologists work to improve prevention and treatment of trauma-related stress disorders.

Children's Common Fears

Parents often wonder whether their young children's fears are normal or something to worry about. Most children develop some fears, so there seems little reason for concern about a child who suddenly screams at the sight of a dog or becomes terrified of the dark if this is an isolated problem. In most instances, such reactions are temporary and dissipate over time, especially if the child develops some skills to handle the feared situation.

Not only is it normal to have specific fears, but there is also a normal developmental progression in the *types* of fears children develop (Gullone, 1999; Vasey, 1993). Babies and toddlers tend to fear things they experience directly, such as loud noises, the appearance of unexpected, surprising objects and images, the threat of falling, and strangers. At around 7 or 8 months of age, infants cry and protest when separated from their mothers or other regular caretakers. However, preschoolers and kindergarten children who can easily distinguish novel events from familiar ones are more likely to display fears of animals, darkness, and injury. They also continue to fear separation from their parents. Fear of monsters and imaginary beings is more typical of younger elementary school children, who are developmentally capable of thinking about threats that aren't actually present. Children this age also begin to worry about school failure, evaluations by others, appearing foolish, and natural events such as thunderstorms or fires.

Some specific fears continue into adolescence. For example, the most frequent fears reported from early childhood through late adolescence concern death and dangers or threats to self or loved ones. Older children, teens, and adults typically worry most about devastating future events, such as street violence, bombings, warfare, political dangers, environmental threats, or inability to find work and earn a living. On a personal level, adolescents are typically worried about peer rejection, school failure, and becoming independent. They particularly dread rejection by other teens or teachers ("I'm going to flunk this test and will have to leave school." "Can everyone see me sweating?" "I hide under long bangs so no one will see my ugly face.").

It appears that many worries plague children, even the youngest ones, and what they worry about is

Table 7-1 Frequent Worries and Fears of Children and Adolescents

Age Range	Types of Worries and Fears
0–12 months	Loss of support, loud noises, unexpected, looming objects, strangers
12–24 months	Separation from parent, strangers, injury
24–36 months	Separation from parent, animals, especially dogs, darkness
3–6 years	Separation from parent, strangers, animals, darkness, injury
6–10 years	Darkness, injury, being alone, imaginary beings
10–12 years	Injury, social evaluations, school failure, ridicule, thunderstorms, death
12–18 years	School failure, peer rejection, family problems, wars and other disasters, future plans (especially in boys)

partly determined by their developmental level (see Table 7-1). Knowledge of the common worries and fears of children of different ages helps parents and psychologists to determine the likelihood that a particular child's fear is normal or clinically significant.

The exact nature of a fear may not indicate whether it is normal or not. Silverman and her colleagues tested both a community sample that contained a mix of children and a clinic sample that consisted of children at an anxiety treatment center. The researchers found that both groups worried most about their health, school, natural disasters, personal harm, and threatening future events (Silverman, La Greca, & Wasserstein, 1995; Weems, Silverman, & La Greca, 2000). These findings suggest that it is not specifically what they fear that separates youngsters with anxiety disorders from the average child. Instead, it is the crippling nature of their worries—the extreme intensity, frequency, and persistence of their distress—that set apart those with anxiety disorders.

The Research Focus box reports on children's sharply increased anxiety levels. It is important to note that the types of things children fear have not changed much over the years, so the historical difference must be in fear frequency and level.

There are many possible sources of children's fears. Young children's physical and cognitive limita-

Research Focus

Why Are So Many Children Afraid?

Anxiety rates among children have increased to truly alarming levels during recent decades, and today the average American child reports feeling more anxiety than disturbed child psychiatric patients in the 1950s (Twenge, 2000). Children's current increased anxiety is particularly striking since high anxiety levels might have been expected because of threatening global events in the earlier time period. The 1950s were the time of the Cold War between the West and the Soviet Union, when devastating nuclear attacks were widely feared, people built home bomb shelters because they thought atomic attacks were imminent, and children were taught "duck and cover" routines to protect themselves at school. World War II, which killed millions of people, was a recent memory. In comparison, we now live in a time of peace and prosperity. (At the time of the study by Twenge on children's fears, the terrorist attacks on New York City and the Pentagon had not yet occurred.) The grim specter of nuclear conflict between superpowers has eased and we enjoy more creature comforts than ever, so why are today's children and young adults more anxious than their parents were?

There are many possible solutions to this puzzle. Perhaps today we have better methods for testing children, or youngsters have become more concerned about their school performance and their future job prospects. There are other possibilities:

- The increase in divorce and family dissolution, which directly affect children
- The explosive growth of the violent and dangerous drug culture
- Increased violence in films, Internet games, and TV shows
- School violence that targets children in mass shootings and bombings
- More graphic news coverage of kidnappings, warfare, and terrorist attacks
- Threats to the world environment
- Personal worries about doing well in school and achieving a comfortable way of life in adulthood

Think about what is making today's children so anxious.

Does their greater apprehension mean that more children than ever before will suffer from anxiety disorders?

There is no clear-cut explanation of these research findings. To begin with, some possible explanations seem unlikely. For example, the increase in anxiety does not seem to come from improved, more sensitive assessment methods since many of the same types of tests, interviews, and observations have been used since the 1950s. And the types of children tested have not changed. That leaves major social changes as the potential sources of the increased anxiety. Economic depressions can increase mental disorders, but no such event has occurred. Anyway, wealth may not control feelings of well-being. As long as people are not desperately poor, more money does not seem to bring greater happiness (Myers & Diener, 1995).

Perhaps the basic changes are closer to home and in the family. A number of changes in family life have occurred since the 1950s. One new development, which most directly affects children, is the increased divorce rate and prevalence of lower-income, single-parent, mother-headed families, as described in Chapter 2. As a group, these single-parent families are among the poorest in the nation, and even the richest of them tend to suffer relative deprivation when compared with two-parent families. The children of divorce most often lose income when their parents split up, but most are still adequately supported. The important thing may be their feelings of relative deprivation, compared with their friends and relations, and not how many dollars they actually have (Collins, 1996). However, living in poverty does not correlate significantly with children's anxiety scores (Twenge, 2000), so lack of money does not, by itself, cause children to become anxious. Jean Twenge (2000), the researcher who discovered the upsurge in childhood anxiety, suggested that part of the problem may lie in decreases in families' social connectedness, or the social and emotional bonds between members. Decreased social connectedness can be seen in the greater number of family break-ups, fewer marriages occurring at later ages, the increasing number of Americans who live alone, fewer people who belong to clubs and other social organizations, and even declines in attendance at films, theater productions, concerts, and other events that bring people together. Many of these changes in family and community life are significantly correlated with increases in children's anxiety.

Perhaps children are more anxious because their environments have actually become more threatening. In that case, their anxiety is functional rather than irrational. That is, there may be legitimate reasons for worrying. The things children say they fear can provide clues to this puzzle. Health concerns, school disasters, personal harm, and future events are high on the list of children's worries (Weems et al., 2000). These seem realistic in today's world. School shootings have received heavy news coverage and rightfully concern children, teachers, and parents. For previous generations, the worst threat at school was bad grades, but that has now been eclipsed by many reports of mass shootings and bombings at schools. It seems reasonable to conclude that at least some portion of the huge increase in fears and worries is reality-based and can be attributed to genuine threats (Twenge, 2000), some of which are new rather than familiar to previous generations. Interestingly, one of the first public responses to the terrorist attacks on September 11, 2001 was an upsurge in Web sites advising parents on how to explain the devastating event to their young children. Adults are clearly aware of the possibility that such attacks can make children feel overwhelmingly anxious and insecure.

There are other possible contributors to children's increased anxiety:

- Adults may have overused scare tactics. Most school children have been exposed to various prevention campaigns aimed at alerting them to the dangers of sexual predators, shootings, bombings, drugs and drug dealers, and tobacco and alcohol use. School and media appeals are offered by groups such as Mothers Against Drunk Driving, D.A.R.E., police and firefighters, and probably others who use similar, fear-based persuasion techniques (but see Chapter 5 for a description of how D.A.R.E. is developing other, more positive tactics). It could be that these well-intended warnings actually scare students and increase their anxiety levels.

- Perhaps children are more likely to admit to fears and worries than they were in the past. The entertainment media offer many self-disclosing models for them to imitate. TV talk shows featuring people revealing the intimate details of their lives lend some support to this interpretation.

- Children have become more experienced test-takers. Will test-wise children score higher on fear scales than children who are less experienced at taking tests? This seems unlikely, but certainly could be evaluated.

This does not exhaust the list of possible reasons for the upsurge in anxiety. All of these alternatives and many more must be empirically tested. Here, again, this book's theme that research protects children is relevant. Only rigorous and objective research can provide the solutions we seek.

tions limit their abilities to solve problems and defend themselves, so they are unable to cope with situations that adults handle with ease. Infants and preschool children can become petrified if they lose sight of their parents in the supermarket, if they are addressed by a stranger, or if an enthusiastic hound bounds up to them and licks their faces. Everyday life presents many intimidating situations for young children, who lack fully developed physical and mental coping skills.

Children also learn specific fears from observing other people's fearful reactions or through adults' warnings to avoid potential threats. Parents can transmit their own fears to their children by showing their fear of thunderstorms, insects, blood, reptiles, or medical treatment. Fearful facial expressions, exclamations, and attempts to escape inadvertently teach children what to fear and how to show it. Playmates and siblings can be fearful models as well and may also enjoy frightening younger children by forcing them into scary encounters. Thus, children can acquire fears directly from frightening experiences with a particular object or situation or indirectly from verbal warnings or modeled fearful reactions of family members or playmates. There are many ways to become afraid, which may help explain why most children develop specific fears.

PHOBIAS

IN FOCUS 1 ▶ Define *phobia*, and explain how a phobia differs from separation anxiety disorder and generalized anxiety disorder.

The DSM-IV-TR diagnostic criteria recognize that children's phobic symptoms may differ from those of adults. The criteria for assessing whether children's fears are normal or pathological include the child's age and the duration, intensity, and type of fear. Intense, unusual fear that persists as the child grows and that interferes seriously with the child's functioning may be a mental disorder, **specific phobia** (also called **simple phobia**). The following are some clues that a child's intense fear may be a specific phobia:

1. *Age of onset.* Fears may be clinically significant when the age of onset is highly unusual, as when a child as old as 10 develops a strong aversion to dogs or strangers. Such fears are common among much younger children. When a fear reaction arises at a developmentally unusual or inappropriate time, it may represent a phobia rather than a normal childhood fear.
2. *Persistence.* A strong fear reaction that persists long after the usual age of occurrence could be a phobia. To qualify as a specific phobia, the fear must be intense, limited to a particular stimulus or situation, and persist for at least 6 months.
3. *Intensity.* Most mild fears are not abnormal. However, even developmentally common fears may be of clinical concern if they are so intense they become incapacitating. When a common fear, such as apprehension about public speaking, is strong enough to limit career choices severely or to prevent school attendance, it becomes pathological.
4. *Prevalence.* Some types of fear are so unusual that their very occurrence signals abnormality, as in some social fears. Social phobia is the incapacitating fear of certain situations from which escape could be difficult or embarrassing (e.g., leaving the safe confines of home and family to attend school or social occasions). This disorder, which is discussed later, precludes school attendance, interferes with social relationships with peers and with holding a job, and is clearly pathological whatever the person's age.

For youngsters under age 18, the phobia must persist for at least 6 months to be diagnosable, so that even if it is intense, a child's short-lived fear will not be mistaken for a clinically significant condition. Further, the fear must be severe enough to interfere with normal activities such as attending school, using public transportation, shopping, or visiting other public places. Unlike adults, children may not recognize that their fears are excessive or unreasonable, and so they rarely complain about them. However, when placed in the feared situation, children may scream and cry, have tantrums, physically freeze, or cling to a parent. In contrast, adolescents and adults are more likely to experience a devastating panic attack, in which they experience several minutes of terror that they are about to die, have a heart attack or stroke, lose control, or "go crazy." Exposure to the phobic stimulus or situation provokes intense anxiety, which leads to active attempts to avoid the feared situation whenever possible, and the distress is relieved when the threat is reduced or removed. To be considered a phobia, the person's fear and avoidance attempts must be sufficiently intense as to interfere significantly with normal functioning at school or home. Thus, for example, a phobic person cannot live next to a neighbor with a dog or cannot attend school or social occasions (American Psychiatric Association, 2000). Further, DSM-IV-TR criteria require the person to experience marked distress about having the phobia or other anxiety disorder.

SEPARATION ANXIETY DISORDER

One of the earliest fear reactions to appear is separation anxiety. Most 1-year-olds are afraid when separated from their usual caretaker, even for a few minutes, but they later tolerate separations as they grow into confident toddlers. However, some children grow less rather than more tolerant of separations from one or both of their parents. In such cases, **separation anxiety disorder** may be diagnosed, either before the age of 6 years, when it is termed *early onset*, or after 6 but before 18 years (DSM-IV-TR; American Psychiatric Association, 2000). Separation anxiety disorder is among the more common childhood problems, affecting approximately 4% of youngsters (American Psychiatric Association, 2000). In separation anxiety disorder, children show excessive, age-inappropriate worries about separation from a usually present loved one, typically their mother, or from their home. Such children are so distressed about separation that they may insist on knowing where their mom is at all times, sometimes phoning incessantly to check on her whereabouts when she is away for a short time or nearby visiting a neighbor or going to the store. This type of anxiety is age-inappropriate since it would be more normal and expected in an infant or toddler than in an older child or adolescent.

Although the DSM-IV-TR combines school refusal with other forms of separation anxiety, many authorities consider these separate, though related, as discussed later in this chapter. It is sometimes difficult to distinguish separation anxiety from a child's attempts to hold the mother's attention and keep her close, which are more related to issues of control and convenience than anxiety. Another contributing feature is the mother's anxiety about being separated from her child. Sometimes a problem in close-knit families is intense mutual dependence of parent and child.

GENERALIZED ANXIETY DISORDER

Some children see threats everywhere, even in the most unlikely situations, and they cannot be comforted or reassured. These children are likely to be suffering from generalized anxiety disorder. **Generalized anxiety disorder** consists of uncontrollable, excessive anxiety and worry, occurring consistently for at least 6 months and extending to many events or activities. It now includes a formerly separate category, *overanxious disorder of childhood* (American Psychiatric Association, 2000). Essentially, the child is anxious almost all the time about nearly everything. The child must also show at least one of the following in extreme form:

- irritability
- restlessness
- fatigue
- difficulty in concentrating
- muscle tension or sleep disturbance

Further, the child's anxiety must be sufficient to interfere with normal school or social activities. In extreme cases, children with anxiety disorders may refuse to eat or drink, and must be hospitalized (Fitzpatrick, 1998). Such children are unrealistic perfectionists about their work and very insecure and unsure of themselves no matter how well they do, even when they are not being evaluated by others (American Psychiatric Association, 2000). This behavior resembles obsessive-compulsive disorder. Generalized anxiety disorder can occur at any age after infancy but typically begins at around 10 years of age. The disorder is marked by physical complaints of respiratory distress, racing pulse, trembling, feeling faint, chills, or sweating. Many adults with generalized anxiety disorder say they have been very anxious all their lives (Kessler, Davis, & Kendler, 1997). This is not a condition that children simply outgrow.

Depression often accompanies generalized anxiety disorder. However, anxiety differs from depression in that anxious children are concerned about a threatened loss, such as the death of a parent, while depressed children are more likely to have already experienced a loss (Eley & Stevenson, 2000). Some researchers believe that fear and anxiety are mediated by different brain systems (Barlow, Chorpita, & Turovsky, 1996). The limbic system of the brain, which is thought to regulate anxiety, includes the hippocampus and the amygdala and is active in regulation of emotional experiences, physical expressions of emotional states, and impulse control. This system mediates activity between the brain stem and the cortex. Children who develop anxiety disorders usually first experience heightened and prolonged stress, then they suffer from severe anxiety, and, finally, some become depressed unless adequately treated. Anxiety and depression are closely associated in that both include a component of negative emotion or negative affectivity (Lerner et al., 1999; Seligman & Ollendick, 1998). However, anxiety and depression each have distinctive features (Murphy, Marelich, & Hoffman, 2000), as described here and in Chapter 8.

Unlike related disorders, generalized anxiety disorder involves widespread anxiety in many different situations, rather than only one or two. The other anxiety disorders are more focused on particular settings, people, or events. Generalized anxiety disorder and specific phobias are the most prevalent of the childhood psychological disorders, while obsessive-compulsive disorder and childhood depression are much less common (Silverman et al., 1995). Posttraumatic stress disorder can be traced to a particular event, in contrast to most of the other conditions covered in this chapter.

POSTTRAUMATIC STRESS DISORDER

People who have experienced a devastating event such as a catastrophic flood, fire, bombing, or criminal assault often develop an emotional disorder known as **posttraumatic stress disorder (PTSD)**. Often the victim or someone close to him was threatened with unavoidable severe injury or death and experienced sheer terror and helplessness. The DSM-IV-TR diagnostic criteria for PTSD include persistent and unwilling re-experiencing of the traumatic event, persistent attempts to avoid all thoughts and acts related to the event, and a high state of arousal evidenced by insomnia, irritability, difficulty concentrating, and exaggerated startle responses. Formerly, PTSD was considered to be uncommon in childhood, but research has indicated that children can and do develop this disorder, even if they were not directly physically threatened but only knew about the event (Vila, Porche, & Mouren-Simeoni, 1999). One study found that children who lost a parent were at particular risk for symptoms of PTSD, even compared to children who experienced a tornado disaster (Stoppelbein & Greening, 2000), testifying to the vital role played by parents in their children's emotional lives. In fact, in one study, a very high rate (24.6%) of children developed PTSD if they were exposed to traumatic events such as violent crime, family violence, accidents, or death or incapacity of a parent or someone close to them (McCloskey & Walker, 2000).

Catastrophic events affect people of all ages, but there are some gender and developmental differences in their reactions. For example, DSM-IV-TR states that for children, sexual abuse and sexually traumatic events can lead to PTSD without involving either threatened or actual physical injury. Girls may be five times more likely to develop PTSD than boys (Davis & Siegel, 2000), and their problems were found to persist at a 6-month follow-up (Tremblay, Martine, & Piche, 2000). The girls' greater vulnerability to PTSD may be because they are much more often the victims of sexual abuse. In addition, girls respond to exposure

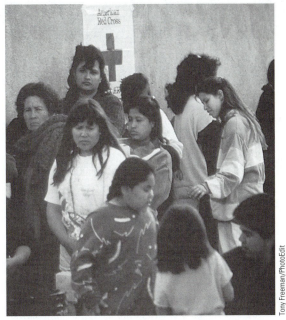

A natural disaster such as a hurricane can leave children with phobias and generalized anxiety disorder, even children who did not experience the disaster themselves but only heard about it.

to domestic and community violence with more PTSD symptoms than boys do (Berton & Stabb, 1996).

Posttraumatic stress disorder may develop immediately or months or even years following the stressful event. Children's major symptoms may include disorganized or agitated behavior. Other symptoms include persistent mental experiencing or play enactment of the traumatic event or the reverse—avoidance of anything associated with it. A child may appear to have little memory of a disaster at one time, but then play kidnapping scenes or storm scenes again and again at another time. Long periods of re-experiencing the event may alternate with long periods of avoidance and emotional numbing, making PTSD difficult to diagnose in children [American Academy of Child and Adolescent Psychiatry (AACAP), 1998]. Children display different symptoms at different ages and developmental levels. Young children are most likely to express some aspects of the traumatic situation in their play; for example, young auto accident victims may repeatedly enact accidents with toy cars. Young children also may have nightmares but be unable to report

Posttraumatic Stress Disorder in a Young Girl

Gail was a healthy, happy 5-year-old before her family's house was engulfed in flames one night. Everyone was asleep, and Gail's mother received second-degree burns over much of her body as she just managed to carry her daughter to safety. Her older brother could not escape and died in the fire. Gail's father was away on a business trip at the time.

Gail responded well to medical treatment after the fire, although she couldn't stay by herself at night and insisted on sleeping with her parents. In fact, she slept fitfully and had terrifying nightmares about being trapped when she did get to sleep. Everyone expected Gail to recover emotionally as her mother's burns healed and the family coped with their grief over her brother's death, but 3 months later, Gail had gotten worse and developed severe separation anxiety. She could not tolerate being left alone, even for short periods of time, and was also irritable, defiant, and hyperactive. She was fascinated by flames from candles and matches and would stare at them, while maintaining a rigid posture,

until someone extinguished them. Her pediatrician checked her thoroughly, but could not find a physical basis for her headaches, frequent stomachaches, and loss of appetite. Since Gail no longer appeared healthy and clearly was unhappy, her parents sought psychological treatment for her.

Gail's therapist used modeling of appropriate safety procedures so that Gail could detect and escape from fires or other emergencies, helping her to feel able to protect herself. Gail was also helped to lose her fascinated fear of candle and match flames through gradual exposure and relaxation training. Her parents were instructed in how to reduce her extreme dependence on them by gradually increasing the periods during which she was separated from them, while providing rewards for tolerating the separations. Other therapeutic techniques, such as play therapy and coping self-talk were used to increase Gail's feelings of self-efficacy and confidence. She may always have some emotional scars from the fire, but Gail is now a much less anxious, better-adjusted child.

their content. They may show difficulty in sleeping, irritability, attention problems, exaggerated startle responses, and some become hyperalert to many potential dangers and terrified by sirens, fire alarms, and other danger signals (American Psychiatric Association, 2000; Davis & Siegel, 2000). Physical symptoms such as stomachaches and headaches may appear, and young children may regress to baby talk, lose their toilet training, and become passive and clinging or defiant (Amaya-Jackson & March, 1995). Gail's Story describes posttraumatic stress disorder in a young child.

Psychologists have just begun to study the coping styles children use in dealing with highly stressful events. One group of researchers (Weisenberg, Schwarzwald, Waysman, Solomon, & Klingman, 1993) found differences in how well children under enemy missile attack during the Persian Gulf war handled the experience. Those who engaged in distraction and avoidance activities ("I talked to the others," "I

thought of things not connected to the situation") were less likely to develop stress reactions than children who focused on their problems ("I kept checking my gas mask," "I constantly checked to see if everyone was okay"). As expected, older children tended to use more effective distraction activities, including anger at those involved, than did younger children (Vernberg, La Greca, Silverman, & Prinstein, 1996). As the terrorist attacks of September 2001 show us, research on ways to counteract PTSD is desperately needed.

The limited research published on treatment of children exposed to disasters indicates that they get some immediate relief from support from teachers and classmates (Vernberg et al., 1996) and small group discussions led by mental health professionals (Weisenberg et al., 1993). Communities commonly bring in teams of counselors to help children when their schools or neighborhoods have been struck by a disaster. Parents and teachers need to convey a sense of calm control and safety to help children to avoid extreme emotional reactions (Davis & Siegel, 2000). The parents' reactions are particularly important in Hispanic and other cultures in which families seldom seek help from professional mental health services (Wasserstein & La Greca, 1998). The treatment approaches that show some effectiveness include cognitive-behavioral therapy, sometimes combined with family or group treatment (Yule, 1998). More research is needed to show the short-term and lasting benefits of treatments for children's PTSD.

However, diagnosis of this and other emotional disorders in children is difficult because: (1) there is overlap in the symptoms of the various anxiety, mood, and other internalizing disorders and (2) diagnosis depends heavily on self-reported anxiety, fear, or depression, and young children are often unable to tell others about their concerns. New, specialized self-rating scales and interviews and increased recognition that children may have an internalizing disorder all help in the detection of these conditions.

SOCIAL ANXIETY DISORDER, OR SOCIAL PHOBIA

Social anxiety disorder (also called *social phobia*) strikes 3.7% of Americans between the ages of 18 and 54 each year (NIMH, 1999). This anxiety disorder is much more common and more debilitating than was previously recognized (Kashdan & Herbert, 2001). Social anxiety disorder strikes many teens and has an average onset of 15 years of age (Schneier, Johnson, Hornig, Liebowitz, & Weissman, 1992). Social anxiety disorder is marked by extreme self-consciousness and incapacitating anxiety in social situations. It can be so severe that people avoid all possible social occasions and are unable to attend school, go to work, or make or keep friends. Like depression, social anxiety disorder occurs twice as often in women as in men, but men are more likely to seek help when they have this disorder.

This condition begins with the child complaining about pervasive fear of being observed and judged negatively by others and constant concern about inadvertently doing things that are humiliating. Children with social phobia worry far in advance about a social situation, such as a party, and, of course, the more

they worry, the less able they are to deal with the situation when it finally occurs. Surprisingly, social anxieties are likely to peak at informal social gatherings rather than at formal presentations, which are highly scripted. People can practice giving a report over and over until it is satisfactory, but they cannot so easily practice what to say when someone asks an unanticipated question. People with social phobia worry most about becoming tongue-tied when they are caught off-guard while everyone else is relaxing and enjoying themselves.

Compared with other children, social phobic children tend to dread social situations, anticipate more negative outcomes for themselves from these situations, and evaluate their own performance more negatively (Spence, Donovan, & Brechman-Toussaint, 1999). Interestingly, they actually are less skillful when they interact with others, and so they draw negative reactions from their peers. In a vicious cycle, their social skills problems lead to negative reactions from others, which in turn undermine their self-confidence, leading to further social failures. Both cognitive-behavioral therapy and medications are recommended for social anxiety disorder; medications that have been used include the SSRIs described in Chapter 8 for treatment of depression, the high-potency benzodiazepenes (minor tranquilizers), and the beta-blockers, which are used to control high blood pressure (National Institute of Mental Health, 1999). Clinical trials of these treatments are just beginning, so their effectiveness in general use remains to be demonstrated (Kashdan & Herbert, 2001).

SCHOOL-RELATED AVOIDANCE DISORDERS

There is growing evidence of co-occurrence of anxiety disorders and conduct disorder, which suggests that it would be misleading to draw a clear distinction between school refusal and truancy (Russo & Beidel, 1994).

School refusal refers to persistent avoidance of school motivated by intense fear and anxiety. This condition can stem from a specific phobia about some aspect of school (school phobia) or can indicate generalized anxiety or separation anxiety disorder. School refusal is not included in the DSM-IV-TR, except as a symptom of separation anxiety disorder. Nevertheless, some children suffer from school refusal, which stunts their academic achievement and social development, even though they do not meet the criteria for phobia or anxiety disorder. School refusers often are perfectionists who display excessive concerns about academic performance (Ficula, Gelfand, Richards, & Ulloa, 1983). The onset of school refusal often follows a set pattern. When the school day dawns, the child wakes up with a painful stomachache or headache. This often occurs when the child goes back to school, either on a Monday after a school vacation, at the beginning of the school year, or after being kept home by a minor illness. Moving to a new school may also set it off. When parents agree that the child can stay home from school, the child's physical complaints diminish dramatically, since avoiding school reduces the anxiety. The child becomes anxious and symptomatic whenever preparing for school, and so stays home, if the parents allow it. School refusal can arise from different causes, such as modeling of anxious and overprotective parents, having an anxiety disorder or specific phobia, or reacting to a frightening experience at school. School refusers can meet diagnostic criteria for one or more emotional disorders, or for none. However, they all share an anxious, insistent avoidance of school.

When the child's fear is centered on some aspect of the school, such as fear of a particular teacher, of being called on in class, or of entering the classroom, a specific phobia is diagnosed (sometimes called *school phobia*). Striking between 1.4 and 17 children per 1,000 (Rutter, Tizard, & Whitmore, 1981), school refusal is a more frequent childhood problem than some other, better known disorders such as childhood autism (see Chapter 13), and it is worldwide. Reported in many countries, school refusal is found wherever there is formal classroom education. By depriving children of an education, school refusal represents a serious social and economic problem.

Types of School Refusal

IN FOCUS 2 ▶ Describe the two types of school refusal, and note the prognosis for children with each type.

There are two types of school refusal: mild acute and severe chronic. In *mild acute school refusal*, which tends to affect younger children, there is little or no family discord and initial onset is sudden. Here, the prognosis is excellent, since the child's primary problem is school attendance. The usual treatment approach for these cases of school refusal is direct and often successful, and recurrences are rare. The principle of returning school-avoidant children to school as rapidly as possible is not a new one. Years ago, Kennedy (1965) recommended that the fearful child should begin by spending just a half hour at school and progressively increase time at school over several days. The child's somatic complaints about headaches, weakness, and stomachaches are dealt with matter-of-factly by scheduling medical examinations before or after school hours. This tactic ensures that possible physical illness receives prompt attention, but the child's complaints do not serve as a means for avoiding school. Rapid return to school remains the most often used treatment for simple school refusal or reluctance (Chorpita, Albano, Heimberg, & Barlow, 1996). Unfortunately, many children suffer from more serious and prolonged cases of school refusal accompanied by other psychological problems that are less easily treated. (See Angie's Story.)

Severe chronic school refusal in older children and teens has a much less favorable prognosis than mild acute school refusal. Chronic school refusal is typically seen in children older than 11 years who come from unstable families. These children may also suffer from depression, negative self-image, and difficulty in getting along with family members (Kearney & Silverman, 1995). Parents of children with chronic school refusal and anxiety disorders tend to be overcontrolling and are reluctant to give their children much independence (Rapee, 1997), which adds to the children's problems. Parents who are behaviorally deviant themselves or who express negative attitudes toward school are unlikely to help their children return to school. Adolescents with chronic school refusal have a poor prognosis and may also develop debilitating panic attacks and *agoraphobia*, or dread of becoming trapped somewhere away from home or unable to get help in an emergency (Rutter & Garmezy, 1983).

Management of School Refusal

As already mentioned, mild acute school refusal is best treated by the parents' firm but supportive insistence that the child gradually resume regular school

A Teenager with Anxiety-Related Disorders

Angie was a model student; her work was good and always turned in on time. She rarely missed a day of school and seemed eager to please her teachers. But this rosy picture changed when she entered junior high school. Her new school presented her with more challenging assignments and she feared she could not continue to do well. She became visibly worried and very concerned about every little thing. Her teachers reported that she would incessantly smooth out her papers and arrange things on her desk, trying to make things perfect, but she never succeeded to the point that it pleased her. So her busy hands kept on smoothing her papers and rearranging things on her desk even though it began to attract stares. Her grades were good, and her achievement test scores indicated that she had the ability to perform well, but she worried incessantly about dropping behind the class and never catching up. The teachers in junior high were more reserved and businesslike than those in elementary school, and they did not know Angie. Her worst fears were having to give a report before the class or go to the blackboard, and the thought of having the teacher call on her unexpectedly made her sit bolt upright in her bed. She worried that she would blush bright red, sweat so everyone could see it, and be totally unable to answer the teacher's questions. She began to complain about physical problems such as blinding headaches, and she woke up many times a night worrying about school.

The family doctor assured Angie's parents that there was nothing wrong and that she would adjust to the school and grow out of the headaches, but they persisted. Her dad said she kept to herself too much and should go out and have fun with her friends, but Angie had only one real friend and couldn't think of anything they would enjoy together. The once active and well-adjusted little girl her parents knew was being replaced by an anxiety-ridden teenager. Her mom knew how Angie felt, because she had gone through the same thing herself and had dropped out of school to marry as soon as she could. So when Angie began to come home early, before school was out, her mom didn't have the heart to send her back. Anyway, she enjoyed having Angie's company. Angie felt relieved on days when she and her mom decided she didn't have to go to Valley View Junior High. Her mother thought that home schooling might relieve the pressure on Angie to go to a school she hated.

Here are some of the clues that Angie could have anxiety disorders. Her attempts to have a perfectly organized desk and completely smooth, uncreased papers could represent compulsive behavior. She could be on the way to developing obsessive-compulsive disorder. She was also worrying too much about ordinary school routines that had not bothered her in the past. This raises the possibility of school refusal, separation anxiety, and even generalized anxiety disorder. Since she no longer attended school regularly and was often miserable, Angie needed professional help. Her mother loved her but was not helping through overprotectiveness and encouragement to avoid school. This pattern of mother-child enmeshment contributes to separation anxiety and school refusal, conditions that seem to run in families. Like many youngsters with school refusal, Angie showed signs of several different anxiety-related disorders and she was probably developing chronic school refusal, the more serious type. If someone at her school failed to spot the problem and initiate a discussion with Angie and her family on the importance of getting help for her, she could face many years of distress and social isolation.

SOURCES: Bernstein, Hektner, Burchardt, & McMillan (2001); Ficula, Gelfand, Richards, & Ulloa (1983).

---

attendance. Severe chronic school refusal is often accompanied by other psychological disorders and almost invariably requires professional attention. Behavioral and cognitive-behavioral interventions are widely accepted treatments (Elliott, 1999), but the complexity and severity of chronic school refusal require assessment and therapy tailored to the individual child. A combination of the tricyclic antidepressant imipramine and cognitive-behavioral therapy had failed to improve the anxiety and depression of many children with severe chronic school refusal who were assessed 1 year after the treatment (Bernstein, Hektner, Burchardt, & McMillan, 2001). These disappointing results suggest that prevention and early intervention programs should be developed. The condition is not easily remedied, so the best course would be to attempt to prevent it and/or to treat it before it becomes chronic.

ETIOLOGY OF ANXIETY DISORDERS

There are two main types of psychological explanations of childhood phobias: psychodynamic theories and social learning and cognitive theories. Both of these general approaches offer similar explanations of the origins of other anxiety disorders as well as depressive and other emotional disorders. Therefore, the following discussion of the origins of phobia formation also generally applies to internalizing disorders.

Psychodynamic Theory: Historical and Modern Forms

Originally, Freud's theory of psychoanalysis (Freud, 1963/1909) attributed phobias to psychologically created tension, anxiety, guilt, sexual jealousy, and rage. In his famous psychoanalytic interpretation of the horse phobia displayed by a 5-year-old boy named Hans, Freud (1963/1909) traced the boy's fear of horses to his presumed Oedipal sexual desires for his mother and his unconscious rage and fear toward his father. Freud argued that all of the child's emotions toward his father were displaced onto a powerful animal that reminded the boy of his father—the horse. His fear also permitted the boy to stay at home with his mother in order to avoid the horses in the streets. Under Freud's direction, the boy's father (who was a patient of Freud's) interpreted the psychological nature of his fear to Hans and the boy's horse phobia was overcome. This case provided the model for the psychoanalytic interpretation of children's phobias.

Sigmund Freud's psychoanalyst daughter, Anna, described children's anxieties as originally diffuse and vague but later becoming compressed into anxiety about one symbolic object, such as a dog, which represents an unconscious fear (Freud, 1977). The child believes she fears the symbolic figure (e.g., the animal),

but actually she fears becoming overwhelmed by sexual and aggressive feelings and probable retaliation from her parents if she acts on those feelings. Once the child's anxiety is redirected toward the symbolic, external object, she can reduce her anxiety to some extent by avoiding that object. Psychoanalysts believe that the choice of phobic object is not random, but depends on some actual or fancied resemblance to persons or events featured in the psychological conflict.

Present-day psychodynamic theory is loosely based on psychoanalysis, but emphasizes the importance of social rather than sexual attachments to parent figures. In this view, the phobic person unconsciously longs to be the center of a parent's attention and exclusive love ("Social phobia," 1994). Since this ideal situation is impossible, real or imagined rivals for the beloved parent's attention become internalized (introjected) images, which are critical and threatening and must be appeased. For example, the child may come to imagine that the father is a rival for the mother's love rather than a source of love. Being internalized and therefore inescapable, the child's fear takes the form of excessive self-criticism. In order to reduce anxiety caused by these internalized images, the child focuses the fear on some external object that has a special, symbolic connection with the fear. The child then develops a specific phobia or generalized anxiety as a way of expressing an unacceptable desire in a disguised form that does not stimulate ridicule or retaliation from others. In the case of social phobia, the unconscious fear of provoking the father's jealous rage is transferred to other people, so the child fears being dependent on or intimate with anyone, and avoids social contacts. Psychodynamic explanations of avoidant behavior continue to draw significant support, especially among practicing clinicians, although research validation of many of the concepts remains sparse.

Social Learning and Cognitive Approaches

Social cognitive theory (also called social learning theory) is largely research-based and emphasizes the role of modeling (observational learning) in the development of fears. The child may never actually encounter a dreaded object such as a tiger or snake, but still comes to fear it mightily. Why? Social learning suggests that the child observes and imitates the fearful reactions of parents, other children, and even of TV characters. People also may give the child verbal instructions (e.g., "Stay away from that snake! Snakes are so slimy; I can't stand them!"), as well as showing dramatic physical reactions such as grimacing, gesturing, or running away. Fears are most likely to be acquired through imitation and verbal instructions to be afraid (Bandura, 1969). However, phobias may arise more from lack of confidence in one's ability to handle a fear-provoking situation than from specific fears acquired from others.

Bandura's (1986) **self-efficacy theory** maintains that people do not develop fears so much from fright paired with the sight of the feared object as from anxiety that they cannot successfully avoid the feared object and protect themselves. Their lack of self-confidence leads them to dwell on the possibility of losing control, being injured, or embarrassing themselves publicly. Their fears can be reduced if they begin to believe that they can successfully manage an encounter with a snake, spider, business client, or audience of more than four people.

Ironically, children do not necessarily fear things that actually could harm them. For example, children are much more likely to be hit by automobiles or to drown than to be bitten by a wolf or a snake. Yet they tend to fear wolves and snakes more than cars or bodies of water. Parents must make special attempts to teach children realistic fears and help them overcome unrealistic ones. Similarly, parents should avoid an attitude of anxious overcontrol of their children, because this is likely to convince children that they are incapable of functioning on their own.

Biological Contributors to Phobias and Anxiety

IN FOCUS 3 ▶ How do a mother's history of anxiety disorder and a child's temperament contribute to the child's risk of developing an anxiety disorder?

Researchers are beginning to find answers to the puzzle of why some people are highly anxious and likely to develop anxiety disorders. There are hints in the research findings that there may be complex, multiple-gene contributions to anxiety and panic disorders (Plomin, DeFries, McClearn, & Rutter, 1997). Also, children of mothers, but not fathers, who have a lifetime history of anxiety disorder have double the risk of developing an anxiety disorder themselves. The

risk triples if the mother has co-occurring anxiety and depressive disorder, which is usually a more severe condition than either anxiety or depression alone (McClure, Brennan, Hammen, & Le Brocque, 2001). Parenting practices did not seem to make a difference in such children's adjustment, suggesting that there may be a genetic basis or some other biological basis for their high risk for anxiety disorders. This does not mean that a genetic tendency to develop anxiety invariably results in a disorder, but that, under certain conditions of stress and threat, a genetically predisposed person is more likely to develop anxiety disorder than the ordinary person is.

People have long noticed that some babies have shy, fearful, and anxious temperaments. These infants and toddlers seem alarmed by novelty, are wary of unfamiliar adults, and hang back rather than initiate normal approaches to new playmates (Fox, Henderson, Rubin, Calkins, & Schmidt, 2001). These shy children have unusual physiological reactions as well. When confronted with a startle stimulus, such as a sudden loud noise or novel visual pattern, they display a fast and stable heart rate (their pulse races). In addition, they react with high baseline cortisol levels (a stress hormone) and exaggerated muscle tension (indicated by EMG amplitude) (Kagan, Reznick, & Snidman, 1987; Schmidt, Fox, & Schulkin, 1999). Their parents describe such babies as anxious or fearful (Rubin, Nelson, Hastings, & Asendorpf, 1999). Children who continue to respond poorly to novelty as toddlers and preschoolers show larger resting activation in right frontal brain areas (right versus left frontal activity as measured by EEG) than other children (Fox et al., 2001). This finding suggests that stable differences in brain activity may characterize certain children, who later prove to be particularly susceptible to specific fears, phobias, and perhaps anxiety disorders when subjected to stress.

PROGNOSIS FOR CHILDREN WITH PHOBIAS AND ANXIETY DISORDERS

Fortunately, most early phobias are quickly and effectively treated. Brief psychotherapy and cognitive-behavioral therapy can produce significant improvement in most simple phobias, and some anxiety disorders are overcome without professional treatment (Last, Perrin, Hersen, & Kazdin, 1996). Thus, the prognosis can be quite positive for children with specific phobias, but not for those with severe anxiety disorders that begin in childhood and may continue into adulthood (Kendall et al., 1992). When they persist, only around 20% of these disorders are finally overcome (American Psychiatric Association, 2000). Fears that tend to continue throughout life include fear of physical illness and social anxiety disorder, which incapacitates people in social situations (Vasey, 1993).

PSYCHOLOGICAL INTERVENTIONS FOR ANXIETY DISORDERS AND PHOBIAS

IN FOCUS 4 ▶ What are four types of psychotherapy used to treat anxiety disorders?

Psychodynamic Therapies

Because psychoanalysts do not view the anxious or phobic behavior itself as the child's central problem, they do not advocate treatments based on encounters with feared situations. Rather, the child is encouraged to act out fears and fantasies in play within the accepting atmosphere of the therapy sessions. The analyst interprets the underlying meaning of the child's fantasies, play themes, and dreams. During analysis, the child's troubling unconscious feelings are transferred from the parents to the analyst and re-experienced as intense rage against or love of the analyst within the safe treatment environment. When treating older, more cognitively mature children and adolescents, the analyst points out the importance and meaning of the transference, which helps the patients to understand and overcome past relationship problems.

Heinecke (1989) offered the example of a young boy named John, who became furious at his mother for being late, making him late for his therapy appointment, thus failing to protect him as he believed a mother should. John's anger became evident when the therapist was also a few minutes late. At first, John said it didn't matter and he didn't want to discuss it, but he then began to throw balls provocatively at the

therapist and at a plant in the office. He seemed to want to communicate some message to the therapist that he could not describe in words. Later, in his free play, John pretended there were two ferocious catlike animals that threatened to destroy each other. This prompted the therapist to interpret John's resistance and the underlying anger as follows: "It is very difficult for you to let me know how angry you were at being kept waiting, because your anger might really destroy me and I would in turn destroy you." John: "NO, no, no. Let's get on with the game." When it occurs at the right time in the therapy process, this type of interpretive therapeutic interchange is thought to free patients from the parental introjections (imagined parental reactions) responsible for their incapacitating feelings of guilt and shame. The child's phobic reaction is expected to disappear without specific intervention when his basic psychological conflicts have been resolved and his troublesome misconceptions have been corrected through the analyst's enlightening interpretations. The parent's role is limited to supplying information that is pertinent to the child's problem, but which the child may be unwilling or unable to discuss. Most parents are also in analysis themselves with another therapist; so treatment of parent and child proceeds in parallel, and both may improve together.

Critique of Psychodynamic Therapies

Psychoanalysis and analytic play therapy are very expensive and time-consuming, sometimes requiring 2 or more years of individual treatment sessions. Health insurance is unlikely to pay for more than a few weeks of therapy, so psychodynamic treatment is prohibitively expensive for most families. Many eclectic psychotherapies for children include some aspects of psychodynamic treatment, such as the therapist's interpretations of the child's feelings, but are much less lengthy and expensive. For example, psychodynamic interpretations of the meaning of a child's play and use of play materials and the idea of releasing the child's emotions in such therapy are components of psychodynamic treatment that have become incorporated into the mainstream of child psychotherapy. There have been a number of case reports of successful psychoanalytic treatment of children with phobias, but, as noted in Chapter 3, uncontrolled case studies do not provide scientifically accepted evidence of treatment success.

Desensitization Therapies

Desensitization methods focus on the child's learning to relax in stress-inducing circumstances. Systematic desensitization was first developed for use with phobic adults (Wolpe, 1958) and later adapted for use with adolescents and children (Kendall et al., 1992). The client is first helped to construct a fear hierarchy, ranking his fears from the least to the most severe. For example, a mild-intensity fear item for a test-anxious child might be "You hear about a friend who has to take a test soon." The most intense fear item on this child's hierarchy might be "You are taking a test, and you don't remember any of the answers and know you won't be able to finish in the amount of time left." Then the therapist teaches the client a set of exercises to deeply relax the different muscle groups throughout the body. Relaxation is used to counteract the muscular tension associated with fear and anxiety, since it is impossible to be tense and anxious and yet relaxed at the same time. Ideally, the client first imagines the least potent of his fears (e.g., seeing a picture of a classroom) while relaxing his body completely. Then he is helped to imagine increasingly frightening scenes while maintaining a state of relaxation. At the conclusion of treatment, the child should be able to maintain relaxation even while imagining or encountering the most intimidating situations.

Although the imagining procedures have successfully treated adults, there is only mixed research evidence for their effectiveness as the sole form of intervention in the treatment of younger children's fears (Morris & Kratochwill, 1983). However, relaxation exercises have been incorporated in many other types of therapy, especially cognitive-behavioral therapy for children as well as adults.

Children may respond better to graded presentation of threats in a real-life setting (in vivo desensitization), in which they practice relaxation in the actual situation they fear. One study found that water-phobic children between the ages of 3 and 8 benefited more from actual exposure to water than from imagining aquatic scenes in a systematic desensitization procedure (Menzies & Clarke, 1993). All desensitization

therapies take place in gradual steps. For example, the child who fears some aspect of school might be presented with the following sequence of experiences:

- A visit to the school building while school is not in session
- A visit to the building for a few minutes during her favorite school activity
- Sitting in on an entire class, for example, a social studies class
- Finally maintaining relaxation during most or all of an actual school day

A drawback of this approach is that neither systematic desensitization nor in vivo desensitization teaches the child how to deal with the situations or objects she fears. Because children so often lack needed social, athletic, or cognitive skills, they may require treatment other than desensitization, such as the approaches based on modeling and imitation that are described next.

Modeling and Guided Participation

Guided participation (also called guided mastery treatment) is a very effective method for treating children's specific fears and phobias, especially ones that are limited to a particular situation or stimulus (Kendall et al., 1992). In this treatment approach, the child's confidence is first built by simply watching someone else deal with the feared stimulus. One or more models demonstrate increasingly closer encounters with whatever the child fears. The child can see that there are no untoward results for the models and nothing to fear. Moreover, the child learns effective methods for dealing with dogs, snakes, injections, or other dreaded stimuli. This treatment method is particularly effective when a variety of adult and child models participate and they encounter and overcome several different examples of the feared stimulus (Bandura, Blanchard, & Ritter, 1969). To illustrate, two adults and three children might act as models and demonstrate how various people interact with dogs of three different breeds. Modeling displays can conveniently and effectively be presented on videotape, making it unnecessary to assemble a large cast of models and snakes, dogs, medical personnel, thunderstorms, or whatever is needed in the child's treatment.

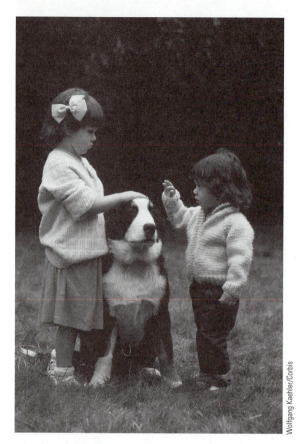

A fearless child teaches an apprehensive younger child to pet a large (and also very brave) dog.

In guided participation, the fearful child engages in carefully supervised confrontations with the feared situations in a natural context, with gradually increasing performance requirements. For example, after viewing fearless models, snake-avoidant children are required to touch the arm of a person who is petting a nonpoisonous snake, to stroke the snake with gloved hands, and finally to lift and handle the reptile (Ritter, 1968). Through guided practice, the therapist teaches the client to do feared tasks without awkwardness, self-imposed restrictions (handling reptiles only with gloves on), or defensive coping rituals (approaching dogs backward in order to be able to run away). Of course, this intervention requires a fearless therapist, who can handle snakes, accompany an apprehensive phobic driver on a high-speed freeway, and undertake other potential dangers (Williams & Zane, 1997).

Guided participation has been employed with highly focused phobias, which makes it especially helpful with younger children. More evidence is needed concerning the effectiveness of this and other stimulus-exposure treatments in relieving less focused types of fears and anxieties, such as generalized anxiety and fear of social situations or social and academic evaluation (King, 1993). Most clinical treatments involve several types of procedures, including systematic modeling and desensitization.

Cognitive-Behavioral Treatments

Anxiety disorders sometimes require complex psychological treatments. **Multifaceted cognitive-behavioral treatment**, which was developed by Phillip Kendall (Kendall, 1993; Kendall et al., 1997), is remarkably effective in overcoming children's anxiety disorders. In fact, having been rigorously tested in controlled research, individual cognitive-behavioral treatment is now considered by the American Psychological Association, Division 12, to be "probably efficacious" in the treatment of anxiety disorders in youth (Kendall et al., 1997). The treatment includes cognitive techniques, such as (1) modifying the child's anxious self-talk (e.g., "I'm helpless, I'm going to throw up or run away and make a fool of myself if I have to go into the swimming pool.") and (2) teaching problem-solving and behavioral strategies, including graded exposure to fear situations, practice in evaluating potentially threatening situations, and reward for successful efforts. The children first imagine (desensitization) and then actively participate in previously avoided situations. Active interventions are then introduced to overcome their persistent worrying and develop adequate coping repertoires in the avoided situation. In problem-solving training, the child is helped to devise appropriate plans for confronting the feared situation, such as recognizing that an unfamiliar teacher will not hurt her, making eye contact with the teacher, and saying hello. When a situation is no longer perceived as dangerous and fear-provoking, the child is free to act constructively and more effectively.

After the treatment, 64% of the children in one study no longer met diagnostic criteria for anxiety disorder (Kendall, 1993). These gains were maintained at a follow-up a year later, and a replication study found the same impressive results for the effectiveness of this cognitive-behavioral therapy (Kendall et al., 1997). Another study of the longer-term effectiveness of cognitive-behavioral therapy found that treatment gains were maintained over a period of 5 to 7 years, as measured by parent and child reports and clinician ratings (Barrett, Duffy, Dadds, & Rapee, 2001). It remains to be seen whether untreated children also improve over an extended time period, as some studies suggest (Last et al., 1996). Like other psychotherapies, cognitive-behavioral interventions require the services of highly trained practitioners, which makes them expensive, even though they may be limited to 16 sessions. Kendall's group recently reported that group cognitive-behavioral treatment is nearly as effective as individual treatment, while being less costly (Flannery-Schroeder & Kendall, 2000).

MEDICATIONS FOR ANXIETY DISORDERS AND SPECIFIC PHOBIAS

Because children suffering from anxiety disorders often have depression as well, they may be given antidepressants that may also relieve their anxiety (discussed in Chapter 8). A recent study of fluvoxamine (Luvox) was conducted with children and adolescents with anxiety disorders who failed to respond to 3 weeks of psychotherapy (Walkup et al., 2001). Fluvoxamine produced improvements in 76% as compared with 29% of those who received placebos. Thus, fluvoxamine may be an effective treatment for children and adolescents with social phobia, separation anxiety disorder, or generalized anxiety disorder. However, studies of possible age and gender differences in responsiveness are needed.

Other drugs have proven useful in reducing anxiety in adults. The benzodiazepines (minor tranquilizers), usually alprazolam (Xanax) or clonazapam (Klonopin), can provide short-term relief of anxiety and thus boost the effectiveness of psychotherapy for adults and younger clients, although additional research support for their use with children is required (Kaplan & Hussain, 1995). Also, the benzodiazapines can impair thinking and physical functioning, making people less alert and interfering with activities such as driving. Worse still, these drugs produce dependency and so can be safely taken for only short periods of time.

Panic disorder occurs infrequently in children, but affects a significant number of adolescents. One drug, clonazepam, has been found to reduce panic attacks and improve school functioning in adolescents (Kutcher & Reiter, cited in Riddle et al., 1999). Adults with panic disorder may benefit from the tricyclic antidepressant imipramine or cognitive-behavioral therapy, or both in combination. Although both imipramine and cognitive-behavioral therapy produced immediate improvement, the therapy had more lasting beneficial effects than the drug (Barlow, Gorman, Shear, & Woods, 2000). The risk of cardiac problems from imipramine and its limited effectiveness in treating separation anxiety disorder (Burns, Hoagwood, & Mrazek, 1999) suggest that cognitive-behavioral therapy is the safer and more promising treatment for younger clients. Psychopharmacology is a rapidly changing and advancing field, and improved medications for a wider range of children's psychological disorders can be expected in the future.

OBSESSIVE-COMPULSIVE DISORDER

Obsessive-compulsive disorder differs markedly from the normal worries and insistence on familiar routines found in most young children. Most infants and toddlers have a familiar, and insisted-on, bedtime routine of being sung to or read to from familiar books, having a pacifier to suck, or hugging a favorite stuffed animal or ragged old security blanket while going to sleep. Children are likely to protest in no uncertain terms if their established routines are not carried out. These common rituals apparently reassure youngsters and provide a sense of security. In contrast, pathological obsessive-compulsive behavior consists of attempts to reduce severe anxiety and involves unusual activities such as repeated hand-washing, bathing, and scrubbing already spotless surroundings. Also, most childhood rituals are abandoned naturally as the child becomes older, while obsessive-compulsive routines often persist. When assessed between 2 and 7 years after they were first diagnosed, 43% of one group of children and adolescents still had obsessive-compulsive disorders, and only 6% were judged to be markedly improved, despite receiving multiple treatments (Swedo et al., 1993). Some young children develop compulsions, apparently without obsessions. Compulsive children are particularly likely to engage in rituals involving washing (Rapoport, Swedo, & Leonard, 1992), and they may also repeatedly place objects in a particular arrangement or check on the presence and location of certain objects over and over again. These children may also develop phobias, depression, and neurological conditions such as Tourette's disorder, which is also marked by compulsive actions. In fact, obsessions more often accompany other problems, such as depression or phobias, than occur alone. Obsessions are likely to persist throughout life, although they may become weaker or more pronounced at different periods.

Obsessive-compulsive disorder shares some symptoms with the previously discussed anxiety disorders, but also has unique features. In order to be diagnosed as obsessive-compulsive disorder, either obsessions or compulsions or both must be present and must constitute the person's major psychological problem (DSM-IV-TR, American Psychiatric Association, 2000). The DSM-IV-TR diagnostic criteria (used by permission of the American Psychiatric Association) indicate that obsessions and compulsions are senseless, repeated thoughts, images, or impulses (obsessions) or repetitive acts (compulsions) that are

1. unrealistic and dysfunctional
2. experienced as unwelcome but irresistible
3. experienced as products of one's own mind rather than external threats
4. ritualistic and stereotyped
5. time-consuming (require more than 1 hour each day)
6. disruptive of everyday activities

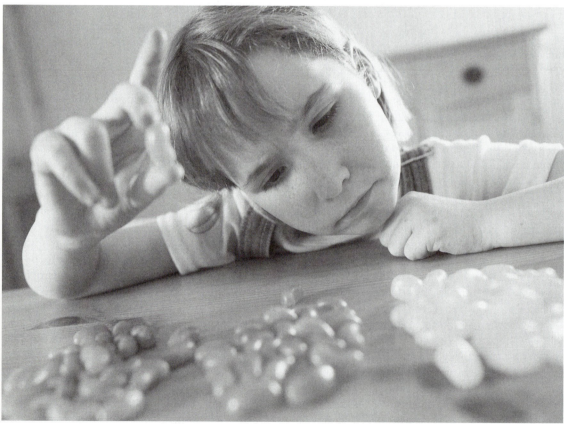

Children with obsessive-compulsive disorder spend inordinate amounts of time arranging objects and trying to control their environment.

Obsessive-compulsive disorder begins in childhood or adolescence in half or more of the cases (Rapoport et al., 2000). Typical obsessive themes of school-age children involve contamination by contact with supposedly unclean objects, aggression, and maintaining ultrastrict order. Many are overwhelmed by fear that their parents or other family members will be killed or injured. Obsessions are unwelcome thoughts that are neither realistic nor constructive and may even prevent the person from engaging in normal everyday activities. In contrast, compulsions are unusual acts that the person cannot stop repeating. Some kids lose sleep because they are compelled to check under their bed endlessly, others must stop and wipe their possessions over and over because they might be contaminated, and yet others cannot stop tapping the wall or a table continually. People are more likely to engage in rituals at home than in public, and many keep their embarrassing ritualistic behaviors hidden; so the prevalence of these acts may be seriously underestimated. Children with obsessive-compulsive disorder often hide their condition, so semistructured interviews by a trained mental health professional are particularly important in diagnosing this disorder (Rapoport et al., 2000).

For many years, psychoanalytic theory provided the generally accepted explanation of obsessive-compulsive disorder. Maladaptive thoughts and rituals were believed to be caused by anxiety resulting from unconscious psychological conflict. Compulsions were seen as avoidance maneuvers engaged in to reduce anxiety and magically prevent some dreaded event such as the death of a parent. In the psychoanalytic view, the patient imagines that performing the compulsive ritual will prevent the threatening event, but the ritual produces only a little relief from anxiety. The compulsive act is construed as the child's attempt to control unconscious hostility toward others, particularly the parents (Breuer & Freud, 1957/1895). More recent psychological explanations stress that compulsive behavior can arise from various sources and can be continued for many different reasons.

Some neuroscientists believe that obsessive-compulsive disorder may have a physical basis. Brain-imaging studies show unusual activation of circuitry between the frontal lobes and basal ganglia in people with obsessive-compulsive disorder. This disorder also co-occurs frequently with disorders of the basal ganglia, such as Tourette's syndrome (Rapoport et al., 2000). These results are stimulating a search for a physiological basis for this puzzling disorder.

Treatment of Obsessive-Compulsive Disorder

IN FOCUS 5 ▶ Describe the most often recommended form of treatment for obsessive-compulsive disorder.

The most highly recommended treatment for pediatric patients with obsessive-compulsive disorder is cognitive-behavioral therapy, either alone or combined with a selective serotonin reuptake inhibitor (SSRI) such as Zoloft or Prozac (March, Frances, Kahn, & Carpenter, 1997). In cognitive-behavioral psychotherapy, obsessive-compulsive clients overcome their compulsive behavior through contact with the situation they dread. Imagined exposure to the anxiety-provoking event may be followed by guided, prolonged exposure to the feared stimulus (March, Franklin, Nelson, & Foa, 2001). Alternatively, the exposure may be in the form of a sudden confrontation with the feared stimulus, without a gradual progression. Treatment may also include physical prevention of compulsive routines (response prevention), such as totally blocking excessive hand-washing or walking in unusual patterns. For example, a 14-year-old compulsive hand-washer might be instructed to think about having a spot on his hand, then think about having his hands covered with mud, and then go on to examine a dirty sink, touch the sink, and clean it, all without washing his hands. Eventually, he must refrain from the ritualistic washing of his hands throughout a 3-week treatment period. Contact with water or other cleaning agents is prohibited, except for a 10-minute shower every fifth day, and the process is closely supervised by family members (McCarthy & Foa, 1988). Alternatively, the water may be turned off, making the ritual impossible to perform. A compulsive object arranger might be deprived of objects to manipulate. The goal is a compelling demonstration to the person that engaging in the compulsive behavior is not necessary and that nothing bad happens if it is not performed. To help the child or teen to endure this uninviting treatment, therapists introduce certain cognitive interventions:

- *constructive self-talk*, or pep talks that the child gives herself

Back to the Beginning
Follow-up on Kidnapping Victim

The 12-year-old girl who was kidnapped showed clear symptoms of PTSD months afterward. Whether she would develop PTSD in full form would depend on several factors, including how well her parents handled the situation emotionally. Family members can serve as steadying, reassuring companions, or they can further alarm the child by anxiously asking questions, showing alarm at each telephone ring, and generally showing their own anxiety. Further, the child's past adjustment history makes a difference; better-adjusted children adapt better following extreme trauma. A child's feelings of self-efficacy will be tested by an uncontrollable event such as kidnapping or a natural disaster, but a child who was self-confident in the past will be more likely to adjust than one who was timid and uncertain. However, it is important for a child who has been through a devastating event to be interviewed by a qualified clinician and followed up in several later interviews, since PTSD can appear after some delay.

- *cognitive restructuring*, or thinking of the task differently
- *nonattachment*, or cultivating a tolerant, noninvolved attitude

Clients must knowingly agree to these relatively restrictive treatment conditions in the expectation that they will improve. Both the youngster and the parent must give written consent. They cannot be assured that even this dramatic form of therapy will successfully remove persistent obsessions and compulsions. Although this is among the best available psychological treatments, much more research is necessary to increase its power.

SSRIs such as domipramine (Anafranil) and fluoxetine (Prozac) are increasingly used to treat children's depression and anxiety disorders. Fluvoxamine (Luvox) has been approved by the FDA for use in treating children with obsessive-compulsive disorder. Fluvoxamine is well tolerated and acts rapidly and effectively in the short term for childhood obsessive-compulsive disorder; in studies by one team of researchers, 42% of those who took this drug improved versus 26% who improved after being given a placebo (Riddle et al., 1999, 2001). The longer-term effectiveness of fluvoxamine is unknown. Because all potent medications have some unintended effects, physicians should use particular caution in administering any type of psychoactive drugs to children. If children are not in immediate danger, the safest rule is to employ drug therapy only after psychological therapies have been tried and failed to give relief (Kaplan & Hussain, 1995).

Overall, psychotherapy and drug treatment seem to be about equally effective in treating anxiety disorders, although more testing is required. Neither the drugs nor the cognitive-behavioral psychotherapy help more than about 60% of children who suffer from obsessive-compulsive disorder. In an attempt to boost treatment effectiveness, some clinicians recommend comprehensive case management, including cognitive-behavioral therapy, family therapy, and medication (McGough, Speier, & Cantwell, 1993). However, it cannot be assumed that if one type of treatment is somewhat effective, adding another type of treatment will be even more effective. Any possible benefits from combining treatments must receive research scrutiny (Kazdin, 2001).

SUMMARY

The internalizing disorders include specific phobias, panic disorder, generalized anxiety disorder, posttraumatic stress disorder, and obsessive-compulsive disorder. Some level of fear, worry, and anxiety is normal, and there is a predictable succession of specific fears during development, beginning with fears of unfamiliar and intense stimuli and progressing to separation anxiety, fears of animals, and, later, fear of threats to physical safety and fear about the future. When fears or anxiety reach an incapacitating level for a prolonged period of time, a phobia or anxiety disorder is diagnosed. Although some anxiety disorders can appear at any age, others are more age-specific; an example is separation anxiety disorder, which overwhelms young children when they are away from their mother or other regular caretaker. While panic disorder is very rare in children, severe specific phobias, anxiety disorders, and school refusal are fairly prevalent. Once diagnosed, children with phobias and other anxiety disorders may receive some type of psychotherapy, especially cognitive-behavioral therapy, modeling and guided participation, or desensitization. Although many children receive various prescription drugs for anxiety-related symptoms, there is little solid research evidence on effectiveness of most medications, and negative side effects are possible.

Various types of trauma can lead to posttraumatic stress disorder. Child trauma victims are often treated in group-counseling sessions in schools, a humane intervention of unknown effectiveness. Posttraumatic stress disorder is insufficiently studied to permit a recommendation concerning its treatment.

Finally, obsessive-compulsive disorder can plague the lives of children for years, making it difficult for them to function normally because of their odd and time-consuming rituals and extreme anxiety. Psychological theories seem insufficient to explain this disorder, and new research suggests a possible physiological origin. Combined psychotherapy and drug treatment is a promising intervention.

Much remains to be investigated about the anxiety disorders, which is important, especially in view of their alarming increase in recent years. That children's emotional problems have increased so much attests to the truth of one of the themes of this book: that children develop in social contexts and respond to major social trends. Changes in marriage and divorce rates, increases in financially stressed single-parent families, threats to children's physical safety at school, growing occupational insecurity, and the failure of government-provided health and economic security nets all add to the worrisome contexts in which some children grow up.

INFOTRAC COLLEGE EDITION

For more information, explore this resource at http://www.infotrac-college.com/Wadsworth. Enter the following search terms:

anxiety in children
posttraumatic stress disorder in children
phobias
fears in children
school refusal/phobia
coping
cognitive behavioral therapy
stress

IN FOCUS ANSWERS

IN FOCUS 1 ▶ Define *phobia*, and explain how a phobia differs from separation anxiety disorder and generalized anxiety disorder.

- A phobia is a severe, incapacitating fear of some specific thing that persists for at least 6 months.
- Separation anxiety disorder is defined as severe, age-inappropriate concern about separation from the mother or home.
- Generalized anxiety disorder is intense, uncontrollable worry about a multitude of events or situations.

IN FOCUS 2 ▶ Describe the two types of school refusal, and note the prognosis for children with each type.

- Mild acute school refusal affects younger children and has sudden onset. Prognosis is good if a quick return to school is encouraged.
- Severe chronic school refusal occurs in older children from unstable families and those with adjustment problems. Prognosis is less favorable than for the milder form.

IN FOCUS 3 ▶ How do a mother's history of anxiety disorder and a child's temperament contribute to the child's risk of developing an anxiety disorder?

- Risk is greatly increased when the mother has a lifetime history of anxiety disorder, especially with co-occurring depressive disorder.
- Children with shy, fearful temperaments and greater right frontal brain activation are at greater risk for anxiety disorders.

- Psychodynamic therapies based on interpretation and resolution of unconscious conflicts
- Desensitization therapies based on relaxing while confronting successively more threatening, feared stimuli
- Modeling and guided participation based on building self-efficacy through mastering successively more feared and avoided activities
- Multifaceted cognitive-behavioral treatment including relaxation, desensitization, skills training, and positive self-talk

IN FOCUS 5 ▶ Describe the most often recommended form of treatment for obsessive-compulsive disorder.

- Cognitive-behavioral therapy featuring confrontations with the avoided situations, used either alone or in combination with medication
- Use of a selective serotonin reuptake inhibitor (SSRI) such as Prozac or Zoloft

Depression and Other Mood Disorders

In the Beginning

Faces of Depression

- Tanya, at age 10, was clearly unhappy, but no one knew why. Her mother took Tanya to the doctor because she refused to eat and would throw up if forced to eat even a little. But her doctor found no physical illness. Furthermore, Tanya was a worry-wart, always afraid of everything, and now she was too nervous to go to her dance class or to play with her friends. She said her dancing stunk, and she didn't like dancing anymore, she had no friends, and no one liked her anyway. She told her mother she hated her when her mother tried to force Tanya to try to smile and cheer up.

- His parents were worried about 13-year-old Dave, because they knew the teenage years could be difficult and because he was having so many problems. His grades had become atrocious, and he just sat slumped at his desk staring vacantly when they forced him to do his homework. He didn't try to do anything at all, and he looked remote and sad all the time. His parents thought the trouble was that he was smoking a lot of dope and running with the wrong crowd, and he had been arrested for shoplifting. His dad had been hospitalized several times for severe depression, and his parents were wondering if Dave was destined to become depressed, too.

- Joe was a tall, thin, serious-appearing high school senior who had worked extra hard in school and earned grades good enough to qualify for some top colleges. Anyway, he was awkward and wasn't good at any sport he had ever tried. His family teased him that he was like a little businessman and never just had fun like a normal kid. He secretly thought that he was dumb and so had to compensate with hard work, that his personality wasn't the greatest, and that he would be lucky to get into a decent college. He felt like a fake and was afraid everyone would find out how hopelessly inadequate he really was. What if he actually got accepted at an Ivy League school? He couldn't possibly do the work. Joe was losing sleep worrying and felt his family would be better off without him, before he brought shame on them. He had been feeling worse and worse for nearly 3 months and nothing made him feel better. He felt trapped.

These three young people illustrate many aspects of depression, including its roots and characteristics. These stories describe danger signals that go beyond normal bad mood and may be symptoms of a depressive disorder requiring professional treatment. It is important that families and teachers recognize these danger signals and get immediate mental health help for such kids.

INTRODUCTION

This chapter describes children's depression and other mood disorders, including the possible causes of these disorders and the outlook for children who develop them. We also survey the availability and effectiveness of antidepressant drugs and psychological treatments, as well as programs aimed at preventing youngsters from becoming seriously depressed.

Depression was once thought to be strictly an adult disorder, believed not to attack children. Now mental health experts recognize that mood disorders, especially depression, do affect children as well as teenagers and adults. Despite popular preconceptions about children being naturally happy, they are vulnerable to depression under adverse genetic and environmental conditions. Long dismissed as trivial and temporary, mood disorders in early life are now considered potentially serious, long-term conditions requiring skilled professional treatment. Perhaps the possibility of childhood depression was downplayed in the past because children's depression symptoms are slightly different from those of adults (as will be discussed later).

Although suicidal thoughts and actions are among the symptoms of adult depression, prepubescent children rarely become suicidal. During adolescence, depression rates increase, and suicide becomes one of the leading causes of death among teenagers. This chapter describes signs of suicidal intent, emergency measures to protect suicidal youths, and programs to prevent future attempts. This information is useful to parents and teachers of kids like Joe, the high school senior introduced at the beginning of this chapter who had begun to think about ending his life.

How did the increased recognition of juvenile depression come about? Several developments in the past few decades made people aware that children can suffer from mood disorders:

- Primary care physicians such as pediatricians and family medicine practitioners began to realize that children could be clinically depressed. Pharmaceutical companies, eager to market psychoactive medications, alerted physicians that children might be depressed and need antidepressant medication. In response, sales of antidepressant medications for children soared.
- Children's rights to mental health treatment, including relief from anxiety and depression, received increased public recognition.
- Research on the genetics of emotional disorders flourished. Increasing depression rates among adults sparked interest in exploring their psychiatric histories to look for a possible genetic basis for their disorders. Research findings that many depressed adults suffered from depression as children stimulated efforts to detect and treat early depression.
- Many reliable measures of depression became available. Behavior checklists and rating scales provide easy and effective methods to screen large numbers of children and identify possible anxiety and depression. Teachers, parents, mental health professionals, and children themselves use well-designed questionnaires and symptom checklists to detect both internalizing and externalizing disorders.

TYPES OF MOOD DISORDERS

IN FOCUS 1 ▶ List the different types of mood disorders.

Mood disorders, including depressive disorders, are considered to be recurrent, but the course is highly varied. Clinical depression may disappear forever

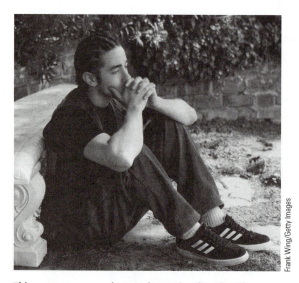

Frank Wing/Getty Images

This young man may have a depressive disorder if he experiences unaccountable, persistent sadness and a loss of pleasure in his usual activities.

Table 8-1 DSM-IV-TR Symptoms of Depression

To qualify for classification as a major depressive episode, many of the following symptoms must occur, represent a deterioration from usual functioning, and interfere with daily activities. Major symptoms are depressed mood and loss of ability to enjoy oneself.

Mood Disruption

Depressed mood, sadness

Loss of pleasure or interest in usual activities

Irritability (particularly in children and adolescents)

Physical and Behavioral Problems

Appetite, weight, and growth disturbances

Underactivity or overactivity (more common in children)

Energy loss and fatigue

Sleep disturbances (less common in children)

Cognitive Changes

Inability to concentrate and focus one's attention

Indecisiveness

Low self-esteem, feelings of worthlessness

Excessive guilt

Hopelessness, helplessness

Thoughts about suicide

SOURCE: Reprinted with permission from the *Diagnostic and Statistical Manual of Mental Disorders*, 4th ed., Text Revision. © 2000 American Psychiatric Association.

within months after a single episode or may endure for years, during which episodes may be frequent or rare. Mood disorders can range from mild (barely meeting diagnostic criteria) to totally debilitating, requiring hospitalization.

A **major depressive episode** is diagnosed when a person's behavior meets a set of diagnostic criteria specifying problem severity and persistence (the DSM symptoms are listed in Table 8-1). Major depressive episodes may follow an identifiable loss or severe stress such as rejection by a loved one or the loss of a close friend or family member. However, in some cases, there is no obvious external precipitating event, as for 10-year-old Tanya, who appeared in the beginning of this chapter. Older teenagers and adults are diagnosed with a major depressive episode when they have either severely depressed mood or very diminished interest or pleasure in their usual activities for most of the time over a minimum of 2 weeks.

Major depressive disorder is diagnosed when a person has had two or more episodes (each at least 2 weeks long) of depressed mood or loss of interest or pleasure in life and other signs of serious distress or impairment, such as marked changes in appetite or weight, bothersome insomnia or prolonged sleeping, dramatic increase or decrease in physical activity, extreme fatigue, inappropriate feelings of guilt or worthlessness, indecisiveness or inability to concentrate, or unwelcome, recurring thoughts of death or suicide. The definition of major depressive disorder excludes very mild or brief symptoms or normal shock or grief reactions to tragic events. Depression and other mood disorders adversely affect a person's social, emotional, cognitive, and physical functioning—in fact, all aspects of life. Depressed people unknowingly make their situation worse by driving other people away with their negative, irritable, and self-critical behavior, just when they need social support the most.

Inability to concentrate or function effectively is a common response to stress, but can also indicate depression. When seriously depressed, a usually efficient and decisive person may become hesitant, confused, troubled, withdrawn, and unable to make simple decisions, such as what to wear or when to take a bath. The quality of the person's academic or professional work tends to decrease, but not as much as the person thinks it has. Friends and family members usually find that it is impossible to talk a very depressed person out of feeling despondent and hopeless.

In **bipolar disorder** (also called *manic-depressive disorder*), the person switches between normal mood, depressive episodes, and hyperexcited manic episodes, which often immediately precede or follow a plunge into depression. Manic episodes are characterized by inexplicable exhilaration, greatly increased, or even tireless, activity, sleeplessness, talkativeness, impulsive behavior, irritability, and grandiose, unrealistic thoughts and plans. At first, the person may appear highly energetic, optimistic, and sociable, but the apparent good mood seems to get out of control. The person becomes irritable, impulsive, and irrational, sometimes gambling away large amounts of the family money or investing in wildly improbable business schemes. While suffering from severe manic episodes with psychotic features, teens have gone without sleep for several days and then become suicidal or assaultive when their wishes were thwarted. Some have leaped from high places, believing they were special beings and could fly. Others have incurred huge debts through buying things they could

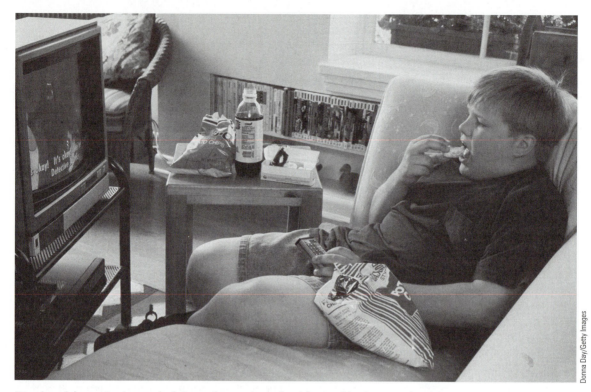

One sign of depression is a marked change in appetite and activity, resulting in unusual weight loss or gain. A depressed youngster may also withdraw from friends.

not use, such as 30 pairs of sneakers, thinking they were millionaires. To make matters worse, when teenagers in a manic state take illicit stimulant drugs, they become even wilder and often require hospitalization because they are dangerous to themselves and others. Bipolar disorder usually appears in early adulthood and is rare in childhood. Although very infrequent, early bipolar disorder is a serious, recurrent condition that should be treated medically to reduce the likelihood of future episodes and the risk of antisocial behavior, accidents, and suicide.

Minor depression, which is sometimes called *subclinical depression*, is a condition in which the person feels and appears depressed, but fails to meet all diagnostic criteria for major depression. The symptoms may also be less severe than in clinical depression. Minor depression typically occurs together with or after extremely stressful events such as the end of a close relationship or the death of a loved one. Over time, minor depression usually fades. In contrast, **dysthymic disorder** (*dysthymia*) is persistent mild depression that interferes with functioning or causes the person significant distress over an extended time period. Dysthymic disorder persists for most of the time for at least 2 years in adults or 1 year in children. Dysthymic disorder may begin in childhood, adolescence, or early adulthood and can develop into more severe depression. About 40% of adults with dysthymic disorder also experience either major depressive disorder or bipolar disorder in any given year (Regier, Narrow, & Rae, 1993). This combination of dysthymic disorder with intermittent episodes of major depression or bipolar disorder is termed *double depression*. Many of the people you encounter in everyday life suffer from either subclinical depression or dysthymic disorder that is never detected or treated.

PREVALENCE OF DEPRESSION

IN FOCUS 2 ▶ Describe how depression rates differ for children, adolescents, and adults.

Depression has sometimes been called the common cold of psychiatric illnesses, because so many people become depressed at some time in their lives. Major depressive disorder is the leading cause of disability in the United States and other technologically advanced countries (Murray & Lopez, 1996). Economists estimate that each year major depression costs the United States almost $20 billion in lost work productivity and treatment-related expenses. The additional toll of emotional suffering is incalculable. According to the U.S. Surgeon General (2001), each year about 9.5% of adult Americans develop some type of depressive disorder, a condition that attacks nearly twice as many women (12.0%) as men (6.6%). Fortunately, diagnosable depression is much less frequent among children.

Very rare before the age of 6 years (less than 1% prevalence), depression gradually increases in prevalence during childhood, climbs rapidly in adolescence, and reaches adult levels by the late teens, as shown in Table 8-2. Depression increases at an irregular rate over the course of development, with prevalence dou-

bling between the ages of 3 and 14 years, when it reaches 1.7%, then dramatically increasing during adolescence to affect 7.6% or more of 18- to 19-year-olds (American Psychiatric Association, 2000). In a large, representative sample of high school students, an amazing 20.4% had been depressed at some earlier time and 2.9% currently met diagnostic criteria for major depressive disorder or dysthymic disorder (Lewinsohn & Rohde, 1993). Other estimates agree that between 15% and 20% of teens will suffer from a major depressive episode by the time they reach voting age (Harrington, Rutter, & Fombonne, 1996).

Teenagers are likely to experience other psychological disorders, particularly substance abuse, together with depression (Aseltine, Gore, & Colten, 1998). As in the case of the 13-year-old boy, Dave, described at the beginning of the chapter, parents and teachers can easily focus on the substance abuse or rebellious behavior and never realize that the child actually suffers from depression. Anxiety disorders and conduct disorder also frequently accompany adolescent depression (Kessler et al., 1994; Regier et al., 1998). This co-occurrence of depression with other disorders is disturbing, because disorders that occur together tend to be more severe and more difficult to treat than isolated disorders (Kessler et al., in press). Depression is a serious threat and relapse rates are

Table 8-2 Prevalence of Mood Disorders at Different Ages

Age Group	Type of Disorder			
	Major Depression	**Dysthymia**	**Bipolar**	**Any**
Early childhood 1–6 years	–	–	–	<1%
Early adolescence 10–14 years	–	–	–	1.7%
Late adolescence 18–19 years	–	–	–	7.6%
Adulthood 18–55 years	5%	3%	1.2%	7.1–9.5%
Late adulthood 55+ years	3.8%	1.6%	0.3%	4.4%

NOTE: Rates for different age groups come from different studies, so are difficult to compare. Nevertheless, large age differences are consistently reported, as shown here.

SOURCE: Adapted from American Psychiatric Association (1994); Garrison, Schluchter, Schoenbach, & Kaplan (1989); Lewinsohn & Rohde (1993); U.S. Surgeon General (2001).

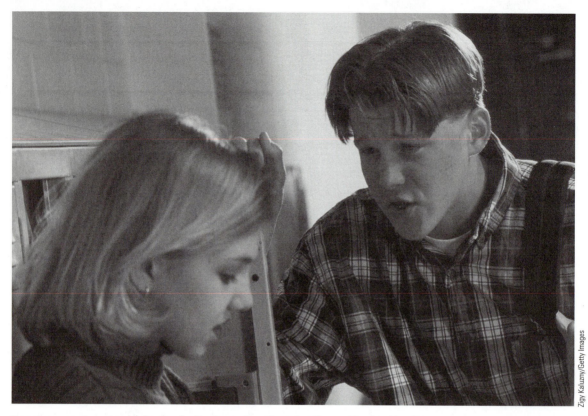

Teenagers are at greater risk for developing depression after a break-up with a boyfriend or girlfriend.

high; some 18.4% of adolescents with major depression will probably have a recurrence (Lewinsohn, Rohde, & Seeley, 1993). Clinical or diagnosable depression is a serious condition that cannot be overcome through will power alone and will not simply go away if untreated. Clearly, the prevention and treatment of depression should be a national priority.

AGE DIFFERENCES IN DEPRESSIVE SYMPTOMS

The DSM-IV-TR diagnostic scheme of the American Psychiatric Association contains no separate category for childhood depression. With minor alterations, adult criteria are used for diagnosing children. Children typically do not know what depression is and fail to realize that they are depressed. Being much less

able than adults to label and report their emotions, young children do not complain about feeling depressed. Because children fail to show this major indicator of depressive disorder, they are difficult to diagnose. Table 8-3 presents some of the distinctive features of juvenile depression. In contrast to adults, children are more likely to express their depression through somatic or physical complaints, such as headache, stomachache, or fatigue. Also, rather than seeming sad, a young child who is depressed may appear highly irritable, anxious, or frantically hyperactive. Anxiety, irritability, physical symptoms, and overactivity are all symptoms of other types of disorders. Depressed children may be more likely to be diagnosed with attention-deficit/hyperactivity disorder (ADHD), anxiety disorder, oppositional defiant disorder, or conduct disorder than with depression. Often their depression goes unnoticed while their other,

Table 8-3 Depressive Behaviors in Children and Adolescents

Age Group	Depressive Behaviors
Infants	Sadness, weeping, apathy, motor retardation, failure to thrive, vomiting, irritability, developmental delays, feeding or sleeping difficulties
Toddlers and preschoolers	Irritability, social withdrawal, negative self-image, peer problems, anxiety, phobias, weeping, loss of interest/pleasure in usual activities (anhedonia), loss of appetite, sleep disturbances, changed activity rates, desire to die, somatic disorders including enuresis, encopresis, asthma, eczema, failure to thrive, aggression, self-endangering behavior
School children	Irritability, anhedonia, fatigue, somatic complaints, sleeping and eating disturbances, changed activity rates, suicidal thoughts, guilt, low self-esteem, sudden schoolwork problems, aggression, decreased ability to concentrate, phobias, anxiety, separation anxiety problems, depressed facial expression
Adolescents	Disturbed sleep, appetite or weight changes, changed activity rates, fatigue, anhedonia, self-devaluation, difficulty in concentrating, indecisiveness, suicidal thoughts or attempts, anxiety, phobias, somatic disorders, excessive emotional dependency, withdrawal, reckless behavior

Sources: American Psychiatric Association (2000); Herzog & Rathbun (1982); Nottelmann & Jensen (1995); Poznanski, Mokros, Grossman, & Freeman (1985).

more disruptive, problems command adults' attention (Seppa, 1997).

Development of Sex Differences in Depression Rates

Why do approximately twice as many women as men suffer from major depression over their lifetimes? Between 10% and 25% of women develop depressive disorder as compared with 5–12% of men (American Psychiatric Association, 2000). It is unclear whether more women truly do become depressed or whether men and women are equally likely to be depressed but show their depression in different ways. Perhaps men's depression is expressed in their greater alcohol and substance abuse or their aggressive, antisocial behavior, whereas women's depression is reflected better by the standard diagnostic criteria for depressive disorder.

The sex differences in depression are not apparent during childhood, when boys and girls are roughly equally likely to be diagnosed with mood disorders (Hankin et al., 1998; Nolen-Hoeksema, 1995). Unaccountably, girls' depression rates increase dramatically during puberty, but boys' rates do not (Hankin et al., 1998). The gender difference in susceptibility to depression seems to emerge around the age of 13. Others' perceptions of girls and their perceptions of

themselves seem to play an important role. While boys generally welcome signs of physical maturation, girls may experience more conflict about their changing bodies. Adolescent girls who express dissatisfaction with their body appearance, diet severely, and have bulimic symptoms (eating binges followed by purging) are at above-average risk for developing major depression (Stice, Hayward, Cameron, Killen, & Taylor, 2000) (see Chapter 14 on eating disorders). This pattern of obsessive concern with weight and appearance may help explain the dramatic rise in depression for teenage girls. Body changes in puberty make it difficult or impossible for many girls to achieve the fashionably thin feminine ideal, and they may therefore feel dissatisfied and depressed (Stice et al., 2000).

Sex differences in how teens cope with stress may also explain girls' tendencies to become depressed. Parents more often expect their sons to attempt to overcome stress on their own and not give way to self pity. Girls are expected to need more comforting. Reassurance from others may act as reinforcement for girls' helpless behavior, and so they express depressive complaints (Sheeber, Davis, & Hops, 2002). These different social expectations for girls and boys could suppress boys' expressions of depression and boost girls' rates of depression. In addition, hormonal and other physical changes of puberty might combine with rigid sex role expectations to strengthen the female tendency toward depression. However, it is important to realize that males are not exempt from depressive disorder. Young men's depression rates are rising (Gotlib & Hammen, 1992), perhaps because of changing social role expectations. In contemporary U.S. society, it is becoming more acceptable for men to see themselves and to be seen as emotionally sensitive and vulnerable to depression, a trend that would naturally appear first among the young who are less bound by traditional sex roles than their elders.

RISK FACTORS FOR MOOD DISORDERS

Growing up under adverse circumstances places children and teenagers at risk for depression. Some types of mood disorders, especially depression and bipolar disorder, seem to run in families. It is probable that both genetic factors and unhealthy family environments are responsible for children's mood disorders. In this section, we review what is known about family environments that may lead to depression, particularly inadequate and harmful parenting; later we will examine the role of biological factors in depression.

Adverse Family Environments

IN FOCUS 3 ▶ How do adverse family environments lead children to become depressed or otherwise disturbed?

First, a word of explanation. Many readers wonder why psychologists who study children's abnormal behavior emphasize the role of mothers so much more than fathers. There are several reasons for the centrality of mothers. Most theories and research on parent-infant relationships have centered on mothers, in part because they are more available for and interested in participating in research than fathers are. Also, at least for infants and young children, the primary parenting role still belongs to the women in the vast majority of families. In contrast, relatively little is known about the parenting practices of fathers, although clearly infants can and do become attached to fathers as well as to mothers. So be prepared for a preponderance of information on the effects of mothers' parenting prac-

tices, because almost all of the reliable data currently available focus on mothers.

Parents' own mental health is often reflected in their children's adjustment. Depressed parents are often worried and preoccupied and so cannot provide good parenting for their children. In particular, mood-disordered parents tend to be inattentive, unresponsive, uninvolved, negative, and not cognitively stimulating for their children. They are preoccupied with their own struggles with depression, which deprives their children of the warm and sensitive parenting that leads to secure attachment. Depressed parents also provide models of depressive reasoning, display chronically sad or irritable facial expressions and body postures, and express a generally pessimistic outlook, which their troubled children sometimes imitate. Parental depression and other forms of psychological disturbance place children at risk of maladjustment. There is little family "togetherness" when a parent is mentally ill. Under these circumstances, children are often inadequately supervised, and family members rarely work together as a team (Johnson, Cowan, & Cowan, 1999). However, these ill effects are not invariable. It is important to recognize that not all depressed people are inadequate parents and that many of their children escape adjustment problems.

Maternal depression affects children surprisingly early in life (Lyons-Ruth, Lyubchik, Wolfe, & Bronfman, 2002). Infants and toddlers typically do not interact with depressed mothers as smoothly and enjoyably as most parents and children do (Jameson, Gelfand, Kulcsar, & Teti, 1997). These early communication difficulties predictably take their toll on infants' social and emotional development (Weinberg & Tronick, 1998). The emotionally ill mothers' lack of confidence (low parenting self-efficacy beliefs) seems to reduce their effectiveness as parents (Teti & Gelfand, 1991). Older children with a depressed mother are also at risk of maladjustment and school difficulties, particularly when the depression is persistent, severe, and began very early in the child's infancy (Wright, George, Burke, Gelfand, & Teti, 2000). We do not yet know whether children's experiences with a depressed parent continue to affect their adjustment as adults, but many psychological theories predict a lifelong effect.

Family violence also relates to children's depression, and in this case, the father may be more likely to adversely influence his children's adjustment. Adolescent girls are more likely to develop depression in early adulthood when: (1) they were exposed to family violence, typically involving a violent father, (2) they are under unusual stress, and (3) they had some prior adjustment disorder other than depression (Daley, Hammen, & Rao, 2000). Causal relationships between family conditions such as maternal depression, marital conflict, or family violence and children's disorders are far from clear. Many unfortunate families have a mix of handicapping conditions that together appear to produce children's adjustment difficulties.

Children's Contributions

Of course, children themselves are unwilling contributors to their own problems, either directly or through the effects of their behavior on others. Some infants are temperamentally negative and present a management challenge for their mothers. These babies readily show fear and sadness, become angry easily, are very fussy and nearly impossible to comfort (Goldsmith, Buss, & Lemery, 1997). Their insistent crying, bad moods, and resistance to being comforted undermine their parents' ability to be good caretakers. An unfortunate child-parent match, such as that of a depressed or anxious parent with a difficult child, can result in emotional disorders in the child. In contrast, children who adjust well in spite of adverse circumstances such as poor parenting tend to have higher levels of verbal ability and are probably brighter than average (Malcarne, Hamilton, Ingram, & Taylor, 2000).

As children grow, the types of risk factors they encounter change and broaden. For example, teenagers encounter romantic relationships for the first time and come to judge themselves partly on their ability to attract a desirable partner. A romantic break-up can be devastating for an adolescent and can lead to a first onset of major depressive disorder (Monroe, Rohde, Seeley, & Lewinsohn, 1999). Having experienced one major depressive episode, the teenager is more likely to have a recurrence when faced with even less severe stress in the future.

THEORIES

IN FOCUS 4 ▶ According to several theories, what types of persistent cognitive patterns are associated with risk for depression?

The many theories of the origins of depression differ in terms of where they place their emphasis: on the effects of early childhood experiences as opposed to current events, on the importance of cognition, and on biological versus social factors. The psychodynamic theories, including psychoanalysis, object relations theory, and attachment theory, focus on the enduring power of early childhood relationships with parents or parent surrogates. These experiences are thought to form the basis for future personality and social characteristics, including a propensity for depression. In contrast, the cognitive theories picture depression as arising from more varied social sources, with prolonged failure producing a pessimistic, unhappy mental style that often leads to depression. Cognitive and social cognitive theories of depression tend to agree that early experiences can lead to mood disturbance, but they place more importance on how people perceive themselves and the world. In contrast, the reinforcement-loss model traces the onset of depression to current events that deprive the person of enjoyable, rewarding activities. This section briefly describes several of these explanations of depression (see Table 8-4, which contrasts these major theories).

Table 8-4 Major Theories of Depression

Theory	Predisposing Event	Precipitating Event
Psychoanalytic theory	Constitutional overreliance on oral stimulation	Real or imagined loss or rejection
Attachment theory	Attachment insecurity, early loss	Major loss or rejection
Beck's cognitive theory	Early rejection, loss, or failure	Major loss or disappointment
Learned helplessness theory	Unavoidable pain or failure	Major loss or traumatic event
Social cognitive theory	Overly demanding parents, inadequate coping	Threat to self-efficacy
Reinforcement-loss model	No necessary predisposition	Massive reduction in reinforcement

Psychodynamic Theories

Psychoanalytic View

The early work of Sigmund Freud (1965/1917) and his colleague Karl Abraham (1968) portrayed adult depression as based on a constitutional predisposition toward overreliance on oral stimulation (such as sucking and biting) as the source of pleasure and reassurance. The person with such a predisposition might be dependent, with excessive needs for physical and psychological contact, touching, and reassurance, or alternatively might overreact and be rigidly independent (Malmquist, 1977). A child's unusually strong need for love and affection makes him highly vulnerable to any form of real or perceived rejection. Events such as the birth of a sibling, being harshly weaned, or experiencing more subtle forms of loss of love and attention from parents could constitute traumatic events and leave a psychological scar. People predisposed to depression fail to develop a strong, positive sense of self and are overly dependent on what others think of them. Desperate for love and recognition, depressives seek to punish those they feel have abandoned them, but they fear expressing this rage and instead turn their anger inward, punishing themselves. Some blow to self-esteem later in life rekindles the basic conflict and results in depression. The psychoanalytic explanation of depression has had many proponents, but is very difficult to verify.

Attachment Theory

British pediatrician John Bowlby (1969/1982) was impressed by babies' total dependence on their mother or other primary caretaker and their severe anxiety if separated from her. Through prolonged interactions with a capable mother, the child forms an internal working model, or mental representation, of her, which provides comfort and stability if some loss occurs in the future. Disorganized/disoriented infant attachment may arise when mothers are severely depressed, cold, or abusive, are substance abusers, or are otherwise psychologically disturbed (Teti, Gelfand, Messinger, & Isabella, 1995). Such dysfunctional early attachment experiences may predispose children to develop depression when they encounter some loss in the future (Cicchetti, Toth, & Lynch, 1995). Several interventions for depressed mothers and their babies and toddlers that are inspired by attachment theory are described later in this chapter.

Cognitive Theories

In psychiatrist Aaron Beck's *cognitive theory of depression* (1967), the individual is predisposed toward depression by experiencing an early rejection or loss of a parent or by holding unrealistic and perfectionistic self-expectations. Kovacs and Beck (1977) described a *cognitive triad* of distorted depressive thinking regarding self, situation, and the future; this triad makes the person vulnerable to depressive mood disorders. A later major loss or disappointment can trigger a depressive reaction in these cognitively vulnerable individuals. As Beck predicted, children diagnosed with depression have negative beliefs about themselves, the world, and the future, perhaps because their parents tend to evaluate them harshly, reject them, and overuse punishment (Stark, Humphrey, Laurent, Livingston, & Christopher, 1993). Thus, early loss and rejection appear to predispose children to depression. Nonetheless, many children with bad family situations do not develop depression, so other factors must also be at work.

The *learned helplessness theory* (Abramson, Metalsky, & Alloy, 1989) maintains that a sense of hopelessness about ever achieving control is the psychological culprit that causes depression. As in Beck's model, hopelessness can result from a pessimistic tendency to attribute negative events to personal shortcomings ("I flunked the test because I'll never understand math" or "I'm too lazy to do the work" or "I'm just plain dumb") (Abramson, Alloy, & Metalsky, 1995; Gotlib & Abramson, 1999). The theory does not specify the age at which a pessimistic or optimistic style first appears. Tanya, the young girl portrayed at the beginning of this chapter, clearly displayed a hopeless, pessimistic pattern of thinking about her popularity and her dancing skills by the age of 10; the older boy, Joe, felt so hopeless about his academic ability and future success that he began to think about suicide. But it is difficult to say just when these youngsters first began to despair. Some longitudinal research evidence is available. One study followed children over a 5-year period and found that stressful life events triggered depressed feelings in younger children regardless of their cognitive style, while older children became depressed if they had a negative cognitive style in addition to stress. These results suggest that younger children become depressed over bad things occurring in their lives, while older children, like adults, become depressed if they already have negative expectations (Nolen-Hoeksema, Girgus, & Seligman, 1992).

Social Cognitive Theories

Bandura's Theory

Bandura's (1986) social cognitive theory attributes depressive feelings to low self-efficacy, or the belief that one cannot succeed in important tasks. One source of these negative self-expectations is parents who set their children up for failure because of their unreasonably high aspirations, which the children cannot fulfill. Ruminating about bad grades, an unattractive appearance, or lack of friends can increase and prolong depression. Also, the worry itself makes the child awkward and hesitant, which is socially unattractive and can lead to rejection. Bandura's remedy for negative expectations and behavior is repeated successful practice of avoided tasks that are essential to the person's positive self-image. This graduated mastery approach to therapy is described in Chapter 15.

Contingency-Competence-Control Model

The contingency-competence-control (CCC) model (Weisz, 1986; Weisz, Southam-Gerow, & McCarty, 2001) also views repeated failure as a key factor in depression. This model portrays depression as arising from a lack of control over events, a personal inability to produce a positive outcome (such as convincing a cold parent to become loving), and low levels of perceived contingency between one's personal efforts and desired outcomes. Thus, depressed people may conclude that trying is useless because "life is unfair" or "trying hard gets you nowhere." Like Bandura's social cognitive theory, the contingency-competence-control model considers negative self-perceptions important in depression because they reduce effort and the likelihood of success. Weisz and his colleagues (Weisz et al., 2001) found that this model accounts well for depression in adolescents, but not in younger and less cognitively mature children.

Reinforcement-Loss Explanation

The reinforcement-loss model maintains that depressed behavior can be produced by a severe reduc-tion in earned outcomes or discontinuation of positive reinforcement for one's effort (Ferster, 1973; Lewinsohn, 1974). An example would be a student at a highly competitive college who no longer gets the good grades she earned in high school. The high grades previously reinforced and maintained the student's hard work. In adolescence, the break-up of a romantic relationship provides a significant risk factor for a first episode of major depressive disorder (Monroe et al., 1999). Psychologist Peter Lewinsohn and his associates (Lewinsohn, Hops, Roberts, & Seeley, 1993) have observed that in addition to their obvious unhappiness, depressed people often become seclusive, ill at ease, and socially inept. Their poor social skills lead other people to avoid them and result in a loss of reinforcement for their efforts no matter how hard they try (the process of extinction). Only energetic, positive, and effective efforts to re-establish old sources of reinforcement and find new ones can terminate the depressive reaction. This may require learning new social skills, perhaps in behavior therapy.

Problems with the reinforcement-loss explanation are that it is not always possible to identify major losses of reinforcement preceding depressive episodes and that drug treatments restore normal social functioning for many depressed people, without success experiences or the provision of a reinforcement-rich environment.

BIOLOGICAL BASIS OF DEPRESSION: GENETIC, BRAIN, AND BIOCHEMICAL FUNCTIONS

IN FOCUS 5 ▶ Describe four difficulties in tracing childhood depression to genetic or biochemical abnormalities.

The many complexities of depression and of genetics make it difficult to answer the seemingly simple question of whether depression has a hereditary basis. The answer depends on many factors, including the interplay between the child's characteristics and the environment, the age at which the depressive disorder first appears, whether the child is female or male, and the particular type of mood disorder under consideration. Much research evidence suggests that there is a substantial genetic contribution to depressive disorder that begins in adulthood (Tsuang & Faraone, 1990). However, for depression with a childhood onset, the evidence for a genetic basis is less clear.

Surprisingly, heritability plays a larger role in the development of less severe forms of childhood depression, and environmental factors seem to have a stronger influence on more severe forms of children's depression. These relationships may be different during adulthood. Further, what is genetically passed down in families may not be depression or another disorder as such, but rather a general propensity to develop one or more disorders that tend to occur together, including depression, alcoholism, substance abuse, and antisocial or conduct disorders (Goodman & Gotlib, 1999). A family history of combined depression and alcoholism is only suggestive of heritability, because the actual transmission process could be totally or partly environmental rather than genetic.

Many people believe that the effectiveness of antidepressant medications proves that at least some types of depression have a biochemical basis. This line of reasoning is faulty. A positive response to an antidepressant drug does not necessarily mean that the person's depression is biologically based. In fact, mood improvement after taking an antidepressant does not even prove that the person is depressed, because some modern antidepressants, particularly the SSRI inhibitors such as Prozac, improve mood even in people who are not depressed. Usually, such nonspecific drug effects fade away over time, leaving the depression to be treated by other means.

Researchers are investigating the possibility that there are sensitive periods in neural development during which biological and environmental influences interact to affect the emerging emotional and behavioral systems. Perhaps a propensity toward depression stems from these early developmental influences. The fetal environment may be affected by the mother's depressive mood disorder through neuroendocrine abnormalities, reduced blood flow to the fetus, or the mother's use of antidepressant medication. These are possible sources of mother-child transmission of depression, but there is no convincing evidence for any of them at this point (Goodman & Gotlib, 2002). Although brain-behavior relationships are under intensive study, the neurobehavioral explanation and other biosocial models of depression remain highly conjectural.

TREATMENT OF CHILDHOOD DEPRESSION

IN FOCUS 6 ▶ Identify the two most promising types of treatment for depressed children.

Antidepressant Medications

Most antidepressant drugs were developed for adults, and their effects on children remain largely untested. Some antidepressant medications show promise in relieving children's depressive symptoms, while others are no more effective than **placebos** (mock medications, or sugar pills) for treating childhood and adolescent depression. Most antidepressants (including the SSRIs) and placebos produce some improvement in approximately half of the cases. (See Table 8-5 for a list of frequently used antidepressants.) Until very recently, children were most likely to receive a tricyclic antidepressant such as imipramine (Tofranil) for their depressive symptoms, but such drugs appear to be ineffective in treating depression in children and adolescents. In addition, tricyclic antidepressants such as imipramine and desipramine (Norpramin, Pertofrane) could prove lethal for children if an overdose were given or taken accidentally or as a suicide attempt. Nevertheless, the tricyclic antidepressants are widely used to treat children's anxieties, phobias, and enuresis.

The selective serotonin reuptake inhibitors (SSRIs) and other fairly recently developed antidepressants were frequently prescribed for children in advance of any demonstration of their effectiveness and long-

Table 8-5 Some Antidepressants Used with Children and Adolescents

Generic Name	Trade Name
Fluoxetine	Prozac
Paroxetine	Paxil
Fluvoxamine	Luvox
Sertraline	Zoloft
Buproprion	Wellbutrin
Citalopram	Celexa
Venlafaxine	Effexor
Clomipramine	Anafranil

term benefits. Three SSRIs have recently received FDA approval to treat obsessive-compulsive symptoms in children and adolescents: sertraline hydrochloride (Zoloft), clomipramine (Anafranil), and fluvoxamine (Luvox) (Rapoport, 2000). This does not mean that they are also effective in cases of depression, however.

There have been remarkably few adequately controlled studies of the use of SSRIs, indeed, any antidepressant drug, with children. Nevertheless, one well-controlled double-blind study of children with major depression found significant improvement with fluoxetine (Prozac) compared to a placebo (56% improved compared to 33% improved) (Emslie et al., 1997). These results are encouraging, but some of the children classified as "improved" showed only modest improvements, and it is necessary to look at long-term as well as immediate drug effectiveness. A more recent open (uncontrolled) research study of adolescents receiving typical treatment in an HMO was less positive. The teenagers, who suffered from major depression, received short-term psychotherapy together with one of the SSRIs. The disappointing outcome was that only 33% of them showed improved mood in the months following the treatment (Hamilton & Bridge, 1999).

Moreover, little is known about potential hazards of prescribing the SSRIs or any antidepressant together with other drugs a child is taking for co-occurring problems. Children are often passed from one health care provider to another and may receive several different diagnoses, for which they take several medications in combinations that could prove risky. Treatment oversight is minimal, often accomplished by separate telephone check-ups by each of several health providers (Jensen et al., 1999; Woolston, 1999). Children are particularly vulnerable to medication side effects, and they are taking more untested medications than ever before. The health care industry and the government have an obligation to protect them. Although progress is being made, we do not yet have a definitive answer to the question of how medications can be used to treat depression in children and adolescents.

Psychotherapies for Juvenile Depression

Psychotherapies vary in their effectiveness in treating depressed children, but the outlook is good—many recent research trials indicate significant improvement for children treated with some type of psychotherapy. Many of the older types of insight-based psychotherapy developed for adults were not very helpful with younger clients. Nondirective, or psychodynamic, forms of therapy are generally aimed at uncovering presumed underlying psychological conflict and are thus difficult to use with depressed children, who have trouble understanding and describing their feelings. Various types of play therapy (see Chapter 15) have been used with depressed youngsters, but with unknown results. Surprisingly little information about the effectiveness of play therapy has been published (Russ, 1995). The most promising developments in child psychotherapy have centered on the newer, more highly structured cognitive-behavioral and interpersonal approaches.

Controlled research indicates that **cognitive-behavioral therapy** can help young people to manage their depression and anxiety effectively. As developed by Lewinsohn and colleagues (Clarke et al., 1992; Lewinsohn, Clarke, Hops, & Andrews, 1990), cognitive-behavioral intervention is conducted in small groups of three to eight adolescents in 16 sessions over an 8-week period. Designed to reduce the adolescents' feelings of being different or mentally ill, the treatment takes place in a classroom setting in which adolescents are taught how to control their depressed mood. Brief readings, structured learning tasks, short quizzes, and homework assignments are familiar activities and are not stigmatizing because they resemble normal classroom routines. Course content emphasizes that depression results from life stress and teaches students to master new skills to deal more effectively with stress and control their moods. Teenage clients are informed that some of the skills taught, such as relaxation or self-control tactics, may not be useful to them personally, and they may select which techniques are the best for them. The intervention teaches adolescents how to relate to peers, how to increase the number and quality of enjoyable activities in their lives, and how to set and how to achieve realistic goals for change. In addition, depressed teens are taught relaxation techniques for use when they are stressed, ways to increase positive thoughts and decrease depressive thoughts, and basic problem-solving skills. The adolescents can practice the skills alone or with their parents. Finally, each adolescent is taught to recognize the signs that depression is returning and how to deal with them.

The content of the teen depression course is research-based, and the results have been excellent. In two research studies, between 54% and 67% of the treated teenagers recovered to the extent that they no longer met DSM criteria for an affective disorder as compared with only 5% to 48% of those in a wait-list control group. The adolescents continued to improve in the months following the cognitive-behavioral treatment, which is remarkable (Lewinsohn & Rohde, 1993). Individualized "booster" sessions are offered at 4-month intervals over a 2-year period in an attempt to prevent relapses, although these sessions did not affect relapse rate. This work indicates the importance of basing therapies on psychological principles, adapting the intervention to the developmental characteristics of the client group, and rigorously assessing treatment outcomes.

The next step is to develop therapies with long-term effectiveness. Although cognitive-behavioral therapy was clearly superior to other psychotherapies in the short term, treatments that confer lasting benefits are needed. What happens over the course of several years? One study randomly assigned over 100 adolescents with major depressive disorder to 12–16 weeks of cognitive-behavioral therapy, systemic behavioral family therapy, or nondirective supportive therapy (Birmaher et al., 2000). Most teens (80%) recovered within about a year from the time they were originally assessed, and there were no significant differences in long-term outcome for the three types of psychotherapy. That is, the cognitive-behavioral therapy did not retain its superiority in the long run. Nearly one-third of the teens had a recurrence within the 2-year study period; many of these were initially more depressed and reported high levels of conflict with their parents. More research is needed to confirm the conclusion that the type of psychotherapy does not matter in long-term follow-ups, because any one study could give misleading results. Nevertheless, it is clearly too soon to conclude that we have effective and long-lasting treatments for juvenile depression.

Prognosis for Depressed Children

Childhood depression is a severe and relatively persistent condition that may recur and worsen over time. Even mild cases of early mood disorder send a danger signal. Preschool children with mild but chronic dysthymic disorder are likely to develop a more serious major depressive disorder by the time they are 5 years old (Kovacs, Feinberg, & Crouse-Novak, 1984). It is quite unusual for a preschooler to be diagnosed with even a mild depressive disorder, which could explain the bad prognosis. A child's long-term outcome probably depends on the type and severity of illness and on family factors such as divorce, marital discord, family violence, and parental physical or mental illness, particularly the mother's depression (Malcarne et al., 2000).

Once established, adolescent depression is not easy to overcome. A recent study of adults who had major depression when they were adolescents raises a red flag (Weissman et al., 1999). As compared with a group free of obvious psychiatric illness, young adults who had been depressed as teens showed a four times greater risk for a first suicide attempt, a doubled risk of experiencing another major depressive episode, increased rates of medical and psychiatric hospitalization, and impaired work, social, and family functioning. These findings suggest that adolescents with major depression should be followed closely and treated promptly if they show signs of recurring depression.

Parents and teachers should follow these tips for helping depressed children:

- Call in a mental health professional if the child feels miserable for a period of 2 weeks or more, cannot cope with usual routines, including schoolwork, and avoids social contacts with others. Get help immediately if children or teens talk about suicide.
- Show you understand that the child is suffering and that you are concerned. Reassure depressed children that you value and love them, even if they sometimes don't act lovable. Tell them that their depressed feelings won't last forever and that they will feel much better later on. Assure them that treatment can help them.
- *Don't* urge depressed children to cheer up and use will power to overcome their unhappiness. They can't. Trying to appear happy in order to please you will only stress them further. Don't attempt to diagnose and treat mood disorders by yourself or rely on friends or family members. Don't underestimate the seriousness of mood disorders in children and adolescents.

- Be a facilitator. Some parents simply cannot admit that their children are depressed, and don't want to hear about it. Tell them what signs of depression you have observed and supply them with pamphlets on depression from your local public health department, public library, or the National Depressive and Manic-Depressive Association (730 N. Franklin St., Suite 501, Chicago, IL 60610-3526; phone, 800-826-3632).

PREVENTION OF DEPRESSED MOOD IN INFANTS AND CHILDREN

Programs for Infants and Toddlers

Because infants of depressed mothers are at particular risk for developing early maladaptive behavior, investigators have begun to devise interventions that might reduce this group's likelihood of developing psychological problems, including depression. Increases in single-parent, mother-headed households (described in Chapter 5) mean that there is a large group of stressed, impoverished, depression-prone mothers. Their depressed mood or other incapacitating conditions render many mothers psychologically unavailable, sad, confused, irritable, or unable to cope with everyday demands (Goodman & Gotlib, 2002). In addition, both the children and the mothers may be genetically vulnerable to depressive illness (Weissman et al., 1997). Whatever the source of the mothers' problems in functioning, their children have a higher than average rate of psychological problems.

Several interventions show promise of improving a disturbed mother's relationship with her child. Home-visiting programs are frequently used for depressed mothers of very young children. In one study (Gelfand, Teti, Seiner, & Jameson, 1996), a course of 29 home visits from experienced public health nurses produced beneficial effects for depressed mothers and their infants. The nurse home visitors showed the mothers more satisfying and effective methods of caring for their babies, supported their efforts to overcome their depression, and encouraged the mothers to visit friends and neighbors. The result was a significantly more rapid reduction in the mothers' depressive symptoms than with regular mental health care alone and a reduced rate of disorganized/disoriented attachments among the babies.

Another intervention (Cicchetti, Rogosch, & Toth, 2000) used toddler-parent psychotherapy, in which a therapist provided the mothers with a warm, supportive, corrective emotional experience so that they could become more nurturing and positive toward their toddlers. The mothers learned to improve their communication and interaction with their toddlers, and this made mother-child interactions more positive and enjoyable. The toddlers' IQ and mental development scores also improved.

Roseanne Clark (1993) has developed a supportive program for mothers with postpartum depression. Each mother is provided with brief relationship-focused group therapy, which assumes that postpartum depression originates largely in the mother's faulty early relationship with her own mother. The mother is helped to resolve her negative and limiting internal working models of relationships (see the earlier discussion of attachment theory) and to understand how her past relationships with her own parents affect how she perceives and treats her baby. With her own emotional needs better satisfied, she can support her infant's healthy attachment to her. Fathers are also included in the treatment, so that they can understand the mother's depression and offer support, and the infants are treated in their own developmental therapy group. Each infant has a therapist, who also watches and coaches the mother and infant as the mother massages the baby and plays interactive games with her. This new mother-infant relational therapy has yet to be thoroughly evaluated.

Powerful interventions are needed to counteract the early and pervasive effects on children's psychological development of maternal mental illness and other extremely stressful conditions. Early intervention programs require more work to increase their general effectiveness and identify their long-term effects. The gains in functioning produced by early interventions may fade and require booster sessions, or they may endure and facilitate cognitive and social development in later years.

Programs for School-Age Children

There is relatively little research on prevention of depression in school-age children. However, two recent studies with late elementary school and middle school students showed some positive but also some negative results. One intervention (Peterson, 2000) taught middle school students cognitive and problem-solving techniques, including how to reduce irrational worries, increase self-confident thoughts, and use techniques such as relaxation training. The intervention seemed to aid coping and general adjustment. However, although the treated girls reported reduced depressive symptoms, the treated boys reported more depressive symptoms than the control group did. Some modification in the intervention is needed in order to benefit both sexes.

The Penn Optimism Program (Gillham, Reivich, & Shatte, 2001), based on the positive psychology initiative of Martin E. P. Seligman, shows promise in reducing depressive symptoms in older school children. The positive psychology initiative is as follows:

> *There are human strengths that act as buffers against mental illness: courage, future mindedness, optimism, interpersonal skill, faith, work ethic, hope, honesty, perseverance, and the capacity for flow and insight, to name several. Much of the task of prevention in this new century will be to create a science of human strength whose mission will be to understand and learn how to foster these virtues in young people. (Seligman & Csikszentmihalyi, 2000)*

The Penn Optimism Program employed training in relaxation and assertiveness skills, together with various other cognitive and social problem-solving skills. The cognitive skills taught to the children included understanding how thoughts interact with mood, identifying negative thinking, generating positive alternatives, and evaluating evidence to support positive and negative thoughts. Children in the intervention program reported significantly fewer depressive symptoms than controls for a 2-year period, but not thereafter (Gillham, Shatte, & Freres, 2000). The program's effects were stronger for boys than for girls, although both groups improved. The longer-term benefits of such interventions have yet to be demonstrated. Also, depression treatment programs need to cope with the possibility of suicide attempts.

SUICIDE

Contrary to popular belief, children do try to commit suicide, and they sometimes succeed. Suicide is very rare in children younger than 12 years, but rises sig-

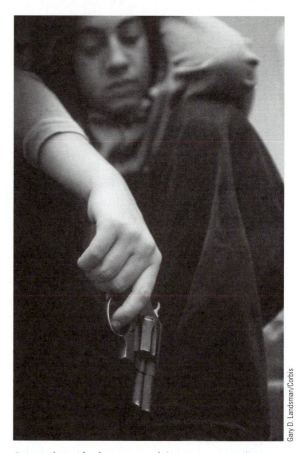

One tragic result of young people's easy access to firearms is their use and lethal effectiveness in suicide attempts.

nificantly in early adolescence beginning around the age of 14. Suicide is the third leading cause of death for 15- to 24-year-olds (National Center for Health Statistics, 1995). Each year about 3% of older adolescent girls and 1% of older adolescent boys make a serious suicide attempt (National Center for Health Statistics, 1995). An alarming statistic is that roughly 1 in 10 college students (around 10%) in a recent survey said they had considered suicide during the past 12 months (Brenner, Hassan, & Barrios, 1999). Of even more concern are their actual attempts.

"Approximately 1 in 10 adolescent girls and 1 in 25 adolescent boys report making some form of suicide attempt" (Lewinsohn, Rohde, & Seeley, 1993). It is important to realize that suicide rates for different age groups are not static, but can change dramatically over time. For example, the suicide rate for 15- to 24-

year-olds *tripled* from 1945 to 1995 (National Center for Health Statistics, 1995). Suicide rates may have increased because depression has become more prevalent in this age group, as previously discussed. Other possible causes include the increasing availability of firearms, especially handguns, and of drugs that can be used lethally and impulsively. Also, more health care providers have become aware that suspicious accidents and deaths may represent suicide attempts and so are more likely to report suicides. With so many young people at risk, it becomes important to detect suicidal tendencies early to avert tragedy.

Warning Signs of Suicide in Adolescents

Adolescents are more likely to attempt suicide if they have several of the following:

- Adjustment problems
- Past psychiatric disorders
- Depressive thought patterns
- Inadequate coping styles
- School or health problems
- Thoughts of death, desire to be dead or to commit suicide, or past suicide attempts

The greater the number of risk factors a teenager has, the more likely he or she is to attempt suicide (Lewinsohn et al., 1993). Adolescent girls have more of these risk factors than boys and are more likely to attempt suicide. However, more males actually kill themselves, perhaps because men tend to use faster and more lethal methods, such as firearms. Suicide methods most often chosen by adolescent boys include cutting, substance ingestion, guns, and hanging. Women and girls more commonly overdose on prescription drugs or cut themselves (Lewinsohn et al., 1996), both of which act slowly, allowing the suicidal person to change her mind and save herself or be discovered and rescued. However, women and girls are increasingly using firearms in suicide attempts, with more lethal results.

During childhood, there is no marked preponderance of male suicides. Children of both sexes younger than 12 tend to choose nonlethal methods in suicide attempts, such as throwing themselves down stairs, jumping from the roof, or eating soap, and extremely few use firearms for suicide. Ironically, gun use and safety classes may familiarize women and children

Table 8-6 Annual Suicides among U.S. Youth (per 100,000 Individuals)

Age Range	Females	Males	Total
10–12	–	1.0	0.5+
13–15	2.27	5.63	3.95
15–19	3.48	16.5	9.5–9.99

SOURCE: National Center for Health Statistics (1999).

NOTE: There were too few suicides among girls younger than 13 and all children younger than 10 to provide official estimates. In comparison, the highest rates, 37.8 suicides per 100,000, were found for white men age 65 and over.

with weapons that can be used in suicide or homicide attempts.

Suicide looms large as a cause of death in young people in part because they are generally very healthy and unlikely to die from other causes such as disease. Suicide rates increase throughout life (see Table 8-6 for juvenile rates), peaking among white men over 65 who are suffering from depression, disability, or disease (National Institute of Mental Health, 2000).

Depression, Alcohol, and Suicide

For troubled college students, the use of alcohol, drugs, and tobacco significantly increases the risk of suicide (Brenner et al., 1999). Drinking a large amount of alcohol preceded the attempt in many cases, either binge drinking at the time of the attempt or heavy drinking over a longer period of time (Hawton, Haigh, Simkin, & Fagg, 1995; Reifman & Windle, 1995). Being depressed is one of the strongest predictors of suicidal thoughts and intentions in adolescents (DiFilippo & Overholser, 2000). Since suicidal thoughts and behavior are symptoms of depressive disorders, the connection between suicide and depression is understandable. However, many suicidal youngsters are not depressed (Reynolds, 1994), and no history of major depression was found in 42% of one large sample of troubled adolescents who attempted suicide (Andrews & Lewinsohn, 1992). The picture is somewhat different for completed suicide. Completed suicide is more often associated with depression, while unsuccessful suicide attempts can reflect a host of different motivations, including craving for attention, revenge, jealousy, self-pity, and other manipulative or hostile intentions (Lumsden, 1980). Young children may imagine that they will be around to see their parents suffer anguish and remorse after they commit suicide. Suicidal thoughts are more likely when a person suffers from several co-occurring disorders (King, Pfeffer, Gammon, & Cohen, 1992), especially depression combined with conduct disorder or drug or alcohol abuse. The combination of depression and borderline personality disorder is dangerous. Borderline personality disorder is a pattern of intense, unstable relationships, unstable self-image, impulsivity, anger, and recurrent suicidal gestures or behavior.

Family Disturbance and Suicide

Family characteristics also play a role in juvenile suicides. If family members are depressed, suicidal, or otherwise disturbed, a child's risk for suicide increases, either immediately or in the future. Child suicide is also linked to the death of someone close, such as a parent, and to the child's own adjustment problems (Reynolds, 1994). Suicidal family members create emotional turmoil at home, and they can unknowingly serve as self-injurious models for children. Alternatively, a child may be unwanted or abused, feel valueless, or be locked in serious conflict with parents. Whatever the reason, the child comes to despair that improvement is possible. The most common problems of suicidal children are depression and hopelessness, but they also may show impulsive anger and hostility (Wilson, 1991).

Because of young children's cognitive immaturity, their beliefs about suicide may appear bizarre, and their attempts are pathetically unsuccessful. Most children younger than 9 years do not understand that death is universal, irreversible, and unavoidable. They may envision returning to enjoy seeing how much their family regret having treated them badly, or they may expect a last-minute magical rescue. Troubled children's hints that they may not be around to enjoy a holiday or that they may not grow up should be questioned as possible indicators that they are thinking about suicide.

Cultural and Social Factors

Where suicide is honored as a tradition, as in Japan, rates tend to be high, even among youth, but in Catholic or Muslim countries where suicide is forbid-

den for religious reasons, suicides are much rarer than in other regions. Suicides are increasing in many parts of the world, especially where religious and cultural prohibitions are loosening and record keeping is becoming more accurate.

Outbreaks of suicide or consistently high rates of suicide occur repeatedly among the youth on Indian reservations in North America (see the Research Focus box). (Some tribes prefer the term *Native American*, others favor *American Indian*, and still others use *Indian*. Since there is no clear choice, this book uses *Indian* to refer to members of the tribes of North America.) The loss of their culture and traditional way of life combined with their exclusion from the prosperous white mainstream culture leave many Indians culturally homeless and bitter about past wrongs. Facing discrimination and poverty if they leave the reservations and even worse poverty and joblessness if they stay, many young Indians feel hopeless, drink excessively, and use illicit drugs heavily. These young people have lost the values and spiritual beliefs of their culture, but are clearly not members of the majority culture. They are outsiders everywhere, and it is not difficult to understand why they lose hope. Children who are too poor, young, and geographically isolated to buy the usual illicit drugs can always sniff gasoline, which leads to brain damage and death for many Innu children in Labrador (Rogan, 2001). At the request of concerned tribal leaders, the Canadian Royal Mounted Police and child protection authorities are evacuating the children from their far northern villages to try to prevent them from attending all-night parties outdoors, then collapsing in snowbanks and freezing to death or accidentally setting themselves on fire. The children are not motivated to change, and no one is sure how to rehabilitate them other than removing them from their community.

America's decaying, violent inner cities also represent pockets of poverty and cultural chaos in which there are high rates of juvenile depression and suicide. Gangs routinely engage in wildly reckless and violent behavior that is self-destructive and dangerous to others. Suicide rates are increasing among African-American and Hispanic-American adolescents, particularly those involved with gangs (Griffith & Bell, 1988; Rotheram-Borus, Piacentini, Cantwell, Belin, & Song, 2000). Although suicide prevention programs are being developed especially for minority youth, little

Where Have All the Children Gone?

American Indians, including Alaska Natives, have the highest suicide rates of all ethnic groups in the United States. Iris Wagman Borowsky and her research team set out to discover some reasons for these many suicide attempts and ways to prevent them. The researchers surveyed a huge number (11,666) of 7th through 12th graders in schools in Indian reservations, looking for adolescents who said they had attempted suicide. This group represented 21.8% of the girls and 11.8% of the boys. They were compared with students who denied ever having made a suicide attempt. A number of problems appeared significantly more often in the lives of the suicide attempters:

- Family or friends who attempted or committed suicide
- Somatic (physical) symptoms to an unusual degree
- Physical or sexual abuse
- Health concerns (e.g., diabetes, tuberculosis)
- Alcohol, marijuana, or other drug use
- Special education class placement
- Treatment for emotional problems
- Gang involvement
- Access to a gun

The greater the number of these risk factors in a child's life, the greater the estimated probability that the child would attempt suicide. Any one risk factor might not increase the probability much, but it would be wise to offer counseling to youngsters with several risk factors and to their parents.

The researchers also found some factors that *protect* youth from making suicide attempts, including:

- Being able to discuss their problems with someone
- Having good emotional health
- Being closely connected to their family

These things may sound trivial, but they are important. Being close to someone is important to children. The researchers were surprised to find that adding protective factors more powerfully reduced the probability of a suicide attempt than did decreasing the number of risk factors. This finding suggests that any program that could strengthen the ties within Indian families and encourage teenagers to confide in family members and friends might also improve the teens' adjustment and decrease their suicide rates. It would also help to give them reason to hope for a future in which their culture would be more widely respected, and they could escape from extreme poverty and lead safer, more rewarding lives.

SOURCE: Borowsky, Resnick, Ireland, & Blum (1999).

---

success has been reported thus far (Summerville, Kaslow, & Doepke, 1996). Perhaps their difficult battles with poverty, inadequate education, poor health care, and discrimination outweigh the relatively weak positive influence of suicide prevention programs.

Alarmingly high rates of suicide have been reported among gay and lesbian youth (also termed *sexual-minority youth*). Between 23% and 42% of them reported that they have attempted suicide at least once (D'Augelli & Hershberger, 1993; Remafedi, French, Story, Resnick, & Blum, 1998). However, it appears that their sexual orientation itself does not cause these young people to become suicidal. Rather, the problem lies more in their social exclusion because of their sexual orientation. As compared with a similar group of heterosexual adolescents, the sexual-minority youths felt greater depression and hopelessness, which could be traced to the discrimination and rejection they experienced (Safren & Heimberg, 1999). When the effects of their greater depression and hopelessness were controlled, gay and lesbian adolescents were no more likely to be suicidal than heterosexual youth.

Suicide Prevention

Suicide is a leading killer of adolescents, and it is important for people who work with them to be alert to risk factors and signs of suicidal intent. Risk factors include depression, severe family strife, a troubled attachment to the mother, substance abuse, romantic relationship problems, school-related problems, and other types of stress (Monroe et al., 1999; Spirito,

Brown, Overholser, & Fritz, 1989). Unfortunately, this is a list of typical teenage problems, none of which clearly points to suicide. Additional factors may indicate that the threat is significant. Severe depression is one of the strongest predictors of suicidal thoughts (e.g., thoughts of death, wishing to be dead, dwelling on suicide, having a plan) and attempts (DiFilippo & Overholser, 2000). Any suicidal statements, threats, past attempts, or suspicious "accidents" should be taken seriously, even if they seem theatrical and improbable, as in superficial cutting. Having a definite plan to commit suicide and making actual preparations, such as gathering a large quantity of sleeping pills, place a person at high risk and call for hospitalization. The situation is less dangerous if the person can easily give a reason for living when asked to do so. A teenager who is severely depressed and cannot offer any reason for living is likely to attempt suicide (Gutierrez, Osman, Kopper, & Barrios, 2000).

Interpersonal problems may motivate self-destructive behavior. Peer relationships are especially important to teenagers, and some become suicidal because of perceived peer rejection, lack of supportive, close friendships, affiliation with deviant peers, and family dysfunction (Prinstein, Boergers, Spirito, Little, & Grapentine, 2000). So people who work with teenagers should be especially alert to suicidal intentions among youth who are depressed, socially rejected, associate with a deviant group, use drugs, and come from severely troubled families. Recent programs have had some limited success in preventing depression, as we noted previously, and combating depression should also reduce suicide (Gillham et al., 2000). However, a successful national program is probably a distant goal. For the present, it is important to know how to intervene when someone becomes suicidal (see Table 8-7).

Suicide prevention requires removing all means to commit suicide until the person calms down, receives professional counseling, and can assess the situation more realistically. The person must be denied all access to weapons of any type, motor vehicles, high places, drugs, poisons, and other means to commit suicide. Ironically, people who attempt suicide are very likely to feel better and abandon the attempt to kill themselves after an unsuccessful attempt. But sometimes the feeling of relief does not last. The ones who are quietly determined to commit suicide are the most difficult to identify and treat, because they are so secretive. Nevertheless, prompt, decisive intervention can save lives, and no one should hesitate to call 911 or a hospital emergency center if a teenager is making serious threats.

People are likely to do the most good if they act decisively to protect the teenager from self-harm. The teenager's family must be notified of the threat, and it

---

Table 8.7 First Aid to Help Prevent Suicide

The general principles of first aid for suicidal people are to put their physical protection first and foremost, secure their environment so that no means of suicide are available to them, and get professional help as quickly as possible. There are several commonsense actions to take:

1. Evaluate the danger. Does the suicidal person talk about a plan and a way to carry it out? Do you see physical evidence of an attempt, such as a weapon, pills, or self-injuries? Does the person admit to thinking about suicide or death or threaten to commit suicide? Are the threats new or usual for this person? Does the person need surveillance or hospitalization? It is better to make a mistake in the form of being overly cautious, because that may save a life.

2. Immediately secure all firearms, potentially lethal drugs, and car keys, and block the person's access to dangers such as high buildings or bodies of water.

3. Call your local suicide hotline or helpline, which is listed in the telephone book. If there is immediate danger, call the police or dial 911. Do not imagine that you can handle a seriously suicidal person by yourself, even if the person says it's all right now and pleads with you to keep it secret.

4. In cases of attempts involving pill ingestion (poisoning) or a wound, get medical help as soon as possible. Call an ambulance or drive the person to an emergency room. Suicidal people require medical treatment. If they cannot protect their own lives, someone else must save them. Hospitalization can prevent suicide and may be the only possible intervention.

SOURCES: Stoelb & Chirboga (1998); Younggren (2001).

Back to the Beginning
When to Seek Professional Help

The three youngsters whose stories began this chapter—Tanya, Dave, and Joe—illustrate the symptoms and treatments for depression:

- Thirteen-year-old Dave was entering adolescence, but was feeling lost. He was alienated from his parents, and his father had been hospitalized for depression, indicating that heredity and environment may have combined to make Dave depressed. His signs of conduct disorder (his drug use and minor criminal behavior) might make his depression particularly difficult to treat, but his previous good grades improve his prognosis.
- High school senior Joe's father was putting pressure on him to get into a highly competitive business school and fight hard to succeed, just when Joe was questioning his own academic ability. He, too, was alienated from his family, and it seemed that no one would listen to his concerns. A son has to achieve.
- At 10, Tanya was experiencing self-image problems, suffering from the notion that she was getting fat, when she was only growing up and entering pubescence. She too viewed herself as a loser, with no friends. Societal expectations about women having perfect, slim bodies and being very popular could produce Tanya's depressive feelings. Being highly popular *and* happy *and* having a perfect body is an impossibility for almost all teenagers.

In all three of these cases, the families are demanding, emotionally unconnected with the child, or help-less to cope with their child's growing depression. Excessive self-criticism marked these children. They felt they were socially and physically unattractive, academic failures, outcasts, and total losers and believed that they caused bad things to happen and always would (helplessness, hopelessness, and depressive cognitions). Their severe and persistent sense of hopelessness, alienation, and irritability should warn family and friends that they need psychological help. They showed other signs of serious depression, too. Eating disorders, anxiety, drug abuse, conduct disorder, and sleeping problems are all frequent accompaniments of depressive disorder.

Joe's hopelessness and self-criticism have reached the point that he should be assessed for suicide risk. His problems have been getting worse for several months, and he needs immediate attention and treatment. His parents must be helped to listen to him and support him. Tanya's serious eating problems should be diagnosed and treated without delay. She might develop anorexia, which sometimes becomes life-threatening (see Chapter 14). Dave also requires professional attention, because he is using drugs, getting into trouble with the law, failing in school, and showing signs of depression, including despondency and inability to concentrate. In all of these cases, a thorough assessment and diagnosis should come first, followed by treatment, probably including cognitive-behavioral therapy or behavioral family therapy and possibly antidepressant medication with periodic follow-ups to adjust type and dosage.

---

may be necessary to take him to an emergency room for medical care, whether he wants to go or not. Saving a life is more important than preserving privacy or sparing someone's feelings. People with acute suicidal urges require immediate professional treatment and many need hospitalization. Many individuals have put suicide attempts behind them and gone on to happier and more productive lives.

SUMMARY

Contrary to earlier views, children can become clinically depressed and are appropriately diagnosed using criteria for adult depressive disorders, with some modifications. Children are more likely than adults to show their depression in the form of irritability, physical complaints, and social withdrawal. Children's depression is often accompanied by anxiety disorders and conduct problems, which may make diagnosis difficult. Recent research indicates a probable genetic basis for some forms of depression, but the specific pathways have not yet been demonstrated.

Various psychological theories trace depression to unconscious conflict originating early in life in interactions with parents (psychodynamic approaches, including interpersonal and attachment theories), to distorted thinking linked with early loss (cognitive theories such as Beck's), or to defeatist attitudes associated with learned helplessness (Seligman's theory). Other approaches trace depression to catastrophic loss of positive reinforcement (Lewinsohn's reinforcement-loss model) or extremely low self-confidence and the conviction that nothing can be done to improve the situation (Bandura's self-efficacy theory and Weisz's contingency-competence-control model).

Depression is rare prior to puberty, then increases rapidly to reach adult rates in the late teens. Older types of antidepressant medication are not useful with children and adolescents, but some of the newer medications such as Prozac show promise and are widely prescribed. Cognitive-behavioral therapy and other forms of psychotherapy have proved effective in both prevention and treatment, but further demonstrations are needed.

Suicide is extremely rare before the age of 12, but rises rapidly in early adolescence and continues to increase into old age. Many problems in addition to depression are related to suicide in young people, especially peer rejection, substance abuse, psychiatric problems, and family discord. Suicide prevention must include treatment of depression, limiting access to potentially lethal means of committing suicide, and detecting and preventing attempts. Professional help is absolutely necessary. Teenagers who are successfully prevented from committing suicide may overcome the inclination and go on to satisfying and productive lives.

INFOTRAC COLLEGE EDITION

For more information, explore this resource at http://www.infotrac-college.com/Wadsworth. Enter the following search terms:

depression in children
mood disorder
bipolar disorder
suicide in children/adolescents
minorities and mental health
antidepressants and children/adolescents
cognitive-behavioral therapy

IN FOCUS ANSWERS

IN FOCUS 1 ▶ List the different types of mood disorders.

- Major depressive episode and disorder
- Bipolar (or manic-depressive) disorder
- Minor depression (or subclinical depression)
- Dysthymic disorder

IN FOCUS 2 ▶ Describe how depression rates differ for children, adolescents, and adults.

- Depression is very rare before the age of 6, occurring in less than 1% of children.
- Depression increases irregularly until the age of 14, then dramatically during adolescence to a prevalence of 7.6% or more for 18- to 19-year-olds.
- Depression occurs in 12% of adult women and 6.6% of adult men.

IN FOCUS 3 ▶ How do adverse family environments lead children to become depressed or otherwise disturbed?

- Depressed parents have poorer interactions with their children and also model depression.
- Family violence, particularly by the father, stresses and depresses children.

IN FOCUS 4 ▶ According to several theories, what types of persistent cognitive patterns are associated with risk for depression?

- Threats to self-esteem and feelings of abandonment—the psychoanalytic and attachment theories
- Negative beliefs about the self, the world, and the future—Beck's cognitive theory
- Overwhelming feelings of hopelessness about controlling one's world—learned helplessness theory
- Low self-efficacy or the conviction that one is doomed to failure—social-cognitive theories

IN FOCUS 5 ▶ Describe four difficulties in tracing childhood depression to genetic or biochemical abnormalities.

- Research points to genetic roots for adult but not childhood depression.
- Heritability appears greater for the less severe forms of childhood depression, not the more severe forms.
- Childhood depression may not run in families but may be related to other disorders that do, such as alcoholism, substance abuse, and antisocial behavior.
- Transmission of depression could be largely or totally environmental.

IN FOCUS 6 ▶ Identify the two most promising types of treatment for depressed children.

- Among drugs, the SSRIs are showing particular promise. Other drugs appear ineffective.
- Cognitive-behavioral and interpersonal therapies have the most research support.

9 Attention-Deficit/Hyperactivity Disorder

In the Beginning

A Case of ADHD

Allen's birth was seemingly routine, and his mother's pregnancy was normal. His early development progressed at a satisfactory rate, although he seemed to show an extremely high level of activity and an inability to attend. In the 1st grade, Allen was diagnosed as having attention-deficit/hyperactivity disorder (ADHD). What follows is a description of Allen's case 3 years later.

Allen is a 4th-grade boy who was referred to the clinic for ongoing reading difficulties despite having had 3 years of special education services. He had been diagnosed with ADHD and had responded favorably to Ritalin. In kindergarten, Allen was first identified as experiencing difficulty with readiness skills. He was very active and had great difficulty staying in a group and participating in activities. He started taking Ritalin in 1st grade and was kept in 1st grade an additional year because of significant delays in academics. Allen was evaluated in 2nd grade and placed in a learning disability program. Behaviorally and socially he was reported not to experience any difficulties, and was well accepted by his peers. He was also reported to be hard working and motivated. (Teeter & Semrud-Clikeman, 1997, p. 244)

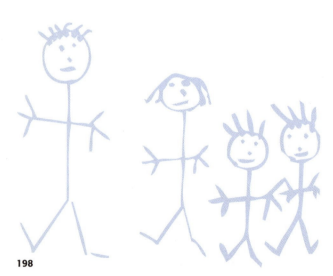

INTRODUCTION

IN FOCUS 1 ▶ Give two prevalence estimates for ADHD that characterize the difference in occurrence by gender.

Allen's circumstances are quite like those of many other youngsters with ADHD. He has substantial academic difficulties, including reading problems, and co-occurring learning disabilities that involve both poor receptive and expressive language performance and subpar memory skills. Allen is hyperactive and has been taking a medication called Ritalin that seems to have helped. Ritalin has been widely used with youngsters having ADHD, and it is not uncommon for the results to be assessed favorably by parents, teachers, and others around these children.

Allen is also different from many children with ADHD. Thus far, he seems to be operating in a socially acceptable manner and is not reported to have significant behavioral problems. Youngsters with ADHD often experience interpersonal and social difficulties that may result from, or at least be related to, some rather prominent and undesirable behaviors. As we examine ADHD in this chapter, it is important to remember that children with this disorder are individuals. Even though we are describing *some* similar characteristics they share, they have as many differences as they have similarities. So you shouldn't be surprised that Allen is like others with ADHD but also different.

Attention-deficit/hyperactivity disorder (ADHD) is one of the most frequently referred psychological disorders of childhood, despite the fact that until the 1990s it was often viewed as a set of symptoms accompanying other disabilities (Barkley, 1998; Hardman, Drew, & Egan, 2002; Voeller, 2001). Many children with ADHD are not referred for professional help until they enter school and experience difficulty in that setting. Services to school children with ADHD increased substantially in the last decade as the U.S. Department of Education determined that these youngsters are eligible for services through the Individuals with Disabilities Education Act under the category of Other Health Impairments. Twenty states in the United States indicated 20% or greater increases in services to children with ADHD under this category between 1996–97 and 1997–98 (U.S. Department of Education, 2000).

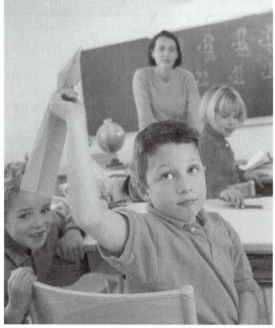

Britt Erlanson/Getty Images

Children with ADHD often present a challenge to teachers because they do not attend to schoolwork and can be somewhat disruptive.

The overall prevalence of ADHD is estimated to be approximately 3–5% of the school-age population, but this estimate varies widely depending on the criteria used to define the condition (National Institutes of Health, 1998; Rhee, Waldman, Hay, & Levy, 1999). However, researchers agree that ADHD is more prevalent in males than in females, with the male-to-female ratio ranging from 2-to-1 to 10-to-1, depending on the sample population (National Institutes of Health, 1998; Rhee et al., 1999). The average male-to-female ratio across all ages is about 3.5 to 1. There is age-dependent variation, with young children showing a higher male-to-female ratio than older groups (American Psychiatric Association, 2000; Barkley, 1998; Bender, 1998).

A sizable minority of mothers (30%) report early difficulties with their infants who later develop ADHD. These infants are described as colicky, irritable, and hard to manage and as having a difficult temperament (Barkley, 1998). It is estimated that about half of those children who develop ADHD in childhood continue to have some adjustment difficulty in adolescence and early adulthood (Austin, 1999; Mancini,

Table 9-1 DSM-IV-TR Definition of ADHD

Criterion	Description
Criterion A	The essential feature of attention-deficit/hyperactivity disorder is a persistent pattern of inattention and/or hyperactivity-impulsivity that is more frequent and severe than is typically observed in individuals at a comparable level of development.
Criterion B	Some hyperactive-impulsive or inattentive symptoms that cause impairment must have been present before age 7 years, although many individuals are diagnosed after the symptoms have been present for a number of years.
Criterion C	Some impairment from the symptoms must be present in at least two settings (e.g., at home and at school or work).
Criterion D	There must be clear evidence of interference with developmentally appropriate social, academic, or occupational functioning.
Criterion E	The disturbance does not occur exclusively during the course of a pervasive developmental disorder, schizophrenia, or other psychotic disorder and is not better accounted for by another mental disorder (e.g., mood disorder, anxiety disorder, dissociative disorder, or personality disorder).

SOURCE: American Psychiatric Association (2000), p. 85. Reprinted with permission from the *Diagnostic and Statistical Manual of Mental Disorders*, 4th ed., Text Revision. © 2000 APA.

Van Ameringen, Oakman, & Figueirdo, 1999; Silver, 1999). It is a myth that ADHD changes dramatically in adolescence.

DEFINING ATTENTION-DEFICIT/ HYPERACTIVITY DISORDER (ADHD)

IN FOCUS 2 ▶ Identify the five DSM-IV-TR diagnostic criteria for ADHD.

IN FOCUS 3 ▶ Identify the three types of ADHD according to DSM-IV-TR.

The condition now known as **attention-deficit/ hyperactivity disorder (ADHD)** historically has had several different labels, including hyperkinesis (high rate of movement) and minimal brain dysfunction (MBD). The variety of names has been unfortunate and confusing. These terms have implied high rates of motor activity, some type of brain dysfunction, and difficulty in paying attention. More recently, the primary focus of the diagnostic criteria for this condition has been on poor attending and hyperactivity-impulsivity. Table 9-1 presents the definition of ADHD as outlined in DSM-IV-TR, and the diagnostic criteria are found in Table 9-2 (American Psychiatric Association, 2000).

CHARACTERISTICS OF ADHD

IN FOCUS 4 ▶ Identify three major characteristics that present challenges for individuals with ADHD.

Inattention

It can be seen from the diagnostic criteria for ADHD that inattention is a central characteristic of this disorder. Descriptions of children with ADHD often include statements like this: "He can never concentrate on his schoolwork because he is staring out the window or disturbing his neighbor," or "She never listens to instructions; it all goes in one ear and out the other." Clearly, when compared to children without disabilities, children with ADHD have more difficulty in both attending to a task for a sustained period of time and working independently (Auerbach, Benjamin, Faroy, Gellar, & Ebstein, 2001; Speltz, DeKlyen, Calderon, Greenberg, & Feisher, 1999; Zillessen, Scheuerpflug, Fallgatter, Strik, & Warnke, 2001). In addition, these children may also have difficulty screening out irrelevant or extraneous stimuli. Even if a child with ADHD tries to attend, he may be distracted by a common noise such as a truck passing outside the school window or a classmate tapping her pencil (Colledge & Blair, 2001; Ralph, Oman, & Forney, 2001).

Table 9-2 DSM-IV-TR Diagnostic Criteria for Attention-Deficit/Hyperactivity Disorder

A. Either (1) or (2):

  1. Six (or more) of the following symptoms of *inattention* have persisted for at least six months to a degree that is maladaptive and inconsistent with developmental level:

  Inattention

    a. Often fails to give close attention to details or makes careless mistakes in schoolwork, work, or other activities.

    b. Often has difficulty sustaining attention in tasks or play activities.

    c. Often does not seem to listen when spoken to directly.

    d. Often does not follow through on instructions and fails to finish schoolwork, chores, or duties in the workplace (not due to oppositional behavior or failure to understand instructions).

    e. Often has difficulty organizing tasks and activities.

    f. Often avoids, dislikes, or is reluctant to engage in tasks that require sustained mental effort (such as schoolwork or homework).

    g. Often loses things necessary for tasks or activities (e.g., toys, school assignments, pencils, books, or tools).

    h. Is often easily distracted by extraneous stimuli.

    i. Is often forgetful in daily activities.

  2. Six (or more) of the following symptoms of *hyperactivity-impulsivity* have persisted for at least 6 months to a degree that is maladaptive and inconsistent with development level:

  Hyperactivity

    a. Often fidgets with hands or feet or squirms in seat.

    b. Often leaves seat in classroom or in other situations in which remaining seated is expected.

    c. Often runs about or climbs excessively in situations in which it is inappropriate (in adolescents or adults, may be limited to subjective feelings of restlessness).

    d. Often has difficulty playing or engaging in leisure activities quietly.

    e. Is often "on the go" or often acts as if "driven by a motor."

    f. Often talks excessively.

  Impulsivity

    g. Often blurts out answers before questions have been completed.

    h. Often has difficulty awaiting turn.

    i. Often interrupts or intrudes on others (e.g., butts into conversations or games).

B. Some hyperactive-impulsive or inattentive symptoms that caused impairment were presented before age 7 years.

C. Some impairment from the symptoms is present in two or more settings (e.g., at school [or work] and at home).

D. There must be clear evidence of clinically significant impairment in social, academic, or occupational functioning.

E. The symptoms do not occur exclusively during the course of a pervasive developmental disorder, schizophrenia, or other psychotic disorder and are not better accounted for by another mental disorder (e.g., mood disorder, anxiety disorder, dissociative disorder, or a personality disorder).

Code based on type:

Attention-Deficit/Hyperactive Disorder, Combined Type: if both Criteria A1 and A2 are met for the past 6 months.

Attention-Deficit/Hyperactive Disorder, Predominantly Inattentive Type: if Criterion A1 is met but Criterion A2 is not met for the past 6 months.

Attention-Deficit/Hyperactive Disorder, Predominantly Hyperactive-Impulsive Type: if Criterion A2 is met but Criterion A1 is not met for the past 6 months.

Coding note: For individuals (especially adolescents and adults) who currently have symptoms that no longer meet full criteria, "In Partial Remission" should be specified.

SOURCE: American Psychiatric Association (2000), p. 92. Reprinted with permission from the *Diagnostic and Statistical Manual of Mental Disorders*, 4th ed., Text Revision. © 2000 APA.

Impulsivity

Inattention by itself does not completely define ADHD. Other characteristics are also important. For example, the diagnostic criteria in Table 9-2 list impulsivity as an important characteristic of the disorder. The word *impulsivity* suggests poor self-control, excitability, and the inability to delay gratification or to inhibit urges (Molina, Smith, & Pelham, 2001; Solanto et al., 2001). Many impulsive behaviors are dangerous and result in accidents, including automobile accidents for adolescents with ADHD. In essence, impulsivity is characterized by acting before weighing alternative responses. Recent literature addresses this characteristic in terms of impulse control and thinking about the consequences of one's actions; the deficit shown in ADHD is presumed to be in what is termed *executive function*, the ability to monitor and regulate one's behavior (Entwistle, 2000; Fleck, 1998; Speltz et al., 1999).

One approach to assessing impulsivity is to have a child scan an array of different line drawings and identify the one that is identical to a comparison drawing. For instance, children would be shown the picture of a bear at the top of Figure 9-1 and would have to pick a bear from the bottom group that exactly matches the sample bear. This test is called Matching Familiar Figures, and children with ADHD generally make decisions faster and with more errors than children without disabilities (Albaret, Soppelsa, & Marquet-Doleac, 2000). (Also see the Research Focus box.)

Overactivity

The terms *hyperactivity* and *hyperkinesis* refer to high levels of activity and energy. Frequently, children with ADHD are described as "always on the move" or "bouncing off the walls" (Barkley, 1998; Goldstein, 1999). ADHD can be diagnosed with hyperactivity-impulsivity as the predominant characteristic. While this high level of activity diminishes in some children as they age, this is not true for others. For some, hyperactive behavior seems to emerge in adolescence and may continue through adult years (Moore & Fombonne, 1999; Stein, Fischer, & Szumowski, 1999; Wood, 1997).

The methodological measurement of hyperactive children's motor activity ranges from simple observa-

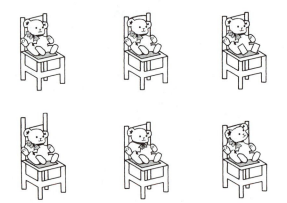

Figure 9-1   Sample Item from the Matching Familiar Figures Test
Source: Kagan (1966).

tions of behavior to the use of sophisticated measuring devices such as ultrasonic sensors, actometers (which take readings from self-winding wristwatches), and pneumatic cushions that measure movement. Interpretation of activity-level measures is difficult because of the lack of norms specifying average rates of activity for children at different ages and the many different types of overactivity (Barkley, 1998). In the absence of clear-cut norms for different types of motor activity, researchers usually compare motor activity of children identified as having ADHD with that of children without disabilities. The results are perplexing. It appears that children with ADHD are generally indistinguishable from their peers without disabilities in unstructured free play situations (Bender, 1998; Smith, 1998). Further, levels of activity of children with ADHD with different diagnostic labels (e.g., combined and primarily inattentive types) do not differ consistently (Dane, Schachar, & Tannock, 2000).

Perceived activity of children with ADHD, however, seems to vary with the type of environment. Situations differ in their structure and the demands they place on the child. As the structure and demand char-

Impulsivity and Mediating Fidgety Behaviors in Hyperactive Boys: A Possible Link

One aspect of impulsivity is the inability to wait in order to earn a reward (reinforcer). Children with ADHD are often described as being unable to delay gratification and needing instant gratification. Figure 9-2 summarizes data from a study with hyperactive and nonhyperactive boys in which participants had to learn to wait and withhold a response to earn a piece of candy. To earn this candy, the boys had to first press a button, then wait a period of time (6 seconds), and then press the button again. If they pressed the button too quickly, they lost the candy. This type of procedure is called *differential reinforcement* of low rates of behavior.

The nonhyperactive boys did much better than the hyperactive boys on the waiting task. The hyperactive boys seemed unable to wait. The nonhyperactive boys (1) made fewer responses than did hyperactive boys, (2) earned more pieces of candy than hyperactive boys, and (3) were overall more efficient in their responding (see Figure 9-2).

One interesting aspect of the study was the behaviors the boys used to help themselves wait between button pushes (mediating behaviors). Ninety percent of the hyperactive boys used one of the following observable motor behaviors to help them wait, but only 30% of the nonhyperactive boys used such behavior mediators:

Circling DRL response button with finger 9 times
Swinging legs 11, 12, or 20 times
Counting with lip movements
Counting out loud—numbers or ABCs
Blowing on reward box
Singing out loud
Shaking reward box 10 times
Hitting knee with right hand 20 times
Foot-tapping 16 times
Tapping finger 10 times on button box
"Walking" fingers around DRL button 9 times
Stomping with foot 9 or 10 times
Running around table once
Hitting side of box

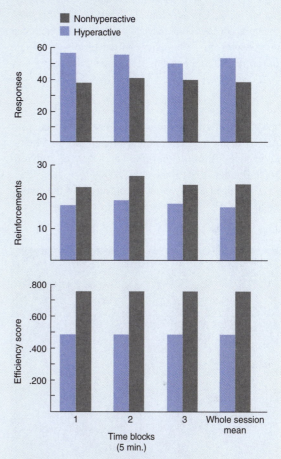

Figure 9-2   The Performance of Hyperactive and Nonhyperactive Groups over Three Time Blocks of a DRL 6-Second Schedule
SOURCE: Gordon (1979). Reprinted by permission.

Jumping jacks 4 times
Hitting collateral buttons (other nonfunctional buttons on console)

Most (80%) of the nonhyperactive boys used nonbehavioral mediators or some type of thinking strategy to pass the time. The more behavioral mediators a child used, the poorer his performance on the waiting task. The more covert or nonbehavioral mediators a child used, the better his performance. The behavioral mediators listed are closely related to the fidgety, restless behaviors commonly used to describe the hyperactive child. It was suggested that such physical mediating responses may be used by hyperactive children to help control their own impulsivity.

SOURCE: Gordon (1979). Reprinted by permission.

acteristics of an environment increase, children with ADHD begin to stand out and be perceived as being overactive (Antrop, Roeyers, Van Oost, & Butysse, 2000; Bender, 1998; Dane et al., 2000).

The type of activity must be considered in the assessment of ADHD. Overall levels of activity may not be the critical element in identifying hyperactive children (Dane et al., 2000; Hardman et al., 2002). Instead, it may be whether children's activities bring them into conflict with their caretakers. A child who fidgets, taps his foot, is unable to keep his hands to himself, and talks out of turn may constantly come to the attention of the teacher and be perceived as overly active. A child who is engaged in the same amount of motor activity but is working diligently is judged to be normally active.

Rather than being primarily overactive, a child with ADHD can be primarily off-task and impulsive, with several associated disruptive behaviors from checklists that are used to identify children with ADHD. Rating scales often have many items addressing behavior problems that are predictive of ADHD, such as quarrelsomeness, emotional reactivity, distractibility, and aggressive behaviors, rather than focusing on activity level (Crystal, Ostrander, Chen, & August, 2001; Johnson & Rosen, 2000). Barkley (1998) has characterized these disruptive behaviors in general as constituting a primary deficit in "rule-governed" behavior. Children with ADHD basically have difficulty in adhering to rules and instructions, which is commonly interpreted as noncompliant, inattentive, impulsive, and disruptive behavior (Tramo, 1999; Tripp, Luk, Schaughency, & Singh, 1999). The disruptive behaviors become more pronounced and problematic as the structure and rule demands of the environment increase, and this increases the likelihood of referral (Merrell, 1999; Shaver, 1999; Venn, 2000). Most children are first identified as having ADHD when they enter school, a structured, rule-bound environment.

There has been some interest in distinguishing ADHD from attention deficit disorder (ADD) in chil-

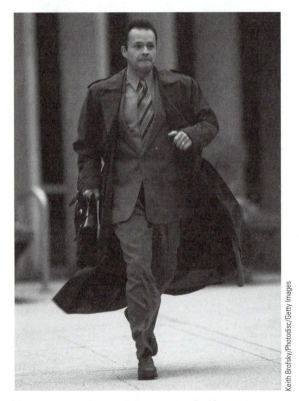

Keith Brofsky/Photodisc/Getty Images

In some cases, characteristics associated with ADHD continue well into adulthood.

dren who have attention problems but do not exhibit hyperactive behavior. Some researchers have conceptualized this condition as representing the inattentive type of ADHD using the DSM-IV-TR framework (Padolsky, 2001). Some research seeks interventions for the attention difficulties of these children while attempting to avoid the medication that has often been used to control hyperactivity (Pozzi, 2000). While there are some reports that 35% of the youngsters identified with attention deficit do not have hyperactivity, such assessment is probably best considered as a part of the ADHD diagnosis. Research with popular assessment approaches has not reliably produced clinically meaningful discriminations between ADD and ADHD as separate disorders (Forbes, 2001; Snider, Frankenberger, & Aspenson, 2000; Stewart, Steffler, Lemoine, & Leps, 2001).

Other Characteristics of ADHD

Although the defining characteristics of ADHD are primarily inattention, impulsivity, and fidgety motor behavior, there are associated characteristics that are also common to this condition. For example, children with ADHD commonly have social difficulties, particularly with peers (Henker & Whalen, 1999; Lochman & Szczepanski, 1999; Weller, Rowan, Weller, & Elia, 1999). They are viewed as being immature, uncooperative, self-centered, and bossy. Most of them have few close friends, they tend to play with younger children, and 50–60% experience social rejection from their peers. Children with ADHD are more often seen as aggressive, annoyingly uncooperative, and easily led by others. Aggressive behaviors are found in perhaps half of children with ADHD (Stahl & Clarizio, 1999;

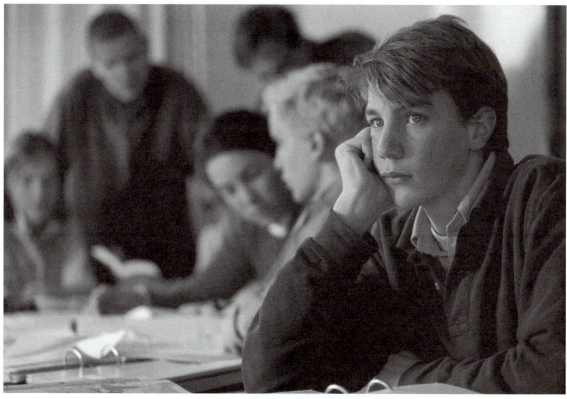

Children with ADHD may be somewhat isolated socially, having few close friends and encountering difficulty in interacting with peers.

Venn, 2000; Weller et al., 1999). Some children with ADHD exhibit antisocial or pathological social behavior, such as cruelty to animals (Luk, Staiger, Wong, & Mathai, 1999). When aggression is associated with ADHD, the prognosis is generally poorer.

Children with ADHD also tend to be academically deficient, and some of this performance deficit may well be due to their poor planning and time management; a substantial proportion have reading deficiencies (Pisecco, Baker, Silva, & Brooke, 2001; Sakelaris, 1999; Tripp et al., 1999). A high proportion (ranging from 40% to 80%) of children labeled as having ADHD or being hyperactive are also identified as having significant problems with learning and achievement (Aro, Ahonen, Tolvanen, Lyytinen, & Todd-de-Barra, 1999; Barkley, 1998; Raggio, 1999).

POSSIBLE CAUSES OF ADHD

IN FOCUS 5 ▶ Identify three possible causes of ADHD.

There is probably no single cause of ADHD. However, in the past decade, a great deal of effort has gone into researching the possible causes of ADHD. Some of the research is highly controversial, such as that on the effects of food additives, fluorescent lighting, and sugar. But most of the work has followed more conventional lines of research, investigating genetics and other biological causes.

Organic Brain Damage

Overactivity and poor impulse control have long been associated with the diagnosis of organic brain damage in children. Some writers described what is now viewed as ADHD as early as 1902 and referred to behaviors such as overactivity, inattention, and aggressiveness, as well as other characteristics now associated with ADHD (Solanto, 2001). In many instances, these behaviors were linked with brain damage caused during birth by injury or deprivation of oxygen. These early injuries often went unnoticed until school age, when increased demands were placed on the child. The brain damage hypothesis received additional support following an encephalitis epidemic that occurred in the United States in 1918. On recovering

from this disease, many children showed a major shift in behavior and general personality changes. Children who had previously been compliant became hyperactive, distractible, irritable, deceptive, and generally unmanageable in school. Other evidence of the possible link between hyperactive behavior and brain damage was provided by brain-injured soldiers and children who had suffered head injuries (e.g., Strecker, 1929; Strecker & Ebaugh, 1924). Since the injury through disease, birth trauma, or head trauma was mostly of a minimal nature and not health- or life-threatening, the term *minimal brain damage (MBD)* was coined. Current research still explores brain injury but also focuses on chemical imbalances related to neurological functioning as potential causes (Faraone et al., 1999; Sagvolden, 1999).

Many children with ADHD do not show "hard" signs or histories of brain damage (Barkley, 1998; Dinn, Robbins, & Harris, 2001). It should be noted that the identification of neurological abnormalities among those with ADHD has advanced significantly with new technology, particularly brain-imaging procedures. In the past, it was not uncommon for a clinician to speculate regarding neurological status based on behavior. In some cases, it is now possible to examine brain function directly. Brain imaging, for example, indicates that many with ADHD seem to exhibit brain abnormalities in three areas: the frontal lobes, selected areas of the basal ganglia, and the cerebellum (Casey, 2001; Castellanos, 2001; Voeller, 2001) (see Figure 9-3).

The neurological involvement noted above is logically consistent with the behavioral impulsivity or lack of self-control in many children with ADHD. For example, some researchers report an association between frontal lobe pathology and impairment of executive function, thought to control impulsivity. The inhibition control of children with ADHD who show damage in this brain area appears deficient (Konrad, Gauggel, Manz, & Schoell, 2000; Ylvisaker & DeBonis, 2000).

Children with ADHD are thought to have a deficiency in the metabolism of neurotransmitters that relates to an impairment in the ability to control impulses (Wendt, 2000). For most of us, a balance generally exists between neurological excitation and inhibition. The child with ADHD is thought to have a defective in-

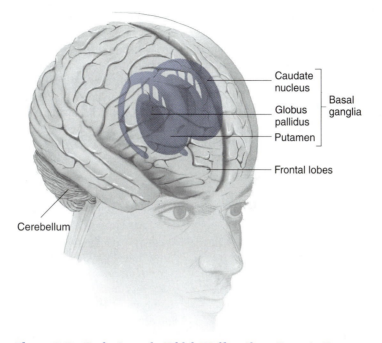

Caudate
nucleus

Globus
pallidus

Putamen

Basal
ganglia

Frontal lobes

Cerebellum

Figure 9-3   Brain Areas in Which Malfunctions Seem to Be Associated with ADHD

hibitory system that makes him or her more active and less sensitive to the effects of positive reinforcement than the normal child. The behavior problems experienced by children with ADHD are thought to be caused by their inability to learn effectively through positive reinforcement. The use of stimulant medication with these children is aimed at restoring the balance between the excitatory and inhibitory systems, which enhances the effects of positive reinforcement so that learning and behavioral adjustment are facilitated (Cunningham, 1999; Elia, Ambrosini, & Rapoport, 1999; Greenhill, 2001). Some writers question the research on neurotransmitter balance with ADHD children, regarding both the effects of stimulant medication and some clinical concerns about the drug use (e.g., Cherland & Fitzpatrick, 1999; Jensen et al., 1999; Vance, Luk, Costin, Tonge, & Pantelis, 1999). Research continues on neurotransmitters and ADHD; some researchers are manipulating levels of neurotransmitters through mechanisms other than medication (Putnam, 2001; Wendt, 2000). Much remains to be examined in this area of ADHD research.

Genetic Factors

Several researchers have sought to explain the behavioral characteristics of ADHD through some type of genetic mechanism. Scientific work in this area is difficult to conduct because the causal effects of heredity and environment are difficult to separate. Researchers have used two basic approaches. First, the incidence of psychiatric disorders in parents of children with ADHD is compared to that in parents of children without disabilities. Researchers assume that a higher incidence of psychiatric disorders in the families of children with ADHD would indicate a possible basis for heritability of the condition (Faraone, Doyle, Mick, & Biederman, 2001; Rapport, 2001). Genetically close relatives of youngsters with ADHD appear more likely to also have the condition or to show multiple symptoms of the condition than do close relatives of children without ADHD. This also appears to be the case with certain other disorders, such as bipolar disorder (Faraone, Biederman, & Monuteaux, 2001; Ross & Campagnon, 2001). Such results require some caution, however, because other influences may also follow family lines. For instance, parents who suffer from psychiatric conditions may provide a marginal home life, which may also contribute to the development of ADHD.

The second approach to the study of genetic causes of ADHD has been to compare identical twins and fraternal twins. Identical twins are genetically the same because the two embryos are formed after fertilization, and thus the two babies develop from the genetic material of a single fertilized egg. Fraternal twins are formed from two separate fertilizations of different eggs by separate sperm; the two embryos develop from different zygotes and therefore are not genetically identical. In twin studies, a genetic linkage is presumed if pairs of genetically identical twins share a characteristic, such as ADHD, more frequently than do pairs of fraternal twins. Current evidence suggests that a genetic linkage does exist, but some characteristics associated with ADHD, such as hyperactivity-impulsivity and reading disabilities, show a stronger genetic relationship than others (Nadder, Silberg, Rutter, Maes, & Eaves, 2001; Rhee, 2000; Willcutt & Pennington, 2000).

Genetic studies of children with ADHD indicate that heredity does play a role in the development of the condition. The exact role of genes, however, is still difficult to determine. Specific genes may cause higher activity levels, inattention, or impulsivity. However, it would not be surprising to find an interaction effect between combinations of genes (Auerbach et al., 2001). Continuing research attempts to sort out the various genetic questions as well as to investigate environmental influences (Eaves et al., 2000).

Environmental Factors

Children today are subject to a number of stresses, such as environmental pollution, exposure to low levels of radiation, ingestion of foods containing chemical additives, and high divorce rates that did not exist 50 years ago. These environmental stresses have all been implicated at one time or another as reasons for the increasing number of children with ADHD. Some environmental influences clearly represent risk factors for developing neurological systems and may be linked to ADHD behaviors. Prenatal exposure to toxins, as in heavy use of alcohol by mothers during pregnancy, is an example of an environmental circumstance that may be seriously detrimental to the developing child (Drew & Hardman, 2000; Trawick-Smith, 2000). Such factors may result in low-birth-weight babies and difficult deliveries, both of which increase the risk of later ADHD (Hardman et al., 2002; Johnson-Cramer, 1999; Levy, Barr, & Sunahara, 1998). Not surprisingly, a mother's health status during pregnancy is vital to the developing fetus and is an important predictor of ADHD. This is true for the mother's emotional health as well as her general physical health; both of these contributing factors may interact in prenatal development to lead to ADHD (Cook, 1999; Eshleman, 1999).

Neurological development occurs very rapidly during the prenatal period and continues at a somewhat slower rate during the childhood years. However, disruption of neurological development during these years may also have serious detrimental effects, resulting in ADHD behaviors (Hardman et al., 2002). For example, ingesting or inhaling toxic substances like lead can result in serious brain damage in children (Brockel & Cory-Slechta, 1998; Drew & Hardman, 2000; Trawick-Smith, 2000). Lead compounds in paint and gasoline have been identified as particular problems for years, and widespread efforts to minimize these sources have met with some success. Even with such efforts, however, the National Institute of Mental Health notes that lead is still found in dust, soil, and some water pipes, and exposure to such sources may lead to ADHD symptoms [National Institute of Mental Health (NIMH), 2001]. Other toxins, such as household poisons in cleaning products, may also present serious risks to children. Because children with ADHD are impulsive and on the move, they are more likely to investigate and experiment with items found around the house; they may even ingest toxic substances though they have been told not to touch such items.

Food additives and diet received a great deal of publicity as causing ADHD over 25 years ago. The "Feingold Diet," which restricted artificial food colorings, flavorings, and natural salicylates (aspirin-like compounds), received the most attention (Feingold, 1975), although the results with this diet were not replicated by other researchers. Currently, diet as a source of environmental causation is not viewed as supported by empirical evidence (NIMH, 2000; Steele, 2000).

Other Family Factors

Some early research investigated parenting problems as a possible contributor to ADHD behaviors (e.g., Battle & Lacey, 1972). However, it is now generally agreed that parental stress is more likely a response to the inappropriate behavior of the child with ADHD rather than the cause of it (Jones, 2001; Morris, 2001). Children with ADHD do seem to leave a significant mark on their families including high stress levels, depression, relationship disruption, and even reduced work productivity (Hankin, Wright, & Gephart, 2001). It is therefore not surprising that behavioral improvements in the child seem to be associated with reduction in some of these problems (Mulsow, O'Neal, & Murray, 2001; Wells et al., 2000). Family dynamics appear to be interrelated with ADHD behaviors, and the influences seem to be bidirectional (Barkley, 1998).

Likelihood of Multiple Causes

As we finish the examination of causes related to ADHD, one of this book's overall themes surfaces strongly—that behavior has biological and genetic roots. This is quite evident in the current research and even in many of the historical theories about the causation of ADHD. Progress in neuro-imaging technology makes the presence of biological (neurological) causes more confirmable than before, even though the soft signs were always suggestive. Genetic contributions to causation of ADHD have long been suspected, and research continues to support this. It is likely that future research may confirm this as progress is made in genome exploration. Even the environmental influences examined in this section are mainly factors that interfere with neurological development or cause neurological damage through physical insults or anoxia. Thus, these environmental causes also have biological connections. In sum, it is likely that an interplay of multiple causes—genetics, biological factors, environmental influences, and family stresses—increases the vulnerability of a child to ADHD (Barkley, 1998).

TREATMENT OF ADHD

IN FOCUS 6 ▶ Identify two broad approaches to intervention that appear to show positive results with children having ADHD.

Few childhood behavior disorders have raised such controversy and heated debate as ADHD. Historically, treatment of this condition has followed a wide range of approaches, including medication, psychotherapy, educational interventions, and diet. Each approach had supporters who were certain that their treatment was the most effective. However, interest in many of these approaches has declined, and most attention currently focuses on two general categories of intervention: medical and behavioral (Hardman et al., 2002). It is important to note that interventions are most effective when individually tailored to the child's needs, which, of course, vary considerably. There is also growing general agreement that effective treatment is often multimodal—that is, employing elements of multiple methods—and often best implemented by a multidisciplinary team (Abikoff, 2001; Greene & Ablon, 2001; Jensen et al., 2001).

Stimulant Medication

Probably the most controversial current treatment for those with ADHD is prescription stimulant medication. Ritalin (generic name, methylphenidate) is the most widely used, although other medications such as Adderall and Dexedrine are also being investigated and prescribed. In 1995, physicians wrote over 6 million prescriptions for stimulant medications (Faraone et al., 2001; NIMH, 2000). From the standpoint of effectiveness, psychostimulant treatment results in behavioral improvement for about 80% of children with ADHD (Cunningham, 1999; Elia et al., 1999). The effect appears to be an enhanced ability to control impulses that, in turn, seems to improve behavior (Johnston et al., 2000; Ohan & Johnston, 1999). The improved impulse control is thought to occur because the stimulant drug arouses the frontal lobes of the brain. These portions of the brain exert regulatory influences that ultimately allow the youngster to better monitor motor activity and distractibility (Barkley, 1998).

Improvements in behavior of children with ADHD are often like a breath of fresh air for teachers and parents. A seemingly high level of activity, perhaps including aggression and general disruption, may be reduced substantially. This quieter demeanor may lead to an expectation that the youngsters are going to perform better in academics—or even a belief that they *are* performing better academically simply because they are not bouncing off the walls. It is important to note that this expectation or belief about academics is not supported empirically. While evidence on the effectiveness of medication in modifying ADHD behaviors continues to grow, such medical intervention does not appear to have similar academic benefits. Academic performance of children with ADHD is a serious concern since many of them exhibit significant academic underachievement (Reddy, Spencer, Hall, & Rubel, 2001; Zentall, Moon, Hall, & Grskovic, 2001). Children with ADHD who receive medication may initially show an improvement in academics because they are more focused, more planful, and less impulsive or active (Evans et al., 2001). However, psychostimulant treatment shows little or no long-term effect on academic performance (Aro et al., 1999; Benedetto-Nasho & Tannock, 1999).

Controversies surrounding the use of drug treatment for ADHD continue to surface in the popular press periodically. Concerns are related to overprescription, side effects, cumulative effects over long-term use, and possible abuse (Beck, Silverstone, Glor, & Dunn, 1999; Buckingham, 1999; Kollins, MacDonald, & Rush, 2001). Side effects that accompany the use of stimulant medication include insomnia, rebound irritability, decreased appetite, and headaches, all of which are relatively minor and temporary most of the time. It should be noted, however, that issues related to side effects are far from resolved, and some believe these effects to be very serious (Bhaumik, Branford, Naik, & Biswas, 2000; Elia et al., 1999). In some cases, side effects may include a progression from hyperalertness through obsessive-compulsive or perseverative behaviors and even seizures as the central nervous system toxicity increases (Breggin, 1999a, 1999b). Another concern that has been raised involves potential abuse, including unauthorized use of the child's psychostimulant medications by other family members or by other juveniles such as classmates (Connors, 2000). Despite its successes, drug treatment for ADHD still raises many questions that require answers, including some that would seem rather basic regarding dosage, side effects, and long-term effects (e.g., Ardoin & Martens, 2000; Evans et al., 2001; Greenhill, 2001).

Behavior Management

A variety of behavior management techniques have been used with children having ADHD, and not surprisingly, some appear more effective than others. For the most part, more narrowly targeted behavior modification strategies seem more helpful for controlling behavioral problems than do those involving cognitive-behavioral interventions (Hardman et al., 2002). Targeted behavior modification techniques vary, of course, but most frequently they include (1) positive reinforcement for on-task behavior, remaining seated, and completing assignments; (2) response cost, or loss of reinforcement, for inappropriate behaviors such as noncompliance, refusal to sit down, and aggression; and (3) cognitive-behavioral modification that emphasizes self-control and self-reinforcement.

Cognitive-behavioral approaches use behavior management techniques combined with components aimed at changing the way a person thinks about his or her behaviors. Use of these approaches attempts to improve the cognitive control a person has over his or her actions (Hoza, 2001). While such approaches are intuitively appealing for use with children with ADHD, research evidence does not consistently suggest beneficial results from cognitive-behavioral interventions with these youngsters [DuPaul & Eckert, 1997, 1998; National Institutes of Health (NIH), 1998]. There are some applications where specific effects appear beneficial, such as increasing on-task behavior (Shimabukuro, Prater, Jenkins, & Edelen-Smith, 1999). However, as with medication alone, simply increasing on-task behavior does not necessarily improve academic performance. Behavioral interventions for children with ADHD are complex, involving interactions of various components (e.g., the child's chemical make-up, interpersonal context, academic capacity, parents, and teachers). The interactions of all of these components mean that behavior therapies are going to be complicated, adding to the challenge for clinicians and researchers attempting to establish their benefits (Greene & Ablon, 2001; Wells, 2001; Whalen, 2001).

Teaching the parents of children with ADHD to execute behavioral programs for their children has been demonstrated to be practically effective, particularly when the target behaviors consist of rather focused activities, such as increases in on-task behavior, compliance, and task completion, and reduction of aggressive or disruptive behavior (Danforth, 1999, 2001; Smith, 2001). Placing simple behavioral targets within the broader family context complicates matters and adds to the challenges of applying research methods in such settings (Ayers, Sellers, Schneider, Gottschling, & Soucar, 2001; Power, Karustis, & Habboushe, 2001). However, parent training and the comprehensive involvement of parents in the behavior management of their children with ADHD receive considerable attention in the literature. Professionals continue to see parent involvement as essential because the family is such a crucial portion of the overall social context affecting the child (Driskill, 2000; Nolan & Carr, 2000). It appears that this involvement is most beneficial when parents receive specific training rather than more generalized, nondirective counseling, a point of little surprise to behavioral clinicians (Sonuga-Barke, Daley, Thompson, Laver-Bradbury, & Weeks, 2001). The core nature of much behavior management involves fairly detailed specification of the behavior changes to be targeted, the management tactics to be used, and the consequences to be implemented to achieve the desired changes.

Behavior management in educational settings is often aimed at imposing structure in the classroom environment and targeting aspects of the child's behavior on which controls are needed. Such combinations of behavior management techniques require enormous effort because of the complexities of managing behavior and imposing structure, but they do seem to be academically productive. A rather high level of structure with rewarded learning experiences is often central to descriptions of effective instructional settings for children with ADHD (Davies & Witte, 2000; Reddy et al., 2001). Educators need to design as many elements of the classroom setting as possible to facilitate the child's ability to respond, attend, and behave. It is important for teachers to monitor their directions to the students, often cuing them that a specific academic instruction is about to be delivered. Often this is accomplished with a simple prompt ("Listen, Greg") or some similar signal. It is important that mechanisms like this are comfortable for the teacher or they won't be used, and they must convey a clear signal to the students that a directive is to follow (Ervin et al., 2000; Folstrom-Bergeron, 1998).

The overall treatment picture for children and adolescents with ADHD suggests that effective intervention should include both medication and behavior management—known as *multimodal intervention*. Combined treatment approaches (such as drug and behavior therapies) tend to be more effective for children with ADHD than any single approach, probably because of the multifaceted nature of their problems (Goldstein, 1999; Harwood & Beutler, 2001). The general treatment effectiveness will be dependent on how well all treatment ingredients are considered and matched to a given child with ADHD (Greene & Ablon, 2001; Harwood & Beutler, 2001; Whalen, 2001). One risk factor that surfaces with multimodal treatment models and may not with a single-treatment approach is the fact that communication and coordination among educational (school-based) and health-related (medical) assessments and services have been noted as poor (Hardman et al., 2002; NIH, 1998). This has posed a long-standing challenge in the treatment of ADHD, where personnel from multiple disciplines are often working with one child (Drew & Hardman,

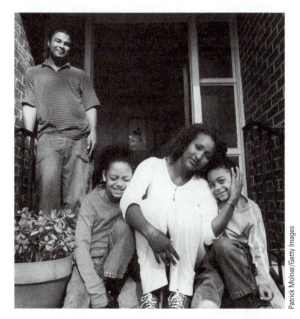

Because the family is a critical part of a child's social context, parents and other family members are frequently involved in behavioral interventions for children with ADHD.

Back to the Beginning
A Comprehensive Plan for Allen

When we met Allen at the beginning of this chapter, it was clear that he has a number of learning disabilities co-occurring with ADHD. Some of his problems were noticed very early, and his assessment has been an ongoing process of tracking progress and watching for further problems that might surface. Allen also has a number of strengths that can be capitalized on educationally. Below are excerpts from a rather comprehensive plan developed to further his education and development. Note that the features of this program are prescriptively designed to address his areas of deficiency and to support his strengths.

Testing of language functions revealed striking weaknesses in both receptive and expressive language skills. Although parental reports indicated that Allen has made a stable pattern of gains since speech therapy was initiated this year, his language problems are of such severity that they are continuing to have an impact on his ability to use and understand language effectively.

Testing of memory and learning indicated that Allen experienced difficulties in encoding and memorizing verbal information, such as stories and lists of words. . . . He does not have difficulty in retrieving and outputting information from memory; that is, once information is encoded into memory, he can retain it for relatively long periods of time. . . . It is important to emphasize that despite his encoding difficulties, Allen has the potential to learn and memorize new information, but he will do so at a rate that is significantly slower than his same-aged peers, and he will require more than the usual amount of repetition. Allen does not appear to have significant difficulty memorizing material that is visual in nature, such as designs and pictures.

Recommendations include an intensive learning disabilities program to work on his phonological coding difficulties while simultaneously strength-ening his sight-word vocabulary. Given Allen's good visual-perceptual and visual memory abilities, it is recommended that teaching strategies focus on a sign-word approach with the high-frequency words he encounters. . . .

It is further recommended that Allen be provided with a computer for rehearsing reading skills. Moreover, a language experience approach should be incorporated into Allen's classroom program. This method, which will encourage Allen to use his own words, includes writing his own book by dictating a story to a teacher or aide who provides him with a written transcript. Allen would then read the story back and accumulate flashcards of unknown words that he encounters. Taped books should also be available for Allen. . . . (Teeter & Semrud-Clikeman, 1997, pp. 246–247)

To foster development of Allen's phonological processing, the plan also recommended use of a particular program that employs multiple sensory approaches to teaching material and heavily focuses on the skills Allen needs to become an effective reader. This program begins with very basic skills and proceeds in carefully designed steps to enhance the child's skill acquisition.

This plan is heavily oriented toward the academic limitations that accompany Allen's ADHD diagnosis. It is important to try to foster growth in these areas as quickly as possible to help him progress and to minimize his academic lags as much as possible. Allen will obviously be the focus of intense effort and scrutiny. As noted before, he is fortunate because he seems to be operating fairly well socially and interpersonally. Although this is an important strength, it is crucial to monitor his interactions to be on the alert for any developing difficulties. While there are substantial challenges for Allen, there are also some significant strengths and a plan of action.

2000). Thus, the already complicated treatment for children with ADHD is further complicated by those who are supposed to help the child. The good news is that, as noted above, progress in effective intervention is evident—the challenge is to coordinate the many complexities presented by individual cases.

SUMMARY

ADHD is one of the most frequently referred psychological disorders of childhood. This disorder is characterized by poor attending, impulsivity, and fidgety motor behavior. It is estimated that about 3–5% of the U.S. school-age population has ADHD, with males outnumbering females approximately 3.5 to 1. ADHD children often have academic problems, perhaps partially because they are poor planners, do not attend well, and exhibit disruptive behaviors that do not endear them to teachers or their peers.

It is likely there are several causes of ADHD, with biological factors playing a significant role. Specific causes of ADHD include brain injury from physical insults, oxygen deprivation at birth, and other neurological anomalies that may include physical abnormalities and chemical imbalances. Causation of ADHD may follow family lines, and a certain risk may be genetically transmitted. Environmental risks for children having ADHD include prenatal exposure to toxic agents such as alcohol that interfere with the developing nervous system during pregnancy. The pregnant mother's general health is a potential contributor to the risk that the developing fetus will later have ADHD.

Treatments of ADHD have been numerous over the years but have settled into two broad categories of medical and behavioral interventions. Medical treatment has most often included the prescription of stimulant medication that can have a beneficial behavioral effect in helping to control activity levels and disruptive behaviors. Drug treatment for ADHD is widespread and quite controversial because of concerns regarding side effects and potential abuse. Behavioral interventions also appear to be effective to the degree that they are focused, systematic, and matched to the individual child's needs. Parent involvement and parent training have received considerable attention, and many parents become important intervention team members.

IN FOCUS ANSWERS

IN FOCUS 1 ▶ Give two prevalence estimates for ADHD that characterize the difference in occurrence by gender.

- Estimates of gender differences in prevalence range from 2-to-1 to 10-to-1, with males outnumbering females.
- On average, the male-to-female ratio appears to be about 3.5-to-1.

IN FOCUS 2 ▶ Identify the five DSM-IV-TR diagnostic criteria for ADHD.

- A persistent pattern of inattention and/or hyperactivity-impulsivity
- Some hyperactive-impulsive or inattentive symptoms that cause impairment and are present before age 7
- Some impairment from the symptoms evident in at least two settings
- Clear evidence of interference with developmentally appropriate social, academic, or occupational functioning
- The disturbance does not occur exclusively during the course of a pervasive developmental disorder, schizophrenia, or other psychotic disorder and is not better accounted for by another mental disorder.

IN FOCUS 3 ▶ Identify the three types of ADHD according to DSM-IV-TR.

- Combined type
- Predominantly inattentive type
- Predominantly hyperactive-impulsive type

IN FOCUS 4 ▶ Identify three major characteristics that present challenges for individuals with ADHD.

- Inattention
- Impulsivity
- Overactivity

IN FOCUS 5 ▶ Identify three possible causes of ADHD.

- Neurological dysfunction caused by organic brain damage
- Hereditary (or genetic) transmission
- Environmental factors that may lead to neurological dysfunction

IN FOCUS 6 ▶ Identify two broad approaches to intervention that appear to show positive results with children having ADHD.

- Stimulant medication
- Behavior management

Conduct Disorder and Related Conditions

10

In the Beginning

With Demolition Dan

He was a preschool version of the "white tornado" in the TV ad for a cleaning product, except he wasn't cleaning things. "Boom! Boom!" he yelled, as he seemingly bounced from the ceiling to one wall to another, his small body quivering with excitement from the destruction he produced. At his feet lay a pile of blocks his classmate had stacked neatly in the shape of a house. Looking up from the drinking fountain, she screamed, adding at least 50 decibels to the noise level in the room. Dan repeated his mantra of destruction as he ran to the next student's play area.

Using her arms to shield her tidy block building, little Caitlin shouted at him, "No Danny! No! No!" It was too late; her building came crashing to the ground. Danny stood over it jumping up and down and continuing to chant. By the time teacher Eileen Hattson had grabbed Danny's arm, he was already on his way to another play site, with the aim of destroying another child's prized block structure.

"Danny, you do not destroy other kids' blocks," Eileen told the boy as she bent down to look at him at eye level. But Danny was intensely uninterested in listening to another lecture about "appropriate" behavior. He looked away and continued his perpetual motion. "Look at me! Look at me!" Eileen insisted. She took his hand, walked over to Caitlin's pile of rubble, and ordered Danny to help build a new house in her most firm tone of voice (also about 20 decibels above normal). "Think about what you did and how sad you made Caitlin feel," she lectured. "You need to learn to not destroy other children's work," she said as she sat him on her lap in front of the blocks. (Adapted from Danforth & Boyle, 2000, p. 72)

Demolition Dan is his nickname, and he is enrolled in Eileen Hattson's preschool class, a program that is affiliated with a university. Danny has been evaluated by school psychologists and diagnosed as having developmental delays in language skills and social competence, although he remains in his preschool class. Dan is frequently involved in confrontations with his classmates and situations like those just described. He is avoided by the other children because he destroys their artwork, tears up their papers, and creates continual classroom management challenges for his teacher.

215

INTRODUCTION

One of several questions for this chapter is whether or not Demolition Dan's problems are serious enough to classify as oppositional defiant disorder. As we examine the diagnostic criteria for this condition a bit later in this chapter, we will see that several do fit. Should his parents and teacher be concerned? For some young children, oppositional defiant disorder is a precursor to more serious conduct disorders. Or is too much being made of this boy's behavior? Is Demolition Dan just a rambunctious little boy? Eileen Hattson's opinion varies somewhat, depending on what he has done most recently.

The potential developmental trajectory from oppositional defiant disorder to conduct disorder raises the developmental theme that has emerged throughout this book. A developmental progression here is a serious consideration. If Dan is diagnosed with oppositional defiant disorder, a red flag is raised and intervention is suggested. This is a positive benefit *if* it interrupts a course of events that might lead to more serious conduct disorders. *If*, on the other hand, Dan is a rambunctious boy prematurely labeled as having oppositional defiant disorder, the result may be detrimental by promoting a self-fulfilling prophecy. In that case, diagnosing (labeling) him is not a good move. Such dilemmas are often faced by psychologists and educators working with youngsters who seem at risk for academic or social failure. The developmental component of oppositional defiant disorder does not mean that there is an inevitable pathway to more serious problems. However, knowledge of the developmental issues must be considered in evaluating behavior and planning programs for young children.

In addition to the developmental theme noted above, others are quite evident in relation to conduct disorder. For example, the theme "research protects children" plays a significant role for youngsters with these problems. It is important for clinicians, parents, and other caregivers to understand how aggressive behavior like Dan's is fostered. As we review the literature on oppositional defiant and conduct disorders, we will find that interactions between children and their caregivers may promote behavioral excesses. Research on treatment is essential in order to learn how best to intervene in such interaction patterns and

establish more productive and acceptable behavior—literally protecting the children involved by informing their parents and others about how to foster positive environments.

Problem behaviors that affect society, the environment, and other people directly are particularly difficult to prevent or to treat. These problem behaviors have been called *externalizing behaviors* because they are directed outwardly toward people in the social environment (Gupta, Nwosa, Nadel, & Inamdar, 2001; Verona & Patrick, 2000). They can be contrasted with *internalizing behaviors* (e.g., anxiety, fears, depression) that primarily affect the child and have less obvious impact on the social environment. A physical attack on a teacher by a student, a deliberate setting of a fire by a child to burn a home, or the robbing of a store by a neighborhood gang are all examples of externalizing behaviors that are likely to bring a strong negative reaction from the community. Frequently, this reaction results in the child or adolescent being expelled from school or enmeshes him or her in a correctional system that may only reinforce the problem behaviors.

Externalizing problem behaviors are among the most common reasons for a child's referral for help by teachers and parents (Kipps, 2000; Serdahl, 2000). But treatment success is modest. Children who are aggressive, argumentative, and noncompliant have poorer long-term outcomes than most children with other behavior disorders (McConnell, 2000; Tremblay, LeMarquand, & Vitaro, 1999). These antisocial behavior problems portend later problems in adulthood, including alcoholism, criminal behavior, marital difficulties, and poor work histories. Yet, many professionals and educators tend to underestimate the long-term seriousness of externalizing social disorders. These children are not likely to outgrow their problems. Actually, the reverse is true because people who were socially disordered as children are more likely to develop adjustment problems in adulthood, such as hospitalization for a mental disorder, arrest, multiple job changes, and divorce (Kazdin, 2001; McConnell, 2000).

The terms commonly used by schools, juvenile courts, and mental health clinics to describe children with externalizing social disorders include *antisocial*, *aggressive*, *oppositional*, *socially maladjusted*, *disorderly*, and *delinquent*. These labels are not mutually exclu-

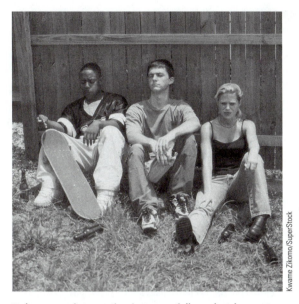

Unless some intervention is successfully undertaken, externalizing disorders in young children are likely to continue into adolescence and even adulthood.

sive but overlap to a great extent. This chapter will review major types of externalizing social disorders, including conduct disorder and oppositional defiant disorder and juvenile delinquency. All of these conditions are related to some extent, and we will note the developmental pathways that connect them. In many cases, reference to conduct disorder also includes oppositional defiant disorder because the externalizing behaviors are often cumulative; that is, a youngster identified with conduct disorder often exhibits behaviors of oppositional defiant disorder along with other, more serious, social transgressions.

CONDUCT AND OPPOSITIONAL DEFIANT DISORDERS

IN FOCUS 1 ▶ Why does the possibility of a developmental trajectory for antisocial behavior concern many psychologists?

Oppositional defiant disorder and conduct disorder are related in some children. Oppositional defiant disorder is less severe and, in certain cases where intervention does not occur, may lead to the development of conduct disorder. Children with **oppositional defi-**

ant disorder exhibit " . . . a recurrent pattern of negativistic, defiant, disobedient, and hostile behavior toward authority figures" (American Psychiatric Association, 2000, p. 100). Children diagnosed with oppositional defiant disorder may argue with authority figures—especially their parents—lose their temper often, and act in a number of ways that make it a challenge to be around them (see Table 10-1). However, these youngsters do not evidence the more serious behavioral excesses found in conduct disorder. Children with conduct disorder often behave in ways that violate the rights of others, destroy property maliciously, or persistently violate rules or age-related societal norms of behavior. The behaviors found in oppositional defiant disorder are less severe than those associated with conduct disorder. Children with oppositional defiant disorder are not characteristically aggressive, destructive of property, or thieves.

Conduct disorder is a broad label used to identify a number of aversive and socially disruptive behaviors in children. Children diagnosed with conduct disorder have exhibited a " . . . repetitive and persistent pattern of behavior in which the basic rights of others or major age-appropriate societal norms or rules are violated" (American Psychiatric Association, 2000, p. 93). The key phrase in this description is "societal norms or rules," which indicates socially determined standards of personal behavior. A breakdown in the social regulation of a child's personal standard of behavior can lead to the behavioral excesses that are referred to as conduct disorder, an externalizing disorder that affects all the people that deal with the child. The types of problem behaviors associated with children having conduct disorder include aggression, antisocial and disruptive behaviors, noncompliance, temper tantrums, stealing, and fire-setting (Crystal, Ostrander, Chen, & August, 2001; Kolko, Day, Bridge, & Kazdin, 2001; Landy & Menna, 2001; McBurnett, Lahey, Rathouz, & Loeber, 2000).

Two general types of conduct disorder are linked to age. Childhood-onset conduct disorder occurs before age 10, generally showing the early characteristics of physical aggression, disturbed peer relationships, and early oppositional or noncompliant behavior. The second type is adolescent-onset conduct disorder, which is characterized by the display of disruptive behavior appearing after age 10. The youngster with adolescent-onset type is less likely to

Table 10-1 DSM-IV-TR Diagnostic Criteria for Oppositional Defiant Disorder

A. A pattern of negativistic, hostile, and defiant behavior lasting at least 6 months, during which four (or more) of the following are present:

   (1) often loses temper

   (2) often argues with adults

   (3) often actively defies or refuses to comply with adults' requests or rules

   (4) often deliberately annoys people

   (5) often blames others for his or her mistakes or misbehavior

   (6) is often touchy or easily annoyed by others

   (7) is often angry and resentful

   (8) is often spiteful or vindictive

   Note: Consider a criterion met only if the behavior occurs more frequently than is typically observed in individuals of comparable age and developmental level.

B. The disturbance in behavior causes clinically significant impairment in social, academic, or occupational functioning.

C. The behaviors do not occur exclusively during the course of a Psychotic or Mood Disorder.

D. Criteria are not met for Conduct Disorder, and, if the individual is age 18 years or older, criteria are not met for Antisocial Personality Disorder.

SOURCE: American Psychiatric Association (2000), p. 102. Reprinted with permission from the *Diagnostic and Statistical Manual of Mental Disorders*, 4th ed., Text Revision. © 2000 APA.

exhibit overt displays of aggressive behavior and to have disturbed peer relations. However, these adolescents may display many of their misbehaviors in the company of other conduct-disordered peers. The children with childhood-onset conduct disorder have a poorer prognosis than those with the adolescent-onset type in that they are likely to maintain their disruptive behavior through adolescence and into adulthood (Hill & Maughan, 2001; Landy & Menna, 2001; Loeber, Farrington, Stouthamer-Loeber, Moffitt, & Caspi, 2001).

Comparing the diagnostic criteria for oppositional defiant disorder (Table 10-1) and conduct disorder (Table 10-2) illustrates the similarities and differences between the two conditions. As noted, oppositional defiant and conduct disorder are related. In some children, the less disruptive oppositional defiant disorder develops into conduct disorder and thus is considered a likely precursor to the more serious disorder (American Psychiatric Association, 2000). Some researchers see the emergence of antisocial behavior as a developmental process, with early deviant behavior developing into more serious antisocial behavior as the child gets older (Dahlberg & Potter, 2001; Loeber et al., 2001). This process may continue well into adulthood, with antisocial behavior in adolescence predicting similar behavior as an adult (Barratt, Felthous, Kent, Liebman, & Coates, 2000; Loeber & Coie, 2001).

It is not always the case that children with oppositional defiant disorder progress to the more serious conduct disorder. As we examine the characteristics of children having these two disorders, we will distinguish between them where the data are available. In some cases, however, the research methodology needs considerable improvement (Cherulnik, 2001; Matsumoto, 2001). Ethical concerns (coercion and potential participant abuse) and methodological limitations (e.g., high dropout rates and comparisons of dissimilar participants) plague many investigations on various behavior disorders (Ladouceur, Gosselin, Laberge, & Blaszczynski, 2001; Regehr, Edward, & Bradford, 2000).

Characteristics of Conduct-Disordered Children

IN FOCUS 2 ▶ Identify several characteristics of children with conduct disorder.

Parents and teachers are annoyed and worried by the antagonistic behaviors of conduct disordered children, but their misdeeds are not unique. Virtually all children have engaged in some of these mean and aggressive

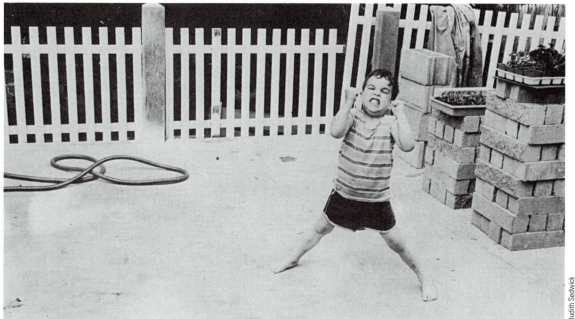

Disruptive and aggressive behavior at a young age may suggest childhood-onset conduct disorder.

behaviors at one time or another during their development. What distinguishes a conduct-disordered child from a child who acts out but is not diagnosed with a disorder is the intensity and frequency of the behaviors. Behavioral excesses involving frequent aggression and noncompliance are the most obvious characteristics of conduct disorder (Costello & Angold, 2001; Pettit, Polaha, & Mize, 2001). Along with the excesses, however, come a series of deficits, such as withdrawal from peer and environmental interaction that may lead to later

Table 10-2 DSM-IV-TR Diagnostic Criteria for Conduct Disorder

A repetitive and persistent pattern of behavior in which the basic rights of others or major age-appropriate societal norms or rules are violated, as manifested by the presence of three (or more) of the following criteria in the past 12 months, with at least one criterion present in the past 6 months:

Aggression to People and Animals

(1) often bullies, threatens, or intimidates others

(2) often initiates physical fights

(3) has used a weapon that can cause serious physical harm to others (e.g., a bat, brick, broken bottle, knife, gun)

(4) has been physically cruel to people

(5) has been physically cruel to animals

(6) has stolen while confronting a victim (e.g., mugging, purse snatching, extortion, armed robbery)

(7) has forced someone into sexual activity

Destruction of Property

(8) has deliberately engaged in fire setting with the intention of causing serious damage

(9) has deliberately destroyed others' property (other than by fire setting)

SOURCE: American Psychiatric Association (2000), p. 99. Reprinted with permission from the *Diagnostic and Statistical Manual of Mental Disorders*, 4th ed., Text Revision. © 2000 APA.

violent behaviors. It is easy for parents, teachers, and professionals to focus on the aversive behavioral excesses and miss treating the behavioral deficits.

One of the most disturbing deficits of children with conduct disorder is their poor moral development and lack of empathetic behavior (Summers, 2000). Many conduct-disordered children show little guilt or conscience concerning their hurtful and destructive behavior. Some have described this flaw as more of a deficit in following rules or in self-management (Angold & Costello, 2001). Typically, a social rule guides a child in how to behave in different situations, particularly unsupervised situations. Social rules are designed to protect people from theft and attack. For instance, a rule might be "honest people do not steal" even when they are unobserved. Children with conduct disorder *do* appear to be governed by contingencies because they respond to the immediate rewards in the environment (e.g., "I will steal it if I can get it now") instead of the social rules prohibiting theft. This contingency orientation is reflected in many conduct-disordered children's questioning what will happen to them if they misbehave (egocentrism or self-focus) rather than considering the effect the behavior may have on some other person.

Other deficits associated with conduct disorder include poor social skills and academic deficiencies, particularly poor reading skills (Hardman, Drew, & Egan, 2002). Researchers have shown that one of the strong correlates of antisocial behavior in adolescents is an academic skills deficiency (Barrera, Biglan, Ary, & Li, 2001; Dumas, Prinz, Smith, & Laughlin, 1999; Klorman, 2000). Poor academic achievement has been shown to be a predictive variable in the relationship between early disruptive behavior and later delinquency (Loeber & Coie, 2001; Loeber et al., 2001). Poor school performance is often linked to disruptive classroom behavior, truancy, suspension, and dropping out. Once a conduct-disordered student is no longer attending school, he or she is often unsupervised, which further compounds social problems. School failure, poverty, and domestic violence are among the several environmental circumstances that seem to increase the risk for youngsters being involved in a continuing cycle of antisocial and often aggressive behaviors that lead to criminal acts and interaction with the criminal justice system (Cottle, 2001; Levitt & Lochner, 2001; Preski & Shelton, 2001).

In their social relationships, children with conduct disorder are frequently described as being inappropriately competitive, uncooperative, bossy, and defensive about criticism. These children do not know how to be an appropriate leader, how to initiate conversations, or how to socially reward other adults and peers. Poor

Table 10-3 Behavioral Characteristics of Children with Conduct Disorder

Behavioral Excesses	Specific Behaviors
Aggression	Physically attacks others (peers and adults)
	Verbally abusive
	Destroys property
	Sets fires
	Vandalizes
	Cruel to animals
	Revengeful
Noncompliance	Breaks established rules
	Does not follow commands
	Argues
	Does the opposite of what is requested

Behavioral Deficits	Specific Behaviors
Moral behavior	Shows little remorse for destructive behavior
	Appears to have no conscience
	Lacks concern for feelings of others
Social behavior	Has few friends
	Lacks affection or bonding
	Has few problem-solving skills
	Acts aggressively and impulsively rather than cooperatively
	Constantly seeks attention
	Poor conversation skills
	Does not know how to reward other peers and adults socially
Academics and school	Generally behind in academic basics, particularly reading
	Has difficulty acquiring new academic information
	Truant

Bobby's Story

A Child with Conduct Disorder

Bobby Jones is the type of boy who makes his teacher regret Mondays and the choice of teaching as a profession. Bobby seems to go out of his way to do the opposite of what is requested. Adults have to repeat what they want multiple times, after which Bobby will argue and fight back. He seems to have a million excuses why he should not have to do the simplest tasks. When pushed, Bobby will respond by fighting or trying to get even. He once destroyed an art project by another boy because he thought he should get the prize. He is also suspected of setting a fire in the classroom last year, although it couldn't be proven. What is most frustrating about Bobby is that he does not seem to care about others. As long as he gets his way, that is all that matters to him. He never shows guilt or remorse for a behavior that hurts another person, even when caught red-handed.

Because he is such a troublemaker, other children in the class don't like Bobby and try not to be associated with him. They simply stay away from him and would rather not include him in any of their activities because he takes charge and tries to push them around. Bobby's schoolwork also suffers. It is so much trouble to get Bobby to do anything that most teachers have given up on him, and he is now 2 years behind in reading.

At home, Bobby rules the household. His mother is permissive and has trouble handling him. She cannot set limits. His father is seldom home, and when he is, he is overly strict, trying to change things immediately. Bobby is a constant source of conflict between his mother and father, and they talk of getting a divorce.

Things have gotten so difficult with Bobby at school that he has been referred to a special education classroom. The incident that triggered the referral involved Bobby beating a smaller boy for a collection of scratch-and-sniff stickers. He will be sent to the classroom next week. Bobby's mother objects to the placement and wants a second chance for him.

---

peer relations and unstable relationships often characterize children and adolescents with conduct disorder (Hill & Maughan, 2001). One problem resulting from their poor social skills development is that these children lack the basic ability to solve many social problems, such as how to resolve simple disputes, formulate rules for games, or enter new play groups. This lack of rudimentary social problem-solving ability and basic interactive social skills leads to peer rejection and loss of self-esteem (Pearce, 2000; Yanof, 1999). Rejection and low self-esteem have several cascading social effects. First, conduct-disordered children are often accepted only by other antisocial-aggressive children, building early social alliances and groups that are deviancy-based and likely to engage in delinquent acts (Levitt & Lochner, 2001; Preski & Shelton, 2001). Thus, rejection and a need to belong socially may be the roots of later gang behavior. Second, there is a high comorbidity between conduct disorder and childhood depression (Rodemaker, 2000; Simic & Fombonne, 2001). It appears that there is an interaction between depression and conduct disorder, although researchers have not yet sorted out whether these youngsters are basically depressed or are depressed about being in trouble (Fombonne, Wostear, Cooper, Harrington, & Rutter, 2001b; Marmorstein & Iacono, 2001). Research will need to further explore some of the apparent gender differences in depression in children with conduct disorder, as well as biological factors, anxiety and guilt levels, and other characteristics that seem to intermittently appear (Fombonne et al., 2001a; O'Koon, 2001; Simic & Fombonne, 2001).

Table 10-3 lists both behavioral excesses and behavioral deficits commonly associated with conduct-disordered children. Although the behaviors listed in the table are many and diverse, the basic definitive characteristics of the conduct-disordered child are excesses in aggression and noncompliance, with deficits in rule-governed, social, and academic behaviors (Bobby's Story provides a case example).

Comprehensive Treatment of Chronic Fire-Setting

Jim was a 10-year-old boy enrolled in a mental health day program that treated severely behaviorally disordered children. In this program he was treated for a major fire-setting problem (Koles & Jenson, 1985). Jim's developmental history was characterized by deprivation, inadequate parenting, chaotic home life, and a series of foster home placements. He was diagnosed as having both conduct disorder and attention-deficit disorder. His list of referral problems included stealing, hyperactivity, tantrumming, learning disabilities, aggression, noncompliance, zoophilia, and fire-setting. The fire-setting had been a problem since Jim was 3, when he burned down the family home. Since his foster placements, Jim had averaged approximately one fire-setting every two weeks.

It was assumed that Jim set fires partly because he enjoyed seeing the fires and partly as a reaction to stress. The stress was related to a series of skill deficits in the social and academic areas. In addition, it was assumed that Jim did not fully realize the dangerous consequences of his behavior. His therapy involved a multiple treatment approach that served to educate, relieve stress, and consequate fire-setting. It included:

1. *Social problem-solving skills* involving positive relationships to others, successful classroom adjustment, peer interaction skills, and problem solving.
2. *Relaxation training* using basic muscle relaxation techniques to help reduce anxiety.

3. *Oversensitization* in which Jim visited a hospital burn unit and interviewed a depressed 10-year-old boy who had suffered burns over 80% of his body while playing with matches. He was also given additional information from the burn unit social worker and a fire investigator.
4. *Fire safety education* in which Jim participated in a program through a local fire department that involved film and lecture materials on the destructive effects of fire.
5. *Overcorrection procedures* in which Jim collected combustible material in a metal container and set it on fire. He recited a series of statements over and over again during the safe fire (e.g., "fires can kill people," "this fire is safe because it cannot spread"). He was then required to scrub the container. The overcorrection procedure served to oversatiate Jim with the fascination of fire-setting.
6. *Behavioral contracts* were used to reward no fire-setting or mildly punish (e.g., going to bed early) when a fire was set.

After treatment, Jim's fire-setting dropped from an average of one every two weeks to virtually zero fires at a 1-year follow-up. Jim improved his basic social skills and appeared better prepared to handle stressful situations, although some of his inappropriate behaviors such as stealing and family problems have continued.

Antisocial-Aggressive Behavior

IN FOCUS 3 ▶ What are some common antisocial-aggressive behaviors of children with conduct disorder?

The American Psychiatric Association definition of conduct disorder (see Table 10-2) emphasizes two categories of aggressive behaviors: aggression to people or animals and destruction of property (as in fire-setting; see Jim's Story).

Aggression and violence can be used as a means of controlling others through coercion, as evidenced in the literature on sexual coercion and family violence (e.g., Forbes & Adams-Curtis, 2001; Hogben, Byrne, Hamburger, & Osland, 2001). The use of aversive behaviors like hitting or other forms of abusive behavior to control others has also been described in terms of power-oriented social interaction and antisocial behavior in children (Poulin & Boivin, 2000; Tedeschi, 2001). An example frequently seen in grocery stores involves a child who wants a particular item but whose parent refuses to buy it. The child may escalate hostilities and start to engage in a screaming and kicking tantrum until the parent buys the item to quiet the child and escape the disapproving stares of other customers.

Here, the child has purposely or unwittingly used a tantrum as an instrument to control the parent's behavior. Coercive control through physical and verbal aggression is much more common in conduct-disordered children and their families than in families without such children (Spillane-Grieco, 2000). Further research is needed on this topic to better understand the development of conduct disorder in young children.

Noncompliance

IN FOCUS 4 ▶ Explain why noncompliance is seen as central to conduct disorder.

Noncompliance is simply refusing to do what is requested; in the context of child disorders, the request is generally made by a parent or teacher. Noncompliance is one of the most common behavior problems of childhood, certainly comprising a significant proportion of children's deviant behavior (Alterson, 2000; Munneke, 2001; Patterson & Forgatch, 2001). Noncompliance is so central to the problems of aggression and antisocial development that it has been termed a core behavior, one that controls many of the behavioral deficits and excesses found in conduct-disordered children (Drabick, Strassberg, & Kees, 2001). If compliance can be increased in these children, then many of the difficult behaviors such as aggression, arguing, and temper tantrums may improve without being directly treated (Martinez & Forgatch, 2001). (See the Research Focus box.)

Noncompliance can take many forms. A child may simply ignore a request made by an adult, often causing the adult to wonder if the child heard or understood the request. Noncompliance can also take the form of delaying, passively resisting, arguing, or giving excuses for not doing something. Frequently, noncompliant and oppositional behaviors that are persistent for at least 6 months can be classified as oppositional defiant disorder (refer back to Table 10-1). The core of this disorder is negativistic, defiant, disobedient, and hostile behaviors toward authority figures such as parents and teachers.

The effects on others of a child's severe noncompliant and oppositional behavior are not difficult to understand; they leave adults with feelings of helplessness and frustration. The expression "out of control" has frequently been used to describe the socially disordered child, and its use stems directly from non-compliance and opposition. A lack of conscience, moral concern for others, and rule-governed behavior may be partially traced to the effects of noncompliance in early development (Martinez & Forgatch, 2001; Stifter, Spinrad, & Braungart-Rieker, 1999). Learning to comply may be the "essential core to morality" in that a child learns to regulate his or her interpersonal behavior by a set of external rules and values that lead to self-managed or rule-governed behavior (Donovan, Leavitt, & Walsh, 2000; Kochanska, Coy, & Murray, 2001). Learning to comply may also affect other areas for both children and adolescents. For example, following teachers' directions and establishing positive interpersonal interactions with peers in academic situations are important elements in enhancing academic performance (Cowart, 2000; McCurdy, Skinner, Grantham, Watson, & Hindman, 2001; McDonnell, Thorson, Allen, & Mathot-Buckner, 2000). If a child is uncooperative and cannot resolve problems with other children, then the development of basic social and interactive skills may be delayed. If a child does not follow simple directions from teachers, then the development of basic academic and study skills may be slowed.

Prevalence Rates of Oppositional Defiant and Conduct Disorders

IN FOCUS 5 ▶ Give prevalence estimates for conduct and oppositional defiant disorders, and note any gender differences.

Boys are far more likely to be diagnosed as having conduct disorder problems than are girls (Modestin, Matutat, & Wuermle, 2001; Robins, 1999; Wakschlag et al., 2000). However, the behaviors displayed differ qualitatively between the sexes. Males frequently exhibit more aggression, stealing, vandalism, firesetting, and school-related problems. Females tend to display more lying, substance abuse, running away, and prostitution (American Psychiatric Association, 2000).

The DSM-IV-TR (American Psychiatric Association, 2000) notes that the prevalence rate of conduct disorder ranges between 1% and 10%, with males substantially outnumbering females. The prevalence estimates for oppositional defiant disorder range from 2% to 16%. More males than females are identified before puberty, but this gender difference disappears after

Behavioral Noncompliance and Its Relationship to Other Problem Behaviors

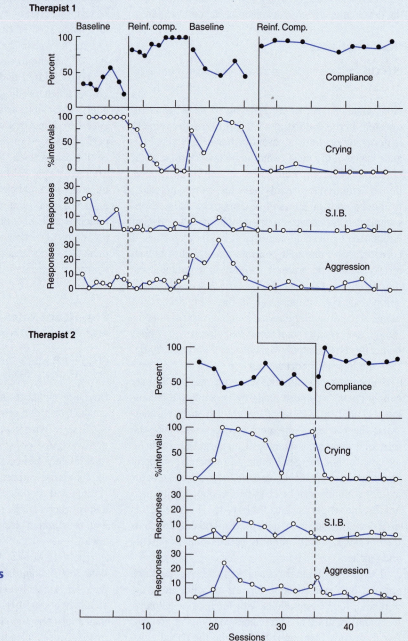

Figure 10-1   Percentage of Compliance and the Three Untreated Corollary Behaviors (Crying, SIB, and Aggression) for Tom across Experimental Conditions and Therapists

SOURCE: Russo, Cataldo, & Cushing (1981). Reprinted by permission.

Problem behaviors of children with externalizing or conduct disorders seem to revolve around a common set of problems that include noncompliance, tantrums, fighting, arguing, and crying. These problem behaviors may be more than slightly related. In fact, they may revolve around one basic behavior, noncompliance. Russo, Cataldo, and Cushing (1981) investigated the effects of successfully changing noncompliance and then observing the covariation in other problematic behaviors that were not treated directly. This study included three children who had been identified as being noncompliant, hyperactive, and uncontrollable with at least two other negative behaviors such as aggression, self-injury (SIB), or tantrums. For example, Tom, who was 3 years and 7 months old, was referred for tantrums, aggression (kicking and biting), and self-injury (head banging and hand biting).

The intervention included having the experimenter give the child a command and waiting 5 seconds. If the child complied, he was reinforced with a small piece of food (e.g., candy, cereal, raisins), physical contact (e.g., hug and a "good boy"). None of the other problem behaviors such as tantrums or aggression were treated. The results of this experiment for Tom are shown in Figure 10-1.

It can be seen that as compliance increased (because it was directly reinforced), the other problem behaviors (crying, self-injury, and aggression) decreased even though they were not directly treated. It appeared for Tom and the other two children in the study that improving compliance also had the side benefit of spontaneously improving the other problem behaviors. This study also showed that "nagging" (repeating a request over and over) made the situations worse by decreasing compliance and increasing problem behaviors.

that developmental landmark. It is likely that males are a bit more confrontational than females, but otherwise the two sexes seem to exhibit oppositional symptoms similarly (American Psychiatric Association, 2000). Some research suggests that the prevalence of conduct disorder has increased over the past 50 years in industrialized countries. Not surprisingly, there are some cultural variations, and some populations show extremely high occurrence of this disorder, as is true for abuse of alcohol and other substances (Robins, 1999; Schubiner et al., 2000). Certain populations have high risk factors for conduct disorder, such as lifetime prevalences of alcohol dependency that exceed 70% for males and 30% for females (Kunitz et al., 1999). By their very nature, both conduct disorder and oppositional defiant disorder represent deviations from cultural and social norms of behavior; consequently, prevalence varies considerably among various subgroups (Atkins & McKay, 2001; Loeber, Green, Lahey, & Kalb, 2000). Both conduct disorder and oppositional defiant disorder are among the conditions most frequently referred to both outpatient and inpatient mental health facilities in the United States (Kipps, 2000; Serdahl, 2000).

Causes of Oppositional Defiant and Conduct Disorders

IN FOCUS 6 ▶ What are three general causes of conduct and oppositional defiant disorders?

Conduct disorder and oppositional defiant disorder probably have several different causes, all of which can lead to similar behaviors. Some of these causes are likely genetically based. These include inherited temperament characteristics that underlie general behavior, as when someone seems to be generally positive or generally negative in emotional tone (Goldsmith, Aksan, Essex, & Vandell, 2001). In addition, some of the causes are undoubtedly social; these include violence modeled on television, divorce, and family stress.

Like many other conditions, oppositional defiant and conduct disorders lack a single cause, but instead are the result of interaction of many factors. A large number of risk factors and their interactive effects increase the vulnerability of certain children to antisocial patterns of behavior.

Biological Factors

Many researchers believe there is an inherited biological risk for temperamental influences in the development of personality disorders and antisocial behavior in children (e.g., Johnson, 2001; Lynn, 2001; O'Connor & Dyce, 2001). However, few believe that the risk is simply a matter of single-gene transmission or even of inheritance alone. The interaction or reciprocal influence of inherited temperament and factors in the environment is believed to produce disruptive social disorders (Bateson & Martin, 2000; MacDonald, Pogue-Geile, Debski, & Manuck, 2001). An interplay between a child's environment, vulnerability factors, and biological risk factors plays a part in the development of antisocial behavior (Auerbach, Benjamin, Faroy, Gellar, & Ebstein, 2001; Barkley, 1998; Eaves et al., 2000). Temperamental characteristics such as aggressive tendencies and lowered levels of anxiety, inhibition, and fear may become problematic only among children raised in families with poor parenting or in neighborhoods where aggression and crime are common. In harmonious families and good neighborhoods, a child's difficult, negative temperament may not lead to oppositional defiant or conduct disorder. It is quite possible that the environmental triggering effect or the interaction between the environment and biology may not occur.

Temperament appears to be an important factor along the entire developmental pathway from oppositional defiant disorder to delinquency in adolescence and criminal behavior in adulthood. Research on antisocial behavior in adoptees suggests that there could be some genetic predisposing factor, possibly the child's temperament (Goldsmith et al., 2001; Johnson, 2001; O'Connor & Dyce, 2001). Although there are no specific genes for criminality or violence, some children may be temperamentally more difficult to socialize than others, likely because of a complex interaction between genetics and environment (Bateson & Martin, 2000; MacDonald et al., 2001). Some authorities view one dimension of temperament—activity level, or hyperactivity—as a critical factor in the etiology of disruptive behavior. Fearless, aggressive, stimulation-seeking children are more likely to engage in

delinquent activities (Antrop, Roeyers, Van Oost, & Buysse, 2000; Dane, Schachar, & Tannock, 2000; Klorman, 2000). However, they may also be more inclined than more passive children to engage in a heroic defense of family and friends, so circumstances may dictate whether their outcomes are negative or positive.

A characteristic called *hypermasculinity* has also been of interest to those studying conduct disorder over the years. This is a personality variable that reflects exaggerated, stereotyped masculine behavior. Most of us have observed assertive, dominant, and competitive behavior in males in various degrees periodically (sometimes called "macho" behavior or other similar terms). There are a number of factors that influence and seem related to hypermasculinity including particular environments, TV shows or films, and ethnicity (Annambhotla, 2000; Scharrer, 2001; Sullivan, 2001). There may also be a link between hypermasculinity and physiological variables related to the aggression and noncompliance found in conduct-disordered children.

It has been theorized that an extra sex chromosome (XYY) may result in hypermasculinity and enhanced aggression in males (Lacayo, 2000). Normally, humans have one pair of sex chromosomes; males have an X and Y chromosome (XY), while females have two X's (XX). The sex chromosomes have a substantial impact on physical and behavioral development (Arnold, 1996). Although there has been considerable conjecture about the relationship between an XYY chromosome pattern, hypermasculinity, and aggression or violence, the evidence is not yet sufficient to establish any connection (Horgan, 1993; Lacayo, 2000). This book's recurring theme regarding the importance of research surfaces here once again. Currently, the research evidence is very mixed: Men with hypermasculinity sometimes exhibit less anger and aggression than others, and XYY men seem to be a bit taller than the general population but differ little in other respects (Horgan, 1993; Norris, 2000; Norris, George, Davis, Martell, & Leonesio, 1999). Such research evidence is certainly insufficient to support what seems to be an intuitively appealing connection between hypermasculinity, XYY, and aggression or violence.

Some researchers have connected the activity level and stimulation-seeking of youngsters with ADHD with conduct disorder (Antrop et al., 2000; Dane et al.,

2000). It is suggested that the need for stimulation and the physiological reaction that conduct-disordered children show may explain some of the behaviors of children with ADHD (Klorman, 2000; Lee, 1999). It may well be that conduct-disordered children are motivated by a high need for stimulation and reward and are less sensitive to punishment (Atkins, Osborne, Bennett, Hess, & Halperin, 2001; Schmeck & Poustka, 2001; Weiner, 2001). Thrill seeking, aggression, and rule breaking may be forms of stimulation seeking that help relieve boredom.

The genetic model of aggression and antisocial behavior is based primarily on the same logic as described in Chapter 9 for ADHD. There is considerable evidence indicating higher similarity rates for pairs of monozygotic (identical) twins than for pairs of dizygotic (fraternal) twins (Nadder, Silberg, Rutter, Maes, & Eaves, 2001; Rhee, 2000; Willcutt & Pennington, 2000). Aggression and other antisocial behaviors seem more similar in identical twins than in fraternal twins or adoptees, and this has commonly focused attention on genetic influence (Seroczynski, Bergeman, & Coccaro, 1999). However, the implication of twin genetic evidence is being questioned. Some researchers find the inference of genetic influence in crime and antisocial behavior not as strong as previously thought (Joseph, 2001; Ridenour, 2000). Effects may be more complex than once thought, and future research will be needed to clarify the relative influences of environmental and biological factors.

Family Factors

The effects of family influence on the development of antisocial behavior in children are well supported by research evidence. Factors such as child-rearing practices, the consistency of discipline, the supportive atmosphere of the family, separation, and divorce all appear to have some effect in producing aggressive, noncompliant children (Feinberg & Hetherington, 2001; Hetherington, 1999b). Child-rearing practices can vary along several different dimensions, and their impact may vary. For example, varying degrees of parental warmth and negativity have a substantial impact on children's adjustment (Feinberg & Hetherington, 2001; Feinberg, Neiderhiser, Howe, & Hetherington, 2001). Two types of child-rearing practices—harsh/abusive parental discipline and parental inconsistency—have been significantly linked to childhood conduct problems

(Cavell, 2001; Spillane-Grieco, 2000). Harsh, punitive discipline that openly reflects parental anger is associated with elevated levels of antisocial and disruptive behavior by children (Denham et al., 2000; Stormshak, Bierman, McMahon, & Legua, 2000). In many cases, this type of disciplinary environment focuses on what the child did wrong rather than on teaching the child what should be done (Bettner & Lew, 2000). Additionally, parents who are habitually *inconsistent* in rule-setting and discipline can leave a child confused about the exact limits on and consequences for various behaviors (Kennedy, 2001; Nichols-Anderson, 2001). Parents who use erratic control and are sometimes inappropriately permissive are more likely to have aggressive and behaviorally disordered children (Collins, Maccoby, Steinberg, & Hetherington, 2000; Gonzalez, Greenwood, & WenHsu, 2001). The impacts of these interactions are complicated, resulting in children who grow up with a significant amount of faulty learning regarding social interactions (Collins et al., 2000; Hetherington, 1999a; Lamb, 1999). In results of studies from behavioral, social, and psychological research, one finding is strikingly consistent—inadequate, highly negative parenting is related to the child's antisocial behavior. The precise manner in which this parenting style impacts a child's development remains to be clarified, but clearly it is influential.

Divorce, separation, substance abuse, depression, and marital conflict are found more frequently in the families of antisocial children than in the families of normally adjusted children. Boys are particularly affected by divorce, and they are more likely than girls to develop noncompliant and aggressive behavior after a divorce (Hetherington, 1999b). Single-parent family environments tend to have high stress levels and parenting that is inconsistent and neglectful, which may contribute to the development of antisocial behaviors (see Chapter 6). Antisocial and delinquent behaviors do not appear to develop as a direct result of divorce or separation, but seem more likely to emerge from the marital conflict and disharmony leading up to the break between parents or from the stressed financial circumstances that follow divorce. It should also be noted that a child's antisocial behavior may promote marital disharmony, which in turn is associated with increased acting-out behavior in the child (Guidubaldi & Duckworth, 2001; Hetherington, 1999a; McDonald, Jouriles, Norwood, Ware, & Ezell, 2000).

Table 10-4 Factors That Contribute to Antisocial Behavior

Psychopathology and criminal behavior in parents: The risk factor for antisocial behavior is increased when either parent has a psychiatric illness. However, alcoholism or criminal behavior in the father is particularly associated with antisocial behavior.

Parent-child interactions: Inconsistent parenting and discipline practices are associated with antisocial behavior. Lax, erratic, or overly harsh punishment practices are related to antisocial behavior. One pattern is especially associated with antisocial behavior: a lax mother and an overly severe punishing father.

Broken homes and marital discord: Divorce and broken homes can be related to antisocial behavior particularly when there is continuing bitter conflict between parents, reduced income, reduction in the quality of living, and decreased child supervision.

Birth order and family size: Delinquency and antisocial behavior are greater among middle children than they are for first and last born children. In addition, family size is related to delinquency, with a greater number of children associated with higher rates of antisocial behavior.

Social class and socioeconomic disadvantage: Delinquency and antisocial behavior are related to poorer living conditions and economic and social disadvantage. However, this effect is not particularly strong across studies.

Source: Adapted from Kazdin (1985).

Family variables are only part of the cause for conduct disorder and delinquency. Many other variables also appear to influence the risk of a child's becoming antisocial. Table 10-4 summarizes a number of these factors. However, there is another powerful contributor to noncompliance and aggression—modeling.

Modeling

Modeling is the acquisition of new behaviors through observation and imitation of other people's behavior. For antisocial children, acquiring aggressive and noncompliant behaviors may involve the imitation of parents, peers, and possibly characters from TV shows and films (Curtner-Smith, 2000; Sanders, Montgomery, & Brechman-Toussaint, 2000). Antisocial parenting seems to have a substantial influence on children's psychopathology and behavior, although the link to criminal violence is not as clear as one might think (Harris, Rice, & Lalumeire, 2001). Modeling by parents may occur in direct interactions with the child in the form of abusive discipline or may occur as the child is exposed to domestic violence between parents (Cavell, 2001; McDonald et al., 2000; Sims, 2001). Such exposure may have a significant effect on youngsters, and although the most prevalent view emphasizes the negative influence on young males, some researchers are beginning to question this limited perspective (McNeely, Cook, & Torres, 2001). This type of parental behavior may model and/or reinforce the youngster's antisocial or aggressive behavior, irrespective of gender (Bettner & Lew, 2000; Denham et al., 2000; Stormshak et al., 2000).

Violent children tend to come from violent homes (McCloskey & Stuewig, 2001). There has been a decline in family violence (also called *intimate violence*) in the United States since about 1993. In the 3-year period from 1993 to 1996, the estimated number of women experiencing family violence decreased from about 1.1 million to 840,000. This is still a significant amount of violent behavior for children to observe and learn from. More than half of the female victims experiencing intimate violence are in households with children under 12 years of age (U.S. Department of Justice, 1998). Such children run a significantly increased risk of experiencing emotional and behavioral problems, including becoming antisocial and aggressive themselves (Lemmey, McFarlane, Wilson, & Malecha, 2001; Mahony, 1999).

Violent films and TV shows can provide negative models for children, teaching them new and more sophisticated forms of physical and verbal aggression (Huesman & Miller, 1994; Murray, 1995; Sanders et al., 2000). There is ample exposure of children to TV programming. Ninety-eight percent of American households have TV sets, and 76% have more than one set, one of which is used primarily by children (Nielsen Media Research, 2000). American children spend a great deal of time involved with media. On average, children in U.S. households watch over 21 hours per week of regular TV programming, not including movie videos, music videos, or video games. This time spent in a relatively sedentary activity often displaces other activities that are more social, active, or creative, and consequently may contribute to an array of problems that are emerging in American youth, such as increasing obesity and declining school achievement (American Academy of Pediatrics, 1999). For example, in a 12-year period, a child in the United States spends approximately 11,000 hours in school but over 15,000 hours watching television (Murray & Lonnborg, 1995). Research has shown a significant and detrimental effect of TV violence on aggressive behavior and on judgments about aggressive acts (Hoffner et al., 2001; Krcmar & Cooke, 2001; Scharrer, 2001).

Violence has not only permeated prime-time television but has also been included in commercial product advertisements, music videos, and cable television. The Saturday morning cartoons, always violent, have become even more so in recent years (Kinder, 1999). A growing body of research indicates beneficial effects of viewing prosocial television (e.g., *Sesame Street*, *Blue's Clues*). Cognitive growth and emotional well-being not only improve, but the effects seem to endure for many years (Anderson et al., 2000; Fisch, Truglio, & Cole, 1999). Unfortunately, the negative effects of violent programming also endure for years, suggesting that the broadcast media can have both detrimental and positive effects (Cantor & Mares, 2001). Hazards of TV viewing pertain to children's development of fears and sexual attitudes as well as to their aggressive and violent behavior (Cantor et al., 2001).

Treatment of Oppositional Defiant and Conduct Disorders

IN FOCUS 7 ▶ Identify three types of treatment for oppositional defiant and conduct disorders, and indicate how effective each has been.

The very diverse nature of the behaviors that make up antisocial disorders makes them difficult to treat. Aggression can take several different forms, ranging from physical and verbal aggression to property destruction such as fire-setting. Noncompliance can range from simply ignoring requests to doing the exact opposite of what was requested. In addition, deficits such as poor social skills, faulty problem-solving skills, a lag in development of rule-governed behavior, and

poor academic skills make each antisocial child a unique and individual case. Clinicians from different backgrounds may set entirely different priorities in treating these problems.

Traditional Treatment Approaches: Is Catharsis Necessary?

Traditional approaches to the treatment of antisocial disorders have involved techniques such as therapeutically induced insight into the origin of the problem, play therapy, catharsis (discharge of pent-up aggressive energies), or the parents' or therapist's trying to rebond with the child so that socialization can begin anew. Psychodynamic approaches to the treatment of these disorders have generally included assisting the older child to develop insight into the development of an underlying conflict, which usually involves the child's parents (Friedlander, 2001; Meloy, 2001). Psychodynamic therapeutic approaches to the treatment of antisocial children have not been well researched, but many of those that have been studied have not been found to be particularly effective (Brestan & Eyberg, 1998; de Brito-Orsini, 2000). Chapter 15 contains a more complete description of these treatment approaches.

Catharsis as a treatment approach has received some attention in public media over the years. **Catharsis** is a therapeutic release of pent-up aggressive drives in a socially acceptable manner. The hypothesis suggests that aggressive energies build up in a child and must be discharged in some form of aggressive behavior. In treatment, the therapist assumes that one form of aggression can be substituted for and is equivalent to other forms of aggression. For example, a frustrated child who is restrained from hitting a peer who has taken his toy can instead release the built-up aggressive impulses by hammering pegs. In this example, hammering pegs is substituted for hitting the other child. The two acts are considered equivalent in that once the pegs are hammered, the aggressive energies are assumed to have dissipated. In treatment contexts, a therapist may urge a conduct-disordered child who is violent to punch a large inflated "Bobo" doll, play with toy weapons, or fight with rubber foam bats.

Although widely accepted, the assumed release of rage in catharsis therapy is probably a therapeutic myth and it may actually make an antisocial condition worse. The research evidence indicates that catharsis does not significantly reduce the aggressive behavior of children (Goldstein, 1999; Wann et al., 1999). There is some evidence that individuals who are involved in catharsis therapy report feeling better, but little to suggest that this results in lowered aggressive tendencies (Bushman, Baumeister, & Phillips, 2001). If confirmed by further investigation, this would certainly help explain why catharsis therapy is widely viewed as effective, despite evidence to the contrary.

Social Learning and Behavioral Approaches

Social learning and behavioral approaches contrast with traditional psychotherapy because they emphasize changing observable behavior through direct interventions. Instead of trying to interpret underlying conflict or release stored aggressive impulses, behavioral methods utilize environmental consequences, parent training, contingency contracting, and problem solving to change disruptive behaviors (Cunningham, 1996; Danforth, 1999; Weisz, Weiss, Han, Granger, & Morton, 1995). Techniques such as point systems, reinforcement, precision request making, and time-out (brief withdrawal from a positive environment) are commonly used to deal with aggressive and noncompliant behavior. A complete cure is often considered unrealistic once antisocial behaviors are well established. Instead, a continued management approach throughout childhood and adolescence may be necessary.

Preventive approaches that combine several different treatment approaches to promote family competence, reduce school failure, and improve social relationships early in a child's life may be an alternative to chronic management. The FAST Track (Families and Schools Together) is a nationwide project designed to identify and intervene with high-risk children when they first enter school. This model, which combines parent training, home visits, social skills training, academic tutoring, and classroom intervention at an early age, is highly promising. While the longitudinal data are still being gathered, research thus far suggests that this comprehensive program is effective and socially beneficial (Conduct Problems Prevention Research Group, 2000; Vitaro, 1998).

Improving compliance and reducing aggression are insufficient in treating children with conduct disorders. The child's other deficits must also be treated if a child with conduct disorder is to make long-term improvements. Social skills training programs that improve problem solving, conflict negotiation, accepting of negative feedback, and giving of positive feedback to others can be effective with behaviorally disordered children (Christenson & Sheridan, 2001; Gumpel & David, 2000). When the children master these skills, they are assigned homework to ensure that they practice them. Similarly, academic problems must be corrected if a child with conduct disorder is going to make a successful adjustment to a school setting.

The nature of the problem behaviors presented by youngsters with conduct disorder focuses considerable attention on social and interpersonal skill areas. Juvenile delinquents often lack a broad array of interpersonal, planning, aggression management, empathy, and other psychological skills (Bodtker, 2001; Eisenberg et al., 1999). Each of these missing skills must be painstakingly taught to the aggressive youngster. Social skills training has been used effectively in a variety of settings to reduce disruptive behavior and enhance a child's ability to adapt to environmental circumstances (Christenson & Sheridan, 2001; Gumpel & David, 2000; Ison, 2001). Various behaviors are targeted, depending on individual need. Targeted training includes highly detailed instruction in matters like controlling anger and aggression, moral reasoning, problem solving, accurate perception of situations, stress management, cooperation, recruiting supportive models, and understanding and using group processes (Escamilla, 2001; Kellner & Bry, 1999). Program components such as anger control training teach specific alternative skills for responding to provocations and aim at improving behavioral self-regulation, which represents a significant challenge (August, Realmuto, Hektner, & Bloomquist, 2001).

Clearly, the skills deficiencies of many aggressive youths are immense, and much training is required. Training in social and interpersonal skills has shown some success, but the challenge is a significant one. Like other treatment programs for delinquents, behavioral programs show a serious limitation: failure of treatment gains to transfer to everyday life and be maintained by children at nearly all ages and in many different contexts (Cottle, Lee, & Heilbrun, 2001; Sigurdsson, Gudjonsson, & Peersen, 2001).

Behaviorally based direct instruction programs have been proven effective in teaching appropriate classroom behavior and basic academic and study skills to conduct-disordered children (Kozioff, LaNunziata, Cowardin, & Bessellieu, 2000; Nelson, Johnson, & Marchand-Martella, 1996). However, deficits in rule-governed and problem-solving behaviors are still problematic for these children. One promising approach that has been developed combines both cognitive and behavioral techniques to teach problem-solving skills to these youngsters (Kazdin, 2001). This approach emphasizes realistic personal situations with siblings, parents, peers, and teachers, and teaches problem-solving skills directly through generating of alternative solutions, consequential thinking, and taking the perspective of the other person. The preliminary evidence from this approach shows that it is significantly superior to traditional therapeutic approaches in its effectiveness (Kazdin, 2001).

JUVENILE DELINQUENCY

Characteristics of Adolescent Delinquents

Legally, any person younger than age 18 who engages in unlawful activities is a **juvenile delinquent**. Delinquent activities can range from occasional illicit drug and alcohol use to a pattern of violence or even murder. Children and teens who are truants from school are considered delinquents, as are juveniles with extensive histories of assault with deadly weapons or drug dealing. As discussed in Chapter 1 on developmental differences in behavior problems, a certain amount of nonconformist, oppositional behavior and minor law-breaking is not uncommon in adolescence.

Developmental Paths to Delinquency

IN FOCUS 8 ▶ Identify three developmental pathways to delinquency.

Certain types of disruptive behavior are more likely at specific ages. As children become older, aggressive behavior decreases but delinquent behavior increases; so they typically go from disobedience and threats to truancy, theft, and substance abuse (e.g., Green, 2001; Nansel et al., 2001). The most serious type of juvenile delinquency is associated with diagnosable psychiatric disorders, most often conduct disorder in children and adolescents and antisocial personality disorder in older adolescents. We have already examined the developmental pathway from oppositional defiant disorder to conduct disorder, and we can now extend that unfortunate trajectory to delinquency and antisocial personality disorder. In the latter condition, the antisocial behavioral patterns beginning in childhood continue into adulthood and are characterized by terms such as *sociopath* in popular and lay media. Table 10-5 summarizes the diagnostic criteria for this condition. With regard to characteristics, causation,

---

Table 10-5 DSM-IV-TR Diagnostic Criteria for Antisocial Personality Disorder

A. There is a pervasive pattern of disregard for and violation of the rights of others occurring since age 15 years, as indicated by three (or more) of the following:

    (1) failure to conform to social norms with respect to lawful behaviors as indicated by repeatedly performing acts that are grounds for arrest

    (2) deceitfulness, as indicated by repeated lying, use of aliases, or conning others for personal profit or pleasure

    (3) impulsivity or failure to plan ahead

    (4) irritability and aggressiveness, as indicated by repeated physical fights or assaults

    (5) reckless disregard for safety of self or others

    (6) consistent irresponsibility, as indicated by repeated failure to sustain consistent work behavior or honor financial obligations

    (7) lack of remorse, as indicated by being indifferent to or rationalizing having hurt, mistreated, or stolen from another

B. The individual is at least 18 years.

C. There is evidence of Conduct Disorder with onset before age 15 years.

D. The occurrence of antisocial behavior is not exclusively during the course of Schizophrenia or a Manic Episode.

SOURCE: American Psychiatric Association (2000), p. 706. Reprinted with permission from the *Diagnostic and Statistical Manual of Mental Disorders*, 4th ed., Text Revision. © 2000 APA.

---

and treatment, juvenile delinquency has many similarities with oppositional defiant and conduct disorders.

Only when antisocial behavior is severe, chronic, and represents a pervasive pattern of disregard for, and violation of, the rights and welfare of others does it constitute conduct disorder or antisocial personality disorder (American Psychiatric Association, 2000). There are different pathways to juvenile delinquency, depending on the youngster's use of violence and illicit drugs:

1. *Adolescent violent criminality path (the aggressive versatile path)*: The antisocial behavior pattern typically has an early onset during the preschool years and includes conduct problems and hyperactivity combined with impulsivity and attention-deficit problems. School achievement problems and a large repertoire of different antisocial problems are other features (Crespi & Giuliano, 2001; McCoy & Reynolds, 1999).
2. *The nonviolent path*: Violence is not a feature during adolescence but property and drug offenses occur; problem onset is later, during late childhood or early adolescence, and the youth often has deviant peers.
3. *The illicit drug use path*: Adolescents who use illegal drugs but are not violent or criminal are more likely to have had internalizing problems such as shyness or anxiety as children.

Frequent commission of any one type of offense, such as stealing, makes it more likely that the youth will progress to committing more serious offenses. There may be a developmental progression from characteristic disobedience, aggression, and destructiveness during childhood to later truancy, stealing, and illicit substance use (Loeber et al., 2001; Vitaro, Brendgen, & Tremblay, 2001; Welte, Zhang, & Wieczorek, 2001). Note, however, that childhood antisocial behavior is common, particularly among boys, and most often is followed by normal adult adjustment.

Onset and Course of Delinquency

Adolescents who committed their first offense at an earlier age have a larger total number of offenses and are more likely to become chronic offenders. Early commission of criminal acts is associated with a worse prognosis than is later initial illegal activity. Nevertheless, other factors are important in delinquent careers, such as the amount of violence or cruelty associated

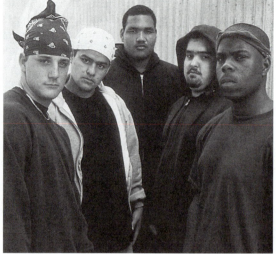

Gang members are expected to support the group's activities and may be required to prove themselves through ritualistic violence or criminal acts.

with the illegal act, whether others persuaded the child to act, and whether the act was motivated by considerations of personal gain or by excitement (Loeber et al., 2001; Patterson, Dishion, & Yoerger, 2000; Vitaro et al., 2001). Juvenile delinquency is related to the same set of characteristics as the externalizing or social disorders already discussed. A large portion of those who are delinquents meet the diagnostic criteria for conduct disorder (Loeber & Coie, 2001; Weist & Cooley-Quille, 2001).

How does this destructive, and self-destructive, lifestyle begin, and what can be done to prevent violence by adolescents? The roots of violent delinquency lie partly in an increasingly violent society. Firearms injury is second among non-natural causes of death for children and adolescents (Centers for Disease Control, 2000). As a group, 18- to 24-year-olds have committed homicides more frequently than other age groups, with the rate doubling from 1985 to 1993. The 14- to 17-year-olds were second in this dubious category. Although homicide rates have declined since their peak in 1993, they are still higher for teens and young adults than they were in the mid-1980s. Deaths due to firearms in the United States number 11.3 per 100,000, while those in Western European nations range from 0.1 to 0.3 per 100,000 (Centers for Disease Control, 2001; U.S. Department of Justice, 2001). The

Gangs: Then and Now

An increase in the number and violence of gangs draws more youths into criminal activities. Gangs seem to have originated as neighborhood play or athletic groups providing a social structure for young people's activities. Some became criminal groups, with an organization, identifiable leadership, territory, and the avowed purpose of engaging in illegal activities (Short, 2001). However, gangs continued to have a social function, and members spent much of their time simply "hanging out," or congregating together, not necessarily engaging in illegal activities. Americans' growing involvement in illicit drug use provided an opportunity for criminal activity in drug dealing, much as Prohibition did in the 1920s when alcohol was outlawed and adult gangs controlled alcohol distribution. Then and now, demand for illegal substances and activities such as drugs and prostitution stimulated the growth of gangs.

A major historical difference, though, is that Prohibition-era gangsters were adults and today's gangs are more likely to be juveniles. Gangs attract many children with their individual hand signs, graffiti, distinctive clothing, and reputations for toughness and adventure. Even if not attracted to a gang, a schoolchild may have little choice but to affiliate with one gang or another in order to seek protection from extortion and physical assault. Once recruited, the boy will be expected to support and participate in the gang's activities, whether harmless, mildly criminal, or physically assaultive. Girls associated with gangs are reported to be involved in the full array of gang activities, although perhaps not as frequently as their male counterparts (Esbensen, Deschenes, & Winfree, 1999). Some research has linked the allure of gang membership to that of terrorist groups and cults, in terms of both activities and internal rhetoric (Levine, 1999). In this respect, affiliating with a gang is somewhat like joining the military: You cannot choose which command to obey. There is no single definition of a gang, because the structure and activities of gangs differ across the country, but today's gangs appear to be more involved in violence, alcohol, and drugs than in previous times (Hunt & Laidler, 2001; Riedel, 2000; Short, 2001).

public taste for violence seems to increase in general terms. Preferences in movies and television programming are for more and more violent aggression, which stimulates both exact imitation of particular violent acts and generalized aggression, especially among aggressive younger viewers (Gupta et al., 2001). With weapons so readily available and people so willing to use them, it is hardly surprising that many young people grow up violent and callous to the needs and rights of others. Groups of such individuals have been around for a long time, as illustrated in the Research Focus box.

Family Factors Associated with Delinquency

Family factors are also important contributors to juvenile violence in ways similar to the ways they contribute to the other disorders reviewed in this chapter. The structure of the family itself appears to affect children's antisocial attitudes and behavior. As though the increasing number of mothers who are single parents did not have enough troubles, their children, especially the boys, may defy them and exhibit increased hypermasculine behavior, including aggression, boasting, and risk-taking (Sullivan, 2001). Many children in mother-only households are well-socialized and achievement-oriented, but the risks of inadequate socialization are greater when children become defiant and the mother alone must bear all responsibility for maintaining the family (McConnell, 2000). In either intact or single-parent families, children are at greater risk for delinquency if there is poor parental monitoring and supervision, harsh and inconsistent discipline, family violence, and parental rejection. Large families in which grandparents, parents, and several siblings have criminal records also place children at risk (Crespi & Giuliano, 2001).

Schooling

Academic skills deficits often precede and accompany delinquency (Barrera et al., 2001; Dumas et al., 1999).

At times, the seriousness of defiant youngsters' academic deficiencies is underestimated because of their more flamboyant oppositional behavior and truancy, which lead teachers to reject them. Reading difficulties are common among delinquent and predelinquent youth (Loeber & Coie, 2001; Loeber et al., 2001). Since children who cannot read cannot master other academic subject matter, they quickly fall far behind the class and may drop out of school altogether. Normal peers tend to shun classmates who are disruptive, aggressive, and academically deficient; thus, children who begin to fail in school find it increasingly difficult to associate with well-adjusted peers. Childhood academic failure may substantially contribute to loss of social status at school, poor self-esteem, discouragement, association with more deviant peers, and delinquent behavior (Levitt & Lochner, 2001; Pearce, 2000; Preski & Shelton, 2001).

Prevention and Treatment of Delinquency

Should juvenile delinquents be punished or given rehabilitative treatment? Should youths who commit serious crimes be punished as adults, or should we assume that they lack the experience and judgment of an adult and treat them as children capable of moral and behavioral education? Society has alternated between giving minors the same type and severity of punishment as adults, which was typical in the 17th and 18th centuries, and treating them as child victims in need of education and socialization. The present juvenile justice and mental health systems recognize the need for both restriction and education of youths convicted of crimes.

Juvenile Corrections Institutions

People demand protection from property destruction, theft, and violence. The punishment of crime in the United States appears to be related to the seriousness or perceived seriousness of the offense rather than the likelihood that the individual will commit another crime. There is also a tendency for the public to seek an expression of remorse on the part of the criminal—even to the extent of making public note of this in discussions of sentencing (Darley, Carlsmith, & Robinson, 2000; Sarat, 1999). There is some evidence that correctional programs are generally effective in reducing repeat offending, but there are many questions regarding

cost-effectiveness and the degree to which rehabilitation is a central goal in criminal sentencing (Cullen & Gendreau, 2001; Farrington, Petrosino, & Welsh, 2001; Grier, 2000). The increased use of firearms by youthful offenders makes them just as dangerous as armed adults, so it is not surprising that the public is demanding harsher punishment and incarceration for violent minors (Braga, Kennedy, Waring, & Piehl, 2001).

Institutional placements include large state training schools, forestry camps, detention centers, long-term youth correctional facilities, and municipal jails. Most institutions hold juveniles awaiting court action, administer diagnostic evaluations, provide temporary housing, and administer correctional punishment. Despite their great expense, the effectiveness of such institutions is questionable. Most importantly, they do not stop crime. The strongest predictor of incarceration in such a facility is previous incarceration (Benda, Flynn-Corwyn, & Toombs, 2001). Training schools for juvenile delinquents too often become "crime training centers" in which juveniles learn new and more serious criminal techniques from fellow inmates (Lyons, Baerger, Quigly, Erlich, & Griffin, 2001; Taylor et al., 2001). It soon becomes a sign of prestige and a rite of passage to graduate to incarceration in a high-security juvenile detention center. Inmates simply expect to be sent to the high-security detention center when they reach the appropriate age and offense level. When they reach that stage, they may find themselves intimidated and physically and sexually assaulted by the other inmates. Nevertheless, institutionalization is a frequent societal response to juvenile crime.

Perhaps there is nothing inherently wrong with the idea of incarcerating youthful offenders, although much is wrong with the way it is presently done. Certainly questions have been posed regarding their potential for unhealthy influences on young detainees and whether their only benefit is moving delinquents out of the societal mainstream where they may do harm (Benda et al., 2001, Lyons et al., 2001). These institutions are typically underfunded, understaffed, poorly managed, and grossly overpopulated, which produces accompanying behavioral control problems. To a considerable extent, inmates' lives are controlled by the fiercest of the other inhabitants rather than by the authorities. In such an environment, antisocial behavior patterns are likely to become stabilized or even exacerbated rather than overcome. Attempts to improve in-

Back to the Beginning

Behavior Management Helps Dan

All of this brings us back to Demolition Dan, the preschooler who was terrorizing his classmates and defying his teacher. As we look back at the research we have explored, there are perhaps more reasons to be concerned about Dan than might be assumed. Clearly, he may be no more than a rambunctious little boy, but there are some other possibilities that are sufficiently serious to warrant a second, serious look. One crucial issue is the developmental component of behavior disorders. For those who ultimately end up as adult criminals, there is considerable evidence that many were previously juvenile delinquents and before that were diagnosed as having conduct disorder, and there is some probability that they exhibited less serious oppositional defiant disorder before that. There are many for whom a traceable developmental trajectory of increasingly serious behavior problems is evident.

Fortunately, for Dan, his teacher, Eileen Hattson, took his behavior seriously. As we noted, he had been evaluated by school psychologists who had found him to be a bit delayed in language and social skills competence. Further observations convinced one of the psychologists that Dan's behavior was related to these delays and that the roots could be traced back to his home. In conference with Eileen Hattson, the psychologist suggested that one of the ways Dan got attention was by causing disruption in the class. During the rare times when he was quiet, everyone was so relieved that they breathed a sigh of relief and focused on the many other elements of the classroom that needed attention. Discussions with Dan's mother suggested that some elements of Dan's behavior may have emerged early at home, when she and her husband had first noticed a bit of slowness in his language development. They were so demonstrative when he began early vocalizations that they may have inadvertently reinforced his loud outbursts, beginning a cycle of reinforcement that led to increasingly disruptive verbal and physical behavior.

Behavior therapists typically don't spend a lot of time exploring causation except when they outline the details of what is reinforcing or maintaining a behavior in a particular environment. A carefully managed program of parent training and collaboration with Dan's teacher was implemented to change the interaction patterns with Dan both at home and in his preschool class. Care was taken to help his parents respond to Dan when he was *not* running around and yelling and to ignore his outbursts—all aimed at decreasing the disruptive behavior and increasing the amount of time he was being quiet or quietly interacting with others. His overall time exhibiting disruptive behavior did begin to diminish at home, leading to a much quieter household.

Dan's quieter behavior at home did not generalize to the classroom at all. Eileen Hattson had to implement a behavior management program for Dan that had several elements in common with what his parents were doing at home. The school environment was a little more challenging because Dan had more sources of reinforcement than at home—his classmates gave him a lot of attention when he was disruptive. Over time, however, the reinforcement cycle was broken, and Dan's behavior pattern at school became much calmer as he received attention for many behaviors other than demolishing the classroom.

This didn't resolve all of Dan's challenges; he still had some language delays that needed attention. But the behavior management program did enhance his social competence and made it possible for his teacher to focus more on his academic work. Perhaps Dan was diverted from a darker developmental pathway that might have led him toward an unfortunate interaction with the criminal justice system.

mates' behavior through special programs of milieu therapy, therapeutic communities, self-government, psychodrama, and confrontation therapy often do not succeed, in part because they are seldom applied appropriately or consistently (Ashford, Sales, & LeCroy, 2001; Goldsmith, 2001; Ziegler, 2001).

Foster Group Homes

Behavior therapy is employed in institutional settings when a determination has been made that a youngster needs to be removed from the home and neighborhood. The introduction of behavioral interventions in institutional settings has yielded somewhat positive outcomes, especially in improving such youths' behavior within the institutions. A community-based, foster family intervention places a small group of six to eight delinquents in a private home with teaching parents who are highly trained behavioral psychologists. Begun in the 1960s, this program continues to show success in decreasing both major and minor behavior problems (Wong, 1999). Assuming that the delinquent's behavior problems are caused by the lack of specific adjustment skills, the model involves rigorous training in social skills. The teaching parents' goal is to train the youths in social, academic, and self-care skills, through acting as appropriate models and providing highly structured direct instruction using prompts and earned response consequences. Each group home features: (1) a motivational system (token economy and level system), (2) a self-government system that allows the boys to participate in decisions that affect them, (3) a behavioral skills training program, and (4) a relation-building program between the youths and the teaching parents. At first, each boy must earn daily privileges such as TV viewing time, sports participation, or extra snacks; later, as he advances through the program, he earns longer-term privileges on a weekly basis. The teaching parents work closely with the children's schoolteachers, and each youngster brings home a daily report card on his school performance and behavior and earns points for positive reports.

SUMMARY

Social disorders are some of the most common behavior disorders for which children are referred for treatment and special education services. The social disorders presented in this chapter included oppositional defiant disorder, conduct disorder, and juvenile delinquency. For some children, there is a developmental progression from oppositional defiant disorder to conduct disorder and in turn to juvenile delinquency. The child with oppositional defiant disorder may challenge authority, argue, and lose his temper, but does not exhibit the persistent behavioral excesses that violate the rights of others. The child with conduct disorder is a rule breaker who is noncompliant and aggressive and exhibits more serious transgressions. The youngster who is a juvenile delinquent has many of the characteristics of the child with oppositional defiant disorder and conduct disorder; however, more serious social rule-breaking has occurred, and the individual has also engaged in some type of law-breaking.

The childhood social disorders stand out because the behaviors that define these disorders are primarily behavioral excesses. All children occasionally fight, are sometimes inattentive, and sometimes break rules. However, children with social disorders engage in these behaviors to an excess when compared to their peers. It is easy, however, to focus on the behavioral excesses of these children and neglect the behavioral deficits. These deficits include poor academic achievement, inappropriate social skills development, and inadequate moral or rule-governed behavior. Some of these children may be withdrawn and socially isolated. If the deficits are not treated along with the excesses, these children are more likely to have a poor outcome in adolescence and adulthood.

INFOTRAC COLLEGE EDITION

For more information, explore this resource at http://www.infotrac-college.com/Wadsworth. Enter the following search terms:

behavior therapy
conduct disorder
juvenile delinquency
divorce
externalizing behaviors
family influences
parenting and child behavior
gangs
genetic etiology

juvenile justice system
institutionalization
violence
modeling
media violence
oppositional defiant disorder
social learning

IN FOCUS ANSWERS

IN FOCUS 1 ▶ Why does the possibility of a developmental trajectory for antisocial behavior concern many psychologists?

- There is significant risk that children with oppositional defiant disorder will progress to the more serious conduct disorder if no intervention occurs.
- There is also significant risk that youngsters with conduct disorder will progress to more serious behavior excesses that may ultimately result in a crime being committed and their becoming juvenile delinquents.

IN FOCUS 2 ▶ Identify several characteristics of children with conduct disorder.

- Frequent aggression and noncompliance
- Withdrawal from peer and environmental interaction
- Poor moral development and lack of empathetic behavior
- Poor social skills and academic deficiencies

IN FOCUS 3 ▶ What are some common antisocial-aggressive behaviors of children with conduct disorder?

- Aggression toward people or property
- Destruction of property
- Deceitfulness or theft
- Serious violation of rules

IN FOCUS 4 ▶ Explain why noncompliance is seen as central to conduct disorder.

- Noncompliance is one of the most common behavior problems in childhood.

- In some cases, it involves delaying or passive resistance, which is difficult to target for intervention.
- Noncompliance often leaves the adults around the child feeling helplessness and frustration.
- Learning to comply may affect other developmental areas.

IN FOCUS 5 ▶ Give prevalence estimates for conduct and oppositional defiant disorders, and note any gender differences.

- Prevalence estimates for conduct disorder range from 1% to 10%, with males substantially outnumbering females.
- Prevalence estimates for oppositional defiant disorder range from 2% to 16%, with more males than females identified before puberty, but this gender difference disappears after that point.

IN FOCUS 6 ▶ What are three general causes of conduct and oppositional defiant disorders?

- Biological causes including genetic inheritance
- Family factors such as child-rearing and disciplinary practices
- Modeling by parents, peers, or others

IN FOCUS 7 ▶ Identify three types of treatment for oppositional defiant and conduct disorders, and indicate how effective each has been.

- Psychodynamic therapy—not shown to be effective
- Catharsis—not shown to be effective in reducing aggression
- Social learning and behavioral approaches—some programs have been effective, although they require specific targeting of behaviors for intervention

IN FOCUS 8 ▶ Identify three developmental pathways to delinquency.

- Adolescent violent criminality (the aggressive versatile path)
- The nonviolent path
- The illicit drug use path

11 | Learning Disabilities

In the Beginning
Mathew's Story

Mathew was a psychology undergraduate student with learning disabilities. Here is his story in his own words, recounting some of his school experiences, his diagnosis, and how his learning disabilities affect his academic efforts:

> In elementary and high school, I was terrified of math classes for several reasons. First, it did not matter how many times I practiced my times tables or other numerical combinations relating to division, subtraction, and addition, I could not remember them. Second, I dreaded the class time itself, for inevitably the teacher would call on me for an answer to a "simple" problem. Multiplication was the worst! Since I had to count on my fingers to do multiplication, it would take a lot of time and effort. Do you know how long it takes to calculate 9×7 or 9×9 on your fingers?
>
> When I was a sophomore at a junior college, I discovered important information about myself. After two days of clinical cognitive testing, I learned that my brain is wired differently than that of most individuals. That is, I think, perceive, and process information differently. The clinicians discovered several "wiring jobs," which are called *learning disabilities*. First, I have a problem with processing speed. To bring information from long-term memory takes me a long time. Second, I have a deficit with my short-term memory. This means that I cannot hold information there very long. When new information is learned, it must be put into long-term memory. This is an arduous process, requiring that the information be rehearsed several times. Third, I have a significant problem with fluid reasoning. Fluid reasoning is the ability to go from A to G without having to go through B, C, D, E, and F. It also includes drawing inferences, coming up with creative solutions to problems, solving unique problems, and the ability to transfer information and generalize. Hence, my math and numerical difficulties.
>
> With all of this knowledge, I was able to use specific strategies that help me in compensating for these neurological wiring patterns. Now I tape all lectures rather than trying to keep up taking notes. I take tests in a room by myself, and they are not timed. Any time I need to do mathematical calculations, I use a calculator.

INTRODUCTION

Many otherwise bright and capable college students are like Mathew, facing an enormous struggle with academic work that other students take for granted. They may have been diagnosed as having a learning disability and may even be among the 1% of the population who have *dyslexia*, a very severe type of learning disability that involves tremendous difficulty in learning to read (Bender, 1998).

Learning disabilities is a relatively new diagnostic label. Although people have had learning difficulties in the past, their problems were likely mistaken for signs of low intelligence, which is incorrect. The term *learning disabilities* was first proposed in 1963 by Dr. Samuel Kirk, one of the pioneers in the field of special education. He used the term to describe a group of problems that had been previously recognized and studied, but had never been given sufficient organized, formal attention to provide a solid information base. The children with these problems did not fit neatly into any major category of disability condition recognized at the time. They did not have mental retardation—in fact, they were often of normal or above average intelligence. They exhibited a wide variety of behavioral characteristics. However, a common theme recurred in the stories that their parents exchanged. Many of these youngsters were failing in school; they were often having difficulty in reading, spelling, and mathematics. Simply stated, these children had learning disabilities; their problems largely defied the existing diagnostic and treatment techniques available at the time the label was proposed.

Most current definitions of learning disabilities include academic performance problems (Kauffman, Hallahan, & Lloyd, 1998; Wong, 1999). Thus, in recent years, the concept of learning disabilities has had an extremely important influence on special education. Today, children with learning disabilities are the largest group of children with disabilities in the United States, and the growth in the number of children diagnosed with learning disabilities has been unparalleled by any other type of exceptionality (U.S. Department of Education, 2000).

With learning disabilities, definitions, causes, and behavioral characteristics often become confusingly intertwined (Shapiro & Kratochwill, 2000). A number of children may exhibit similar behavior, such as not following directions, but each child's behavior stems from a different cause. In other cases, the reverse is true—the same cause may generate different behaviors. Perhaps nowhere is the complexity of the human organism as evident as it is with learning disabilities.

PREVALENCE OF LEARNING DISABILITIES

IN FOCUS 1 ▶ What is the current estimated prevalence range for learning disabilities, and what does that mean in numbers of children?

Imprecise use of the label *learning disabilities* has made it difficult to determine how many children actually do have these disabilities. Epidemiological studies, which would provide empirical evidence concerning the prevalence of learning disabilities, have not been undertaken to the same degree as for other types of disabilities. As we will see later, definitions of learning disabilities have varied greatly over time and between geographical locations. This imprecision, of course, makes even gross estimates of frequency unreliable.

In addition, the estimated prevalence of learning disabilities has always varied greatly, with some estimates being so high as to be alarming and questionable. For example, Smith (1998) noted prevalence estimates ranging from 2% to 20% (1 in 5) of all school children. Regardless of which prevalence rate one accepts, learning disabilities clearly affect a very large proportion of all exceptional children served in U.S. schools. During the 1997–1998 school year, over 5.4 million exceptional children were being served, and over 2.7 million (or about 51%) of these were labeled as having learning disabilities (U.S. Department of Education, 2000).

DEFINING LEARNING DISABILITIES

IN FOCUS 2 ▶ Why have definitions of learning disabilities varied?

There has also been considerable variation in the definition of *learning disabilities* over the years. Kirk (1963) introduced the term in response to growing pressure for a *commonly accepted term* that would focus efforts in research and program funding. He was very cautious in the language he used as he was extremely concerned about the intended purpose—the need for a label that would be useful for research, behavior management, and personnel training. In spite of his caution, the field expanded in an uncontrolled fashion. Children with a wide variety of problems were labeled as having learning disabilities, and definitions were often either very loose and vague or tailored to cover those who were already being served in order to justify their special treatment.

As learning disabilities became recognized as a childhood disorder, parents of children with such disabilities organized nearly overnight and demanded services for their children. Previously, many parents blamed their underachieving children's school failures on lack of application. The existence of the label *learning disabilities* provided a more socially acceptable and nonjudgmental explanation.

Unfortunately, society's demand for services for children with learning disabilities appeared before effective instructional technology had been developed. The growth of the field of learning disabilities was so rapid that it was undisciplined. There was no solid, systematic program of scientific investigation on which to base programs of teacher and therapist preparation. Because of the increasing demand for qualified personnel, the individuals pressed into service frequently had little or no training. This occurred in all institutions and professional groups—teachers, psychologists, and university faculty. Consequently, instructors were often hired more on the basis of their interest in the field than for actual knowledge or experience. This situation led to some very predictable outcomes. Programs were more often based on misconception than solid principles of instruction or diagnosis derived from research. And the children involved suffered. Classes for students with learning disabilities quickly became dumping grounds for children with all types of difficulties.

A number of problems arose from developing a massive program of activity without a firm conceptual base to facilitate scientific knowledge acquisition. The field of learning disabilities is still plagued with the residue from these early problems. Research design and measurement problems continue to trouble investigators working in the area (Drew, Hardman, & Hart,

1996; Swanson, 2000b). Such difficulties have unfortunate consequences for the growth of a reliable knowledge base about people with learning disabilities. They also substantially detract from progress in interventions and treatment (Halfon & Newcheck, 1999; Kaplan, Wilson, Dewey, & Crawford, 1998).

Perhaps the most widely accepted legal definition of *learning disability* is presented in the Individuals with Disabilities Education Act (IDEA) as part of the rules and regulations:

Specific learning disability is defined as follows:

General. *The term means a disorder in one or more of the basic psychological processes involved in understanding or in using language, spoken or written, that may manifest itself in an imperfect ability to listen, think, speak, read, write, spell, or to do mathematical calculations, including conditions such as perceptual disabilities, brain injury, minimal brain dysfunction, dyslexia, and developmental aphasia.*

Disorders not included. *The term does not include learning problems that are primarily the result of visual, hearing, or motor disabilities, of mental retardation, of emotional disturbance, or of environmental, cultural, or economic disadvantage.* (U.S. Department of Education, 1999, p. 51)

This definition resembles Kirk's early description in that it is clearly very broad and quite vague in many respects. It would certainly make a behaviorist or diagnostician uncomfortable, for it fails to specify the behaviors characteristic of learning disabilities. However, it is important to remember that this definition is set in the form of a federal law—which must necessarily be broad in order to apply to many different settings, children, and purposes.

Although it may serve certain school administrative purposes satisfactorily, the general term *learning disabilities* is insufficiently specific for research purposes and even for instructional uses. The term can be effectively used only as a generalized referent or umbrella term, since it encompasses a variety of specific types of problems (Hardman, Drew, & Egan, 2002; Smith, 1998). In fact, some of the types of learning disabilities, such as dyslexia, are still too broadly defined and have been characterized as collections of different syndromes or subcategories. This view is reflected by the American Psychiatric Association in

DSM-IV-TR, where the term *learning disorders* encompasses more specific categories, such as disorders in reading, mathematics, and written expression, as well as a general category "learning disorder not otherwise specified" (American Psychiatric Association, 2000). Table 11-1 presents the DSM-IV-TR descriptions of learning disorders.

DESCRIBING AND CLASSIFYING LEARNING DISABILITIES

IN FOCUS 3 ▶ List several characteristics attributed to those with learning disabilities, and explain why it is difficult to characterize this group.

Children with learning disabilities have often been described as having mild disorders that include many different behaviors (Smith, 1998). As isolated incidents, behaviors such as reversing letters or not focusing attention may not be abnormal; if they recur or occur in combinations that substantially handicap children's daily performance, such behaviors are problematic. It has been said many times that all of us have some type of learning disability in that our perceptions and memory are fallible. This may be an attempt to make learning disabilities seem less threatening by viewing them as variants of normal functioning.

There are some striking differences between the literature on learning disabilities and that focusing on other disorders. It is not uncommon for descriptions of children with learning disabilities to make no reference to actual research; they often seem to be based on unsystematic clinical observations that are presented as "common knowledge" but are marked by ambiguities. In some cases, the actual behavior of the children is not described, but instead stereotypes are referred to. On the other hand, since parents, teachers, and psychologists often agree on many elements of behavioral descriptions for children with learning disabilities, it appears that these disorders do exist. This section describes behaviors that are commonly reported by those who are working with children labeled as having learning disabilities. Often these syndromes do not have a firm empirical base, but any research support that exists will be noted. Further, it is useful to remember that normalcy is socially defined in many different ways.

As noted earlier, learning disabilities have often been viewed as mild disorders (Hardman et al., 2002). There has been little empirical study of their severity, although the topic has continued to appear in the literature (e.g., Bocian, Beebe, MacMillan, & Gresham, 1999; D'Amato, Dean, & Rhodes, 1998). The literature in learning disabilities has also begun to address subtypes and co-occurrence (comorbidity) with other disabilities (e.g., Johnson, Altmaier, & Richman, 1999; Naglieri, 1999; Tirosh & Cohen, 1998). Research on co-occurrence indicates the degree to which individuals exhibit evidence of more than one disability or condition. Certainly there are multiple subtypes of learning disabilities, both because the definitions have been so broad and because the general category is so heterogeneous. Additionally, many students with learning disabilities also exhibit characteristics of other disorders such as ADHD or depression or other emotional difficulties (e.g., Badian, 1999; Heath & Ross, 2000; Moss et al., 2000; Pineda, Ardila, & Roselli, 1999). Students with learning disabilities also exhibit impulsive behavior and attention problems in many, but not all cases. These are also characteristics found in ADHD—a condition that co-occurs with learning disabilities rather frequently (Hardman et al., 2002; Snider, Frankenberger, & Aspenson, 2000).

As we consider various behaviors and characteristics found in youngsters with learning disabilities, it is important to remember that individuals may exhibit some, but not all, of these attributes. These behaviors have been observed in children with learning disabilities often enough to be associated with the condition, but they do not always appear.

Hyperactivity

Hyperactivity is frequently one of the first behavioral characteristics mentioned in descriptions of learning disabilities by teachers (Hardman et al., 2002). It is often reported that such children cannot sit still for more than a very short time, fidget a great deal, and are, in general, excessively active. Such behavior has been viewed as one of the "soft" signs (indirect indicators) of neurological dysfunction. Hyperactive behavior is examined elsewhere in this book, especially in the chapter on ADHD (Chapter 9). However, hyperactivity must be briefly considered here, because it is perhaps the most common behavioral characteristic of

Table 11-1 DSM-IV-TR Descriptions of Learning Disorders

Diagnostic Features

Learning Disorders are diagnosed when the individual's achievement on individually administered, standardized tests in reading, mathematics, or written expression is substantially below that expected for age, schooling, and level of intelligence. The learning problems significantly interfere with academic achievement or activities of daily living that require reading, mathematical, or writing skills. A variety of statistical approaches can be used to establish that a discrepancy is significant. *Substantially below* is usually defined as a discrepancy of more than 2 standard deviations between achievement and IQ. A smaller discrepancy between achievement and IQ (i.e., between 1 and 2 standard deviations) is sometimes used, especially in cases where an individual's performance on an IQ test may have been compromised by an associated disorder in cognitive processing, a comorbid mental disorder or general medical condition, or the individual's ethnic or cultural background. If a sensory deficit is present, the learning difficulties must be in excess of those usually associated with the deficit. Learning Disorders may persist into adulthood. . . .

Differential Diagnosis

Learning Disorders must be differentiated from *normal variations in academic attainment* and from scholastic difficulties due to *lack of opportunity, poor teaching,* or *cultural factors.* . . . *Mathematics Disorder* and *Disorder of Written Expression* most commonly occur in combination with *Reading Disorder.* When criteria are met for more than one Learning Disorder, all should be diagnosed.

Reading Disorder

Diagnostic Criteria

A. Reading achievement, as measured by individually administered standardized tests of reading accuracy or comprehension, is substantially below that expected given the person's chronological age, measured intelligence, and age-appropriate education.

B. The disturbance in Criterion A significantly interferes with academic achievement or activities of daily living that require reading skills.

C. If a sensory deficit is present, the reading difficulties are in excess of those usually associated with it.

Mathematics Disorder

Diagnostic Criteria

A. Mathematical ability, as measured by individually administered standardized tests, is substantially below that expected given the person's chronological age, measured intelligence, and age-appropriate education.

B. The disturbance in Criterion A significantly interferes with academic achievement or activities of daily living that require mathematical ability.

C. If a sensory deficit is present, the difficulties in mathematical ability are in excess of those usually associated with it.

Disorder of Written Expression

Diagnostic Criteria

A. Writing skills, as measured by individually administered standardized tests (or functional assessments of writing skills), are substantially below those expected given the person's chronological age, measured intelligence, and age-appropriate education.

B. The disturbance in Criterion A significantly interferes with academic achievement or activities of daily living that require the composition of written texts (e.g., writing grammatically correct sentences and organized paragraphs).

C. If a sensory deficit is present, the difficulties in writing skills are in excess of those usually associated with it.

Learning Disorder Not Otherwise Specified

This category is for disorders in learning that do not meet criteria for any specific Learning Disorder. This category might include problems in all three areas (reading, mathematics, written expression) that together significantly interfere with academic achievement even though performance tests measuring each individual skill are not substantially below that expected given the person's chronological age, measured intelligence, and age-appropriate education.

SOURCE: American Psychiatric Association (2000), pp. 49–56. Reprinted with permission from the *Diagnostic and Statistical Manual of Mental Disorders*, 4th ed., Text Revision. © 2000 APA.

children who are labeled as having learning disabilities (Aro, Ahonen, Tolvanen, Lyytinen, & Todd-de-Barra, 1999; Snider et al., 2000; Speltz, DeKlyen, Calderon, Greenberg, & Fisher, 1999).

It is important to note that not all children labeled as having learning disabilities are hyperkinetic (Hazell et al., 1999; Willcutt & Pennington, 2000). Additionally, the stereotype of hyperactivity seems to have led many to expect and consequently to see it in children with learning problems. Although hyperactivity is commonly viewed as involving a *general excess* of activity, evidence suggests that this may be incorrect and that it might be more fruitful to look at the *appropriateness* of a child's behavior in particular settings. Hyperkinetic children seem to exhibit higher inappropriate activity levels than their normal counterparts under structured circumstances, such as might be found in the classroom (Bender, 1998; Smith, 1998). However, most research indicates no difference between hyperactive and other children in unstructured situations such as play and other nonacademic settings. That is, hyperactivity is most apparent in situations in which sitting and attending to a task are required.

Clearly, hyperactivity is common in children with learning disabilities. However, observations of hyperactivity alone are not sufficient to lead to a diagnosis of learning disabilities, and not all children with learning disabilities are hyperactive (Aro et al., 1999; Johnson et al., 1999; Kovner et al., 1999). Further, a generalized superficial view of hyperactivity is not likely to be of great value in treatment since it seems to be somewhat situation-specific, as noted above. Research aimed at clarifying the relationship between hyperactivity and the other constellation of attributes associated with learning disabilities is essential if we are to advance our understanding and treatment of children with these problems.

Academic Achievement Problems

Many individuals with learning disabilities encounter significant problems in academic achievement (e.g., Meyer, 2000; Taylor, Anselmo, Foreman, Schatschneider, & Angelopoulos, 2000). In fact, the emergence of learning disabilities as a recognized type of exceptionality was driven by the continuing academic problems that such youngsters experience. Academic difficulties experienced by students with learning disabilities seem to be accompanied by a number of related problems that may also contribute to poor performance (Bryant, Bryant, & Hammill, 2000). Academic achievement difficulties are typically the reason why children with learning disabilities are identified in the primary grades. Such difficulties persist throughout their formal schooling, including college (Ward & Bernstein, 1998), although the ranks of college graduates and successful adults contain many with learning disabilities.

Reading

It is estimated that 85–90% of students with learning disabilities have reading disabilities (Bender, 1998). The specific nature of these reading problems varies greatly. In some cases, children lack basic word knowledge and have difficulties with word recognition. When most readers encounter a familiar word, they recall it readily. However, unfamiliar words require special attention. Consequently, it is important to know some basic rules regarding spelling patterns and pronunciation to derive meaning from new material. Using such knowledge, a reader can often sound out the letters, search her memory for similar words, and roughly determine the meaning of novel words. This process is particularly difficult for many students with learning disabilities (Hardman et al., 2002). While good readers understand the rules of syntax, recognize the common prefixes and suffixes, can generalize letter patterns, and are able to draw analogies rather flexibly, children with reading disabilities are not so fortunate. Many can read only slowly and laboriously when they can accomplish it at all. This doesn't necessarily mean they are not intelligent in other ways. On a positive note, students with reading disabilities can often be taught the necessary skills through specific training, which improves their reading substantially (Gardill & Jitendra, 1999; Wanzek, Dickson, Bursuck, & White, 2000).

The ability to use contextual cues to derive meaning is another important component of reading, one that distinguishes good from poor readers. Skilled readers tend to be quite proficient at inferring the meaning of an unknown word from the contextual information around it. For example, when reading a story about a farm, good readers easily fill in the word *horse* when they encounter a blurred word beginning with *h*. Poor readers, on the other hand, experience difficulty using context to facilitate word recognition.

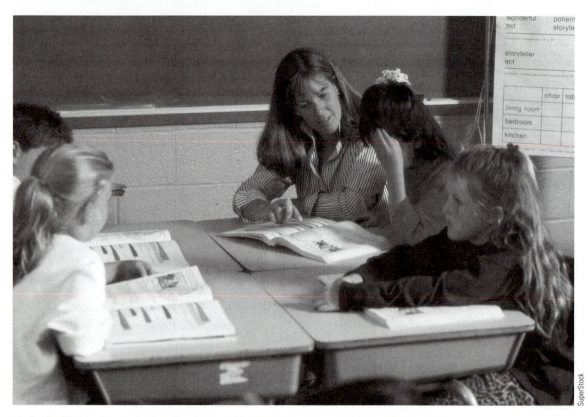

Students with learning disabilities often have problems with word recognition, making reading a significant challenge.

However, specific instruction on using contextual clues improves their performance (Rankin-Erickson & Pressley, 2000; Smith, 1998).

Effective use of contextual information requires that a person be able to perceive what the context is—that is, be able to discern and use the important ideas in the text. Students with learning disabilities encounter considerable difficulty perceiving and using the organization of important ideas in text material, frequently concentrating instead on peripheral details and information. For instance, they may focus on supporting characters in a piece of literature, seemingly exaggerating their importance in the overall plot far beyond what was intended by the author (and perhaps not remembering much about the central character). This problem can also be addressed by focused instructional intervention. Teaching specific learning strategies such as organizational and summary skills, use of mnemonics, and problem solving can counter

such difficulties and substantially enhance reading and other academic performance (Jitendra, Hoppes, & Xin, 2000; Mastropieri, Sweda, & Scruggs, 2000).

Writing and Spelling

It is not unusual for children with learning disabilities to exhibit problems in their writing performance that affect their academic achievement. Handwriting may be very labored and slow, and children may have problems with forming and spacing letters. Additionally, such students often have poor spelling skills and rather immature compositional ability (Ferretti, MacArthur, & Dowdy, 2000; Smith, 1998). Some researchers connect the handwriting proficiency of students with learning disabilities to their reading ability (Simner & Eidlitz, 2000). Part of this logic derives from evidence indicating that children with learning disabilities do *not* write more poorly than their normally achieving classmates who are reading at a comparable level. However, further research is needed to more fully investigate the relationship between poor writing skills and reading ability (Swanson & Sachse, 2000; Vadasy, Jenkins, & Pool, 2000).

Poor spelling abilities are often attributed to children with learning disabilities (Silliman, Jimerson, & Wilkinson, 2000). These youngsters seem to commit numerous errors such as letter omissions, extraneous letter inclusions, and letter-order errors. Some of their spelling seems to reflect developmentally immature mispronunciations (e.g., "spilt" for *spilled*) (Smith, 1998; Vadasy et al., 2000). Research suggests that the spelling abilities of children with learning disabilities generally follow the developmental patterns of their nondisabled peers, although they progress at a slower rate (Bender, 1998). Again, additional research is needed in order to more clearly understand the spelling abilities of students with learning disabilities.

Mathematics

Students with learning disabilities often experience difficulties with some very basic arithmetic skills. They frequently encounter problems with simple counting, writing numbers, and mastering fundamental math concepts (Jordan & Hanich, 2000; Naglieri & Johnson, 2000). Some students omit numbers when counting, while others can count but do not grasp what the numbers mean (their values). Predictably, students with learning disabilities encounter problems in circumstances where more than one digit is involved (i.e., working with numbers greater than 9), which requires an understanding of place value. Many of the math difficulties encountered by students with learning disabilities are not isolated from the difficulties they experience in other academic areas. Identifying spatial and size relations between objects is a consistent problem for such students, and a central skill in math performance. Math problems that look different at first glance may have the same answer (e.g., 3 + 3 and 4 + 2) and those that may appear very similar have different answers (e.g., 3 + 3 and 3 + 2). Furthermore, many arithmetic problems are word problems that require significant reading skills, which results in poor math performance for poor readers (Smith, 1998). Understandably, math anxiety appears to be rather high in such youngsters. The Research Focus box summarizes an investigation of a coping strategy aimed at reducing math anxiety in children

with learning disabilities. This intervention appeared to improve students' math anxiety and also moderately improved their math performance. Research on the difficulties encountered by students with learning disabilities in mathematics is badly needed, as is research on the effectiveness of various interventions.

Perceptual Problems

Children labeled as having learning disabilities often have a **perceptual disorder**. Such difficulties may result in interpreting incoming stimuli incorrectly or not perceiving all of the stimulus features. Abnormalities of perception have played an historic and prominent role in clinical and research descriptions of such youngsters. In fact, the field of learning disabilities seems to have grown out of the early work of Werner and Strauss (e.g., 1939, 1941) and Goldstein (1936, 1939), who were studying the perceptual, cognitive, and behavioral effects of brain injury. The notion that perceptual disorders are related to learning disabilities enjoyed considerable popularity over the years. Interest in this view has diminished somewhat recently because of failure to establish a clear connection between perceptual problems and neurological dysfunction. However, attention to perceptual difficulties in children with learning disabilities has not completely dissipated, and some research continues to focus on neurological bases of learning difficulties (e.g., Kraus & Cheour, 2000; Nicholls, Schier, Stough, & Box, 1999).

It is important to note that perceptual dysfunction cannot be observed directly, but is inferred from the child's behavior. Such behavioral deficits have often been reported by teachers and clinicians working with children. However, explanatory theories such as neurological dysfunction are largely deduced by analogy and are not directly provable. Certain children exhibit various constellations of behaviors that are similar to the behavior of adults with known cerebral injury. However, these children also behave more like younger children than like youngsters their own age, suggesting that general physical immaturity may play a role. With learning disabilities, knowledge is mainly inferential and diagnoses are subject to more error than is the case for conditions such as conduct disorder, anxiety, or phobias.

Despite the assessment and conceptual difficulties, perceptual and neurological problems represent a

Self-Instruction on Coping with Math Anxiety

This study investigated the efficacy of a coping strategy for reducing math anxiety in children with learning disabilities. The coping strategy was based on cognitive behavior modification (CBM). Twenty children from grades 4 through 7 participated; half were children with learning disabilities, and the remaining were normally achieving children. The two groups were balanced for age and sex. The categorization of learning disabilities was primarily based on a discrepancy between measured intelligence and achievement. All of the subjects with learning disabilities had average to above-average intelligence (WISC-R) and evidenced academic deficits of 1 to 2 years, but did not have sensory handicaps, mental retardation, or cultural or environmental disadvantage. The normally achieving students were randomly selected and had an overall average academic performance profile.

An instructor provided participants with directions for completing the mathematics tasks and modeled the completion of sample problems. In the process of modeling the sample problems, three levels of self-talk were demonstrated that focused on affect-laden (emotional) statements designed to inhibit or enhance performance. The first type of self-statement was a neutral or task-specific statement: "I have to carry that number here." The second and third types of self-talk were two levels of task-approach statements: a positive statement ("I'm doing just fine, I got that part finished") and a negative statement ("I'll never get this, I'm too dumb"). Following the modeling procedure, the students engaged in a 10-minute discussion that focused on the kinds of things they said to themselves while completing a mathematics task. After the discussion, participants were assigned to desks and taught how to operate a tape recorder and a clip-on microphone. Once they were comfortable with the equipment, they were provided with a math task and instructed to think out loud, verbalizing everything that occurred to them.

The design for the study included a pretest, intervention, and posttest. Pretest data were collected during two 45-minute sessions on two consecutive days following the first instruction described above. The second pretest period was preceded only by a verbal reminder to think aloud throughout the entire time of working on the mathematics test. The intervention procedure was applied to the students with learning disabilities only and involved six weekly sessions. In-

tervention included presentations on the role played by self-talk in performance. Cue cards were provided that outlined stages in the coping process and sample self-statements to assist in applying the strategies (see Figure 11-1). Posttest data were collected twice from both groups of students, once on the day following the last intervention session and a second time as a maintenance check two weeks later.

The dependent measures were self-talk data and performance data on fraction problems. Typewritten transcripts of the recorded audiotapes were produced following the completion of each session. Coders who knew nothing about the children rated them on the three levels of self-talk (posi-

Cue Card 1: Steps in the Coping Process

(a) Assessment of the situation
     Label and plan
(b) Recognizing and controlling the impulse of negative
     thoughts
       Recognizing that negative thoughts hurt my work
       Controlling by replacing
(c) Reinforcing
       Pat yourself on the back for a good job

Cue Card 2: Coping Self-Statements

(a) Assessment of the situation
       What is it that I have to do?
       Look over the task and think about it.
(b) Recognizing and controlling the impulse of negative
     thoughts
     Recognition:
       Okay, I feel worried and scared . . .
       I'm saying things that don't help me. . . . I can stop and
         think more helpful thoughts.
(c) Confronting/Coping/Controlling
       Don't worry. Remember to use your plan.
       Take it step by step—look at one question at a time.
       Don't let your eyes wander to other questions.
       Don't think about what others are doing. Take it one
         step at a time.
       When you feel your fears coming on . . . take a deep
         breath, think "I'm doing just fine. Things are going well."
(d) Reinforcing
       I really did well not letting this get the best of me.
       Good for me. I did a good job.
       I did a good job in not allowing myself to worry so much.

Figure 11-1   Cue Cards 1 and 2

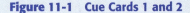

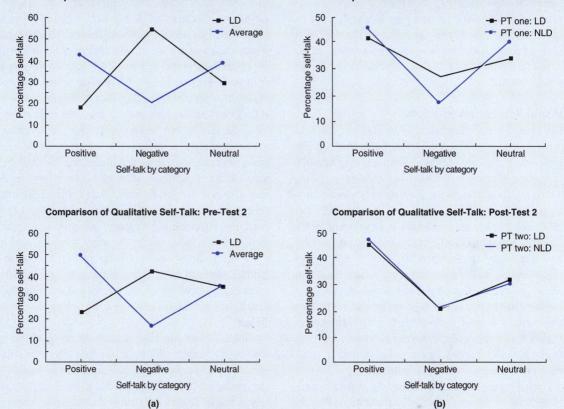

Figure 11-2   Comparisons of Qualitative Self-Talk
(a) Pretests 1 and 2; Comparisons of Self-Talk for Learning Disabled and Average Achievers.
(b) Posttests 1 and 2.

tive, neutral, negative) in operational terms. These raters achieved a very high (93%), level of agreement. Self-talk data are summarized for the two pretest and posttest sessions in Figure 11-2.

Although both groups generated similar amounts of total self-talk in both pretest sessions, normally achieving students produced significantly more *positive* self-statements than did the children with learning disabilities. Conversely, students with learning disabilities produced significantly more *negative* self-statements than normally achieving students during both pretest sessions. Pre-post comparisons indicated that the children with learning disabilities improved their self-talk. That is, after training, these children engaged in significantly more positive and signifi-

cantly less negative self-talk during posttest sessions. As illustrated in Figure 11-2, the patterns of self-talk by children with learning disabilities more closely approximated those of their normally achieving peers during posttest sessions. Additionally, the students with learning disabilities significantly improved their percentage of correct math problems from pretest to posttest measures. Correlation coefficients between all subjects' positive self-talk and math performance were found to be moderately positive (.60 and .61 for pretests 1 and 2, and .43 and .54 for posttests 1 and 2). That is, when subjects engaged in positive self-talk, their math performance tended to improve.

SOURCE: Kamann and Wong (1993).

rather appealing explanation for some of the behaviors exhibited by children with learning disabilities (e.g., the inability to copy from a chalkboard or to recognize properties that distinguish geometric shapes like circles and triangles). In a general sense, and regardless of the particular etiology involved, children with learning disabilities do exhibit behaviors that suggest some disruption in sensory processing, either in the interpretation of sensory information or in the input of stimuli.

Visual Perception Problems

Humans receive information from the environment through a number of sensory systems that vary in efficiency and accuracy. Children with learning disabilities often display difficulties in visual perception, which has ramifications for a variety of academic functions (e.g., Boden & Brodeur, 1999; Kavale & Forness, 2000; Rose, Feldman, Jankowski, & Futterweit, 1999). Children with visual perception problems may exhibit a variety of specific deficiencies. They may see a visual stimulus as unconnected parts rather than as a whole or integrated pattern. For example, a child may see unrelated lines rather than an integrated pattern representing a letter in the alphabet, as illustrated in Figure 11-3. Consequently, such a child may have difficulty identifying letters, inescapably leading to academic performance problems (Smith, 1998).

Visual perception problems may also take the form of deficits in figure-ground discrimination. *Figure-ground discrimination*, which most of us acquire easily, is the process of distinguishing a visually presented object from its background. In school, a child with this type of deficit may have problems focusing on a given word or line on a printed page or recognizing objects (Humphreys & Riddoch, 1999). This particular example raises a question that has plagued the perceptual theorists specifically and workers in learning disabilities generally: Does the inability to focus on or identify a particular word provide substantive evidence of a perceptual problem—specifically a deficit in figure-ground discrimination? It is conceivable that the child merely has an attention problem (another characteristic often attributed to children labeled as having learning disabilities). It is also possible that the child cannot remember the word (memory problems have also been frequently attributed to such children). Perhaps the child has not been effectively taught the word (an instructional deficiency). All of these may be reasonable explanations for the same behavior, and it is difficult to determine which are operative in an individual case (Bender, 1998). Clearly, to answer this question, research efforts in the area of learning disabilities must become more analytical than has been the case.

Children with learning disabilities are frequently described as having difficulty in visual discrimination (the ability to detect objects visually or to discriminate one visual stimulus from another). Such problems may result in several behaviors that are often shown by these youngsters. The children may not be able to discriminate between certain letters or words (e.g., *W* and *V*, *sit* and *sat*). They may exhibit letter reversals that logically relate to a visual discrimination problem (e.g., horizontal reversals of such letters as *b* and *d* or vertical reversals of letters such as *b* and *p*). Discrimination errors such as those noted above are not unusual in all younger children and normally decrease with age, so it may not be easy to determine whether a disability exists. Generally speaking, frequent letter reversals and transpositions in children who are beyond the age of 7 or 8 may suggest a potential problem warranting investigation (Hardman et al., 2002).

Auditory and Haptic Perception Problems

Auditory perception involves the ability to recognize, organize, and interpret stimuli that are received through the sense of hearing. Difficulties in four com-

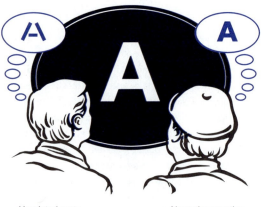

Unrelated parts   Normal perception

Figure 11-3   Example of a Visual Perception Problem

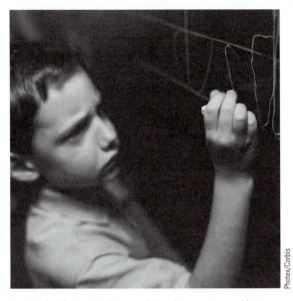

Reversal of letters is characteristic of some types of learning disabilities.

ponents of auditory perception have often been reported, singly or in various combinations, in children with learning disabilities (e.g., Gomez & Condon, 1999; Most & Greenbank, 2000). These components are discrimination, association, memory, and blending. Since auditory stimuli represent a substantial source of information in school (as do visual stimuli), problems in auditory perception may place a significant handicap on learning. For example, children with difficulties in **auditory discrimination** may not be able to distinguish between the sounds of certain syllables or words. Young children with this problem may also have difficulties in identifying particular other sounds, such as the sound of the doorbell, and in distinguishing between one sound and another. Children who have difficulties with **auditory blending** may be unable to blend the phonic elements of a word together into a consolidated whole as they say the word (e.g., an inability to blend the phonemes *m–a–n* to form the word *man*). Auditory association and memory are of obvious significance because of the way in which much modern schooling occurs. A child who has difficulty in **auditory memory** may not be able to recall information that is presented verbally, as is often the case when children are learning the alphabet, the days of the week, and the months in the

year. Children with deficits in **auditory association** often cannot make simple associations between ideas or pieces of information that are presented verbally (e.g., simple analogies).

Children with learning disabilities may also have problems in **haptic perception**, which involves recognizing objects or obtaining information through both tactile sensation (touch) and kinesthetic sensation (body sensation from movement and/or position). These deficiencies are not common, but are thought to play important roles in certain school-related activities (Smith, 1998). Handwriting is thought to rely partially on haptic perceptual abilities, in that a child must receive tactile information from holding the pencil and kinesthetic sensation regarding movement during the process of writing. Children with difficulties in this area may write unusually slowly, may have problems with regard to spacing and forming letters, may not be able to stay on the lines, and may show a variety of other difficulties. It can be difficult to discriminate haptic perception problems from clumsiness or carelessness, however, which makes misdiagnosis likely.

Memory/Information-Processing Problems

Children labeled as having learning disabilities have long been informally characterized as having memory and other information-processing problems (Lorsbach, 2000; Swanson, 2000a; Weiler et al., 2000). Frustrated teachers continually bemoan the fact that such children may learn something one day and have forgotten it by the next. This type of behavior occurs so often in children with learning disabilities that some consideration is clearly warranted here. The clinically reported memory difficulties have been so prevalent that they have led to a variety of common-sense theories (e.g., the "leaky bucket" hypothesis, in which the child is taught a fact, but memory failures result in performance failure later). All of these factors make the study of memory in those with learning disabilities fascinating but also make the problems of such individuals more perplexing.

It is paradoxical that memory problems have been so evident in the clinical descriptions of children with learning disabilities and yet formal research on this topic has been rather scanty. This research deficit is even more striking since memory research on normal and other deviant populations has been so intense.

The limited number of studies of memory characteristics of children with learning disabilities have yielded conflicting findings. Some research has found no differences between the memory performance of youngsters with learning disabilities and their nondisabled counterparts; other investigations have shown that those with learning disabilities perform more poorly (Swanson, 1999; 2000a; Taylor et al., 2000). Thus, the continuing clinical reports of poor memory are not clearly confirmed by research results. The evidence has led some writers to suggest that children labeled as having learning disabilities may have different rather than generally deficient memory and cognitive abilities (Lorsbach, 2000; Swanson, 2000a; van Strien, 1999), a notion that has gained considerable popularity. This perspective has led to the development of specific instructional emphases that are highly focused on children's specific learning problems rather than viewing the children as generally cognitively deficient (e.g., McLean & Hitch, 1999).

Attention Problems

It was suggested earlier that children with learning disabilities may have an attention problem that limits their information-processing abilities. Teachers frequently report that these children are unable to sustain attention to lengthy tasks (short attention span), are distractible, daydream often, and do not plan ahead (Naglieri & Johnson, 2000; Warner-Rogers, Taylor, Taylor, & Sandberg, 2000). However, some experimental research related to cognition has addressed *selective attention*, that is, the ability to focus attention on important stimuli and screen out or ignore irrelevant stimuli (Escera, Alho, Schroeger, & Winkler, 2000; Rothenberger et al., 2000). This has been examined by studying what is known as *incidental learning*. In most learning tasks, certain stimuli are important, central to acquiring the information (e.g., the idea presented in the narrative on a printed page). Other stimuli are unimportant, in fact, irrelevant to acquiring the information (e.g., the page numbers, the location of a certain passage on a page, or the color of the book cover). Using selective attention, the skilled reader tends to ignore the irrelevant stimuli (or at least attends to them to a lesser degree) and focuses on the stimuli that are central to the task, the words in the text. Evidence suggests that some children having learning disabilities do not employ selective attention

to the same degree that normal children do (Kehrer, Sanchez, Habif, Rosenbaum, & Townes, 2000). Normal children tend to recall more of the central information than their peers with learning disabilities, while children with learning disabilities often equal or surpass their normal classmates in recalling irrelevant information, which does not aid them in school tasks. Delineating problems with attention continues to be of significant interest in research on information-processing difficulties of children with learning disabilities (Naglieri & Johnson, 2000).

Social and Emotional Characteristics of Children with Learning Disabilities

Much of the literature on learning disabilities spotlights difficulties in academically related skills and abilities. However, it is not unusual for these youngsters to experience emotional and interpersonal difficulties as well (Allen, 2000; Cordell, 1999; Hagborg, 1999; Heath & Ross, 2000). In a rather circular fashion, learning difficulties seemingly contribute to emotional difficulties and low self-esteem, which, in turn, may affect motivation and academic efforts (Gersten & Baker, 1998; Jenkins, 1999; Palladino, Poli, Masi, & Marcheschi, 2000). (This type of relationship between math struggles and self-esteem is described in Jeanne's Story.) Such students may also have difficulty interacting with others because of misperceived social cues and problems in discriminating some of the subtle nuances of interpersonal interaction.

There has been increasing research interest in the social and emotional dimensions of learning disabilities. Although social and emotional factors have not been included in definitions of learning disabilities, which typically affect funding for research and intervention, there has been some research attention to these dimensions and their treatment (Persinger & Tiller, 1999; Prior, Smart, Sanson, & Oberklaid, 1999). Much remains to be investigated regarding the emotional side of these disabilities. The serious emotional components of learning disabilities include adolescent depression, suicide, and even possibly psychosis and serious violence (Allen, 2000; Cordell, 1999; Hagborg, 1999; Heath & Ross, 2000). There is also some indication that there is substantial emotional residue for these individuals in adulthood (Gralton, James, & Crocombe, 2000).

A Case Involving Math Anxiety

A psychology undergraduate student who has a learning disability tells in her own words how she is coping with this condition and succeeding in college:

Throughout elementary school I sensed a problem but never understood what this problem was.

I watched as the teacher would do math problems on the board totally understanding exactly what was going on. An assignment would be given and I'd start my work. The only problem was I couldn't remember anything I had just been taught. It was gone—there was no memory of it.

I would try and try but for some reason I could not retrieve the concepts I understood previously. Too embarrassed to ask for help I would sit at my desk and write numbers at random, pretending to be finishing my assignments. Every night I would bring home my math and ask my father to help me. Sometimes with his help I could figure it out (after being told the same thing over and over again). Other times I would get upset, he would get upset and it was a disaster that followed. Dad just couldn't figure out why something so easy caused me such difficulty.

After awhile I quit bringing my math book home and found other ways of compensating for my problems. I just felt stupid.

Another problem I experienced was often times I would transpose numbers and end up getting problems wrong. I would switch 27 to 72 and that looked right to me.

My self-esteem was lowered and anxiety would take over. I didn't want anyone to see how "stupid" I was so I used a lot of energy trying to convince teachers and friends of my good strengths.

I learned early what these strengths were and focused attention to the strengths trying to hide my weaknesses.

I remember on one occasion a test the whole class was taking. It was a math test with multiple choice answers. We figured out the problems and then filled in the bubbles. I did very well at guessing and ended up in the top math group. The only reason I made it

through that year was due to a boy in the class. I confided in him that I didn't understand and he allowed me to copy his homework every day.

To be honest I have no idea how I made it through math in junior high and high school. In high school my algebra teacher was also one of the football coaches. The class was the last period of the day and the football team practiced then also. He would come in, give the assignment, give a few examples and usually leave. There was a group of us who would stay in the room and work out the problems together. Thinking about it I realize that group is what helped me the most. Many times they would go over and over problems and some times I just had to copy someone's work and try to figure it out.

I was on the high honor roll all 3 years in high school and no one realized how much I really struggled.

College was never a thought of mine. It actually never crossed my mind.

I married, had 3 children, and 10 years later decided to attend college for the first time. In the back of my mind I told myself, "I'll go as far as I can then when it's time to take my math requirements I'll quit."

When I first started college I bought a mini tape recorder and taped the lectures. I would review the tape when I returned home and fill in missed material in my notes. I made cards to review the material by testing myself. I was doing well, much to my surprise.

It seemed as though I had learned to compensate well and I had strengthened myself in other areas.

I heard about a program at the university about math anxiety and decided to call. I met with a counselor and signed up for a math class with a group called Student Support Services. They offered tutoring and support.

I tried to bluff my way through this class only to realize this couldn't be done in college. Many times I asked myself what I was doing there.

I met with my math instructor after class almost every day doing problems. He would work them out on a board while explaining every step along the way. Sometimes he would ask me to do the problem. "I can't" I would answer and he followed with "Yes you can, I'll help you." He would have me explain why I was doing each calculation and tell me if it was right or wrong. This man had a lot of patience with me and we worked many hours together.

Finally I went in to his office one day and admitted to him that I see some things backwards. He said he could tell something was wrong. I asked how he knew and he said several times he witnessed me switching numbers around.

From that time on he would read the problem to me to copy. That really helped a lot.

It is important to restate here a notion that was mentioned previously: The term *learning disabilities* is a broad label that encompasses many different, specific problems. Clinicians and researchers may observe any of a variety of difficulties, in combination or singly, in an individual child carrying such a label. This section has discussed several characteristics that have been attributed to and studied in children with learning disabilities. It would not, however, be appropriate to *characterize* such individuals because learning disabilities vary so widely in their nature and severity.

DEVELOPMENTAL FACTORS

This book's continuing theme of human development surfaces prominently once again in considering learning disabilities. Theories of human development have played an important role in the study of learning disabilities for many years. For example, theories regarding developmental delays have been involved in researchers' frustrated attempts to derive a single, comprehensive theory about the causation of learning disabilities (i.e., that all learning disabilities can be explained in terms of developmental delays). Developmental theory has been appealed to because performance of children with learning disabilities often resembles that of younger normal children (e.g., Samango-Sprouse, 1999; Smith, 1998). Children with learning disabilities have also often been described as exhibiting extremely uneven abilities across skill areas. Their mental and behavioral development pro-

gresses in an irregular fashion and very unevenly in some cases. It has been suggested that youngsters with learning disabilities show differences and delays in neurological development (Nicholls et al., 1999). In some cases, evidence supporting such a developmental lag has been found as a peripheral result in studies focusing primarily on other topics (e.g., language, handedness, attention, visual impairment), which is not surprising since neurological status is often inferred from behavior in studying many disorders or conditions (Schallert et al., 2000; Shamir, Rotenberg, Laudon, Zisapel, & Elizur, 2000). Other researchers, however, have assessed behavior with the basic intent of studying neurological involvement (e.g., Livingston, Gray, Haak, & Jennings, 2000; Yanez et al., 2000). Although the few studies that have been done seldom examine precisely the same behaviors, there is evidence suggesting neurological immaturities and developmental lag in children with learning disabilities. It also appears that these youngsters are most dissimilar from their normal counterparts at younger ages and converge more with their classmates as they become older.

ETIOLOGY OF LEARNING DISABILITIES

IN FOCUS 4 ▶ Identify three causes thought to be involved in learning disabilities.

Given the range of performance deficits shown by children with learning disabilities, it is hardly surprising that a variety of known and hypothesized factors may cause or contribute to these conditions. Hypothesized causes of learning disabilities have included such factors as birth injuries, nutritional abnormalities, poor self-image, developmental delay, poisoning by environmental elements, genetic defects, and poor teaching. As we discuss causes of learning disabilities, it is important to remember that precise knowledge is often absent and that much of the available information represents theory, hypotheses, analogies, and inferences drawn from other populations or situations. Thus, conclusions are tentative and subject to change as improved information becomes available.

Neurological Damage

We already noted the assumption by some that learning disabilities may be caused by brain damage or some other type of neurological problem (e.g., Hardman et al., 2002; Yanez et al., 2000). Opinions regarding this explanation vary greatly. In most cases, the existence of neurological damage as a cause is presumptive, and credible supportive evidence is lacking (Bender, 1998). This has led many professionals to discontinue the pursuit of neurological bases of learning disabilities. Until technological advances permit more precise assessment of neurological status, determination of a specific neurological problem for the vast majority of children with learning disabilities remains unlikely. Most likely, there are some children labeled as having learning disabilities whose problems are based on neurological damage. It is also probable that others with the same global label and similar abnormal behavior do not have any neurological dysfunction.

There are a variety of factors that could result in the neurological damage suspected in some children with learning disabilities. For example, such damage could arise as a result of difficulties encountered as a child is developing prenatally, such as low birth weight or inadequate gestational age at birth, Rh blood incompatibility between the mother and fetus, or serious maternal infection (Johnson & Breslau, 2000). Similarly, abnormalities during the birth process (inadequate oxygen supply to the baby or abnormal positioning of the fetus during delivery) may also result in neurological damage, or damage may occur after birth, as when a child has convulsions from a high fever (Drew & Hardman, 2000). These are some examples of factors that may have a significant impact on the neurological status of an individual. They are also relevant to childhood disorders other than learning disabilities and are discussed more completely in Chapter 12, which examines mental retardation and poverty-related developmental risks.

Genetic Influences

The possibility that learning disabilities are inherited often concerns parents. There is some evidence that genetic factors may play a role since learning disabilities tend to run in families; however, it is unlikely that any genetic cause can be identified for most or all learning disabilities (Culbertson, 1998; Silver, 1999; Smith, 1998).

Part of the support for genetic causation is derived from research on identical and fraternal twins (Alarcon, Knopik, & DeFries, 2000; Willcutt, Pennington, & DeFries, 2000). Such research has suggested that identical twins share learning disabilities more often than do fraternal twins. The higher incidence rate for identical twins suggests that there may be some genetic contribution to the development of learning disabilities. However, the problems of separating the influence of genetics and environment always persist. A case could also be made that abnormal behaviors in one family member may be reflected by other family members as a result of learning or family expectations and standards. Even the results reported for identical twins could be caused by their very similar environment. Such children not only have the same genetic composition, they also share the same environment, even prenatally. Identical twins most often share chorionic membranes and the same placenta. Consequently, prenatal damage, such as that caused by oxygen insufficiency, could easily affect both twins similarly. With fraternal twins, such damage might not impact both babies to the same extent since they have two chorions and two placentas. If pairs of twins are selected for such twin studies because one has a learning disability and if that condition was due to a prenatal accident of some sort (e.g., oxygen deprivation, nutritional abnormality), the identical sibling of that fetus would likely have been subjected to the same condition, whereas a fraternal twin may have developed in a different environment. There has also been some speculation that the postnatal environment of identical twins is also more similar than that encountered by fraternal twins (Krueger, 2000). Any or all of these possibilities *might* explain the results of twin studies. Although the evidence suggests some genetic influence, environmental factors certainly cannot be ignored.

Environmental Influences

From the discussion of child behavior disorders throughout this book, it is clear that the environment influences children in many significant ways. Thus, environment must be viewed as a potentially important contributor to learning disabilities. In this sense, the environment is conceived quite broadly. Certain maternal activities are significant during the prenatal period (e.g., dietary intake, smoking, alcohol and drug consumption), and these factors affect the environment of the unborn child. A number of environmental influences after birth have also been mentioned as potential causes of learning disabilities (e.g., poverty, neglect, food additives, ingestion of lead, inappropriate or poor school instruction). Deficient general sensory stimulation has also been implicated as a cause of learning disabilities (Smith, 1998). Thus, both prenatal and postnatal environmental influences have been identified as causative of learning disabilities (Bender, 1998; Codina, Yin, Katims, & Zapata, 1998; Lefrancois, 1999).

The environment also appears to play a significant role in learning disabilities with regard to the motivation with which such youngsters approach much of their schoolwork. Poor motivation has long been ascribed to these children, with characterizations of inattentiveness, poor concentration, and minimal task persistence. Such behavior has led to descriptions of some children with learning disabilities as learners who, because of long-term, repeated academic failures, develop a helpless feeling (learned helplessness) about schoolwork and do not see themselves as in control of their own learning (Smith, 1998). It is difficult to determine whether this is a cause (etiology) or effect (resulting behavior). These children likely entered school with certain difficulties, and their environment has contributed to a vicious cycle of failure and poor motivation that exacerbates the problems. Motivational considerations are of vital concern in the schooling of all children, although they are even more

crucial in teaching youngsters with learning disabilities, many of whom have experienced repeated failure—whose effect becomes more prominent as they grow older (Jenkins, 1999; Palladino et al., 2000; Renninger, 2000). Motivation, learning strategies, self-reliance, and social competence all appear in discussions of the school environment and its interaction with students having learning disabilities (e.g., Brown, 2000; Jenkins, 1999; Wong, 2000).

TREATMENT OF LEARNING DISABILITIES

IN FOCUS 5 ▶ Identify three types of interventions or treatments employed with people diagnosed as having learning disabilities.

Learning disabilities have sorely tested the definitional and explanatory capacity of education and behavioral science. However, this testing process has also provided a substantial service to the field. Throughout history, behavioral scientists and educators have often sought single-concept theories that efficiently explain all of the behaviors exhibited by a particular group of individuals. In most cases, such efforts are destined to fail, a point that is perhaps more evident with learning disabilities than any other behavior disorder. The conceptual and explanatory problems associated with learning disabilities have served as a constant reminder to behavioral scientists that it is probably not useful to search for *a single* theory or *a single* treatment for use with a diverse group of individuals.

Developmental Considerations

Treatment of individuals with learning disabilities requires careful consideration of the age of the person being treated (Hardman et al., 2002; Swanson & Sachse, 2000). Interventions that are effective with adolescents and adults having learning disabilities will differ somewhat from those that succeed with children. The specific components of a suitable intervention for a youngster of 7 will clearly be different than those employed for someone who is 13, 16, or 20 years of age. Individuals with learning disabilities who are in their adolescent or young adult years are likely to resemble others of the same age in their social and be-havioral characteristics, such as alcohol consumption, recreational interests, and sexual activity (Blanchett, 2000; Cambridge & Mellan, 2000; Watson, Franklin, Ingram, & Eilenberg, 1998). All of the factors compli-cating the lives of nondisabled adolescents (e.g., achieving individuality, romance, sexuality and hor-monal development, occupational choices) are present for those with learning disabilities. These young peo-ple are also susceptible to antisocial peer pressure and the prospect of gang activities, related misconduct, and violence (Mangina, Beuzeron-Mangina, & Grizenko, 2000). Clearly, it is important to include age considerations in the equation when determining in-tervention plans.

Medications

Drug treatment has frequently been used for learning disabilities, especially to control hyperactivity. Some type of psychostimulant, such as Ritalin (methylphen-idate) or Dexedrine (dextroamphetamine), or any of a number of different drugs may be administered, de-pending on the response of the individual child (Elia, Ambrosini, & Rapoport, 1999). Medication is effective in some areas, such as in improving children's class-room behavior, but not as effective in others, such as enhancing academic achievement or social adjust-ment on a long-term basis (Snider et al., 2000). Fur-ther, medication may have unfavorable side effects, and concern has been expressed regarding potential abuse, including unauthorized use of the child's psy-chostimulant medications by other family members (Connors, 2000).

Despite the frequent prescription of drugs for learning disabilities, the difficulty of determining which medication to administer highlights our poor understanding of both the disorders and the actions of the drugs. It is not always possible to predict which specific medication will perform properly for a given child, sometimes resulting in the need to undertake trial sessions with more than one medication. Identify-ing an effective medication and an appropriate dosage level can prove difficult. In some cases, psychostimu-lants have been administered to children in very high doses, which raises serious concerns regarding poten-tial toxic effects or undesirable side effects (Bhaumik,

Branford, Naik, & Biswas, 2000; Elia et al., 1999). More typical doses may result in only minor side ef-fects such as insomnia, some headaches, and mild irri-tability. For the most part, these side effects are insignificant and temporary, although there is considerable variation among individuals.

Most current literature suggests that there appear to be distinct benefits to the use of medication. How-ever, parents' and physicians' expectations regarding *generalized* improvement are often exaggerated far be-yond what the existing research evidence will support. While children's classroom behavior seems to be im-proved by medication, long-term academic enhance-ment is not evident (Snider et al., 2000). Thus, medica-tion may control the hyperactive behavior, but administering the drug certainly has not "cured" the learning disability. The children most likely still have learning problems, if for no other reason than that they have already lagged academically.

Behavioral Treatment

Behavioral interventions are also used extensively with individuals having learning disabilities. Such treatment programs may be aimed at enhancing acad-emic skills or modifying other behavior in some fash-ion. In many cases, behavioral procedures are used to supplement medical treatment, although they are also widely used as a primary therapy tool. Distinguishing between behavioral and instructional interventions is not always easy and often unnecessary. Both types of interventions entail altering behavior and acquiring skills, and those that are most effective typically em-ploy the most fundamental principles of learning—strategic use of stimuli and controlling the conse-quences of behavior, such as by reinforcement (Hardman et al., 2002). For some students, it is also important to teach them to take increased responsibil-ity for their own learning, which is often accomplished through self-monitoring and the use of learning strate-gies (Bender, 1998; Wong, 1999). Learning strategy interventions may be packaged in formats that have considerable appeal to young students with learning disabilities; an example is described in the Research Focus box.

Behavioral treatment procedures are frequently employed to intervene in social skills areas for some

The GET IT Strategy—Teaching Responsibility for Learning

The GET IT strategy is characterized by its developers as a cognitive learning strategy for reading comprehension, although it can easily be modified for use in a number of instructional contexts. This program is a video-mediated package developed with the clear intent of appealing to the student. It is patterned after TV game shows and incorporates real-life situations from the perspective of the student. Part of the presumed appeal of the GET IT package is that it portrays life through the eyes of the student rather than as adults conceive it.

The GET IT program attempts to teach basic learning strategies and responsibility to the student. The title is a mnemonic supplied to assist students to remember the components and associated tasks as follows:

Gather the objectives (or Get objectives).
Execute the search for objectives.
Take notes.
Inspect inventory of objectives.
Test your comprehension.

GET IT accentuates interactive student participation (Welch & Sheridan, 1995). It has been employed effectively with students in a number of settings. Larsen-Miller (1994) studied the program with 6th-grade students identified as having learning disabilities in an integrated setting. Her data suggested that students made significant gains in reading comprehension and knowledge about the parts of a textbook, and they demonstrated more positive attitudes toward reading after use of the program.

youngsters with learning disabilities who suffer frustration and anxiety from failure (Shapiro & Kratochwill, 2000). For example, Bender (1998) describes a young student with learning disabilities named Thomas, who began swearing loudly at his academically successful classmates who walked by him to retrieve their assignments. Researchers determined that Thomas was receiving considerable attention from both his peers and the teacher, who felt forced to respond to his outbursts. In Thomas's case, observations (baseline data) led to a decision to remove the attention for his swearing by placing him in an out-of-the way place (a time-out corner) when he swore and by instructing his classmates not to respond to his swearing in any fashion (e.g., no giggling or laughing). It worked. Thomas's swearing was reduced to very low levels over a 10-day period of intervention, and it remained at an acceptably low rate even when the intervention program was discontinued (returning to preintervention conditions). In this example, a relatively simple behavioral intervention was very effective in making the classroom environment much less frustrating for the teacher and potentially more effective

for all students. An even better intervention would also provide generous attention for Thomas's appropriate behavior and academic success. It should also be noted that for some individuals, residual emotional problems require a more comprehensive treatment program that includes supplementary counseling and other mental health assistance (Boucher, 1999; Hollins, Perez, Abdelnoor, & Webb, 1999).

Instructional Interventions

From an instructional perspective, perhaps the most empirically based treatment approach involves the use of applied behavior analysis principles, which means the precise use of specific stimuli and consequences. Applied behavior analysis permits identification and modification of a wide range of behaviors, but is best suited to simple, easily observed, and countable behaviors. Based on the pioneering work of B. F. Skinner, this approach focuses on observable performance (behaviors) and de-emphasizes unobservable underlying causes such as internal mental, anatomical, or biochemical abnormalities. Such a treatment approach has great appeal in educational settings since its specific format can be modified and applied to a wide variety of problems and many contexts.

There has been a considerable shift in approaches to instructional interventions for students having learning disabilities in the past few years. The treatment of learning disabilities has been one of the most controversy-ridden areas in education and psychology. The various theories of causation have had enthusiastic proponents, who have often comprised "warring" factions competing for funding and public favor. Although this tendency continues, a movement has begun toward focusing on each child's distinctive instructional problems rather than forcing a generalized concept of learning disabilities.

Teachers may encounter children who have a particularly difficult time with information presented through either the visual or the auditory sensory systems. When such problems are identified, it often becomes necessary to teach material using alternate modes of presentation. Depending on the nature of the child's disorder, a teacher may choose to present material predominantly in an auditory mode (such as using tape-recordings of books for an individual who has visual perception problems) or predominantly in a visual mode. Unfortunately, individuals seldom have a "pure" deficit in only one perceptual system, which complicates instructional interventions (Bender, 1998; Rose et al., 1999).

Literature on interventions for learning disabilities is now beginning to address treatments aimed at specific problems such as deficits in writing, mathematics, reading, spoken language, and attention (Gardill & Jitendra, 1999; Naglieri & Johnson, 2000). Some instructional interventions have pinpointed precise difficulties within these areas, such as problem solving, and devised specific interventions, such as problem-attack strategy training (Welch, Brownell, & Sheridan, 1999). Such academic intervention is clearly more directed and narrow than that previously employed with individuals having learning disabilities, all of whom were once thought to need training in physical coordination or letter recognition. However, thorough intervention also includes attention to students' nonacademic needs and will often include treatment of problem behaviors and instruction in social skills in order to help the child enter the academic mainstream.

PROGNOSIS FOR CHILDREN WITH LEARNING DISABILITIES

IN FOCUS 6 ▶ How are the services and supports for adolescents and adults with learning disabilities different from those used with children?

The prognosis for those with learning disabilities as adults is brighter than ever before, even though significant life challenges remain. For one thing, research literature on adults with learning disabilities is increasing. As for many other long-lasting disability conditions, the literature on learning disabilities has historically focused more on childhood than on adolescence and adulthood. Now research on learning disabilities is increasingly investigating long-term outcomes in adulthood (e.g., Gralton et al., 2000; Moss et al., 2000; Wren & Einhorn, 2000) and addressing matters related to postsecondary schooling. Learning disabilities often persist in college (Ward & Bernstein, 1998), and there is heightened interest in designing instructional programs to meet the needs of college students with these disabilities (Olivier, Hecker, Klucken, & Westby, 2000). Although the world has not magically opened up to accept people with learning disabilities in all fields, there is clearly more potential than a few years ago (Bender, 1998).

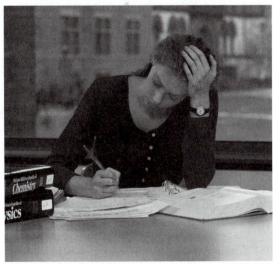

Learning disabilities often persist in college.

The Americans with Disabilities Act of 1990 (ADA) requires that appropriate academic adjustments be provided for college students who are diagnosed as having learning disabilities. The aim of this legislation is that reasonable accommodations (e.g., longer time on an exam) must be made to ensure meaningful access to higher education for these students (Gordon & Keiser, 1998; Hadley, 1998). The language of the ADA is broad and offers little guidance regarding how accommodations are to be considered in individual circumstances. Requests for adjustments are evaluated on a case-by-case basis, with consideration given to the individual's abilities. In many cases, time limits may be adjusted, extra tutorial assistance may be provided, or examination conditions may be altered (e.g., using verbal examinations).

The adolescent and adult years are not without trials for those with learning disabilities, and some of the research does not suggest an optimistic prognosis.

There is considerable evidence that our instructional system fails a substantial portion of adolescents with learning disabilities. For example, the dropout rate of these youngsters is quite high. For those who make it through secondary school and attend college, there is also a tendency to discontinue schooling prematurely, prior to completion (Dole, 2000; Murray, Goldstein, Nourse, & Edgar, 2000; Rojewski, 1999). For those who do continue, there is constant pressure to adapt to the usual academic environment, as well as the ongoing need to request reasonable instructional accommodations. Often, requests for such accommodations are met with great skepticism by faculty and administrators who know little about learning disabilities. While most college students only have to manage the process of learning the required information, students with learning disabilities clearly have a much more demanding task. With understanding and practical assistance from family, friends, and teachers, however,

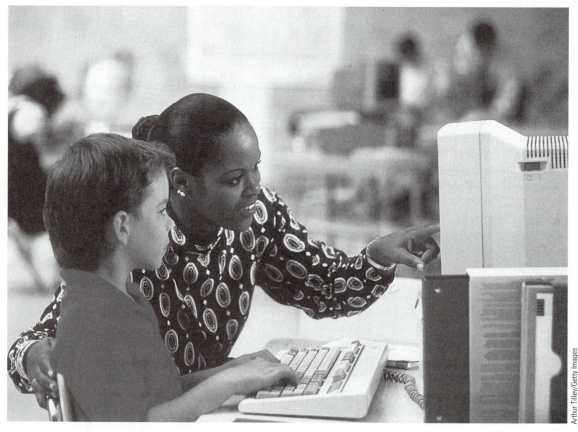

Many students with learning disabilities can benefit significantly from tutorial help.

Arthur Tilley/Getty Images

Back to the Beginning

Mathew's Determination Pays Off

At the beginning of this chapter, it was clear that Mathew had thought a lot about having learning disabilities and had found a number of personal strategies to cope with the demands of academic life. Mathew did graduate with his bachelor's degree, which is a momentous event for most people but was particularly satisfying for him given the additional challenges he experienced. And that wasn't the end of it. He applied and was accepted to a graduate program at a well-known university in the Midwest. A few years later, he received his master's degree. While it didn't get any easier for him, he did well and attacked his higher-level studies with the same determination he had always shown.

---

they can succeed. The stories of both Jeanne and Mathew provide glimpses of what life is like for such students with learning disabilities, who, by most people's standards, are experiencing substantial success in life. Their stories show that, with accurate diagnosis and help from student disabilities services and instructors, learning disabilities can be dealt with and students with them can succeed—even in academically demanding colleges and universities.

SUMMARY

Learning disabilities is an umbrella label that was devised within the past 40 years and has generated considerable confusion and controversy. The individuals so labeled exhibit an extremely diverse set of learning and behavioral problems beyond those typical for people at the same level of tested intelligence. They may be average or above average in intelligence but often have pronounced difficulties in reading, math, and other school subjects. They are often, but not always, characterized as hyperactive as children. People with learning disabilities have also been described as having perceptual difficulties, memory problems, and attention deficits. They may exhibit various combinations of these characteristics and may be impaired to varying degrees, depending on the nature of their problem(s), their age, and the setting. Interventions for people with learning disabilities include medication, behavioral treatments, and/or specially designed instructional programs developed to address acade-

mic problem areas. School-based learning is challenging for individuals with learning disabilities, often requiring extraordinary effort and application. In many cases, a comprehensive treatment program will involve multiple interventions aimed at addressing emotional and social problems as well as academic ones.

INFOTRAC COLLEGE EDITION

For more information, explore this resource at http://www.infotrac-college.com/Wadsworth. Enter the following search terms:

  articulation disorder
  learning disorder
  learning disability
  perceptual disorder
  reading disorder
  dyslexia

IN FOCUS ANSWERS

IN FOCUS 1 ▶ What is the current estimated prevalence range for learning disabilities, and what does that mean in numbers of children?

- From 2% to 20% of the U.S. school-age population has a learning disability, depending on the source.
- During the 1997–1998 school year, over 2.7 million exceptional children were labeled as having learning disabilities.

IN FOCUS 2 ▶ Why have definitions of learning disabilities varied?

- The field expanded in an uncontrolled fashion, and children with a wide variety of problems were labeled as having learning disabilities.
- Parents of children with learning disabilities created a massive focus of activity nearly overnight and demanded services for their children.
- *Learning disabilities* is a general educational term that includes many different specific problems.
- Partially because of definitional challenges, there has been no solid, systematic program of scientific investigation on which to base diagnoses or programs of teacher and therapist preparation.

IN FOCUS 3 ▶ List several characteristics attributed to those with learning disabilities, and explain why it is difficult to characterize this group.

- Often other disorders co-occur with learning disabilities.
- Many children with learning disabilities exhibit impulsive behavior and attention problems.
- Hyperactivity is common in students with learning disabilities.
- Academic achievement deficits, especially in reading, are common in this group.
- Many children with learning disabilities have perceptual problems, such as visual and auditory discrimination problems.
- Cognition deficits, such as memory and other information-processing problems, are associated with some learning disabilities.
- Many of these youngsters experience emotional and interpersonal difficulties.
- The group of individuals included under the umbrella term *learning disabilities* is so varied that it defies simple characterization by a single concept or term.

IN FOCUS 4 ▶ Identify three causes thought to be involved in learning disabilities.

- Neurological damage, malfunction, or maturational delay
- Genetic factors
- Environmental factors

IN FOCUS 5 ▶ Identify three types of interventions or treatments employed with people diagnosed as having learning disabilities.

- Medical treatment, in some circumstances involving medication to control hyperactivity
- Behavioral interventions aimed at improving social skills or remediating academic problems
- Academic instruction and support specifically aimed at building particular skill areas

IN FOCUS 6 ▶ How are the services and supports for adolescents and adults with learning disabilities different from those used with children?

- Services and supports for children focus primarily on building the most basic skills.
- Instruction during adolescence may include skill building but also may involve assistance in developing compensatory skills that permit circumvention of deficit areas and transition skills that will prepare students for adulthood, employment, and further education, based on their own goals.
- Information for adults with learning disabilities should include an awareness of how invisible their disability is to others and how their requests for accommodations might be viewed with skepticism.

Mental Retardation

In the Beginning

Kelly's Challenges

The following case study is based on a real person, but her name and other details have been changed for reasons of confidentiality, consistent with the guidelines of the World and American Psychiatric Associations (Clifft, 1986).

Kelly was a beautiful 16-year-old with golden-brown eyes. Because of her large extended family and supportive friends, she had a full schedule with many community activities. Her family and friends hoped that Kelly would someday have a home of her own. Kelly had severe mental retardation and mild cerebral palsy. The greatest challenges to her family, friends, and future dreams were in the areas of home and personal living skills. After 11 years of training in using the toilet and washing her hands, she still needed help with both skills. Although her parents and friends took her to a wide variety of social settings, they didn't always know what to do about her eating problems. They also did not know how to address the more complex issues of how she would help take care of a home. As an older teen, Kelly needed the opportunity to take charge of her own personal life—to make decisions about her own likes and wants. (Browder, 2001, p. 277)

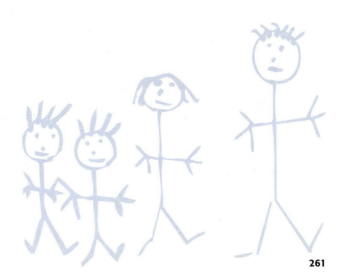

INTRODUCTION

Mental retardation is a disorder that has been recognized perhaps longer than any other currently studied in psychology. Written documents from ancient Egypt made oblique reference to the condition as early as about 1500 B.C., and it may have been implicit in law codes of Babylonia nearly 1,000 years earlier. Particularly in early history, mental retardation was often viewed as part of mental illness, and treatment approaches reflected this social perspective (Dickinson, 2000; O'Brien, 1999). In addition to having a lengthy history, mental retardation is relatively common. It occurs in the families of the wealthy and prominent (including that of late President John F. Kennedy), as well as in less advantaged families. Although prevalent, mental retardation is often misunderstood. Many have a stereotyped notion that all children with mental retardation are extremely dull and look different physically. This is the case with certain individuals with mental retardation (e.g., some with hydrocephalus and Down syndrome), but certainly not all. Many individuals with mental retardation can cope with the demands of daily life and have no distinctive physical characteristics that set them apart from others.

Three of the themes in this book play particularly significant roles in studying mental retardation: social context, biology, and human development. The causes of mental retardation are both social and biological. In some cases, an individual with mental retardation has a condition that can be clearly linked to a biological influence, perhaps a genetic accident or some other biological factor that leads to a lowered intellectual functioning. However, in many more

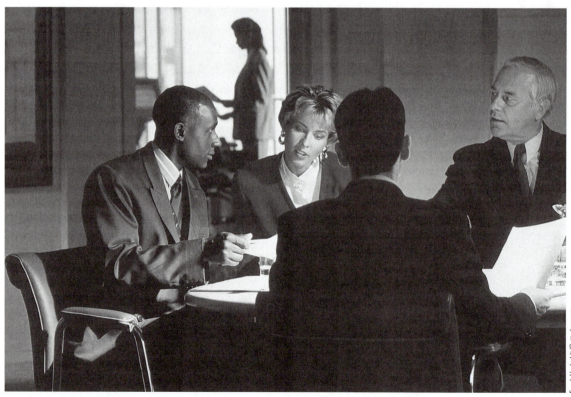

Developing appropriate plans for young children with mental retardation involves multidisciplinary teamwork as well as collaboration with parents.

cases (perhaps as high as 30–40%), environmental and social influences are more likely culprits (American Psychiatric Association, 2000; Hardman, Drew, & Egan, 2002; The ARC, 2000). Environmental circumstances, such as poverty, can have enormous impact on a child's developing intellect. Finally, the theme of human development is perhaps more useful in understanding mental retardation than for any other childhood disorder.

DEFINING MENTAL RETARDATION

IN FOCUS 1 ▶ List the four assumptions outlined by AAMR as essential to application of the definition of mental retardation.
IN FOCUS 2 ▶ What are the ten adaptive skill areas used by the AAMR for assessment of adaptive behavior?

Defining mental retardation is not as simple as it might seem on the surface, and the definition continues to evolve (e.g., Luckasson & Reeve, 2001). In the past, many definitions became popular and then faded into scientific obscurity as others emerged. Part of the difficulty in defining the condition relates to the central role of intelligence. It has been commonly accepted that those with mental retardation have a lower level of intelligence than is typical in the general population. Consequently, definitions of mental retardation have reflected many of the controversies about the nature of intelligence and to what degree it can be altered by experience. Additionally, many disciplines have adopted different perspectives and terminology regarding mental retardation, further complicating the definition. Psychologists, sociologists, anthropologists, educators, medical personnel, and others have undertaken research on mental retardation, but only relatively recently have serious efforts been made to conceptualize it from a multidisciplinary viewpoint. As we will see later, classification systems still vary to some degree from one profession to another; each system emphasizes the treatment orientation or scientific perspective associated with the specific profession.

Perhaps the most widely accepted definition of mental retardation is that of the American Association on Mental Retardation (AAMR) (1992), which has a multidisciplinary membership. This definition has undergone many revisions and refinements over the years, leading to the following formulation:

> **Mental retardation** *refers to substantial limitations in present functioning. It is characterized by significantly subaverage intellectual functioning, existing concurrently with related limitations in two or more of the following applicable adaptive skill areas: communication, self-care, home living, social skills, community use, self-direction, health and safety, functional academics, leisure, and work. Mental retardation manifests before age 18.* (AAMR, 1992, p. 1)

Some of the terminology in this definition is rather general and abstract. However, the AAMR manual includes explanations of key terms and extensive commentary on the concepts, as well as four assumptions that are are considered essential to application of the definition. This material is reproduced in Table 12-1.

The 1992 AAMR definition departs from earlier efforts in several ways. One important difference involves the manner of viewing intelligence measures. The AAMR definition focuses on intellectual functioning primarily at the time of diagnosis and mainly considers an individual's adaptive skills and needed environmental supports for classification and program planning. From a measured intelligence standpoint, a person either has mental retardation—a standard score on an intelligence test of 70 to 75 or below—or does not. This level of intellectual functioning, coexisting with limitations in two or more of the specified adaptive skill areas, fulfills the requirement for a diagnosis of mental retardation.

Adaptive behavior has been part of the conceptualization of mental retardation for over 35 years, although assessment of this aspect has always been troublesome (Balboni, Pedrabissi, Molteni, & Villa, 2001; Flynn, 2000). The 1992 AAMR definition uses specified adaptive skill areas rather than referring more generically to adaptive behavior (see Table 12-2). Although these designated adaptive skill areas are more specific, they continue to present measurement challenges (e.g., Bell & Espie, 2000; Mervis, Klein-Tasman, & Mastin, 2001).

Table 12-1 AAMR Definitional Explanations

Mental retardation refers to substantial limitations in present functioning . . . Mental retardation is defined as a fundamental difficulty in learning and performing certain daily life skills. The personal capabilities in which there must be a substantial limitation are conceptual, practical, and social intelligence. These three areas are specifically affected in mental retardation whereas other personal capabilities (e.g., health and temperament) may not be.

It is characterized by significantly subaverage intellectual functioning . . . This is defined as an IQ standard score of approximately 70 to 75 or below, based on assessment that includes one or more individually administered general intelligence tests developed for the purpose of assessing intellectual functioning. These data should be reviewed by a multidisciplinary team and validated with additional test scores or evaluative information.

Existing concurrently . . . The intellectual limitations occur at the same time as the limitations in adaptive skills.

With related limitations . . . The limitations in adaptive skills are more closely related to the intellectual limitation than to some other circumstances such as cultural or linguistic diversity or sensory limitation.

In two or more of the following applicable adaptive skill areas . . . Evidence of adaptive skill limitations is necessary because intellectual functioning alone is insufficient for a diagnosis of mental retardation. The impact on functioning of these limitations must be sufficiently comprehensive to encompass at least two adaptive skill areas, thus showing a generalized limitation and reducing the probability of measurement error.

Communication, self-care, home living, social skills, community use, self-direction, health and safety, functional academics, leisure, and work . . . These skill areas are central to successful life functioning and are frequently related to the need for supports for persons with mental retardation. Because the relevant skills within each adaptive skill area may vary with chronological age, assessment of functioning must be referenced to the person's chronological age.

Mental retardation manifests before age 18 . . . The 18th birthday approximates the age when individuals in this society typically assume adult roles. In other societies, a different age criterion might be determined to be more appropriate.

The following four assumptions are essential to the application of this definition . . . These statements are essential to the meaning of the definition and cannot be conceptually separated from the definition. Applications of the definition should include these statements. Each statement has clear implications for subsequent assessment and intervention.

1. *Valid assessment considers cultural and linguistic diversity as well as differences in communication and behavioral factors* . . . Failure to consider factors such as the individual's culture, language, communication, and behaviors may cause an assessment to be invalid. Sound professional judgment and the use of a multidisciplinary team appropriate to the individual and his or her particular needs and circumstances should enhance the validity of assessments.

2. *The existence of limitations in adaptive skills occurs within the context of community environments typical of the individual's age peers and is indexed to the person's individualized needs for support* . . . Community environments typical of the individual's age peers refer to homes, neighborhoods, schools, businesses, and other environments in which persons of the individual's age ordinarily live, learn, work, and interact. The concept of age peers should also include consideration of individuals of the same cultural or linguistic background. The determination of the limitations in adaptive skills goes together with an analysis of supports that can include services that the individual needs and supports in the environments.

3. *Specific adaptive limitations often coexist with strengths in other adaptive skills or personal capabilities* . . . Individuals frequently have strengths in personal capabilities independent of mental retardation. Examples include: (a) an individual may have strengths in physical or social capabilities that exist independently of the adaptive skill limitations related to mental retardation (e.g., good health); (b) an individual may have a strength in a particular adaptive skill area (e.g., social skills) while having difficulty in another skill area (e.g., communication); and (c) an individual may possess certain strengths within a particular specific adaptive skill, while at the same time having limitations within the same area (e.g., functional math and functional reading, respectively). Some of a person's strengths may be relative rather than absolute; thus, the strengths may be best understood when compared to the limitations in other skill areas.

4. *With appropriate supports over a sustained period, the life functioning of the person with mental retardation will generally improve* . . . Appropriate supports refer to an array of services, individuals, and settings that match the person's needs. Although mental retardation may not be of lifelong duration, it is likely that supports will be needed over an extended period of time. Thus, for many individuals, the need for supports will be lifelong. For other individuals, however, the need for supports may be intermittent. Virtually all persons with mental retardation will improve in their functioning as a result of effective supports and services. This improvement will enable them to be more independent, productive, and integrated into their community. In addition, if individuals are not improving significantly, this relative lack of improvement should be the basis for determining whether the current supports are effective and whether changes are necessary. Finally, in rare circumstances, the major objective should be to maintain current level of functioning or to slow regression over time.

SOURCE: American Association on Mental Retardation (1992), Copyright 1992 by the American Association on Mental Retardation. Reprinted by permission.

Table 12-2 AAMR Adaptive Skill Areas

Skill Area	Description
Communication	The ability to understand and communicate information by speaking or writing, through symbols, sign language, or nonsymbolic behaviors such as facial expressions, touch, or gestures
Self-care	Skills in such areas as toileting, eating, dressing, hygiene, and grooming
Home living	Functioning in the home, including clothing care, housekeeping, property maintenance, cooking, shopping, home safety, and daily scheduling
Social	Social interchange with others, including initiating and terminating interactions, responding to social cues, recognizing feelings, regulating own behavior, assisting others, and fostering friendships
Community use	Appropriate use of community resources, including travel in the community, shopping at stores, obtaining services such as at gas stations or medical and dental services, using public transportation and facilities
Self-direction	Making choices, following a schedule, initiating contextually appropriate activities, completing required tasks, seeking assistance, resolving problems, and demonstrating appropriate self-advocacy
Health and safety	Maintaining own health, including eating, identifying and treating or preventing illness, basic first aid, sexuality, physical fitness, and basic safety
Functional academics	Abilities and skills related to learning in school that also have direct application in life
Leisure	Developing a variety of leisure and recreational interests that are age- and culture-appropriate
Work	Abilities that pertain to maintaining part- or full-time employment in the community, including appropriate social and related work skills

SOURCE: Adapted from American Association on Mental Retardation (1992), pp. 40–41. Copyright 1992 by the American Association on Mental Retardation. Reprinted by permission.

DESCRIBING AND CLASSIFYING MENTAL RETARDATION

IN FOCUS 3 ▶ Identify the five DSM-IV-TR severity classifications for mental retardation.

Because of the use of different definitions of mental retardation over the years, there have been varied bases for describing and classifying such individuals. Chapter 4 addresses classification of child behavior disorders in a more complete and general fashion. This section specifically examines descriptive classifications of mental retardation, emphasizing the complex nature of the mental retardation diagnosis. Remember that all descriptions and classifications are useful in some circumstances but may be dysfunctional in others, in which case they should not be used.

The term *mental retardation* is an extremely general label that covers a heterogeneous set of conditions with different developmental paths and causes (Miller-Loncar, Winter, & Whitman, 2001). Scientifically, it is

necessary to specify the type of individual being studied. From a practical standpoint, there is also a need to be specific about the type of mental retardation, since different types require different approaches to treatment and service delivery. Classification schemes for mental retardation provide a common vocabulary and serve as a convenient means for communication about the work underway, whether it be research or clinical treatment.

Historically, the characteristic most typically associated with mental retardation has been reduced intellectual functioning. The *severity* of the intellectual impairment has long been a common means of describing and classifying those with retardation. As mentioned earlier, the AAMR (1992) uses measured intelligence as one part of its definition of mental retardation, but employs it only in the initial diagnosis.

AAMR (1992) employs four broad dimensions for the diagnostic-classification process as well as for planning interventions: (1) Dimension I, intellectual functioning and adaptive behavior; (2) Dimension II, psychological/emotional considerations; (3) Dimension III, physical/health and etiology considerations; and (4) Dimension IV, environmental considerations. The diagnostic process concentrates on Dimension I (intellectual functioning and adaptive skills). This process involves consideration of three criteria, which, if met, result in a diagnosis of mental retardation. To receive such a diagnosis, an individual must have an IQ of 70 to 75 or below as measured on an appropriately standardized instrument, significant deficiencies in at least two of the adaptive skill areas (see Table 12-2), and be under 18 years of age.

Once a diagnosis of mental retardation is determined, the classification process then turns to the other dimensions. For Dimension II, an assessment of the person's mental health is undertaken and strengths and limitations are assessed. This evaluation is based on behavioral observations and clinical assessment using multiple sources of data, such as interviews, psychometric instruments, and structured observation. Dimension III evaluation provides a description of the individual's general physical health and the etiology of the mental retardation if known. Finally, under Dimension IV, the classification provides a description of the environmental considerations for the individual—both the current circumstances and those that would be optimal for promoting the person's growth and development. The last element of the AAMR model involves developing a profile of supports needed for the person's individual intervention plan. These supports are outlined in four levels: (1) intermittent support needed (episodic, often crisis-related), (2) limited support needed (time-limited but consistent, not episodic), (3) extensive support (regular in some environments), and (4) pervasive support (continuous and intense, across environments). Throughout the process of diagnosis, classification, and intervention planning, the AAMR model requires the involvement of an interdisciplinary team to provide the most thorough evaluation possible. Attention is directed to cultural differences in both assessment procedures and intervention planning, although some concerns have been raised that this definition may exacerbate the overrepresentation of minorities in the population diagnosed with mental retardation (Drew & Hardman, 2000).

The American Psychiatric Association has revised its definition of mental retardation in DSM-IV-TR to be nearly identical with that of AAMR (American Psychiatric Association, 2000). However, the DSM-IV-TR classification model continues to use measured intelligence to group those with mental retardation, including four severity classifications plus a fifth for circumstances where the individual's intelligence is untestable. The classifications are as follows: (1) IQ 50–55 to approximately 70, *mild mental retardation*; (2) IQ 35–40 to 50–55, *moderate mental retardation*; (3) IQ 20–25 to 35–40, *severe mental retardation*; (4) IQ levels below 20 or 25, *profound mental retardation*; and (5) *mental retardation, severity unspecified*, for situations where there is a presumption of mental retardation but the person's intelligence is not testable with standardized instruments (because the individual functions at too low a level, is not cooperative, or is too young) (American Psychiatric Association, 2000, pp. 42–43).

Etiology (causation) has traditionally provided a basis for classification of mental retardation that has addressed medically related matters. The DSM approaches etiology in terms of factors that predispose a person to having mental retardation. As Table 12-3 summarizes, there are six general predisposing factors, with a notation that "etiological factors may be primarily biological or primarily psychosocial, or some combination of both" (American Psychiatric Association, 2000, p. 45).

The AAMR (1992) examines etiology from two major standpoints: the type of factor involved and the timing of the influence. From the first perspective (type of factor), four categories are involved: (1) *biomedical*, associated with biological process (genetic disorders, nutrition); (2) *social*, matters related to social and family interaction (e.g., poverty and limited schooling); (3) *behavioral*, possible causal behaviors (e.g., maternal substance abuse); and (4) *educational*, influences related to the availability of educational resources that foster mental growth and adaptive skills. The second major perspective (timing of the influence) is addressed primarily from a prevention or intervention position and is arranged in three levels: (1) primary prevention, which is undertaken before the problem begins or that prevents the occurrence of mental retardation (e.g., maternal substance abuse programs); (2) secondary prevention, which reverses the effects or shortens the duration of a problem that already exists (e.g., nutritional treatment programs for

Table 12-3 DSM-IV-TR Etiological or Predisposing Factors for Mental Retardation

Predisposing Factor	Examples
Heredity	Chromosomal aberrations (e.g., Down syndrome, fragile X syndrome), inborn metabolic errors (e.g., Tay-Sachs), single-gene abnormalities (e.g., tuberous sclerosis)
Early alterations of embryonic development	Chromosomal changes (e.g., trisomy 21 Down syndrome), prenatal toxic damage (e.g., infection, maternal alcohol consumption)
Pregnancy and perinatal problems	Fetal malnutrition, prematurity, trauma, viral and other infections
General medical conditions acquired in infancy or childhood	Infections, traumas, and poisoning (e.g., lead)
Environmental influences	Deprivation of nurturance or social, linguistic, or other stimulation
Mental disorders	Autistic disorder and other pervasive developmental disorder

SOURCE: Adapted with permission from American Psychiatric Association (2000), pp. 45–46. From the *Diagnostic and Statistical Manual of Mental Disorders*, 4th ed., Text Revision. © 2000 APA.

phenylketonuria); and (3) tertiary prevention, which restricts unfavorable effects of a problem and improves the person's functioning (e.g., habilitation or education programs) (AAMR, 1992, pp. 71–72).

Each of these classification systems has certain strengths and weaknesses. Clearly, each has a different purpose, and its usage may be limited to a particular discipline or situation. Although there may be some overlap, the systems differ in many ways. An individual with mental retardation may be classified in several different fashions at different times, depending on the system employed, the situation, and any of a multitude of other contingencies (e.g., the services available in a particular community, evaluation by a psychologist as opposed to a physician). Some who would prefer a single approach to classification have criticized this practice. However, a single approach to classification is not possible given all of the different reasons for classifying mental retardation (e.g., legislative, administrative, instructional).

PREVALENCE OF MENTAL RETARDATION

IN FOCUS 4 ▶ What are the general estimates of prevalence for mental retardation, and what does this mean in terms of numbers of individuals receiving services under IDEA?

How many children have mental retardation? Again, answering this question is not as simple as it may

seem on the surface. First of all, a complete census of all those with mental retardation would be neither simple to conduct nor economically feasible. Although some direct census investigations have been undertaken over the years, for the most part estimates based on expected percentages of retardation in the general population have been used. The definition of retardation plays a central role here. Obviously, whenever the definition is altered, there may be a substantial difference in the number of individuals considered to have mental retardation.

As we examine the magnitude of mental retardation, recall the distinction between incidence and prevalence (*incidence* is the number of new cases identified in a specific period, and *prevalence* is the total number of cases present at a given time). This is important here because much of the literature about mental retardation has either ignored the distinction or used the two terms loosely and interchangeably. The number of people considered to have retardation is therefore somewhat variable. Particularly among those with mild disabilities, a person may be identified as having retardation at one point in time (e.g., school years) and no longer be functioning at that level at a later time (e.g., during adulthood).

Estimates of the prevalence of mental retardation have typically ranged from 1% to 3% of the general population (Drew & Hardman, 2000; Larson et al., 2001). The U.S. Department of Education estimated that 11% of all children with disabilities in the U.S. public schools (ages 6–21) have mental retardation. Translating these estimates into actual numbers, over 603,000 individuals with mental retardation received services under the Individuals with Disabilities Education Act (IDEA) during the 1998–1999 school year (U.S. Department of Education, 2000). Using the 3% prevalence figure, Hardman and his colleagues (2002) estimated the population of Americans with mental retardation to be in excess of 7 million people. Clearly, we are faced with an imprecise answer to the question regarding mental retardation prevalence. Prevalence rates differ depending on the definitions being used, the assumptions employed, and even the geographical locale (e.g., in different states). The prevalence estimate depends on the frame of reference (i.e., distinction between incidence and prevalence), the environmental setting, and perhaps other unknown factors.

DEVELOPMENTAL FACTORS

IN FOCUS 5 ▶ Explain how development plays a role in mental retardation.

As was mentioned before, human development is very important in the field of mental retardation—one can hardly examine mental retardation without discussing child development. Study of the causation, classification, treatment, and prognosis of mental retardation directly involves the developmental process (Drew & Hardman, 2000). The purpose of this section is to examine how development plays a role in mental retardation. The next section examines the etiology of mental retardation during prenatal, neonatal, and childhood periods. The prenatal period is vital to normal development. During gestation, toxins, accidents, or other unfavorable events can place the unborn baby at risk for mental retardation. These factors or events often involve maternal health problems or genetic abnormalities that influence fetal growth and development.

In diagnosing child psychopathology, it is important to establish *when* the onset of a particular condition occurred. Very often the timing of an infection or a chromosomal or physical accident will determine the impact of that incident (Dykens & Hodapp, 2001). For example, when a pregnant woman contracts German measles (rubella) determines the impact of the disease on her unborn child. If the mother contracts rubella during the first 3 months of gestation, there is

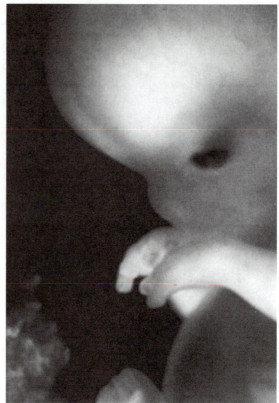

Petit Format/Photo Researchers Inc.

Prenatal development is a crucial period for preventing mental retardation.

considerable risk that the developing fetus will develop mental retardation. There is somewhat less danger later in the pregnancy, although even then such diseases usually involve some risk.

During the first trimester (the first 3 months) of pregnancy, the tissue development of an unborn baby is progressing very rapidly. It is during this time that the foundation of physical development is primarily established. The basic material for what will later become the central nervous system (e.g., brain, spinal cord) is rapidly being established, along with such vital organs as the visual and auditory systems and many other parts of the baby that are extremely important to its ability to function. When the tissue is developing at its most rapid rate, it is most vulnerable to the effects of detrimental influences such as maternal infection by rubella. If the central nervous system tissue is damaged by infection, genetic accident, or factors such as inadequate maternal nutrition as it is first being formed, all such tissue that subsequently develops may be damaged. For example, if a mother contracts German measles at the time that her unborn child is first (and most rapidly) developing tissue related to visual organs, the child has a much higher probability of being born with a visual defect than if the mother contracts the disease at a later time. Thus, the prenatal basis for the physiological development of a child is crucial and is affected by the timing of both fortunate and less fortunate events.

Mental retardation also may arise during early childhood. Physiologically, the baby or young child is obtaining essential substances for life such as food and oxygen from the environment. The child is also affected by environmental stimulation (noises, light, persons), which has great importance for subsequent development of mental functioning, speech, and social development. If the child's environment is basically supportive and stimulating, there is a high likelihood that he or she will develop normally. However, if the early environment is insufficiently supportive or stimulating, mental retardation may result. As before, the timing of unfortunate circumstances (or accidents) may have serious consequences. For example, if an infection is contracted by a newborn or young child and causes deafness prior to development of language, all subsequent language development and acquisition of language may be affected.

ETIOLOGY OF MENTAL RETARDATION

The causes of mental retardation are many and varied. In some cases, pathology of a physiological or biological nature can be identified. However, as noted earlier, for as many as 30–40% of those with mental retardation, causation is unknown. This section provides an overview of the origins of mental retardation.

Prenatal and Neonatal Causation

IN FOCUS 6 ▶ Identify factors that may cause mental retardation during the prenatal and neonatal periods.

Genetic Factors
Genetic abnormalities are discussed in Chapter 2 in relation to a variety of disorders, including certain types of mental retardation. Some gene anomalies (abnormal genetic make-up) can ultimately result in mental retardation. **Down syndrome** is one of these prenatal conditions. Overall, Down syndrome occurs in about 1 in every 1,000 live births (National Information Center for Children and Youth with Disabilities, 2001). Actually, there are three types of Down syndrome, each resulting from a different type of chromosomal error. The most common cause of Down syndrome is known as *nondisjunction*, in which an extra chromosome exists with the 21st pair. This condition is also known as *trisomy 21* because of these three chromosomes. Figure 12-1 illustrates a chromosomal configuration for a Down syndrome female with trisomy 21.

Nondisjunction occurs because of improper cell division during the formation of the egg or the sperm. Because the chromosomal error occurs prior to fertilization, its impact on the developing embryo is substantial and the damage severe. The probability of a nondisjunction error resulting in trisomy 21 is dramatically elevated for mothers over 40 years of age. Evidence suggests that the risk of a Down syndrome birth for women over 40 is approximately 18 in 1,000 births, whereas it is less than 1 per 1,000 for women in their early 20s (Drew & Hardman, 2000). Recent years have witnessed intensified research on improving fetal

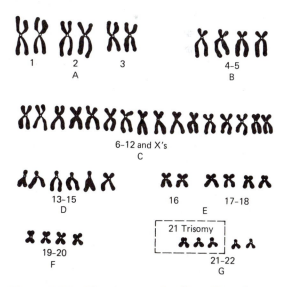

Figure 12-1   Chromosome Configuration of a Down Syndrome Female with Trisomy 21

diagnostic techniques and increased caution related to pregnancies among older women. There has been a resulting decline in the incidence of Down syndrome births.

Down syndrome may also be caused by a second chromosomal aberration involving the 21st pair. This condition is known as *translocation* and occurs when material from the 21st pair of chromosomes detaches (actually breaks off) and fuses to another chromosome pair. For example, the material may fuse with the 14th or 15th pair. This imbalance of genetic material is responsible for about 9% of all Down syndrome infants born to mothers under 30 years of age and 2% of those born to mothers over 30 (Drew & Hardman, 2000). This represents a very different incidence pattern than that for trisomy 21. Nondisjunction may well be a genetic accident that occurs as a function of age or health. Translocation has been demonstrated to be inherited in about one-third of cases.

The third type of genetic abnormality resulting in Down syndrome is known as *mosaicism*. This error is distinctly different from nondisjunction and translocation in that it occurs after fertilization and produces an infant with a mixed chromosomal make-up; some tissues have cells that are affected, whereas others have the normal genetic configuration. The tissues that are involved and the extent of the damage are highly dependent on when the error occurs during prenatal development. The level of mental retardation may vary from mild to more severe. Some children with mosaic-type Down syndrome have even been reported to have a normal range of functioning, which may illustrate dramatically the interaction between genetic and environmental influences.

Down syndrome has historically received a great deal of attention in the research literature on mental retardation. Interest continues on a variety of related topics, such as behavioral treatment and social behavior (Hall & Oliver, 2000; Kasari & Freeman, 2001), functional speech and language development (Bochner, Outhred, & Pieterse, 2001; Kumin & Adams, 2000), and co-occurrence with other conditions (Bosner & Belfiore, 2001; Klinger & Dawson, 2001).

Fragile X syndrome is another genetic abnormality that results in mental retardation about once in slightly over 1,000 newborns, more frequently in males than in females. The name derives from the fact that the X chromosome of an affected individual will show a fragile spot when grown in an experimental culture. Like individuals with Down syndrome, those with fragile X syndrome may vary in measured intelligence, with some functioning in the lower range of average, and may have working-memory performance lower than their age-mates (Cornish, Munir, & Cross, 2001). Individuals with fragile X syndrome exhibit a broad array of aberrant characteristics, including behavioral problems (e.g., hand-flapping, biting, hyperactivity), some difficulties with aggression, language deficiencies, and, potentially, learning disabilities (Dykens, Hodapp, & Finucane, 2000; Kau, Reider, Payne, Meyer, & Freund, 2000; Roberts, Mirrett, & Burchinal, 2001). Males with fragile X syndrome also appear to have autistic-like behaviors and show a number of schizophrenic features. Fragile X syndrome is receiving growing attention in the research literature on behavior and personality characteristics, although there is some concern that intervention methods are based more on clinical observation than on controlled studies (Bailey, Hatton, Mesibov, Ament, & Skinner, 2000; York, von Fraunhofer, Turk, & Sedgwick, 1999).

One genetic disorder that overlaps the prenatal and early stages of infant development is *phenylketonuria (PKU)*, an inherited metabolic disorder that occurs in about 1 of every 10,000 live births. Affected infants lack the ability to process phenylalanine, an amino acid found in certain foods such as milk. This results in an accumulation of toxic levels of phenylpyruvic acid, which severely damages the central nervous system. If the condition remains untreated, dramatic and serious intellectual impairment results (Dion, Prevost, Carriere, Babin, & Goisneau, 2001; White, Nortz, Mandernach, Huntington, & Steiner, 2001). Most individuals with untreated PKU have IQs below 50 and are unable to speak. Many cannot master such basic tasks as bowel control and walking; they often exhibit generally aberrant behavior.

Prenatal damage due to PKU occurs during pregnancy in mothers who themselves have the disorder (Brock, 2000). In such circumstances, the fetus is exposed to a high level of phenylalanine, which damages the fragile developing nervous system. Prenatal diagnosis of PKU is now possible, although the technique is not widely used. Neonatal PKU presents a different situation, one for which great treatment progress has been achieved. In these circumstances, the mother is a carrier but does not have PKU herself. A child with

PKU born to such a mother develops symptoms after birth. The enzyme deficiency prevents proper processing of phenylalanine in the diet, and toxic-level accumulations occur. As was already noted, the resulting damage will be severe if the condition is untreated. Fortunately, such outcomes are unnecessary today because of advances in early diagnosis and treatment through dietary management.

Maple syrup urine disease is another genetic disorder that results in metabolic deficiency. In this case, the diagnostic label is more indicative of a symptom than of the disease process. Affected infants tend to excrete urine that has a distinctive odor of maple syrup. Maple syrup urine disease may cause severe intellectual impairment, although more often than not the condition is fatal. Menkes, Hurst, and Craig (1954) described a family in which four out of six infants died of the disorder during the first few weeks of life. These babies exhibited a variety of difficulties, and their urine had the distinctive odor of maple syrup. The cause of this condition has been linked to metabolic deficiencies of three separate amino acids causing extreme CNS damage in the newborn. As with PKU, treatment may require dietary control although it is complicated by the fact that three amino acids found in many different foods are involved in the problem. Untreated maple syrup urine disease is fatal; few untreated infants survive more than a few weeks. Even treatment is risky since so little is known about the disease.

Galactosemia is another genetically linked metabolic disorder that may produce mental retardation during early infancy. This condition involves difficulty in carbohydrate (sugar) metabolism, rather than amino acid metabolism. Infants with galactosemia are unable to properly process certain sugar components in milk. The results of such a condition, if untreated, are toxic damage to the infant's liver, brain, and other tissues. Again, treatment consists of dietary control (elimination of milk and other foods containing milk sugars) at a very early age, which may successfully prevent substantial damage. Untreated, galactosemia may cause permanent and serious intellectual impairment (Drew & Hardman, 2000).

Not all genetic disorders are metabolic in nature. Some are sex-related, in that the aberration occurs in the sex chromosome portion of the genetic material (e.g., Turner's syndrome, Klinefelter's syndrome,

Lesch-Nyhan syndrome). Other genetic disorders may produce a variety of physical and functional manifestations. You can consult a medically oriented volume for more complete information (e.g., Dykens et al., 2000), since a comprehensive examination of genetic disorders related to mental retardation is quite technical and is beyond the scope of this chapter.

Maternal Characteristics

Maternal age seems to be associated with aspects of the baby's health other than Down syndrome. Spontaneous abortions occur more frequently in women who are very young (under 15), particularly if there have been multiple pregnancies. The risk is also substantially increased for pregnant women over 35. Spontaneous abortion is *least* likely to occur between the maternal ages of 20 and 30, which has been translated by many to mean that these are the prime child-bearing years (Drake, Engler-Todd, O'Connor, Surh, & Hunter, 1999; Wakschlag et al., 2000). Although the mother's age is certainly important, other maternal influences also appear related to infant prematurity. For example, adequate nutrition may be one of the most important factors influencing general fetal health and well-being. Maternal nutritional deficiencies may have a significant impact on fetal development, as discussed in Chapter 5. Such problems become especially severe when expectant mothers do not have access to health care advice or to prenatal medical care (Drew & Hardman, 2000). Logic and the most fundamental knowledge of physiology suggest that poor maternal nutrition endangers early mental development. However, the specific relationship between nutrition and mental development remains unclear.

Sometimes the unborn fetus may be inadequately nourished regardless of the mother's nutritional status. Maternal conditions such as thyroid deficiency, chronic diabetes, and anemia may substantially affect the development of the fetus and result in premature birth. Prematurity substantially increases the possibility of intellectual impairment. The impact of such conditions is mainly dependent on the severity of the mother's condition and on the effectiveness of medical treatment she receives. However, maternal diabetes is always considered to create some degree of risk for the baby, who should be monitored for birth weight and gestational age (age of a fetus) as well as for other complications (Picard, Del-Dotto, & Breslau, 2000).

Serious damage to the fetus may be caused if mother and fetus have incompatible blood types. Perhaps the best-known form of this condition involves the *Rh factor*. Difficulty may be encountered if the mother's blood is Rh negative and the fetus has Rh positive blood. The mother's system may become sensitized to the fetus's Rh positive blood and begin to produce antibodies that cause serious damage to the fetus. Sensitization of the mother may occur if the Rh positive blood from the fetus enters her circulatory system, which commonly happens during delivery, or if Rh positive blood has been used in a transfusion given to the mother. Typically the first born is not at risk unless maternal sensitization has occurred following a transfusion (Drew & Hardman, 2000). However, subsequent pregnancies present considerable fetal risk unless the mother receives treatment. The babies in these successive pregnancies may be damaged in the later stages of gestation as the mother's antibodies seek to destroy the Rh positive red blood cells, which are essentially a foreign substance in the maternal system. This can result in several conditions, including *erythroblastosis fetalis* (a severe form of anemia) and *hyperbilirubinemia*. The latter condition occurs because of accumulating bilirubin from red blood cell hemoglobin, which may be so concentrated that it damages the brain tissue and causes mental retardation.

Fortunately, treatment for Rh incompatibility has advanced substantially and few babies are at risk today. Perhaps the most commonly used treatment involves injecting an Rh negative mother with Rh immune globulin (commercially known as RhoGAM). In pregnancies involving incompatibility, the mother is injected with RhoGAM during gestation (usually at 28 weeks) and then again within the first 72 hours after she gives birth to her first baby. She will then be desensitized, and no antibodies will be present to complicate subsequent pregnancy.

A variety of maternal infections may also increase the risk of harm to the unborn fetus, particularly if they occur during the first trimester of pregnancy. The likelihood of spontaneous abortion or severe defect in the infant is considerably greater when the mother has an infection accompanied by a fever (a febrile infection). Such conditions may be especially problematic since the mother's illness may be mild or even not recognizable but still may result in serious harm to the fetus. This makes both research and treatment difficult. Also,

viral infections may result in serious difficulties during pregnancy, although they do not always damage the fetus. German measles (rubella) is perhaps the viral infection most widely recognized as causing mental retardation. There is a significant risk to the fetus if the mother has rubella during early pregnancy (first trimester), and continued but lesser risk during the later months of pregnancy. It should be noted that mental retardation is not the only damage that results from congenital rubella. Deafness is the most frequent outcome; others include cerebral palsy, cardiac difficulties, blindness, seizures, and other neurological problems (Drew & Hardman, 2000).

Syphilis is an infection caused by a bacterium (the spirochete) transmitted by sexual contact. Maternal infection with syphilis may have a serious impact on the development of a fetus, particularly if the infection continues past the 18th week of gestation. The bacteria cross the placenta and actually infect the developing fetus, causing damage to the tissues of the central nervous and circulatory systems. Although treatment of syphilis has progressed over the years, venereal disease in general remains a serious problem. Often it is unreported, either because of embarrassment or because the symptoms are mild and subside. The danger to the unborn fetus remains, however, and may result in spontaneous abortion, stillbirth, mental retardation, and many other difficulties for the infected baby. Treatment of the mother may prevent such outcomes *if* implemented prior to the 18th week; the damage inflicted after this time is likely to be permanent.

Toxoplasmosis is another infection that may result in severe problems for the unborn fetus. This condition is caused by a protozoa that is carried in raw meat and fecal material. One of the major hazards of toxoplasmosis is that the infection may be so mild in the mother that it does not cause serious concern, perhaps no more so than a common cold. Fetal impact may be dramatic, however. It should be noted that if the mother is exposed prior to conception, the danger to the fetus is minimal; toxoplasmosis is a more serious problem if the exposure occurs during pregnancy (Drew & Hardman, 2000).

Clearly, maternal infection may cause a wide variety of complications leading to mental retardation, other defects, and even stillbirth. The fetus may also be endangered by any of a number of other substances introduced into the mother's system from the outside. Chemicals, drugs, alcohol, and smoking (discussed in Chapter 5), as well as radiation, may cause difficulties for the fetus (Espy, Francis, & Riese, 2000). In some cases, the detrimental effects are well known; in others, the data may only be suggestive. For example, a possible consequence of maternal alcohol abuse during pregnancy is fetal alcohol syndrome (FAS) or the less severe fetal alcohol effects (FAE). FAS is a leading cause of mental retardation and is particularly unfortunate because it is preventable (Adnams et al., 2001; Schonfeld, Mattson, Lang, Delis, & Riley, 2001).

Clinical Defects

One event of great importance in prenatal development is the development of the neural tube that eventually becomes the spinal cord and brain. This occurs quite early, with a groove being evident by the 17th or 18th day (gestational age); closure of the tube is normally completed between the 25th and 28th day. Substantial deviations in the closure process can result in serious outcomes that are typically labeled *clinical defects* because the causes of such problems are unclear.

One closure-related clinical defect is known as *anencephaly*, which appears when the head end of the neural tube does not close normally. Anencephaly occurs early and results in incomplete development of the forebrain portion of cerebral tissue (in fact, the tissue often degenerates as gestation proceeds). Infants born with anencephaly typically die shortly after birth. Improper closure at other parts of the neural tube may also cause damage to the central nervous system in the form of a condition known as *spina bifida*. In such cases, incomplete closure of the spinal column may permit the spinal cord tissue and meninges (tissue covering) to protrude or bulge from their normal position. The type and extent of damage may vary depending on the longitudinal position of the affected area. Paralysis of the body below the damaged area is not uncommon and may prevent control of excretory functions. Infections may result and progress through the spinal cord tissue to the brain causing brain damage. Although typically not as serious as anencephaly, any incomplete closure of the neural tube may produce mental retardation as well as other disabilities.

Hydrocephalus is a clinical defect that is sometimes related to improper closure of the neural tube. In a generic sense, hydrocephalus refers to an increase in cerebrospinal fluid volume in the skull from any cause. With incomplete neural closure, the cerebral tissue does not assume its proper position in the skull cavity and is replaced by fluid. This excess of fluid in the skull is merely a symptom, however, and not the major cause of brain damage. The primary problem, resulting from the improper neural closure, is that the spinal cord begins to fuse with surrounding tissue at the opening. As the body grows in length, cerebral tissue is actually pulled into the spinal area.

Hydrocephalus in the neonatal or infancy period more commonly results from defects in the production or absorption of cerebrospinal fluid. The central nervous system has a circulatory system for the distribution of this fluid, which plays a number of important roles, one of which is to provide a protective layer between the brain tissue and the bones of the skull and spine. As this fluid circulates, a certain amount is replenished and a similar amount is absorbed. If more fluid is produced than is absorbed, an excess accumulates, putting pressure on the brain and causing brain damage and mental retardation. This may occur in two fashions, depending on the extent of skull development. During early infancy, the skull is in sections and is not solid. An excess of fluid accumulating in the skull cavity at this time will place outward pressure on the skull, spreading the sections and enlarging the head. The fluid production-absorption imbalance may instead occur after the sections of the skull lines begun to fuse. In such circumstances, expansion of the skull cavity is not possible. Hydrocephalus from both of these situations places excess pressure on the brain, typically resulting in damage and mental retardation. The degree of impairment may vary from very severe to only mild. In some cases, treatment is possible if the condition is discovered early and immediate surgery is undertaken to implant devices to drain excess fluid.

Atypical Birth

Thus far we have discussed several factors that may operate during the prenatal period to increase the risk of mental retardation. A comprehensive examination of all possible influences that may operate during this period is far beyond the scope of this chapter; many other works provide information on this crucial part of development (e.g., Minde, 2000). The end of this period, the birth process, also subjects a baby to risk of mental retardation. Historically, certain schools of thought viewed the process of birth, even an easy birth, as an extremely traumatic psychological event. Early psychoanalysts (notably Otto Rank and Sigmund Freud) attributed many difficulties in later life, such as anxiety and depression, to repercussions from the shock of birth trauma. Birth is stressful to mother and infant alike. However, current thinking focuses much more narrowly on the physical trauma of atypical births than did earlier theories.

The position of the fetus *in utero* is very important in terms of potential birth complications. Figure 12-2 illustrates a normal fetal presentation with the head positioned toward the cervix and the face down (the mother is lying on her back). Other fetal positions substantially raise the probability of damage. For example, the problematic *breech presentation* occurs when the baby's buttocks (rather than the head) are positioned toward the cervix (see Figure 12-3). Several difficulties may result from a breech birth. Unless the fetus can be turned, the head will exit through the birth canal last rather than first. At that point, the mother is in the later stages of labor, when the contractions are stronger and more rapid than during early stages. Breech birth may place a great deal of stress on the head of the baby. In a normal delivery,

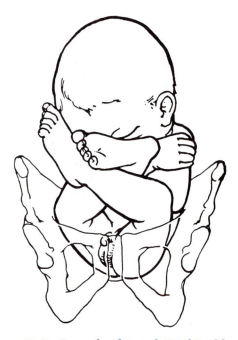

Figure 12-3   Example of Breech Fetal Position
SOURCE: Dorland (1974), p. 1253. Copyright 1974 by Saunders. Reprinted by permission of the publisher.

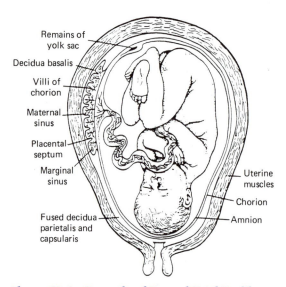

Remains of yolk sac

Decidua basalis

Villi of chorion

Maternal sinus

Placental septum

Marginal sinus

Fused decidua parietalis and capsularis

Uterine muscles

Chorion

Amnion

Figure 12-2   Example of Normal Fetal Position
SOURCE: Chinn (1979).

the head moves through the birth canal slowly, permitting a gradual process of molding of the skull. This molding is possible since the fetal skull is not solid. There are seams in the bony structure that have yet to grow together and that facilitate the molding process (thus, the temporarily misshapen heads often observed in newborn infants). The lower intensity of early labor permits the molding to occur gradually. But in a breech presentation, molding of the head may be rather rapid and perhaps incomplete, causing mechanical damage to the brain tissue. Damage may also occur because of the abnormal pressure (it is more intense and it is brought to bear on a head that is in a reversed position).

The breech position may cause difficulties other than possible mechanical damage. Since the head is the last portion to exit, the baby must obtain its oxygen solely from the umbilical cord until delivery is completed. This may cause two difficulties. First, the cord may be too short to remain attached while the head is expelled. Under such circumstances the placenta may become detached from the uterine wall, eliminating the oxygen supply to the fetus. This becomes particularly problematic if the head does not pass through the pelvic girdle fairly easily and quickly. The head will be tightly confined in this portion of the birth canal. If such difficulties arise, the baby may become *anoxic* (oxygen-deprived) and experience severe tissue damage. Anoxia may also occur if the cord is long enough but becomes pinched between the baby's head and the pelvic girdle. In such circumstances, the oxygen supply can be cut off in the same way as if the placenta had detached. In current medical practice, a breech baby is seldom delivered through the birth canal because of the risks described above. Even turning the fetus is dangerous, both because it is difficult and because of the possibility of entangling the umbilical cord and the body. A breech position baby is generally delivered by Cesarean section.

Figure 12-4 illustrates another abnormal fetal position that results in serious difficulties. In the *shoulder presentation*, a shoulder or arm proceeds through the pelvic girdle before the rest of the fetus. This type of presentaton makes delivery through the birth canal difficult or impossible. Sometimes it is possible to reposition the fetus, which may make delivery routine. However, as noted previously, *in utero* repositioning may prove difficult; Cesarean section is often favored when unusual fetal positions are present.

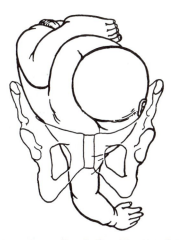

Figure 12-4   Example of Shoulder Fetal Position
Source: Dorland (1974), p. 1253. Copyright 1974 by Saunders. Reprinted by permission of the publisher.

Even if the fetal position is normal, the *time required for delivery* can be another source of risk. It was noted previously that during early stages of labor, contractions are typically less frequent and intense than those occurring later in delivery. This progression of intensity and frequency serves a very important purpose. In the early stages of labor the fetus begins to move into the birth canal and the pelvic girdle begins to stretch. For a normally positioned fetus, the head also begins to be molded to fit through the birth canal. The pressure of molding is absorbed by fluid surrounding the baby's brain, protecting it from injury. However, if labor proceeds very rapidly, time may not permit adequate molding of the skull. Generally, a delivery following a labor of less than 2 hours is considered *precipitous birth*. In these instances, there is an increased risk of brain injury and mental retardation.

The average labor time for a normal delivery is about 7–12 hours, although there is great variation. Difficulties may also result in deliveries in which labor is unusually prolonged. One of the complications that may accompany prolonged labor is similar to that associated with precipitous birth. If advanced labor (intense and frequent contractions) continues for a long period, a great amount of pressure is placed on the skull of a fetus. This pressure may rupture membranes and blood vessels, causing tissue damage and mental retardation. A second danger of prolonged labor is oxygen deprivation (anoxia) to the fetus or even stillbirth. Labor that continues substantially beyond the normal time-span may place a fetus at risk if the placenta begins to detach, cutting off the baby's oxygen supply before delivery is completed.

Neonatal Characteristics

Two neonatal characteristics are highly related to a child's risk of developing retardation: *birth weight* and *gestational age*. **Gestational age** refers to the age of a fetus calculated from the time of conception. Low birth weight and inadequate gestational age at birth (prematurity) are perhaps the most common neonatal risk factors (Minde, 2000; Nadeau, Boivin, Tessier, Lefebvre, & Robaey, 2001; Picard et al., 2000). Infants with these two characteristics may be endangered in a wide variety of ways. They may have mental retardation or be retarded in their physical development; they may be highly vulnerable to infections or other diseases and have a higher probability of dying as an infant.

The preceding discussion may have been anxiety-provoking for the reader who is studying mental retardation for the first time or who is a prospective parent. Anxiety may be unavoidable and could even be helpful. The student of mental retardation cannot ignore these topics but must maintain an appropriate objective perspective. *The vast majority of pregnancies proceed normally and produce normal babies.* Today, more than ever, medical advances have increased the safety of both mother and baby. You will recall that the prevalence of mental retardation is estimated as between 1% and 3% of the total population. Mental retardation that is caused by prenatal influences, including abnormalities in the birth process, is quite infrequent and sometimes preventable, as we shall see later in this chapter.

Causation during Infancy and Childhood: Psychosocial Factors

IN FOCUS 7 ▶ Identify factors that may cause mental retardation during infancy and early childhood periods.

In some cases, a newborn infant may already be in serious difficulty even though damage is not apparent at birth. A number of genetic disorders we have already discussed cause problems during infancy and later in a child's development. But the main cause of mental retardation in infants and children is psychosocial factors.

Infancy and early childhood are an extremely important period in an individual's development in a number of ways. Certain aspects of physiological development must be completed during these years or they will never occur. Additionally, during this time, the individual is acquiring many of the skills and behaviors essential to intelligent behavior (Lacerda, von Hofsten, & Heimann, 2001). This period of child development is enormously affected by a complex interaction between the environment and the physiology of child development. For example, the stimulus provided to an infant through language interaction with adults (e.g., the mother) appears to have enormous positive benefits to infant development (Yoder & Warren, 2001). Developmental effects of a stimulus-rich or stimulus-impoverished environment during infancy may be more potent and lasting than at other times in the developmental cycle (Berk, 1998; Keogh, Garnier, Bernheimer, & Gallimore, 2000; Smith, Groen, & Wynn, 2000). An estimated 90% of all individuals with mental retardation are considered to have mild retardation, and the cause of their disability is not generally evident (Hardman et al., 2002). The vast majority of these individuals are thought to have experienced unfortunate environmental influences that contributed to their condition. Those influences range from poverty and various types of stimulus limitations that deter cognitive growth to malnutrition and other sociological and cultural factors that can inhibit developmental growth (Drew & Hardman, 2000; Larson et al., 2001; Oswald, Coutinho, Best, & Nguyen, 2001).

The most solid evidence of environmental influence has been found in situations where there is severe abuse and neglect. Such adverse circumstances clearly have a serious impact on the young child's development and may result in severe developmental lag and mental retardation (see Chapter 6). Knowledge about the precise influence of less extreme environmental conditions is more limited. During the postnatal period, a complex constellation of social and physical factors are significant in the child's environment. These include socioeconomic status, verbal and teaching interactions within the family, exposure to toxic substances such as lead, and nutrition, to name only a few (Guralnick, 2000; Kessler & Dawson, 1999).

The list of psychosocial risk factors for retardation is huge, and many occur together, making it difficult to trace the origins of mild retardation. This is particularly unfortunate since, as noted earlier, the majority of mental retardation cases fall into this group. These children may be only 1 or 2 years behind their age-mates and are often not identified until they enter school (Hardman et al., 2002). (Youngsters with mild retardation are unlikely to exhibit a learning difficulty that is evident until they enter formal schooling.)

Many individuals who have mild retardation come from low socioeconomic environments. In the absence of other evidence (e.g., identifiable physiological abnormalities) and because of the sheer numbers of such cases, it is difficult to avoid drawing strong conclusions regarding environmental causation. However, investigation of such causes is very complex

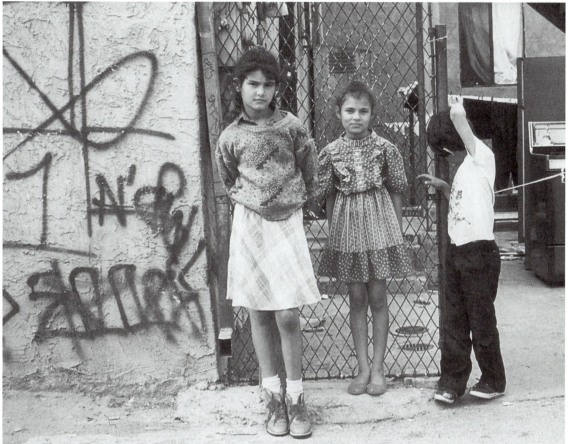

Poverty and related environmental influences, such as lack of health care and poor nutrition, may have significant developmental impact and lead to mental retardation.

since they involve both sociological and psychological influences. Additionally, satisfactory resolution of the nature-nurture debate remains forthcoming.

TREATMENT OF CHILDREN WITH MENTAL RETARDATION

This section examines a variety of techniques employed in working with children and adolescents having mental retardation. The term *treatment* should not be interpreted in a literal sense, for it does not necessarily lead to a cure. Substantial progress has been made in preventing certain types of mental retarda-

tion, notably those with biomedical causes. (As previously noted, prevention of retardation where there appears to be an environmental cause remains a serious societal problem.) Additionally, in some cases, we are now able to arrest the progress of damage that would become more serious if untreated, as in the case of dietary treatment for PKU. However, although some prevention is possible, mental retardation is not amenable to cure as the term is generally interpreted; that is, it cannot be reversed.

The medical profession has played a significant role in the treatment and prevention of mental retardation. This is particularly true for cases that are identified prior to the beginning of formal schooling. Sev-

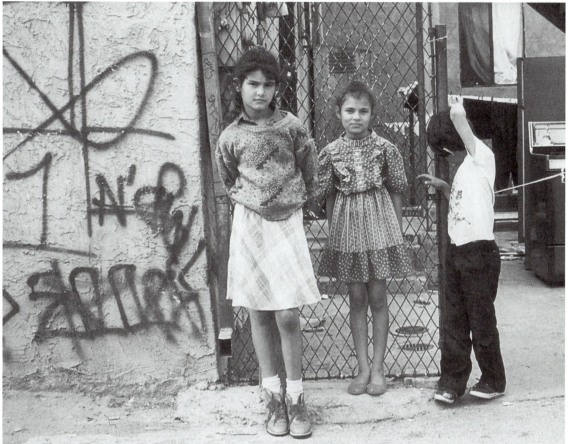

eral factors contribute to this involvement. First, mothers are typically under the care of physicians during pregnancy, and newborn infants are also under close medical scrutiny. Difficulties that arise during this time naturally come to the attention of physicians, since they usually stem from physiological problems of some nature. Medical personnel are influential during a child's early years for yet another reason. Prior to the time the child enters school, the family is more likely to have a relationship with a physician than with a representative of any other discipline (Nickel & Desch, 2000). Whereas it is not uncommon to have a family doctor, it is rather unusual to have a family psychologist and, unless a family is very poor, highly unlikely to have a family social worker. Consequently, if a child of 3 or 4 years of age seems a little slow in mental development, the family physician is probably the one who will be consulted even if the condition seems more mental than physical.

Prenatal Intervention

IN FOCUS 8 ▶ What are three types of prenatal intervention that may prevent mental retardation?

Earlier we discussed Down syndrome, a form of mental retardation caused by chromosomal abnormalities that can be diagnosed *in utero*. This is accomplished by drawing a sample of the amniotic fluid (amniocentesis) and performing a chromosomal analysis. Such procedures carry some risk to the baby and are not recommended on a routine basis for every pregnancy. Amniocentesis may, however, be undertaken with certain high-risk pregnancies (e.g., advanced maternal age, prior birth of a child with Down syndrome).

Using the term *treatment* in the context of Down syndrome arouses a certain amount of controversy. If diagnosis indicates that the fetus has Down syndrome, nothing can be done to *treat* the baby to prevent retardation. The genetic error exists in the cell structure, and cell division will yield more cells that include the chromosomal aberration. The parents may decide to terminate the pregnancy through a therapeutic abortion in order to avoid giving birth to a child with Down syndrome. A decrease in the prevalence of Down syndrome babies in recent years has been partially attributed to the availability of amniocentesis and legal abortions. These preventive measures have become increasingly popular because of the emotional distress and great continuous financial outlay involved in rearing a permanently disabled child.

The issue of abortion is, of course, highly controversial. Even more debatable are practices of allowing such children to die once they are born by withholding medical treatment (unrelated to their retardation) that would permit them to continue living (e.g., surgery to correct an intestinal obstruction). These practices, as well as others (e.g., active termination of life of nonviable neonates), are not uncommon (Drew & Hardman, 2000). A decision involving such alternatives raises many moral and legal questions and is agonizing for both parents and professionals. The physical and emotional outcomes of a decision to terminate life in such circumstances must be carefully measured against the impact of giving birth to and raising a child with Down syndrome or other serious disability that is identifiable at or before delivery. Medical personnel must be extremely sensitive to the needs of the parents during the decision-making process; the parents should also be made aware of the resulting medical actions and potential legal ramifications. In many cases, other professionals (e.g., psychologists, clergy) are called in to assist in this difficult time.

As was noted earlier, Rh incompatibility between mother and fetus can lead to mental retardation. Injection of RhoGAM during pregnancy is certainly a prevention mechanism that is used as a prenatal intervention. Ongoing health monitoring during pregnancy is essential first to detect the Rh incompatibility and then to ensure that treatment is undertaken early enough to avoid antibody development and fetal damage.

PKU can also be diagnosed early through routine screening procedures. If a baby is identified as having PKU early (prenatally or within the first few days after birth), the level of phenylalanine in the system can be *controlled* through dietary restrictions. If initiated in time, dietary control may prevent an accumulation of the phenylalanine from seriously damaging the central nervous system. If, however, this treatment is not initiated promptly, irreparable damage may occur (White et al., 2001; Widaman, 1999). Although PKU may be one of the most studied metabolic disorders related to mental retardation, the exact manner in which accumulated phenylalanine damages the CNS tissue is currently unclear. However, research on this disorder has led to an effective clinical diagnosis and treatment program and a consequent reduction in the number of impaired individuals.

Postnatal Intervention

IN FOCUS 9 ▶ What are some postnatal interventions that may prevent mental retardation or at least facilitate future growth?

There is a great deal of interest in infant stimulation programs as interventions for mental retardation. In some cases, such interventions are used with children who are at risk because of prenatal or later environmental circumstances. In others, the infants may be clearly identified as having retardation because of a condition present at birth (e.g., Down syndrome). This type of treatment often involves psychologists, behavioral therapists, educators, and parents. Although each program has different characteristics, the basic notion is to provide the infant with a stimulus-rich environment through systematic, planned stimulation of all sensory modalities. The goal of such treatment is to accelerate development beyond what may be expected in the normal environment. Research on infant stimulation is logistically difficult, and there is limited evidence regarding its lasting impact. However, the concepts have great intuitive appeal, and some results appear promising (Golbeck, 2001; Hardman et al., 2002; McWilliam, 2000). One of the most prominent projects, the Carolina Abecedarian Project, involved comprehensive intervention in a variety of family environmental areas as well as direct stimulation of infants (Campbell, Pungello, Miller-Johnson, Burchinal, & Ramey, 2001). As with most research of this nature, results are still emerging, but they seem to be favorable with respect to improving intellectual and social functioning.

Children with mental retardation frequently show distinct deficits in language development. Treatment efforts in this area have emphasized establishing an imitative repertoire of language skills as well as generalizing language skills from one environment to another (Drew & Hardman, 2000). Although results have varied to some degree, language treatment appears to offer promise as a potential treatment, and more children with mental retardation are learning to speak appropriately than was thought possible in the past. Teaching procedures have included demonstrating the required sounds and then rewarding children's closer and closer approximations to normal speech. Although effective, the process is extremely tedious and requires devoted teachers and parents who are willing to spend a great deal of time teaching the children. The Research Focus box presents a study investigating the effectiveness of an augmented language system in promoting peer-directed interactions between youngsters with mental retardation.

Treatment takes on a different character as the child with mental retardation begins formal schooling. As mentioned earlier, many children are not identified as having retardation until they enter school. This is particularly true for a large portion of those who are mildly handicapped. These youngsters may be able to adapt and perform at a reasonably acceptable level in most other settings. Even when they are first identified, their slightly lower level of performance may be attributed to mere immaturity. Although their development may have been somewhat slow, their skills are adequate to adapt (if only marginally) in the preschool environment. However, as they enter school, they are expected to perform in those skill areas which are most difficult for them. It is not uncommon for these children to need some level of support or specialized assistance throughout school and they may experience some challenges in the routines of daily life but can generally manage.

People with a moderate level of mental retardation are likely to surface earlier and experience greater levels of challenge in broader areas of life. Their performance limitations are certainly more evident in social circumstances, though they often have some challenges in nearly all aspects of life. In addition to difficulties with some of the concepts taught in school, they often experience problems with interpersonal matters, particularly where some rather subtle social nuances are involved. As children, they are likely to need more academic assistance sooner and for longer periods. These youngsters will also be more likely to have other conditions of disability such as emotional problems or some sensory limitations.

Depending on the type and extent of the child's mental retardation, some of the medical and behavioral treatments discussed earlier may continue during the school years. Medication may be administered on a continuing basis if the child has difficulties that warrant such treatment. A behavioral therapist may continue working with children of school age to shape

Can Youth with Severe Mental Retardation Be Taught to Speak?

Thirteen young males (aged 6.17 to 20.42 years, mean age of 12.25) with moderate to severe mental retardation served as participants in this study. They all had little or no functional speech at the beginning of the investigation. They participated in a 2-year study learning symbols and using a system of augmented language (SAL) designed to supplement their severely limited language abilities. The SAL included a symbol-embossed computerized keyboard that produced synthesized speech, a symbol vocabulary, and teaching procedures to encourage communicative attempts on the part of the participant. The symbol vocabulary was individualized for each participant based on information from parents and teachers. Teachers and parents were trained in the use of the SAL device in three 1-hour sessions. The device was then integrated into each participant's ongoing activities at home and school. Data were collected via 30-minute observation probes during two school years (18 in the first year and 19 in the second); both home and school settings were employed for data collection. Data were collected by a nonparticipant observer using a coding log designed to record the content and context of each communication event. Audiotapes were used to supplement the data collected by observer recording. Communication success was the primary dependent variable.

Figure 12-5 summarizes a portion of the results relating to peer-directed utterances. These data indicate that the

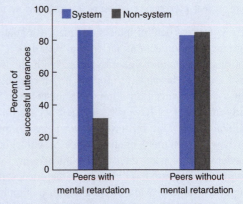

Figure 12-5 Success of Peer-Directed Utterances by Peer Status, with and without SAL
SOURCE: Adapted from Romski, Sevcik, & Wilkinson (1994).

use of the SAL increased the percentage of successful peer-directed utterances when the target students interacted with peers having mental retardation, but not when they interacted with peers who did not have mental retardation. The difference between the percentage of successful utterances directed to peers with mental retardation when using the SAL (87%) and when not using the SAL (31%) underscores the usefulness of the SAL for peers with mental retardation.

SOURCE: Adapted from Romski, Sevcik, & Wilkinson (1994).

social skills or to teach them to speak appropriately. The type of treatment and instructional programming will largely be determined by an assessment of individual needs.

One of the traditional approaches to instructing children with mental retardation in school has been to separate them from their nonhandicapped classmates. This has been accomplished by the use of both special schools and self-contained classes in regular schools. In the former arrangement, children having retardation receive instruction in a separate school, operated exclusively for children with disabilities. Self-contained classes are operated within a school that also houses children without disabilities. In past years, these arrangements were the primary service delivery patterns for most, if not all, children identified as having mental retardation. Recent trends have substantially altered the use of such segregated approaches. Investigations over the past decade suggest that students with mental retardation benefit substantially from placement in regular classes and interaction with their nondisabled peers (e.g., Schwartz & Armony-Sivan, 2001).

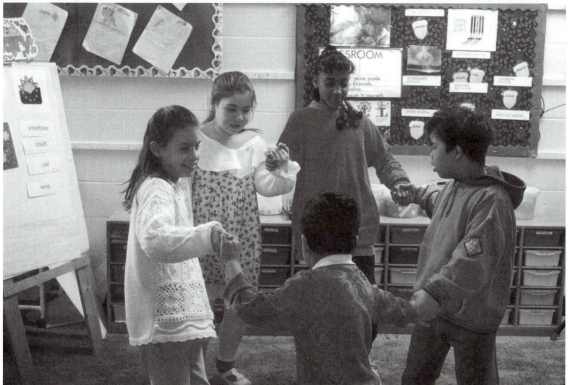

A popular model for teaching children with mild mental retardation is to include them in educational settings with their peers who do not have disabilities.

The currently favored means of instruction aims to minimize separation of handicapped and nonhandicapped children. Those with mental retardation are instructed with their normal classmates to the degree that is feasible, based on each child's level of functioning. Children with mild retardation may receive instruction in a regular classroom with additional special assistance, or they may be in the regular class part of the time and receive specialized instruction part of the time in what is known as a resource room. In general, the more severely the child is disabled, the greater is the likelihood that instruction will be undertaken in a setting apart from the regular educational environment. However, most recent thinking and practice has advocated working with even severely affected youngsters in instructional settings as close as possible to those of their peers without disabilities (Mank, O'Neill, & Jensen, 1998; Slininger, Sherrill, & Jankowski, 2000).

The more integrated pattern of instruction has become a major focus of attention for educators since the mid-1970s. The popularity of this perspective is often attributed to the enactment of Public Law 94-142, federal legislation that was supplanted by the passage in 1990 of the Individuals with Disabilities Education Act (IDEA). Although the idea was promoted by federal legislation, the integration movement predates P.L. 94-142 significantly. In fact, the federal legislation is probably best viewed as the culmination of a trend that began long before the law was conceived. Billy's Story provides a brief sketch of one young man who made it out of special education but likely would have never been placed there if IDEA had been in force earlier.

Educational service delivery for students with disabilities has long been conceived as including a variety of options, ranging from more to less restrictive environments. The placement of each child in the continuum of services is based on the functioning level of

He Probably Would Not Have Been in Special Education

Billy Hawkins is an exception. He moved *out* of the world of special education before federal law required that disabled students be educated with their nondisabled peers to the degree possible. Hawkins spent the first 15 years of his life labeled as having mental retardation. Now he holds a Ph.D. and is an administrator in higher education in Michigan. Dr. Hawkins is African American. During the time that he was classified as having mental retardation, Billy Hawkins was in a special education class separate from his peers in general education. If IDEA had been in force, he would most likely not have been in special education to begin with.

IDEA is aimed at including youngsters with disabilities in the educational mainstream and guarding against racial discrimination. Overrepresentation of children of color in special education is still a concern in the 21st century. According to a 1993 report in *U.S. News & World Report* (Shapiro et al., 1993), minority children continued to be placed in special education classes at a level beyond what would be expected based on population demographics. According to this report, nearly 80% of the states in the country have an overrepresentation of African American students in special education. The passage of IDEA in 1990 was a hopeful move toward rectifying this problem. And Billy Hawkins and others are exerting great effort to see that children receive an appropriate education.

---

the child. Figure 12-6 illustrates this model as conceived for all students who are exceptional, ranging from those with severe disabilities to those who are gifted and talented. The basic concept suggests that children with mental retardation should receive the least restrictive possible instruction and placement; that is, their schooling should be like that of normal children to the degree possible. As this notion gained popularity, the terms *least restrictive alternative* and *mainstreaming* began to emerge, and the term *inclusion* is now commonly found in the literature. Furthermore, integration efforts with more severely disabled children that would not have been even considered a decade ago have been undertaken (Hardman et al., 2002).

In examining the least restrictive alternative concept, it is important to realize that it has many legal connections outside the context of education for children with mental retardation. The least restrictive alternative principle has its basis in criminal law (e.g., *Jackson v. Indiana*, 1972) holding that it is cruel and inhuman to dispense punishment that is disproportionately harsh in relation to the crime committed. The link between criminal law and education of children with mental retardation may seem tenuous at first glance. However, legal scholars have placed a great deal of emphasis on the relationship of this law to the treatment of those with mental retardation. Throughout the years, there has been a great deal of litigation involving education of those with mental retardation. Furthermore, federal legislation such as IDEA is not as innovative for educating those with disabilities as some would suggest.

Dramatic changes such as integrating instruction for disabled individuals into the educational mainstream never occur without controversy. The movement toward educational integration was prompted by two major influences occurring during the past 25 years: (1) shifts in social policy that aligned education of students having disabilities with the general social integration of people of color, and (2) research showing the beneficial effects of integrating disabled and nondisabled youngsters (Hardman et al., 2002; Schwartz & Armony-Sivan, 2001). Educational integration of normal children with those having mental retardation is part of a larger trend called *normalization*. The normalization principle goes far beyond the context of education and refers to placement, residential arrangements, and treatment for individuals with mental retardation of all ages. Normalization essentially broadens the integration effort into the daily lives of those with mental retardation, making their condi-

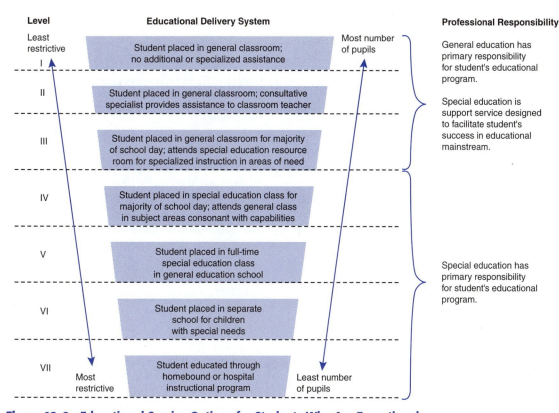

Level	Educational Delivery System	Professional Responsibility

Level

Least restrictive

I

II

III

IV

V

VI

VII

Most restrictive

Educational Delivery System

Student placed in general classroom; no additional or specialized assistance

Student placed in general classroom; consultative specialist provides assistance to classroom teacher

Student placed in general classroom for majority of school day; attends special education resource room for specialized instruction in areas of need

Student placed in special education class for majority of school day; attends general class in subject areas consonant with capabilities

Student placed in full-time special education class in general education school

Student placed in separate school for children with special needs

Student educated through homebound or hospital instructional program

Most number of pupils

Least number of pupils

Professional Responsibility

General education has primary responsibility for student's educational program.

Special education is support service designed to facilitate student's success in educational mainstream.

Special education has primary responsibility for student's educational program.

Figure 12-6 Educational Service Options for Students Who Are Exceptional

SOURCE: From Hardman, Drew, & Egan, *Human Exceptionality*, 7th ed., Allyn & Bacon, Boston, MA. © 2002 by Pearson Education. Reprinted by permission.

tions and circumstances as close as possible to the norms of mainstream society. This notion has been used in arguments against mass institutionalization of large segments of those with mental retardation.

Debate regarding the placement of individuals with retardation in residential institutions has been and continues to be intense. Often the arguments have been based on compassion or on practicality. There is great variation from one institution to another—some provide good treatment and others are quite dismal. Much of the opposition to institutional placement for people with mental retardation has been based on the institutions with extremely bad conditions and treatment. The trend toward deinstitutionalization raises the immediate question of how those with mental retardation will fare in a more integrated setting. It is not surprising that some individuals with mental retardation manage rather well, whereas others encounter some difficulties (Keith & Schalock, 2000). Successful

placements depend on community circumstances as well as on the personal competencies of the individual with mental retardation. Community integration of those with mental retardation has many unresolved issues. Topics of concern emerging in the literature include questions about life expectancy of those with mental retardation who live in the community, their health care, and their sources of supports as family caregivers become aged (Felce et al., 1999; Joyce, Ditchfield, & Harris, 2001).

PREVENTION OF MENTAL RETARDATION

Prevention of mental retardation has been a goal of professionals in the field for many years. Because of the varied causes, prevention efforts have been extremely diverse, and some approaches have involved extremely

Back to the Beginning

Kelly's Skills Development Program

Kelly's story highlights a situation that faces many parents of children with serious disabilities. It is likely that Kelly will need help with daily care throughout her life. However, Browder (2001) outlines a rather comprehensive program to help Kelly become an active partner in her life skills development. The analysis of Kelly's status is presented below, and Table 12-4 outlines elements of the personal living intervention program.

Kelly could become not only active, but more "in charge" of her daily routines as she made the transition to adult living. Kelly could become more self-

determined by making choices in her routines. For example, she would learn to choose clothing, lunch entrees, and toiletry items. Kelly would also begin the process of directing her own care. For example, she would be taught to ask for help in dressing and to nod when ready to be dressed. She would find her own seat in the lunchroom, and would put her glass down to show when she was finished with lunch. . . .

When asked about sex education, Kelly's parents were wary about what the teacher would address. They had strong personal values in this area related to their religious heritage. Kelly's 18-year-

---

Table 12-4 Curriculum Items in the Home and Personal Living Domain for Kelly

Dressing
- Choose shirt or jacket by nodding
- Ask for help with dressing by taking clothing to assistant (e.g., coat to teacher)
- Nod to indicate when ready for help in dressing (e.g., to put coat on or tie shoes)
- Lift legs and arms to assist when being dressed
- Keep shoes on at school
- Wear glasses all day at school

Eating
- Use spoon without spilling
- Spear appropriate foods with a fork
- Put glass on table to indicate when finished (not throw it)
- Choose entrée in lunch line
- Find favorite seat
- "Dump" tray contents in garbage can while holding silverware

Using the toilet/grooming
- Use toilet every 2 hours without accidents
- Request use of toilet by patting side
- Wash hands with assistance to turn on/off water
- Choose (by reaching for) "body mist" or flavored lip gloss

Food preparation
- Microwave a hot dog (favorite food)
- Make air-blown popcorn (low-calorie snack)
- Take dishes to sink
- Rinse dishes (loves water)

Housekeeping and laundry
- Put soiled clothes in bag or hamper
- Wipe table area after eating
- Use feather duster to dust
- Put clothes in washer/pull out of dryer

Sex education
- Shake hands or give "high fives" versus giving tight body hugs
- Avoid physical contact in public settings (especially with strangers)
- Help change sanitary pad (pull adhesive strip, throw old pad in trash)
- Learn receptive language for "private zones," "period"
- Keep "private zones" of body covered when around other people
- Refrain from touching genital area except when on toilet or in own bedroom

SOURCE: Browder (2001), p. 304. Table and Kelly's excerpts are reprinted with permission.

old sister, Heather, who accepted these family values, dressed modestly and valued sexual abstinence. Heather was the one who expressed concern that Kelly might give people the wrong impression with her close-contact body hugs and indifference about whether her clothes covered her. (Browder, 2001, pp. 304–305)

The skills development curriculum outlined for Kelly in Table 12-4 focuses on functional skills that are most useful in her daily life. Aimed at achieving incremental progress toward enhancing Kelly's ability to function as a young adult, these components will require ongoing modification as she develops.

controversial methods. In some cases, preventing mental retardation requires courses of action that are unacceptable to some segments of the population.

As we have seen, there are a number of prenatal causes of mental retardation. In some cases, these involve health problems or disease states that affect the developing fetus through the mother. Certain causes (e.g., rubella) have become less problematic than they once were because of immunizations routinely administered to a large portion of the general population. To the extent that such efforts are effective in reducing the occurrence of maternal difficulties during pregnancy, they become important steps in preventing mental retardation.

A close relationship between medical personnel and new parents is important in the prevention of mental retardation. As we have seen, a number of conditions may lead to neonatal development of mental retardation unless they are recognized through monitoring, assessment, and early intervention. For example, PKU screening is now routinely undertaken when a baby is born. When a baby is identified with PKU, treatment can be successfully undertaken through dietary control, thereby preventing damage to the central nervous system.

Prenatal screening and diagnosis can also lead to preventive intervention that may be highly controversial from a moral and ethical perspective. Procedures are available that permit detection of certain types of fetal damage in utero; discovery of such damage may present those involved with a difficult decision regarding continuation of the pregnancy. Although therapeutic abortion is legal and is much more accepted than it once was, such action still presents dilemmas for many people. In addition, there is greater public awareness of the problems attendant to intervening or withholding treatment from newborn babies who are grossly defective at birth. Decisions to withhold treatment and thereby "prevent" mental retardation are difficult and have many ramifications beyond any specific case being considered.

SUMMARY

Mental retardation has been recognized and studied scientifically for many years. However, problems regarding definition and classification have persisted even into recent times. Although definitional differences significantly affect prevalence figures, estimates of the number of those with retardation have generally ranged from 1% to 3% of the general population. Classification schemes for mental retardation have involved considerations of etiology, adaptive behavior, severity of intellectual deficit, and educational expectations. Each definition and classification system has certain advantages and limitations.

Causes of mental retardation are varied. Mental retardation may result from abnormalities during pregnancy, birth, and infancy. During the prenatal period, mental retardation may result from genetic aberrations or environmental factors that influence the health of the mother and the fetus. Also, the birth process may result in damage that can cause mental retardation. After birth, mental retardation may be caused by environmental influences that limit the opportunity to develop or by trauma or physical accident.

Treatment of mental retardation has been as diverse as its causes and behavioral characteristics. Some treatments have involved biological and medical interventions, whereas others have focused on psychological and behavioral methods. A variety of medical interventions are employed to prevent mental retardation arising from prenatal events or conditions. Psychological and behavioral interventions may include intense stimulation during infancy to promote mental growth, special training in language skill development, and special education once a youngster enters school. Current research supports instruction of children with mental retardation in settings with their peers who do not have mental retardation as much as possible.

INFOTRAC COLLEGE EDITION

For more information, explore this resource at http://www.infotrac-college.com/Wadsworth. Enter the following search terms:

mental retardation
hydrocephalus
Down syndrome
phenylketonuria (PKU)
fetal alcohol syndrome
prematurity
fragile X syndrome
toxoplasmosis
galactosemia

IN FOCUS ANSWERS

IN FOCUS 1 ▶ List the four assumptions outlined by AAMR as essential to application of the definition of mental retardation.

- Valid assessment considers cultural and linguistic diversity as well as differences in communication and behavioral factors (all of which can affect performance).
- The existence of limitations in adaptive skills occurs within the context of community environments typical of the individual's age peers and is indexed to the person's individualized needs for supports.
- Specific adaptive limitations often coexist with strengths in other adaptive skills or other personal capabilities.
- With appropriate supports over a sustained period, the life functioning of the person with mental retardation will generally improve.

IN FOCUS 2 ▶ What are the ten adaptive skill areas used by the AAMR for assessment of adaptive behavior?

- Communication, the ability to understand and communicate information
- Self-care skills such as toileting, eating, hygiene
- Home living, including clothing care, housekeeping, etc.
- Social skills, including interchange with others
- Community use, including shopping and obtaining services and use of community resources
- Self-direction, such as making choices and following a schedule
- Health and safety, including eating and basic first aid
- Functional academics, skills related to learning in school that have direct application in life
- Leisure, developing a variety of leisure and recreational interests
- Work, the ability to maintain part- or full-time employment

IN FOCUS 3 ▶ Identify the five DSM-IV-TR severity classifications for mental retardation.

- Mild mental retardation—IQ of 50–55 to about 70
- Moderate mental retardation—IQ of 35–40 to 50–55
- Severe mental retardation—IQ of 20–25 to 35–40
- Profound mental retardation—IQ below 20 or 25
- Mental retardation, severity unspecified—where there is a presumption of mental retardation but the person's intelligence is not testable with standardized instruments

IN FOCUS 4 ▶ What are the general estimates of prevalence for mental retardation, and what does this mean in terms of numbers of individuals receiving services under IDEA?

- Prevalence estimates have typically ranged from 1% to 3% of the general population.
- About 11% of all children with disabilities in the U.S. public schools (ages 6–21) have mental retardation; slightly over 600,000 individuals received services under IDEA in 1998–1999.

IN FOCUS 5 ▶ Explain how development plays a role in mental retardation.

- During pregnancy, the unborn baby is developing very rapidly and is consequently very vulnerable to diseases, maternal nutritional status, and accidents.
- During infancy and early childhood, a child is dependent on his or her environment for nutrition,

oxygen, protection from disease and trauma, and environmental stimulation. Disruptions in any of these environmental inputs at this time may cause serious developmental problems and result in mental retardation.

- Particularly during the time of most rapid development (prenatal and early childhood), a child may be at risk for developing metabolic disorders (PKU) or other conditions that are genetically transmitted.

IN FOCUS 6 ▶ Identify factors that may cause mental retardation during the prenatal and neonatal periods.

- Genetic inheritance
- Maternal characteristics such as age, nutrition, incompatible blood types, infections, and substance abuse
- Clinical defects, where part of the nervous system does not progress normally (neural tube problem or anencephaly) or becomes vulnerable to damage because a system fails to operate properly (hydrocephalus)
- Birth problems due to delivery position or extremely atypical labor periods (either too short or too long)
- Low birth weight and inadequate gestational age

IN FOCUS 7 ▶ Identify factors that may cause mental retardation during infancy and early childhood periods.

- Genetic disorders that cause developmental damage to the neurological system

- Psychosocial or environmental factors, where adequate stimulation to promote intellectual and social growth does not exist

IN FOCUS 8 ▶ What are three types of prenatal intervention that may prevent mental retardation?

- Chromosomal analysis for Down syndrome or other genetic abnormalities may result in a decision to abort the unborn fetus, but this may be controversial because abortion is controversial.
- Treatment for Rh blood incompatibility between mother and fetus may prevent fetal damage.
- Prenatal identification of a PKU problem may result in maternal dietary restrictions.

IN FOCUS 9 ▶ What are some postnatal interventions that may prevent mental retardation or at least facilitate future growth?

- Infant stimulation programs provide a positive developmental environment for very young children who are at risk because of prenatal or later environmental circumstances.
- Specific instruction for young children in language skills appears promising and probably should be implemented as early as possible.
- Inclusion of young children of school age in classrooms with their nondisabled peers to the extent possible may have educational benefits.

13 Autism, Childhood Schizophrenia, and Related Conditions

In the Beginning
Finding Jake—A Mother's Story

"Your child has autism," he said matter-of-factly.

When I'd found my son lying face down on the driveway at his second birthday party, I stopped believing what our family pediatrician had been telling me over the past few months—that I worried too much. The next week I took Jake to the first of many specialists.

Jake's diagnosis came a month after that birthday. I guess I should have felt relieved that my fears about Jake's development were not imagined. I didn't. . . . [The] diagnosis provided little comfort to me as I looked at my silent son who could barely make eye contact with his mother. No matter what label the doctors gave his condition, the word *autism* resonated through my head. Autism meant my son had entered into a realm of hopelessness and withdrawal from reality. I'd seen it in the movies, I'd read about it in books. . . .

Jake developed normally until he was 17 months old. He reached all of the typical developmental milestones—he walked, talked, and played just like the other kids his age. Gradually over the next few months, he stopped talking. He stopped playing. It was as if one by one, his circuit breakers began shutting down. My once energetic and spirited toddler was developing into a listless, disconnected boy. . . .

Ultimately, my husband Franklin and I chose ABA [applied behavior analysis] as the foundation of Jake's therapy. Our decision was based on all of the scientific evidence coupled with conversations with parents of autistic kids who had been successfully mainstreamed as a result of intensive ABA.

"It's a huge commitment," one of the ABA therapists explained to me and Franklin. "It's not just about his therapy sessions. You'll have to adjust your entire lifestyle to accommodate your son." (Siff, 2001)

INTRODUCTION

IN FOCUS 1 ▶ Identify the five categories of pervasive developmental disorders according to DSM-IV-TR.

The disorders discussed in this chapter include some of the most damaging and debilitating of all childhood disability conditions. Autism is one of a category of disorders known as *pervasive developmental disorders*, which typically become apparent in a child's early years of life. Autism may include severe developmental disturbances in communication and social skills as well as evidence of stereotyped behavior such as manipulating objects for prolonged periods and apparently meaningless repetitive body movements.

Included among **pervasive developmental disorders** in DSM-IV-TR are autism, Rett's disorder, childhood disintegrative disorder, Asperger's disorder, and pervasive development disorder not otherwise specified (American Psychiatric Association, 2000). Children diagnosed with one of the pervasive developmental disorders may exhibit combinations of bizarre, incomprehensible behaviors that seem extremely abnormal, such as a child living entirely in a fantasy world and completely screening out reality. The term *pervasive developmental disorder* suggests that the condition emerges early in the child's development and often affects many or all (pervasive) of the child's developing systems (e.g., interpersonal/social, language, cognitive). With some types of pervasive developmental disorders, the child is never really normal, but is either born with the condition or develops it very early. With other types, there is a period of apparently normal development followed by a regression or the emergence of abnormal behavior.

Childhood schizophrenia is not included in the category of pervasive developmental disorders. Schizophrenia tends to emerge between 7 and 15 years of age and often involves hallucinations, delusions (unreasonable false beliefs), and thought disorders (e.g., illogical or disturbed thinking). DSM-IV-TR does not include a specific category for childhood schizophrenia, relying on the adult criteria and applying them when the disorder strikes a child. Childhood schizophrenia is examined in this chapter because of its interesting comparisons with autism. For example, like children with autism, children diagnosed with schizo-

phrenia may exhibit behaviors that are extremely abnormal. Those with both types of disorders display withdrawal or peculiar social interactions. However, children with schizophrenia may be affected by hallucinations. Although there are certain similarities between autism and childhood schizophrenia, there are also a number of distinctions, which we will examine later.

PERVASIVE DEVELOPMENTAL DISORDERS

A number of areas of functioning are affected by pervasive developmental disorders. DSM-IV-TR notes that "severe and pervasive impairments" are evident in social interaction and in communication skills and are often accompanied by very narrow stereotyped interests, behavior, and activities. An individual often focuses on one object or set of objects and repetitively plays with it or compulsively manipulates it. These impairments reflect substantial deviation from what would be expected given the individual's mental age or developmental level (American Psychiatric Association, 2000, p. 69). Autism is the most widely recognized and most frequently occurring of the pervasive developmental disorders, and Asperger's disorder is a relatively new diagnosis that has received increased public attention recently.

Early conceptions of autism were focused on children with a severely impaired level of functioning. Over time, however, scientists began to realize that children with autism exhibit a far broader range of skill levels than once thought. Some of these children may be relatively high functioning, with normal or near-normal intelligence. This has led to use of the term *autism spectrum disorders*, suggesting that there is a *range* of functioning *in several skill areas* (e.g., communication and language, social interaction, intelligence) (Nesbitt, 2000; Sheppard, 2000; Wing & Shah, 2000). This concept of a spectrum of disorders also emerges as we examine Asperger's disorder. Considerable disagreement has emerged regarding whether Asperger's is a distinct disorder or a type of higher-functioning autism (Bishop, 2000; Mayes, Calhoun, & Crites, 2001; Volkmar & Klin, 2001). While the arguments are heated, many believe that the existing data are inconclusive as to whether or not these are separate disorders (Ozonoff & Griffith, 2000).

Autism

IN FOCUS 2 ▶ What is the general prevalence estimate for autism?

IN FOCUS 3 ▶ Identify four areas of functional challenge often found in children with autism.

Autism is a widely recognized condition even though it develops rather infrequently. Most sources note about 4 to 8 occurrences in 10,000 individuals, although some recent estimates based on the range of functioning concept suggest a prevalence that is substantially higher—ranging from 6 to over 20 per 10,000 (American Psychiatric Association, 2000; Kielinen, Linna, & Moilanen, 2000; Magnusson & Saemundsen, 2001; Patterson & Rafferty, 2001). Autism was specified by federal legislation as a category of disability in the Individuals with Disabilities Act of 1990 (IDEA), but the condition was first described in the early 1800s (Ward & Meyer, 1999).

Autism has received a great deal of public attention in the past few years. Popular awareness of the disorder was enhanced substantially by the release of the award-winning film *Rain Man* in the late 1980s and other compelling descriptions in popular books and other mass media, such as the story of Jake presented (Siff, 2001). An extraordinary example is found in the autobiographical account by Donna Williams (1992), which provides a rare, personal view of autism. Donna' Story is a short excerpt from that work, which describes aspects of Williams's early world. Clearly, Donna Williams is functioning so well that she is not typical of those with autism, although accounts such as hers educate all of us regarding the disorder.

Federal regulations in IDEA define **autism** in the following manner:

Autism means a developmental disability significantly affecting verbal and nonverbal communication and social interaction, generally evident before age three, that adversely affects educational performance. Characteristics of autism include—irregularities and impairments in communication, engagement in repetitive activities and stereotyped movements, resistance to environmental change or change in daily routines, and unusual responses to sensory experiences. (U.S. Department of Education, 1991, p. 41271)

The severity of autism varies considerably, with more serious involvement including significant deficiencies in intellectual functioning, language development, and interpersonal skills (Folstein et al., 1999; Liss et al., 2001; Tjus, Heimann, & Nelson, 2001). The social or interpersonal impairments are frequently pronounced. People with autism are often characterized by a somewhat flat affect (they rarely laugh, cry, or express other emotions) and extreme isolation or detachment from the social world around them. Parents of infants with autism regularly note that their babies are unresponsive to affection and avoid eye contact. The

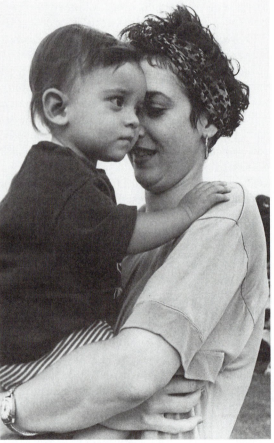

Gale Zucker/Stock Boston

Youngsters with autism often do not return their parents' affectionate gestures or eye contact.

A View from the Other Side

I discovered the air was full of spots. If you looked into nothingness, there were spots. People would walk by, obstructing my magical view of nothingness. I'd move past them. They'd gabble. My attention would be firmly set on my desire to lose myself in the spots, and I'd ignore the gabble, looking straight through this obstruction with a calm expression, soothed by being lost in the spots. *Slap*. I was learning about "the world."

I learned eventually to lose myself in anything I desired—the patterns on the wallpaper or the carpet, the sound of something over and over again, like the hollow thud I'd get from tapping my chin. Even people became no problem. Their words became a mumbling jumble, their voices a pattern of sounds. I could look through them until I wasn't there, and then, later, I learned to lose myself *in them*.

Words were no problem, but other people's expectations for me to respond to them were. This would have required my understanding what was said, but I was too happy losing myself to want to be dragged back to something as two-dimensional as understanding.

"What do you think you're doing?" came the voice.

Knowing I must respond in order to get rid of this annoyance, I would compromise, repeating "What do you think you're doing?" addressed to no one in particular.

"Don't repeat everything I say," scolded the voice.

Slap. I had no idea what was expected of me.

For the first three and a half years of my life this was my language, complete with the intonation and inflection of those I came to think of as "the world." The world seemed to be impatient, annoying, callous, and unrelenting. I learned to respond to it as such, crying, squealing, ignoring it, and running away.

SOURCE: Williams (1992), pp. 3–4.

---

social impairments often associated with autism can seem like a self-imposed social isolation, with young autistic children seeming to prefer interacting with objects rather than with people (Ratey et al., 2000; Weiss & Harris, 2001; Wing & Shah, 2000). Youngsters with autism interact with the environment around them in ways that most of us do not understand. They frequently seem to provide their own stimulation by flicking their hands in front of their eyes, physically rocking their body, or spinning objects on the floor for hours. This self-stimulation and perseverative behavior occasionally resemble or even evolve into apparent obsessive-compulsive activities (Baker, 2000; Klauber, 1999; Shu, Lung, Tien, & Chen, 2001). There are also circumstances when self-stimulation appears to become more pronounced or evolves into self-injurious behavior such as head-banging, self-inflicted bites or slaps, and other similar actions. These, of course, become a serious source of concern for parents and other caretakers—as if they didn't have enough to worry about from the child's other problems (Dennis et al., 1999; McKerchar, Kahng, Casioppo, & Wilson, 2001).

A child with autism places an enormous burden on a family. Specific stressors may take many different forms as the youngster's behavior changes with age (Hecimovic, Powell, & Christensen, 1999; Randall & Parker, 1999). Parents experience numerous physical challenges in addition to the emotional drain. Some of these children go through periods of sleeping *very* few hours a night, making physical fatigue and sleep deprivation a constant part of life. Additionally, parents may desperately need information to help them make decisions about treatment options, and they may have serious need for respite from the increasing demands of caring for a child with autism. Not only is it a challenge to obtain information, it may also be difficult to examine the information thoughtfully in the context of daily activity (Freedman & Boyer, 2000; Hardman, Drew, & Egan, 2002).

Children with autism often have impaired intellectual functioning, with about 75% having measured IQs below 70, which is within the range of mental retardation (Kauffman, 2001; Mastropieri & Scruggs, 2000). However, some children with autism have an exceptional cognitive ability (splinter skills) in one area such as memory for calendar dates over hundreds of years or production of artwork. In some of these cases, there is significant developmental retardation across many or most cognitive areas, and the splinter skills may stand out because they are so notable among other deficits (Hardman et al., 2002; Heaton, Pring, & Hermelin, 1999; Hermelin, Pring, Buhler, Wolff, & Heaton, 1999).

Serious language impairment is one of the characteristics of autism that accompanies the lower intellectual level (Kjelgaard & Tager-Flusberg, 2001; Tjus et al., 2001). Some authors suggest that as many as 40–50% of children diagnosed with autism never develop reliable and functional speech (Conti-Ramsden, Botting, Simkin, & Knox, 2001; Kjelgaard & Tager-Flusberg, 2001; Rode, 1999). Echolalia (repeating back or echoing what has been said) is frequently found among those with autism or mental retardation (Broderick & Kasa-Hendrickson, 2001; Karmali, 2000; Wootton, 1999). Language skills appear to develop more completely in autistic youngsters who are higher functioning (Dennis, Lazenby, & Lockyer, 2001; Parisse, 1999). These children resemble children who do not have autism in grammatical complexity, other matters of sentence structure, and even tonal quality (Botting & Conti-Ramsden, 1999; Hardman et al., 2002). These fairly subtle elements of language and communication are important for adaptation to mainstream environments.

The DSM-IV-TR diagnostic criteria for autism, summarized in Table 13-1, include most of the characteristics found in historic descriptions of the disorder, such as abnormalities in social interaction with others, impaired communication skills, and unusual responses to many facets of the environment. The DSM-IV-TR criteria also note that the condition is characterized by an onset occurring before 3 years of age, although a diagnosis of autism may also be appropriate if the characteristics are apparent after the age of 3. Under such circumstances, the category *atypical autism* is used.

Asperger's Disorder

IN FOCUS 4 ▶ Identify several differences in language or communication between autism and Asperger's disorder.

IN FOCUS 5 ▶ What are some abnormal social interactions that are characteristic of those with autism but not those with Asperger's disorder?

We noted earlier that experts disagree on whether **Asperger's disorder** is distinct from autism or is a type of high-functioning autism (see discussions in Klin, Volkmar, & Sparrow, 2000; Volkmar & Klin, 2001). Table 13-1 summarizes the diagnostic criteria for Asperger's disorder used by the American Psychiatric Association (2000). This table reveals the similarities in diagnostic criteria for autism and Asperger's disorder.

The questions about distinguishing between autism and Asperger's disorder are more than academic, though they may seem so on the surface. Determining the exact status of disorder conditions often has real consequences. For example, whether a group of disorders are distinct or variations of the same condition may affect insurance coverage for diagnosis and treatment—a matter of immediate and significant concern to affected families. Distinct disorders may also have different causes and respond to different treatments—again a consideration that has practical implications for both clinicians and those affected by the disorders (Ozonoff & Griffith, 2000). Research focusing on Asperger's disorder is all relatively recent, since a description of the condition was first widely disseminated only about 20 years ago (Wing, 1981).

Asperger's disorder is characterized by severe impairment in social interaction accompanied by the emergence of an atypical pattern of behavior and activities. Terms used to describe some of these characteristics are evident from Joseph's Story and include pedantic and repetitive language and behavior. In Joseph's case, how many youngsters do you know who would decline a treat by saying it is "not my preferred mode of snacking"? The language of these youngsters is characterized as pedantic, but it is not delayed. Asperger's disorder is not characterized by clinically significant delays of language development (American Psychiatric Association, 2000). Some of the subtle aspects of common language use may be affected, such as reciprocal social interaction between individuals. As illustrated by Joseph's Story, some youngsters with Asperger's disorder use rather pedantic language rather than more common speech forms when they talk about daily topics.

Despite limited and atypical social interactions, a child with Asperger's disorder may progress satisfactorily through school because of his or her reasonable language proficiency. In some cases, the use of pedantic language may suggest a higher level

Table 13-1 Diagnostic Criteria: Autism and Asperger's Disorder

Autism	Asperger's Disorder	Criteria
		Social Interaction
*	*	Qualitative impairment in social interaction manifested by:
X	X	• marked impairment in using multiple nonverbal behaviors such as eye-to-eye gaze, facial expressions, body postures, and gestures to regulate social interaction
X	X	• failure to develop peer relationships appropriate to developmental level
X	X	• lack of spontaneous seeking to share enjoyment, interests, or achievements with others
X	X	• lack of social or emotional reciprocity
**		Delay or abnormal functioning with onset prior to age 3:
X		• social interaction
X		• language used in social communication
X		• symbolic or imaginative play
	X	The disturbance causes significant impairment in social, occupational, or other important functioning
		Stereotyped Behavior Patterns
**	**	Restricted repetitive and stereotyped behavior patterns, interests, and activities manifested by:
X	X	• preoccupation with one or more stereotyped, restricted interest patterns, abnormal in either intensity or focus
X	X	• inflexible adherence to specific, nonfunctional rituals
X	X	• stereotyped, repetitive motor mannerisms (e.g., hand flapping or twisting, whole body movements)
X	X	• persistent preoccupation with parts of objects
		Language/Communication
**		Qualitative impairment in communication as manifested by:
X		• delay or total lack of spoken language development (not accompanied by alternative communication modes)
X		• marked impairment in initiating or sustaining conversations by those with adequate speech
X		• stereoptyped and repetitive use of language or idiosyncratic language
X		• lack of varied, spontaneous play or social imitative play at appropriate developmental level
	X	No clinically significant general delay in language (i.e., single words used by age 2, phrases by age 3)
		Cognition
	X	No significant delay in cognitive development or age-appropriate self-help skills, adaptive behavior (other than social interaction), and curiosity about the environment
		Exclusions
X		Disturbance not better accounted for by Rett's or childhood disintegrative disorder
	X	Criteria are not met for another specific pervasive developmental disorder or schizophrenia

NOTE: A diagnosis of autism requires six (or more) identified behaviors from the social interaction, stereotyped behavior, and language/communication areas, with at least two from social interaction and one each from stereotyped behavior and language/communication.

*Requires at least two of these symptoms

**Requires at least one of these symptoms

SOURCE: American Psychiatric Association (2000), pp. 75, 84. Reprinted with permission from the *Diagnostic and Statistical Manual of Mental Disorders*, 4th ed., Text Revision. © 2000 APA.

A Boy with Asperger's Disorder

Joseph always seemed like a brilliant child. He began talking before his first birthday, much earlier than his older sister and brother. He expressed himself in an adult-like way and was always very polite. When his mother offered to buy him a treat at the movies, for example, Joseph said, "No, thank you, M&M's are not my preferred mode of snacking." He showed a very early interest in letters, and by 18 months could recite the whole alphabet. He taught himself to read before his third birthday. Joseph wasn't much interested in typical toys, like balls and bicycles, pre-

ferring instead what his proud parents considered "grown-up" pursuits, like geography and science. Starting at age 2, he spent many hours lying on the living room floor, looking at maps in the family's world atlas. By age 5, he could name anywhere in the world given a description of its geographical location ("What is the northernmost city in Brazil?"). Just as his parents suspected, Joseph *is* brilliant. He also has Asperger syndrome.

Source: Ozonoff, Dawson, & McPartland (2002), p. 1.

---

of intellectual functioning than is actually the case and may serve the individual well, depending on the circumstances (e.g., an unknowing teacher may think such a child is highly intelligent and will promote the youngster based on this perception). Ozonoff et al. (2002) characterizes such children as "eloquent but inarticulate" in school—they use precocious language and lengthy and complex vocalizations to express ideas that could be stated much more simply. Although not exactly incorrect, their language is sufficiently out of the ordinary as to be contextually strange. The development of cognitive skills and self-help or adaptive behavior skills are also not significantly delayed. These children are simply socially unresponsive and display what most would term eccentric behaviors that interfere with schooling and adult life (Jolliffe & Baron-Cohen, 2001; Kim, Szatmari, Bryson, Streiner, & Wilson, 2000; Szatmari, 2000). Circumstances may have a lot to do with the degree to which those with Asperger's disorder are disadvantaged by their condition. Their young age-mates may view them as odd because of their language patterns, while some teachers may see them as academically intelligent.

Children with Asperger's disorder also may exhibit emotional instability, inappropriate or poor social functioning, and facial expressions that are exaggerated or do not reflect appropriate affect (Carrington & Graham, 2001; Koning & Magill-Evans, 2001; Safran,

2001). Although motor delays and clumsiness are occasionally included in descriptions of children with Asperger's disorder, this is not a reliable distinguishing characteristic (Rinehart, Bradshaw, Brereton, & Tonge, 2001; Weimer, Schatz, Lincoln, Ballantyne, & Trauner, 2001). Asperger's disorder is associated with some general medical conditions, but their causal factors or any associated physical abnormalities remain unclear (American Psychiatric Association, 2000; Manning, Baron-Cohen, Wheelwright, & Sanders, 2001). Available knowledge suggests that Asperger's disorder is a lifelong disorder.

The American Psychiatric Association (2000) notes that data regarding the prevalence of Asperger's disorder is currently unavailable. Others place the occurrence of Asperger's disorder at 2 to 5 individuals per 1000 (Ozonoff et al., 2002). Continued investigation of the condition will clarify its prevalence as well as other aspects.

Other Pervasive Developmental Disorders

Autism and Asperger's disorder are the most common of the pervasive developmental disorders, which also include **Rett's disorder** and **childhood disintegrative disorder**. These two disorders occur infrequently but are devastating when they strike. The Research Focus boxes present brief examinations of Rett's disorder and childhood disintegrative disorder.

Rett's Disorder

Rett's disorder is classified as one of the pervasive developmental disorders and is characterized by the emergence of multiple deficiencies after a period of seemingly normal development, typically at an age between 5 months and 4 years. For children affected with Rett's syndrome, there is a diminishing of some skills that previously developed in a normal fashion. Purposeful hand skills are often replaced with stereotyped movements that resemble hand-washing (American Psychiatric Association, 2000; Umansky et al., 2001). Growth of the head, which appears normal at first, decelerates, and seizure disorders may appear. Children with Rett's disorder also tend to have serious impairments in language development and retardation in motor skills, often exhibiting poor coordination in walking (Mount et al., 2001). Poor social skills and challenges in social interactions are frequently associated with Rett's, not surprisingly given the multiple affected areas (Evans & Meyer, 2001). Some evidence is surfacing that suggests intense, specific training in affected skill areas may result in improvement, although research that more completely explores interventions in general is certainly needed (Jacobsen, Viken, & Von Tetzchner, 2001; Koppenhaver et al., 2001).

Although little is presently known about causation, children having Rett's disorder typically have rather severe mental retardation, and the degeneration seems progressive. Some reports suggest neurological and neurochemical abnormalities among those having Rett's disorder, although further research on this aspect is essential (Satoi et al., 2000). There has also been recent interest in the study of genetic mutation among children with Rett's syndrome, although again substantial trends have yet to surface in these data (e.g., Auranen et al., 2001; Erlandson, Hallberg, Hagberg, Wahlstroem, & Matinsson, 2001).

Rett's disorder occurs infrequently, with some estimates suggesting a prevalence rate of 1 in 15,000 infant females, and to date has been reported only in females (American Psychiatric Association, 2000; Fombonne, Simmons, Ford, Meltzer, & Goodman, 2001). This level of occurrence makes large-scale investigations quite difficult. Research to date is following a familiar trajectory: studying characteristics and causal influences and beginning to move into intervention and improvements in assessment protocols (e.g., Demeter, 2000; Moldavsky, Lev, & Lerman-Sagie, 2001; Roane, Piazza, Sgro, Volkert, & Anderson, 2001).

For more information on these conditions, you can consult more detailed presentations (e.g., Hendry, 2000; Malhotra & Gupta, 1999; Mount, Hastings, Reilly, Cass, & Charman, 2001).

One of the recurring themes in this text is human development—how skills and neurological systems develop as a child matures. The Research Focus box on childhood disintegrative disorder portrays a unique developmental trajectory. With this disorder, a child develops normally until about 3 or 4 years of age. At this point, the disorder surfaces and the youngster's functioning begins a downward trend—with a loss of skills that had emerged to that point. The child's functioning disintegrates, as the diagnostic label suggests. In this case, human development undergoes an unsavory reversal, which cannot be arrested or treated.

CHILDHOOD SCHIZOPHRENIA

DSM-IV-TR does not include a separate, specific category for schizophrenia occurring in childhood, although there is a peripheral observation that the condition rarely has an onset prior to adolescence (American Psychiatric Association, 2000, p. 307). The preponderance of the literature acknowledges the difficulties of studying **childhood schizophrenia** using the criteria and characteristics of adult schizophrenia (e.g., Dunn & McDougle, 2001; Volkmar, 2000). Since children do not have the language complexity, intelligence, or maturity of adults, their psychotic symptoms are often represented in different forms. Their delusions, hallucinations, disorganized speech, and behavioral and affective disturbances may differ from those

Research Focus

Childhood Disintegrative Disorder

Childhood disintegrative disorder is characterized by an initial period of normal development lasting at least 2 years (but not more than 10 years). The developmental regression most often begins between 3 and 4 years of age. The period of normal development is marked by typical social relationships, communication skills, and adaptive behavior. As the condition surfaces, the child begins to regress in skills that were previously acquired. Language, social interaction, and physical matters such as motor skills and bowel or bladder control are all marked by diminished proficiency as the condition progresses. In many cases, the condition ultimately results in disintegration of skills in nearly all areas of development (American Psychiatric Association, 2000).

The behavioral features and social interaction levels resemble those found in youngsters with autism. Despite these similarities, the literature continues to distinguish between the two disorders, although some researchers struggle with the question of whether they are actually different disorders. Previously known as Heller's syndrome or disintegrative psychosis, childhood disintegrative disorder is very rare, which presents a significant challenge to those wanting to conduct research on the condition (Hendry, 2000; Malhotra & Gupta, 1999; Zwaigenbaum et al., 2000). It occurs less frequently than autism and appears to occur equally often in males and females.

The very low prevalence rate of childhood disintegrative disorder suggests to some researchers that genetic transmission plays a notable role in etiology (Zwaigenbaum et al., 2000). Most information on causation remains speculative, however, perhaps because of the disorder's infrequent occurrence. In some cases, the condition has been associated with medical conditions although this association is even less common than the disorder itself and it is certainly not clear that any disease is a triggering mechanism in causation (American Psychiatric Association, 2000).

of adults. According to DSM-IV-TR, "The essential features of the condition are the same in children, but it may be particularly difficult to make the diagnosis in this age group. In children, delusions and hallucinations may be less elaborated than those observed in adults, and visual hallucinations may be more common" (American Psychiatric Association, 2000, p. 307). The DSM-IV-TR diagnostic criteria for schizophrenia are summarized in Table 13-2.

SIMILARITIES AND DIFFERENCES BETWEEN AUTISM AND CHILDHOOD SCHIZOPHRENIA

IN FOCUS 6 ▶ What are the primary differences between autism and childhood schizophrenia?

Researchers continue to examine similarities and differences between autism and childhood schizophrenia (e.g., Eliez & Reiss, 2000; Pilowsky, Yirmiya, Arbelle, & Mozes, 2000). It appears that the primary difference between autism and childhood schizophrenia is reflected in the defining characteristics of the two conditions. Autism is defined basically as a condition in which social relationships are greatly disturbed. Childhood schizophrenia, on the other hand, is primarily characterized by thought disorder and hallucinations. It should be noted that both autism and childhood schizophrenia can occur in the same child, although this co-occurrence is rare.

Other fundamental differences between the two conditions also exist. First, there is a marked difference in the time of first occurrence. Autism appears early in life and has a typical age of onset before age 3, while schizophrenia appears in later childhood and early adolescence (from 7 to 15 years of age). If a child has not developed autism by 5 years of age, he or she probably never will. Autism develops early, disrupts most areas of basic development (i.e., social, language, and intellect), and continues into adulthood with little change in its clinical course. Child-

Table 13-2 DSM-IV-TR Diagnostic Criteria for Schizophrenia

A. *Characteristic symptoms*: Two (or more) of the following, each present for a significant portion of time during a 1-month period (or less if successfully treated):

(1) delusions

(2) hallucinations

(3) disorganized speech (e.g., frequent derailment or incoherence)

(4) grossly disorganized or catatonic behavior

(5) negative symptoms, i.e., affective flattening, alogia, or avolition

Note: Only one Criterion A symptom is required if delusions are bizarre or hallucinations consist of a voice keeping up a running commentary on the person's behavior or thoughts, or two or more voices conversing with each other.

B. *Social/occupational dysfunction*: For a significant portion of the time since the onset of the disturbance, one or more major areas of functioning such as work, interpersonal relations, or self-care are markedly below the level achieved prior to the onset (or when the onset is in childhood or adolescence, failure to achieve expected level of interpersonal, academic, or occupational achievement).

C. *Duration*: Continuous signs of the disturbance persist for at least 6 months. This 6-month period must include at least 1 month of symptoms (or less if successfully treated) that meet Criterion A (i.e., active-phase symptoms) and may include periods of prodomal or residual symptoms. During these prodomal or residual periods, the signs of the disturbance may be manifested by only negative symptoms or two or more symptoms listed in Criterion A present in an attenuated form (e.g., odd beliefs, unusual perceptual experiences).

D. *Schizoaffective and Mood Disorder exclusion*: Schizoaffective Disorder and Mood Disorder with Psychotic Features have been ruled out because either (1) no Major Depressive, Manic, or Mixed Episodes have occurred concurrently with the active-phase symptoms; or (2) if mood episodes have occurred during active-phase symptoms, their total duration has been brief relative to the duration of the active and residual periods.

E. *Substance/general medical condition exclusion*: The disturbance is not due to the direct physiological effects of a substance (e.g., a drug of abuse, a medication) or a general medical condition.

F. *Relationship to a Pervasive Developmental Disorder*: If there is a history of Autistic Disorder or another Pervasive Developmental Disorder, the additional diagnosis of Schizophrenia is made only if prominent delusions or hallucinations are also present for at least a month (or less if successfully treated).

Classification of longitudinal course (can be applied only after at least 1 year has elapsed since the initial onset of active-phase symptoms):

Episodic with Interepisode Residual Symptoms (episodes are defined by the reemergence of prominent psychotic symptoms); *also specify if*: **With Prominent Negative Symptoms**

Episodic with No Interepisode Residual Symptoms

Continuous (prominent psychotic symptoms are present throughout the period of observation); *also specify if*: **With Prominent Negative Symptoms**

Single Episode in Partial Remission; *also specify if*: **With Prominent Negative Symptoms**

Single Episode in Full Remission

Other or Unspecified Pattern

SOURCE: American Psychiatric Association (2000), p. 312. Reprinted with permission from the *Diagnostic and Statistical Manual of Mental Disorders*, 4th ed., Text Revision. © 2000 APA.

hood schizophrenia develops late, leaves many of the developmental areas untouched, and runs a varied course, with episodes of improvement and relapse. Additional differences between autism and childhood schizophrenia are listed in Table 13-3, and their characteristics in terms of social skills, language, intelligence, and self-stimulatory behavior are discussed below.

These two conditions are both rare. As mentioned earlier, research has shown the general prevalence of autism to be approximately 4 to 8 cases per 10,000 individuals (American Psychiatric Association, 2000; Magnusson & Saemundsen, 2001). Some evidence suggests a much higher prevalence ranging from 6 to over 20 cases per 10,000 (Kielinen et al., 2000; Sturmey & James, 2001). Such broad variation in

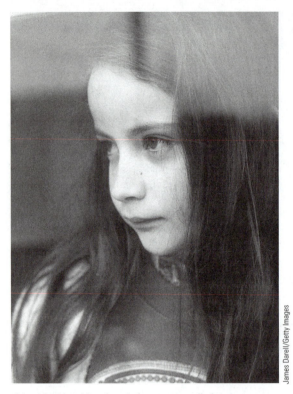

This girl with schizophrenia has an IQ well above average, but suffers from continuing episodes of hallucinations.

some gender difference in prevalence, with males having autism outnumbering females by a ratio between 2 to 1 and 4 to 1, with a greater proportion of males than females at higher levels of functioning (Sturmey & James, 2001). Schizophrenia is relatively rare in childhood and early adolescence. The incidence for schizophrenia in adulthood and adolescence is 2 to 4 individuals per 1000, contrasted with approximately 1 in 1000 for children.

Social Sensitivity and Social Skills

The inability to form personal relationships and to relate socially to other human beings is considered the core characteristic of children with autism (Baker, 2000; Weiss & Harris, 2001; Wing & Shah, 2000). Infants with autism are frequently described by their mothers as being uncuddly babies who seldom laugh, who often become stiff and rigid when they are picked up, or who are unresponsive to physical contact and affection (Hardman et al., 2002). Before these babies were diagnosed as having autism, some mothers described them as exceptionally "good" babies because they were so undemanding and did not need constant attention. This lack of social relatedness is reflected in the child's later social development. Many children with autism do not develop appropriate play skills. For instance, they would rather spin the tires on a toy than play with it appropriately, and they are deficient in pretend or fantasy play. Most children with autism also do not form normal friendships with other children. They are social isolates (Ratey et al., 2000).

prevalence estimates is most likely attributable to differences in the diagnostic criteria employed; some researchers employ the concept of autistic spectrum disorders, while others use a more narrow definition (Patterson & Rafferty, 2001). There also appears to be

Table 13-3 Differences between Autism and Childhood Schizophrenia

Autism	Childhood Schizophrenia
Early onset (before 30 months)	Late onset (late childhood–adolescence)
Early abnormal development	Develops normally and then withdraws into fantasy world
Poor social interaction skills (poor eye contact, social avoidance, lack of play skills)	Dependency on adults but interacts socially
No hallucinations or delusions	Hallucinations and delusions
Mentally retarded	Normal intelligence
Language disturbances (muteness, pronoun reversals, echolalia)	Good language development
Steady course of the disorder	Variable course
Concrete thinking	Thought is disordered (illogical, jumps from one topic to another)

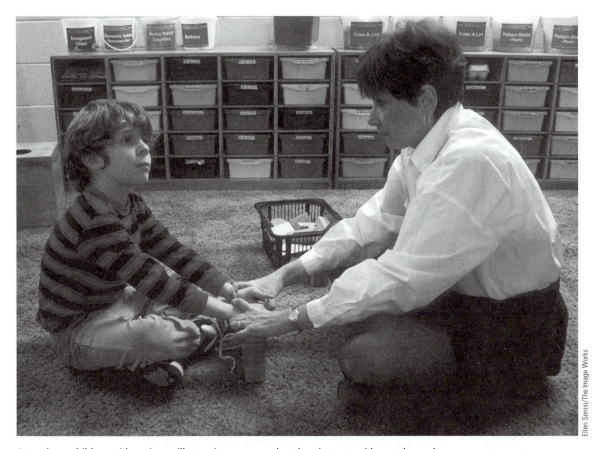

Sometimes children with autism will stare into space rather than interact with people or play with toys.

The research on social behavior and autism has expanded in the past few years. Much of this research has focused on atypical patterns of eye contact and gaze aversion, approach and avoidance tendencies, play skills, and social skills training. However, social interactions of children with autism remains one of the more challenging research areas because of the difficulty in explicitly defining and reliably recording social behaviors. Social interactions are complex, involving perspective-taking abilities as well as turn-taking in play and conversation. Even a small error in social interaction, such as failing to make eye contact with someone, can disrupt the smooth flow of dialogue. A child without autism will frequently initiate social contacts and prolong them with interesting and positive bids for attention. However, children with

autism systematically avoid play situations and engage in solitary and uncooperative activities. These children do not show the necessary social imitation skills needed to engage successfully with other children. Many autistic children relate to other people as "objects," often pushing or pulling them by the hand to get what they want rather than making requests verbally (Baker, 2000; Shu et al., 2001).

The social behavior of schizophrenic children is also characterized by social withdrawal and avoidance of others. However, the nature of this social withdrawal differs from that of autism. The withdrawal occurs later in the child's development and is not a direct, overt avoidance of all social contact, as often described with autism. Children with schizophrenia may be bizarre in their social interactions or may withdraw into their own world (Dunn & Mc-Dougle, 2001; Volkmar, 2000).

Language

Disturbance of language is a basic symptom of childhood autism (Kjelgaard & Tager-Flusberg, 2001; Tjus et al., 2001). The exact nature of the language disturbance distinguishes autistic children from nonpsychotic children who have language difficulties. For example, many prelanguage skills are absent in children who are later diagnosed with autism. Patterns of babble that normally occur in children before 2 years of age frequently do not develop in children with autism. Many of these children who do not babble or respond to sound have intact auditory systems. Similarly, many children with autism do not show age-appropriate gesturing skills and verbal imitation skills, both of which are considered to be prelanguage skills in most children. A significant percentage (40–50%, depending on the study) of autistic children do not develop language and are mute at some point during their childhood (Conti-Ramsden et al., 2001; Kjelgaard & Tager-Flusberg, 2001; Rode, 1999). If a child with autism develops language, it is generally late, and the child shows a poor vocabulary, unusual speech content, and simple speech structure and speaks in a monotone. Many children with autism seem to use language as a noncommunicating self-stimulatory behavior (Hardman et al., 2002). For example, they may repeat TV commercials verbatim or make sounds repetitively to themselves—when alone or in a group of people. In some cases, they interpret language in a very concrete manner, as when the mother of a young boy with autism asked him to "crack a window" to let some air in the room and the youngster broke the window.

Frequently, children having autism exhibit **echolalia**—they repeat sentences or questions addressed to them (Broderick & Kasa-Hendrickson, 2001; Rode, 1999). A child might engage in *immediate echolalia*, or "parrot speech" in which the most recently heard sounds or words are repeated, as illustrated in the account by Donna Williams. Another example of immediate echolalia is when a child with autism is asked his or her name, and instead of answering, simply repeats "What's your name?" Some children with autism demonstrate *delayed echolalia*, in which something heard hours or days ago is repeated. In such cases, a child might repeat something that is unresponsive and totally out of context. Expressions of happiness, sadness, and excitement are typically absent from the language of many children having autism. Inflection and change of emphasis for certain key words containing emotional meaning are missing, which results in a flat, monotonous manner of speaking, reinforced by the child's unemotional facial expression.

The type and quality of language of children with autism can be sharply contrasted with the language of children having schizophrenia. First, the language of children with autism is generally delayed or disrupted in its normal development. The language of children with schizophrenia does not consistently show impaired development (Dunn & McDougle, 2001; Volkmar, 2000). Second, the language of children with autism is often confused and the content is impoverished; that is, speech may be telegraphic and lack normal elaboration. Children with schizophrenia generally use correct language structure but may communicate bizarre thoughts. Children with autism are often set apart by mutism or strange use of language. Children with schizophrenia exhibit more normal language forms, but the content is abnormal—with bizarre meanings and fantasies.

Intelligence

The majority of children with autism perform very poorly on standard intelligence tests (Kauffman, 2001; Mastropieri & Scruggs, 2000). Many cannot be tested accurately because they throw tantrums, refuse to look at the testing materials, and are mute in the testing setting. While early research suggested that these youngsters had difficulty with imitation, more recent work suggests that they may have deficits in many aspects of information processing (Parisse, 1999). Intellectual capacity varies considerably among those with autism. About 75% have measured IQs below 70, while others, such as Temple Grandin, have a much higher intellectual capacity (Hardman et al., 2002). Such high functioning individuals are rare, however, and do not represent the general population of those with autism. Further, even with individuals like Temple Grandin, there are hints that something is different about their functioning (see Temple's Story).

It is easy to be fooled by some autistic children's abilities. From 10% to 15% of individuals with autism

An Adult with Autism

I phoned Temple from the Denver airport to reconfirm our meeting—it was conceivable, I thought, that she might be somewhat inflexible about arrangements, so time and place should be set as definitely as possible. It was an hour and a quarter's drive to Fort Collins, Temple said, and she provided minute directions for finding her office at Colorado State University, where she is an assistant professor in the Animal Sciences Department. At one point, I missed a detail, and asked Temple to repeat it, and was startled when she repeated the entire directional litany—several minutes' worth—in virtually the same words. It seemed as if the directions had to be given as they were held in Temple's mind, entire—that they had fused into a fixed associa-

tion or program, and could no longer be separated into their components. One instruction, however, had to be modified. She told me at first that I should turn right onto College Street at a particular intersection marked by a Taco Bell restaurant. In her second set of directions, Temple added an aside here, said the Taco Bell had recently had a facelift . . . and no longer looked in the least "bellish." I was struck by the charming, whimsical adjective "bellish"—autistic people are often called humorless, unimaginative, and "bellish" was surely an original concoction, a spontaneous and delightful image.

SOURCE: Sacks (1993), p. 110.

---

exhibit what are known as *splinter skills*, fairly narrow areas of functioning in which they seem to excel. For example, some demonstrate a high level of music ability (e.g., perfect pitch) without any training, and others excel in memorization of trivia in rather narrow content areas. Such splinter skills are particularly notable because they represent islands of relatively high capacity surrounded by low functioning in other areas (Hardman et al., 2002). Historically, the presence of splinter skills led to descriptions of people with autism as having advanced cognitive or artistic skills in isolated areas and to terming them "idiot savants."

In contrast to the lower IQs typical of children with autism, those who develop schizophrenia later in childhood tend to show intelligence in the near-normal range (Kauffman, 2001). The majority of children with autism have mental retardation, with particular deficits in verbal and reasoning skills. Children with schizophrenia, however, show less retardation and overall better intellectual development in all areas.

Self-Stimulatory and Self-Injurious Behavior

Self-stimulatory, or stereotypic, behavior is repetitive, apparently purposeless behavior that occurs in nor-

mal, psychotic, and developmentally disordered children. Self-stimulatory behavior is not confined to those with childhood behavior disorders. Everyone self-stimulates at times, and it is interesting to watch people who are unaware they are doing it. Some people without disabilities unconsciously pull their hair, bite their fingernails, wiggle their feet, or tap a pencil. What distinguishes these common forms of self-stimulatory behavior from abnormal self-stimulation is that the latter is exaggerated in form and frequency and is often inappropriate for a particular environmental setting. For example, a child with autism may spend hours spinning coins, gazing at lights, rocking, twirling, or flapping hands (Ratey et al., 2000; Shu et al., 2001; Weiss & Harris, 2001). Such behaviors have a social and educational cost for such children.

In some cases, self-stimulatory behavior may become self-injurious, which is much more destructive (McKerchar et al., 2001). Common forms of self-injurious behavior in autistic children include head-banging, face-slapping, scratching, hair-pulling, and biting oneself. The motivation for self-injurious behaviors is similar to that for self-stimulation. For example, the sensory feedback received from self-inflicting a wound may be reinforcing, leading to further self-injury, in some cases approaching compulsion (Baker,

2000; Shu et al., 2001). Other important factors that may motivate self-injurious behavior include inappropriate but well-intended concern and attention from others, which may serve to reinforce the behavior, and the desire to avoid complying with requests (Kauffman, 2001).

A number of problems are associated with self-stimulation and self-injury, and some of these arise because other people are frightened or repelled by the behaviors and overreact. Self-stimulatory behaviors may also interfere with a child's learning new tasks. They may disrupt previously learned behaviors and displace socially acceptable behaviors of various types.

Differences in self-stimulatory and self-injurious behavior between children with autism and those having schizophrenia have not been thoroughly investigated. Both types of behaviors can occur in both types of conditions. One basic difference is the frequency of occurrence. Generally, children with autism engage in self-stimulatory and self-injurious behaviors at much higher rates than do children with schizophrenia. However, certain types of self-stimulation appear with both autism and schizophrenia. For example, *hand regard*, or hand gazing, is not an uncommon form of self-stimulation for both types of children.

Stimulus Overselectivity

Stimulus overselectivity is a perceptual disability in which a child focuses on only a part of a stimulus, perhaps an irrelevant cue or at least one that is not a central feature, and ignores other important features (Hardman et al., 2002). This disability has been studied mostly in children with autism (e.g., Matthews, Shute, & Rees, 2001). Although it has been found to be particularly evident in those with lower IQs, it also appears in those who are considered to be high-functioning. Stimulus overselectivity interferes with the learning of many of the basic stimulus discriminations needed to adjust to the environment. For example, normal children use a number of cues (e.g., the context or setting, facial expression or tone of voice) to learn discriminations between correct and incorrect responses. For the most part, they focus on the cues that are most vital to the particular discrimination. Some children with autism, however, focus on irrelevant or peripheral cues that are not distinctly different between the alternatives and therefore are not central to discriminating between correct and incorrect responses.

Stimulus overselectivity hinders children with autism as they attempt to learn complex discriminations in language and the subtle choices involved in developing social skills (Weiss & Harris, 2001; Wing & Shah, 2000). This disability may also help explain a common characteristic of autistic children—their marked need to keep their environments the same or unchanging. This "insistence on sameness" characteristically involves requiring that the furniture arrangement stay exactly the same or the daily schedule or travel route remain unchanged (Hardman et al., 2002; Nally, Houlton, & Ralph, 2000). If something is changed, the child may throw a wild tantrum and persistently try to reinstate the original status. Stimulus overselectivity may account for this need for sameness in that the child has learned to rely on an irrelevant characteristic (e.g., a chair's position or a particular arrangement) to help discriminate and map the environment. Stimulus overselectivity has not been studied extensively in schizophrenic children, although there is some indi-

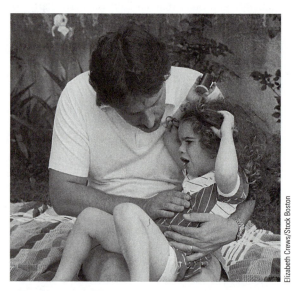

This child is throwing a tantrum because her father has altered her usual routine.

cation that it is present in chronic adult schizophrenics (Kauffman, 2001).

Family Characteristics

There has long been speculation concerning the families, especially the parents, of children with autism and schizophrenia. Some early theorists characterized the mothers of children with autism as being cold and rejecting (e.g., Bettelheim, 1967), which was thought to cause the child to wall off the world mentally. Although some researchers continue to explore psychodynamic theories related to autism, most focus on specific features of the disorder (e.g., Kim et al., 2000; Wheatcraft & Bracken, 1999). The view that parents of children with autism, as a group, are characteristically rejecting and cold receives little research or clinical support.

Family members of children with schizophrenia and autism are quite often faced with considerable stress, which may result in emotional distress (Dewey, 1999; Hardman et al., 2002; Rungreangkulkij, 2001). Even the child's physical demands are significant. For example, a child with autism may sleep for only a few hours per night, making physical fatigue a substantial contributor to family members' emotional stress levels. The family routine is likely to be significantly disrupted, and high stress levels leave parents depressed and anxious (Dominigue, Cuttler, & McTarnaghan; 2000; Piven & Palmer, 1999; Symon, 2001). It is not easy to have a sibling with autism. Siblings may be negatively affected by their parents' stress levels and the amount of parental attention required by the disabled child and may manifest symptoms of depression (Barry & Singer, 2001; Bauminger & Yirmiya, 2001).

CAUSATION THEORIES FOR AUTISM AND CHILDHOOD SCHIZOPHRENIA

Theories regarding the causes of autism and childhood schizophrenia can generally be divided into two broad categories: psychodynamic (or psychoanalytic), and biological. Despite considerable research, these two disorders are not yet fully understood. In both, many symptoms appear to have potential biological and environmental causes (e.g., Brushwick, 2001; Glidden, 2001; Munk-Jorgensen & Ewald, 2001).

Psychodynamic Theories

Freud contributed some of the earliest theoretical work in attempting to explain schizophrenia. Later work by Abraham (1955) maintained that the development of schizophrenia was caused by a fixation of the *libido* (sexual energy) at an early stage. This stalling of normal development presumably produced a withdrawal of personal and object relationships into a sexual state of self-stimulation. As noted earlier, some have portrayed the parents of children with autism as highly intellectual, cold, rejecting individuals showing little interest in other people and little human warmth (Bettelheim, 1967). This view suggests that causation of autism is related to the child's withdrawing from such rejection and erecting defensive barriers to the outside world to avoid psychological pain. Such reasoning is used to explain behavior that appears primarily to involve interactions with an inner world and little attention to the outside environment involving other people. Little recent attention has been given to psychodynamic explanations of etiology because they lack research support and do not correspond with clinical observations (Willick, 2001). Psychodynamic research currently explores the emotional and social interactions of these children (e.g., Dissanayke & Sigman, 2001; Fein, 2001).

Biological Theories

Children with autism and schizophrenia behave so bizarrely that many people believe they are afflicted with some physical disorder. Biological theorists view the causes of autism and schizophrenia as functions of birth trauma, viral infections such as German measles, and metabolic problems. Genetic factors have also attracted considerable attention as a cause of both autism and schizophrenia, although establishment of a solid database is still in progress (Herken & Erdal, 2001; Wassink, Piven, & Patil, 2001). Many of these presumed biological conditions correspond with these children's increased incidence of seizures, low birth weight, abnormal neurological measures such as electroencephalograph (EEG) and computer tomograph (CT), mental retardation, and poor motor development (Drew & Hardman, 2000).

In recent years, major advances in computer-guided imaging have given scientists the ability to view how different parts of the brain function under various conditions, such as mental problem-solving. Magnetic resonance imaging (MRI) and computer tomography (CT) scans are used to examine sizes and volumes of brain structures and produce pictures at different depths within the brain. Individuals with autism have shown some abnormal brain structures, including a larger cerebellum or hindbrain, a region associated with body movement, respiration, and other automatic functions (Hardan, Minshew, Harenski, & Keshavan, 2001; Purcell et al., 2001). One area of the brain, known as the *vermis*, has appeared abnormal, but not larger; it is located in the cerebellum, which might account for some of the cognitive anomalies found in autism (Hardan et al., 2001). The vermis appears to receive, organize, and distribute information (nerve signals) that controls automatic responses in the body (e.g., breathing, sweating, artery constriction) (Henderson et al., 2002; Nunneley et al., 2002). Research on the brain is continuing to clarify the practical effects of abnormalities in structures such as the vermis. MRI scans of patients with schizophrenia show some functional differences from those of individuals without the condition, such as reduced brain activity while performing motor tasks and lower blood oxygenation in the brain (Kodama et al., 2001; McDowell & Clementz, 2001). Figure 13-1 shows MRI scans of normal and schizophrenic brains. Further

study is needed, and continued advances in technology will likely facilitate this line of investigation.

Diseases affecting the central nervous system have been suspected of causing autistic-like symptoms in children. Prenatal infections are high on the list of suspects because of the neurological damage they can inflict (Drew & Hardman, 2000; Fatemi, Cuadra, El Fakahany, Sidwell, & Thuras, 2000). For example, exposure to rubella or influenza has been investigated as a risk factor for autism and childhood schizophrenia. Some researchers report evidence supporting such a linkage (Bagalkote, Pang, & Jones, 2001; Brown et al., 2001; Munk-Jorgensen & Ewald, 2001). However, further study is in order. Some have claimed that immunizing children for measles, mumps, and rubella has actually triggered the emergence of autism, but research evidence for this claim is not supportive (Dales, Hammer, & Smith, 2001). The herpes simplex virus has also been suspected of attacking the neurological system, resulting in symptoms of both autism and schizophrenia. As with other specific disease states, results are mixed. No single disease has been consistently identified as being the causative agent for either autism or schizophrenia (e.g., Oezcankaya, Mumcu, & Istanbullu, 2000).

Genetic factors can be involved in the development of a clinical condition in basically two ways. First, direct damage to the genetic material itself (the chromo-

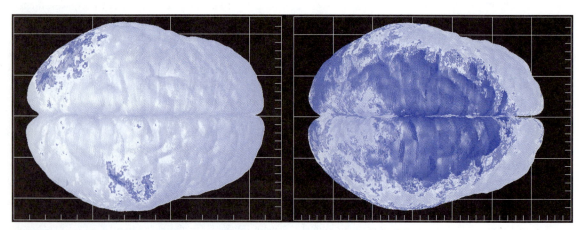

Figure 13-1   Magnetic Resonance Image Comparison: Normal Brain (left) and Schizophrenic Brain (right)
A full-color version of this figure appears on the inside front cover of this book.
SOURCE: Image courtesy of Paul Thompson, Ph.D., UCLA School of Medicine.

somes) can cause a defect. Second, an abnormality can be coded in the genetic material and passed on as an inherited characteristic. In the late 1960s, a new condition that was thought to have a major association with autism was discovered. The condition, known as *fragile X syndrome*, plays a role in causing mental retardation and also appears in a percentage of males having autism (Hatton & Bailey, 2001; Wassink et al., 2001). Although earlier research suggested that fragile X syndrome might be a significant causative factor for autism, more recent literature indicates that it appears in a relatively small percentage of youngsters with autism (5–8%) (Roberts, Mirrett, & Burchinal, 2001; Sudhalter & Belser, 2001). Current research on fragile X syndrome is investigating a variety of developmental differences associated with autism, rather than focusing on a causative relationship (Bailey, Hatton, Skinner, & Mesibov, 2001; Sabaratnam, 2000).

Substantial advances have been made in researching the roles of genetic factors in autism and childhood schizophrenia (e.g., Herken & Erdal, 2001; Wassink et al., 2001). Considerable information has been gained from twin studies, where pairs of identical (monozygotic) twins are compared to pairs of fraternal (dizygotic) twins to determine if there are differences in incidence of the disorders. These twin studies reveal a higher incidence of the two disorders in identical twins than in fraternal twins, which suggests a genetic link for both autism and childhood schizophrenia (Cardno, Sham, Murray, & McGuffin, 2001; Constantino & Todd, 2000; Rutter, 2000). However, this cannot and should not be interpreted to suggest that a single gene causes either condition. Here, as before, the data indicate polygenic influences. A great deal of work remains to be done in order to clarify the causative mechanisms involved and the way they operate. For example, chemical imbalances such as an excess of dopamine may contribute to schizophrenia; this is sometimes termed the *dopamine hypothesis*. The excess is observed because the dopamine receptors are overly sensitive or because an actual excess of dopamine is present (Balla, Koneru, Smiley, Sershen, & Javitt, 2001; Depatie & Lal, 2001). In either case, the condition is seen as genetically transmitted. Identifying a genetic factor is important, but it will be more difficult to explain how such a factor developmentally results in autism or childhood schizophrenia (e.g., Green, 2001).

Genetic studies of both autism and childhood schizophrenia suggest a polygenic model (involving many recessive genes from both parents) as causative in some of the cases. It also seems that these disorders exist as a *spectrum*, evidencing varying levels of severity as well as appearing in one member of a family while others are often unaffected (Herken & Erdal, 2001; Stodgell, Ingram, & Hyman, 2001). Although biological evidence is mounting, it would be incorrect to suggest that all cases of autism and childhood schizophrenia are genetically based. Many researchers now believe that there are multiple biological causes, especially for autism.

TREATMENT OF AUTISM AND CHILDHOOD SCHIZOPHRENIA

Treatments for autism and childhood schizophrenia are varied and many are controversial. Some of the controversy arises from the use of treatment approaches that seem to be based on questionable evidence (Hardman et al., 2002). This is the case with the treatment described in the Research Focus box. Other treatments seem to be very controlling and invasive or to involve punishment techniques. It is not difficult to understand why one would try almost any reasonable approach to save a child from self-injurious behavior or to teach a child to communicate with a parent. All the major types of approaches—including psychoanalytic, behavioral, and medical—have been used with children having autism and schizophrenia.

Psychoanalytic Approaches

Psychoanalytic approaches to treating autism and childhood schizophrenia were early pioneering efforts. However, their overall effectiveness in improving a severely impaired child's behavior is questionable (Willick, 2001). The length of time required for such treatment is very long and thus not considered cost-effective by most hospitals and social services agencies. Most important, the psychoanalytic assumption that parents cause the conditions is fundamentally in error. Such an assumption adds a great burden to a family's problems and separates parents from the treatment process. It is reasonable to conclude that apparent rejection and coldness is likely produced by

How Facilitated Is the Communication?

One of the most controversial treatments emerging in the early 1990s was used with individuals having autism, focusing specifically on their communication problems. Known as *facilitated communication*, this procedure was developed initially in Australia and employs typing as the means of communication in response to questions from others (Biklen, 1990, 1992). The therapist-facilitator provides interpersonal support by touching the student's arm, providing physical feedback through light pressure. The advocates of facilitative communication have been enthusiastically supportive although other researchers have not been able to obtain results suggesting its effectiveness. A number have raised serious questions regarding the soundness of facilitative communication and the research evidence supporting its use (Gresham, Beebe-Frankenberger, & MacMillan, 1999; Huebner & Emery, 1998; Witte-Bakken, 1998). Challenges have included suggestions that the therapist-facilitator is doing the communication rather than the person with autism. Clearly, further objective research using sound scientific methodology is needed to clarify the effectiveness of facilitative communication (Cormier & Cormier, 1998; Ivey & Ivey, 1999).

the child's relentlessly bizarre behavior rather than the reverse. Parents can be valuable assets to a comprehensive treatment approach.

Behavioral Approaches

Behavioral treatment appears attractive to many clinicians and educators because it is based on a thorough observation and evaluation of the child's behavior, treats problem behaviors directly, and includes parents as part of the treatment team (Clarke, 2001; Kauffman, 2001; Weiskop, Matthews, & Richdale, 2001). The basic behavioral approaches follow a consistent pattern. First, the child is closely observed, and empirical data on his or her behavior are recorded objectively for an extended period before treatment is initiated. This pretreatment data sample (baseline) is then used as a standard to evaluate the treatment effects. If the treatment is not effective, it is either stopped or changed. Behavioral excesses, such as self-stimulatory behavior, tantrums, self-injury, bizarre speech, and aggressive behaviors, are treated by ignoring the behavior, by reinforcement of an incompatible behavior, or by direct punishment techniques, such as a loss of tokens or the use of time-out. Behavioral deficits such as poor eye contact, failure to speak, and impoverished social skills are remedied by teaching and reinforcing appropriate replacement behaviors (e.g., Frea & Vittimberga, 2000; Ziedonis & Stern, 2001).

The most dramatic effects of the use of behavior management techniques have occurred in the treatment of severe self-stimulation, self-injury, and other discrete, targeted behaviors (Frea & Vittimberga, 2000; Goldstein, 1999). Behaviors such as head-banging, scratching, biting, and face-slapping can lead to disfigurement and blindness. Behavioral techniques such as time-out, overcorrection, and differential reinforcement of zero rates of behavior (DR0) or of other types of behavior have been effective in reducing self-injury.

Central among the important gains in treating autistic children has been the inclusion of parents as active members of the treatment team. Parents participate in goal-setting for their children and learn therapeutic and behavior management skills. Including parents is important because it gives them skills to successfully manage their child's behavior in the home setting, which decreases the probability that the child will be institutionalized. Parental participation in behavioral treatment programs has shown promising results (Ayers, Sellers, Schneider, Gottschling, & Soucar, 2001; Weiskop et al., 2001); such programs make parents important partners in their child's improvement rather than identifying them as causative agents in the child's disorder. Such approaches represent an important step toward normalization for both the youngster and the family. Family members have an enormous interest in intervention that shows *any* promise for improving the long-term status of their children who are diagnosed with autism. For example, the work of Lovaas and his colleagues in the Young Autism Project is promising in that participants appear to be functioning at a vastly improved level many years later, when some were 20 and 30 years old (McIntosh, 1999). Scientists are always skeptical, however, and research on this intervention approach is continuing.

Techniques employing the basic principles of applied behavior analysis are effective, but they do not cure children with autism or schizophrenia (nor does any other intervention). They effectively manage problematic behaviors (e.g., sleep problems) and teach needed survival behaviors (Clarke, 2001; Weiskop et al., 2001). The main effects of such treatments are teaching children some self-help skills and successfully keeping the children in the community with their families and not in institutions. These techniques are also more humane since they involve whole families in the treatment process.

Medical Approaches

Medical treatment of children with autism and schizophrenia has included a number of different therapies, including psychosurgery, electroconvulsive shock, and drug therapies. The more drastic approaches such as psychosurgery and electroconvulsive shock have mostly been abandoned because of the possible harmful side effects and doubtful therapeutic effects (Hardman et al., 2002; Kauffman, 2001). Controversial drug therapies fruitlessly used with autistic and schizophrenic children include D-lysergic acid (LSD-25) and megavitamin treatment with vitamin B.

The major advances in medication-based treatment for schizophrenic children have involved the use of antipsychotic and other medications directed at controlling behavior and managing symptoms (Allison & Casey, 2001; Remington, Sloman, Konstantareas, Parker, & Gow, 2001). Antipsychotic medications work well with psychotic adults and are more effective with older children with autism and schizophrenia than with younger ones (Posey & McDougle, 2000; Romera & Gurpegui, 2001). These medications help reduce bizarre speech and aggressive behaviors and appear to help "organize" the child's behavior. An-

tipsychotic medications have also been found to be effective in reducing self-injurious behavior, particularly if they are part of a treatment program that includes other elements (e.g., behavioral techniques) and is designed for the individual's contextual circumstances (Moes & Frea, 2000). However, problems with using antipsychotic medication with children include side effects and overuse. Side effects include weight gain, drowsiness (which reduces the ability to learn), and, if the medications are used for an extended period of time, troublesome involuntary motor movements (dyskinesia) (Allison & Casey, 2001; Remington et al., 2001) Most authors agree that no single medication can effectively treat the heterogeneous symptoms found in autism or childhood schizophrenia (e.g., Posey & McDougle, 2000).

Medications often used for treatment of autism include antipsychotic, serotonergic, and dopaminergic drugs (Posey & McDougle, 2000). As with schizophrenia, specific symptoms tend to be treated with particular medications, such as clomipramine for obsessive-compulsive behaviors. Decreasing self-injurious behavior, managing obsessive-compulsive behaviors, and diminishing social withdrawal have been effectively accomplished with medication (Aman, Arnold, & Armstrong, 1999; Remington et al., 2001). Despite evidence for successful treatment in some children, medication is not universally effective across ages or individuals with the same diagnosis, emphasizing again that both autism and schizophrenia encompass a great deal of variability (Posey & McDougle, 2000). Continued research on the use of medication with those having autism is important, and the medications must be improved in safety and efficacy (Schreibman, 2000; Wolery, 2000).

As a treatment for children with autism and schizophrenia, medication is relatively inexpensive, less time-consuming than psychological interventions, and easily administered. These benefits are also the drug's most damaging drawbacks. It is too easy to medicate a difficult child and let him or her languish in the back room of a treatment facility. States of stupor induced by high doses of drugs reduce aggression and bizarre forms of behavior. However, such drug-induced stupor interferes with learning and wastes precious time during which a child might be acquiring new skills. Also, medication has no long-lasting effects. Once the drug is withdrawn, the symptoms often reappear.

Drugs are best used in moderate dosages, under close medical supervision, and in conjunction with other forms of therapy that are designed for the individual in his or her context (Moes & Frea, 2000).

PROGNOSIS FOR CHILDREN WITH AUTISM OR SCHIZOPHRENIA

Without adequate treatment, children with autism or schizophrenia will not improve a great deal as they develop and grow older. Although specific treatment programs may substantially improve functional skills and independent functioning, what is functional for one individual may include traditional academics, while for another it may be basic self-help or self-protection skills. Interventions certainly lead to some successes, although those advances may not be permanent and support networks are not as available for adults as they are for afflicted children (Moxon & Gates, 2001; Sperry, 2001; Walton, 2000).

Intelligence level is one of the most important predictors of future outcome for children with autism. Intelligence is a very stable characteristic that typically does not improve with treatment or special education programs. Near-normal intelligence in young childhood predicts better adjustment in adulthood, although even higher-functioning individuals with autism tend to retain some self-stimulatory behavior and exhibit concrete thinking and inadequate social adjustment. Language seems to be a critical element when IQ is above 50. If the child's IQ is above 50 but the child does speak, then the prognosis is fair. If the child has only a mild language disorder and normal nonverbal intelligence, the prognosis is good. Unsurprisingly, the long-term prognosis for individuals with autism is as variable as the unique characteristics they present (Howlin, 2000). Long-term planning by parents of children with autism requires a great deal of foresight and effort, typically with help and involvement from multiple agencies (Hardman et al., 2002; Moxon & Gates, 2001). School placement and living arrangements are very important and considerably influence the constellation of services available. As with other disability conditions, placement in large institutions frequently harms children with autism or schizophrenia, again with substantial varia-

Table 13-4 Factors Related to Poor and Good Outcomes for Children with Autism and Schizophrenia		
	Poor Outcome	Good Outcome
Autism		
Language before age 5		X
IQ normal		X
IQ below 50	X	
Placement in institution	X	
Placement with trained parents		X
Early intervention		X
Comprehensive treatment services		X
Childhood Schizophrenia		
IQ above average		X
IQ below average	X	
Onset before age 10	X	
Acute onset		X
Slow onset	X	
Identifiable precipitating event		X
Good social skills		X

tion between individuals (Evans et al., 1999; Friedman et al., 2001; Lenior, Dingemans, Linszen, deHaan, & Schene, 2001). Individual treatment programs and educational opportunities are often much more limited in large institutions.

The course and outcome of childhood schizophrenia differ for those with early onset compared to those whose symptoms emerge later. Youngsters with earlier manifestations of symptoms appear to be more severely affected and have a relatively poor prognosis (Consenza, Bruni, & Muratori, 2001; Karp et al., 2001). The earlier the onset, before age 10, the lower the chance of a favorable outcome. Additionally, a slowly developing condition, which takes a great deal of time to manifest itself completely, appears associated with a poor adjustment in childhood. This slow, or insidious, onset is contrasted with an acute onset, which is often precipitated by a stressful event, such as a family member's death or parental divorce. Table 13-4 summarizes the prognostic indicators for both autism and childhood schizophrenia.

Back to the Beginning

Jake's Progress

Jake has been through 2 years, 700 days, 4,160 hours, and thousands of trials of ABA therapy. Gradually, his language began to come in, as did his social and developmental skills. He potty trained at 3. He had his first friend at $3\frac{1}{2}$. At 4, he sang "Happy Birthday" to me.

We began to mainstream Jake at a "typical" preschool last year, and with the aid of shadows (trained therapists), Jake is beginning to thrive in the school setting. The shadows work closely with his teachers, who report that Jake is fitting in. To his classmates, Jake is just like them. I know that my son still needs help—not in the same way that I knew two years ago when I found Jake lying face down in the driveway. I can see it in his eyes. He doesn't understand story time the way the other kids do. And his language skills are still behind his peers.

Jake's circuit breakers, which gradually shut down after 17 months, have almost all clicked back on. But until all of them are on, Franklin and I are committed to continue with his therapy. We'll do it until we are sure that Jake can make it on his own.

The son we thought we'd lost has come back to us. We don't want to lose him again. (Siff, 2001)

Were Jake's parents wise to follow the plan they did? There are several facts that suggest they did pretty well in taking this route. One is the research base for applied behavior analysis (ABA). This is a general term for a broad protocol that was developed and promulgated based on data—something that certainly cannot be said for some other therapies. One foundation principle of ABA therapy is that it is data driven; if the data from observations do not suggest something is working (resulting in improvement), the procedure is modified or terminated in favor of another tactic that does work.

Jake's parents should be praised for another aspect of their therapy plan. This has not been an easy road—2 years, 700 days, 4,160 hours, and thousands of trials! They did not succumb to some of the easier, seemingly "silver bullet" therapies that promise cures. This has not been nor will it be an undemanding undertaking. But these parents did elect a strategy with a higher probability of success than some alternatives.

SUMMARY

Pervasive developmental disorders, as defined in DSM-IV-TR, include autism, Rett's disorder, childhood disintegrative disorder, Asperger's disorder, and pervasive developmental disorder not otherwise specified. This chapter has examined autism and childhood schizophrenia in depth, with some attention given to Asperger's disorder.

Most researchers and clinicians now consider autism and childhood schizophrenia to be separate disorders with several basic differences. The same cannot be said for autism and Asperger's disorder. Current literature focuses considerable attention on whether autism is a disorder distinct from Asperger's disorder or whether the two represent variations along a spectrum of conditions. This issue has some potentially important practical ramifications for diagnosis and treatment.

There are a number of similarities and differences between autism and childhood schizophrenia. Autism is primarily characterized as a disorder in relating to other people that generally develops before 30 months of age. Problems in social behavior can include poor eye contact, avoidance of social interactions, and a lack of basic social skills such as smiling or showing empathy. Along with problems in social relations, children with autism also have language problems. They exhibit high rates of self-stimulatory behavior or self-injurious behavior, and 75% of them have mental retardation. High rates of self-stimulatory behavior, poor intellectual functioning, and a lack of language skills limit a child's ability to relate to other people.

In contrast to autism, childhood schizophrenia is characterized primarily as a thought or cognitive-emotional disorder that develops late in childhood. Hallucinations, an inability to connect thoughts logically, and a withdrawal into a fantasy world are common for the schizophrenic child. Unlike many children having autism, children with schizophrenia generally develop good language skills and have near-normal intelligence. Periods of marked improvement and relapse are characteristic of the child with schizophrenia; autism runs a more steady course, with smaller irregularities in the behavioral symptoms from childhood through adulthood.

Like most of the severe child behavior disorders, autism and childhood schizophrenia appear not to have a single cause but are complex in their origins. Birth complications, diseases, and genetics are suspected of contributing to the development of autism and schizophrenia. The origins of these conditions appear primarily biological in nature, although environmental factors can interact to improve or worsen the course. Inadequate parenting does not cause autism or childhood schizophrenia.

Effective treatment approaches for autism and childhood schizophrenia have been slow in coming. These children typically do not profit from long-term separation from their families and community due to placement in large institutions. Promising new approaches for these children emphasize getting them into treatment at a young age and including family members as part of the treatment effort. Structured behavioral approaches are effective in reducing many bizarre behaviors and teaching more appropriate and adaptive behaviors. Medication may also be effective in reducing problematic behaviors in some cases. However, it should be emphasized that both medication and behavior therapy only manage the behavioral symptoms of these conditions and do not produce cures. The long-term effectiveness of these approaches is promising but only if treatment continues. Variables that best appear to predict later adjustment include the child's intelligence, language usage, and age of onset of the condition.

INFOTRAC COLLEGE EDITION

For more information, explore this resource at http://www.infotrac-college.com/Wadsworth. Enter the following search terms:

Asperger's disorder
autism
childhood disintegrative disorder
childhood schizophrenia
pervasive developmental disorder
behavior therapy for children
drug therapy

IN FOCUS ANSWERS

IN FOCUS 1 ▶ Identify the five categories of pervasive developmental disorders according to DSM-IV-TR.

- Autism
- Rett's disorder
- Childhood disintegrative disorder
- Asperger's disorder
- Pervasive development disorder not otherwise specified

IN FOCUS 2 ▶ What is the general prevalence estimate for autism?

- Most sources suggest 4 to 8 cases per 10,000 individuals.
- Some estimates based on the autistic spectrum concept range from 6 to over 20 per 10,000.

IN FOCUS 3 ▶ Identify four areas of functional challenge often found in children with autism.

- Language
- Interpersonal skills
- Intellectual functioning
- Emotional or affective behaviors

IN FOCUS 4 ▶ Identify several differences in language or communication between autism and Asperger's disorder.

- Asperger's disorder is characterized by no clinically significant general delay in language whereas autism often has a delay or total lack of spoken language development.

- Autism has a marked impairment in initiating or sustaining conversations (by those with adequate speech) whereas Asperger's disorder does not show this impairment.
- Autism often involves a stereotyped and repetitive use of language or idiosyncratic language—this is not so with Asperger's disorder.

IN FOCUS 5 ▶ What are some abnormal social interactions that are characteristic of those with autism but not those with Asperger's disorder?

- Those with autism may not engage in social communication at all, while those with Asperger's disorder may have limited or atypical social interactions.
- Autism is characterized by a lack of varied, spontaneous play or social imitative play at an appropriate developmental level; Asperger's is not.

IN FOCUS 6 ▶ What are the primary differences between autism and childhood schizophrenia?

- Autism is defined as basically a condition in which social relationships are greatly disturbed; childhood schizophrenia, on the other hand, is characterized by thought disorder and hallucinations.
- There is a marked difference in the time of first occurrence. Autism tends to appear early in life (peak age of onset is before age $2\frac{1}{2}$). Schizophrenia appears later in childhood and early adolescence (the greatest risk period is from 7 to 15 years of age).
- Children with autism often have mental retardation, whereas those with schizophrenia tend to have normal intelligence.
- Children with schizophrenia often have hallucinations, while those with autism do not.
- Children with autism often exhibit early abnormal development, whereas those with schizophrenia tend to develop normally and then withdraw into a fantasy world.

14 Psychology and Children's Health

In the Beginning

Serious Eating Problems

- Scott is 11 years old. Although he has inherited his large frame from his over 6-foot father, he is still very overweight and has a waddling walk. And he is teased about his weight. The other boys call him Jumbo and joke that no peanut is safe around him. Scott laughs good-naturedly, but it hurts, and he just tries to avoid them as much as possible. That's easy, because he is now too fat to run much or play any sports, so he sits on the sidelines and comforts himself with something to drink or eat. His favorite lunch is a couple of corn dogs and a few chocolate doughnuts, washed down with a cola, which he and his mom enjoy together. Lately, he has become drowsy, dropping off to sleep during class or in front of the TV set. Perhaps he will just grow out of it when he becomes a teenager—or perhaps not.

- Tina, aged 18, is just the opposite. She would be horrified at the thought of eating high-calorie snacks or drinks and, in fact, tries to limit her food to 700 calories a day. If she doesn't begin to eat more very soon, she will have to be hospitalized for supervised, or forced, eating. She has studied ballet for years, and she thinks her weight is still high by dance standards. Tina is 5 feet 7 inches tall and weighs less than 100 pounds, and her weight is dropping. In addition to her ballet classes twice a week, she tries to exercise and run several miles a day, but she is beginning to have dizzy spells. Last week, she fainted in her dance class and her instructor will not allow her to come back until she gets treatment.

What these two youngsters have in common is a serious eating problem. Scott's problem is not officially listed as a mental disorder, because obesity is not reliably associated with any particular psychological problems (American Psychiatric Association, 2000). However, childhood obesity is a very ominous threat to later health and heightens the risk of diabetes, cardiovascular disease, and muscular and skeletal damage. A child's quality of life is definitely endangered by obesity. In contrast, Tina's anorexia nervosa is recognized as a mental disorder, and it presents an even more immediate threat to life than obesity. Expert professional intervention is required for both of these young people and their parents so that they will enjoy a full and healthy life.

INTRODUCTION

The health-related disorders examined in this chapter have been viewed in different perspectives in the child psychopathology literature (Steinhausen & Verhulst, 1999). Some authors view them as primarily physiological (e.g., Scott's obesity is genetic and shared with the rest of his family), others as psychological (e.g., Scott eats to feel better about being rejected). Similarly, Tina's anorexia and associated disturbances could be shared by other family members, and so could be largely hereditary. However, her problems could also be mainly psychological, since anorexia rates are increasing along with social pressures to be thin and physically active. Since they cannot be distinguished as purely physical or completely psychological, this group of disorders is now most often viewed as having both physical and mental components. All three of these etiological views (biological, psychological, and both) are correct to some degree because the disorders presented here have varying elements depending on the patient and the social and family context. In many cases, research has indicated that the most effective treatment is a combination of physiological and behavioral interventions. Drugs can address a physiological imbalance or suppress unwanted behaviors, while psychotherapies alter faulty cognitive and behavioral patterns.

This chapter points out the causes and adjustment difficulties associated with conditions such as eating disorders, elimination problems, sleep disorders, and speech disorders. In each instance, we describe the types of interventions that are helpful in preventing or treating the disorder.

EATING DISORDERS

Most of us try but often fail to maintain a healthful weight and get an adequate amount of exercise. Many people surrender to the constant temptation to eat too much rich food, often while parked in front of the TV set or the computer for hours at a time. So, a very large portion of the U.S. population fails to maintain a healthy routine despite the wide availability of nutritious food, recreational activities, and sound health advice from schools, physicians, government agencies, and news media. The national tendency is to eat richer foods, become less physically active, and put on weight. Worried about this, some young people try drastic calorie-reduction programs that can slip out of their control. We discuss these dangers in this chapter.

In fact, most people are dissatisfied with their bodies, and few parents are totally happy with the eating habits of their children. Food is an essential part of our lives, and we hold strong beliefs about what, when, and how much we should eat and how much we should weigh. Food is also big business. Restaurants, supermarkets, and food processors and distributors prosper by offering a wide variety of calorie-rich processed foods and fast foods laden with salt, sugar, and fat. For health-conscious consumers, there are natural foods, organic foods, and diet foods. There is a massive economic stake in people's food preferences. Food and food advertising are everywhere and inescapable. Eating is a huge issue in our culture, and it relates closely to our psychological needs ("Food is love." "Thin is beautiful."), as well as our physical and emotional health.

We examine three abnormal eating conditions in this section: anorexia nervosa, bulimia nervosa, and obesity. All three involve a persistent inability to regulate food intake and result in significant health risks. Anorexia is a form of self-starvation that is particularly puzzling because it occurs in a culture of abundance. In a land of plenty, anorexic youngsters deny themselves food until they are actually starving, all the while insisting they are fat. Bulimic teenagers try to maintain a slender appearance by resisting overeating as long as they can, but then consume thousands of calories in eating binges and induce vomiting and/or diarrhea so that the food is not digested. All this suffering is in the service of an impossible dream of achieving physical perfection (Halmi et al., 2000). There are too many obese children like Scott, who buy super-sized soft drinks to sip all day long, eat giant burgers complete with fries, and then go on to overeat at regular meal times. Too obese to exercise, such a child has sacrificed a social life, normal activities, and long-term health because of the love of eating. Food is the one addictive substance we cannot avoid, and overeating is one of the more difficult addictions to manage.

Anorexia Nervosa

IN FOCUS 1 ▶ Identify four characteristics that are often observed in victims of anorexia nervosa.

The typical victim of anorexia nervosa first shows signs of the disorder when she is between the ages of 14 and 18 years, the period when most girls have entered puberty and become acutely aware of fashion trends and their own maturing sexuality. **Anorexia nervosa** is a condition of self-inflicted starvation accompanied by compulsive exercising. Anorexia nervosa is primarily a female disorder, with 90% or more of the victims being female (American Psychiatric Association, 2000). Rather than viewing normal body changes associated with puberty, such as accumulation of fatty tissue in thighs, buttocks, and breasts, as a sign of physical maturity, the anorexic girl views them with alarm, as evidence that she is becoming fat. To avoid this imagined fate, the girl begins to restrict her calorie intake severely and to increase her exercise in a frantic effort to reduce. She feels compelled to be perfect, and the thinner she is, the more nearly perfect she will be. Never satisfied with her weight, the anorexic young woman may reduce her food intake further and eat an unbalanced diet featuring only certain foods, often vegetables. She shows physical signs of starvation, all the while complaining that she has fat thighs and buttocks and needs to reduce. Her sexual appeal and interests diminish along with her weight, which has led to speculation that anorexic youngsters are conflicted about sex and want to continue to be children. She will listen to no one about the damage she is doing to her body by her self-starvation. Meanwhile, the dangers of starvation are real. Uncontrolled anorexia nervosa can result in premature death. If the victim becomes so severely malnourished that she must be hospitalized, her long-term mortality risk is over 10%, a highly significant danger (American Psychiatric Association, 2000). When all cases of anorexia are considered, including milder ones, the overall death rate drops to 5.9%, which is still excessive for young people. Suicide accounts for 27% of those deaths (Sullivan, 1995).

The sheer numbers of news stories about anorexia nervosa and famous personalities who died of its complications, such as singer Karen Carpenter, may mistakenly suggest that the condition is extremely common. Although anorexia nervosa continues to be very

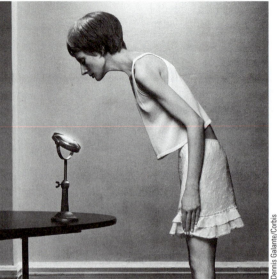

Anorexia nervosa is a life-threatening condition for a significant proportion of those affected.

rare, it is diagnosed increasingly often in recent years. Still, very few people develop all of the symptoms of the disorder. The estimated prevalence varies from 0.5% of women having diagnosable anorexia nervosa sometime in their lives (American Psychiatric Association, 2000) to much higher estimates: For example, 1% of teenage girls will develop a full case of anorexia, with an additional 5% having a mild case (Andersen, 1999). Milder forms of eating restriction are common in a society that prizes thinness and discriminates against people who are noticeably overweight. There is some evidence and considerable anecdotal reporting of a very high prevalence of anorexia nervosa for those involved in activities such as modeling, ballet, and gymnastics, although it should be noted that this is difficult to investigate and empirical data are sketchy (de Jonge & van Furth, 1999; Neumaerker, Bettle, Neumaerker, & Bettle, 2000). As their anorexia proceeds, young women may develop the binge-purge patterns characteristic of bulimia nervosa (Bulik & Sullivan, 1997). They are then diagnosed as having the binge-eating/purging type of anorexia nervosa described in DSM-IV-TR (American Psychiatric Association, 2000). The other type of anorexia nervosa is the restricting type, which involves self-starvation but not bingeing and purging. According to DSM-IV-TR, to be diagnosed with anorexia nervosa, a person must have a weight at least 15% below normal (calculated by life insurance tables or body mass index), although the weight deficit may be much higher in individual cases. The DSM-IV-TR diagnostic criteria for anorexia nervosa are summarized in Table 14-1.

Social History of Anorexia Nervosa

When the hourglass, well-fleshed figure was in fashion a century ago, anorexia nervosa was much less prevalent. However, in the 1920s, with the advent of form-fitting "flapper" styles and ready-made clothing, women became aware of dress sizes. Smaller sizes became desirable, and with this trend came eating disorders (Brumberg, 2000). This line of reasoning is persuasive because of the predominance of style-conscious women among anorexic patients and the increasing prevalence of restrictive eating disorders in the 20th century, particularly in the richer, more industrialized countries with thriving fashion industries (Jimerson & Pavelski, 2000; Lai, 2000; Thomsen, McCoy, & Williams, 2001). Within these societies, families from what might be considered the more fashionable and exercise-conscious upper socioeconomic classes contribute more than their share of the anorexics (Brumberg, 2000). Ironically, true anorexia nervosa is extremely rare in economically deprived groups and during wars and famines, when food is scarce and survival is uncertain.

Personality Traits Associated with Anorexia Nervosa

Certain personality traits are strongly associated with anorexia. Perfectionists are at especially high risk for developing this disorder (Halmi et al., 2000). Levenkron (2000) says, "A child who becomes anorexic is using her body to express her need for perfectionism" (p. 22). These young women are also likely to suffer from excessive self-criticism, guilt, depression, and anxiety (Westen & Harnden-Fischer, 2001). They are typically very hard on themselves and conscientious to a fault, appearing to be good daughters and exemplary students.

Anorexics seem to be driven by a need to be thin or, more specifically, by an obsession to avoid being fat, which they equate with being bad. Ironically, few anorexic patients actually have a history of being overweight, though many are convinced that they once were. In fact, most descriptions of them as children include terms such as "problem-free," and they may defer to others almost to a point of being overly docile about non-food-related matters. (See Tracy's Story.)

Family Factors

Eating disorders often run in families, and first-degree relatives of anorexic individuals are also likely to have mild forms of eating disorders, major depressive disorder, and obsessive-compulsive disorder. Anorexia is calculated to have a moderately high heritability of 58%, although some family resemblances could be due to environment rather than to shared genes (Wade, Bulik,

Table 14-1 DSM-IV-TR Diagnostic Criteria for Anorexia Nervosa
A. Refusal to maintain body weight at or above a minimally normal weight for age and height (e.g., weight loss leading to maintenance of body weight less than 85% of that expected; or failure to make expected weight gain during period of growth, leading to body weight less than 85% of that expected).
B. Intense fear of gaining weight or becoming fat, even though underweight.
C. Disturbance in the way in which one's body weight or shape is experienced, undue influence of body weight or shape on self-evaluation, or denial of the seriousness of the current low body weight.
D. In postmenarcheal females, amenorrhea, i.e., the absence of at least three consecutive menstrual cycles. (A woman is considered to have amenorrhea if her periods occur only following hormone, e.g., estrogen, administration.)

Specify type:

Restricting Type: during the current episode of Anorexia Nervosa, the person has not regularly engaged in binge-eating or purging behavior (i.e., self-induced vomiting or the misuse of laxatives, diuretics, or enemas)

Binge-Eating/Purging Type: during the current episode of Anorexia Nervosa, the person has regularly engaged in binge-eating or purging behavior (i.e., self-induced vomiting or the misuse of laxatives, diuretics, or enemas)

SOURCE: American Psychiatric Association (2000), p. 589. Reprinted with permission from the *Diagnostic and Statistical Manual of Mental Disorders*, 4th ed., Text Revision. © 2000 APA.

Tracy's Story

Overcoming Anorexia

Tracy came to therapy at the age of 19, in her sophomore year of college, where she was getting good grades. She had a boyfriend from high school but had made few friends at college. Tracy stood 5'6" tall and weighed about 98 pounds. She had started losing weight deliberately about 2 years earlier, although she had been thin even then, weighing about 120. She just started eating less and less; losing weight became the most important thing in her life, although she couldn't explain why. When she came to me, Tracy was frankly unhappy about the prospect of gaining weight, but she was also frightened by feelings of fatigue, the loss of her period for over 6 months, and her difficulty in being able to concentrate on school work.

As the younger sister of an unpredictable, rebellious, angry girl, Tracy felt obligated to be a "problem-free" child for her parents. She had witnessed countless fights between her parents and sister and listened endlessly to her parents complaining about her sister. Tracy was praised by her parents for being a good student, responsible, and considerate. Tracy had become entirely oriented toward pleasing others. She learned to hide her negative feelings, conceal different opinions, and had become exceptionally intuitive about other people's wishes and needs.

Whenever possible, Tracy kept her problems to herself. She carried her silence even to the point of telling no one when she was attacked and raped on the way home from school when she was 14.

As high school graduation grew closer, Tracy began to restrict her food intake. She counted calories constantly, began to eliminate whole food groups from her diet, and spent hours inspecting her body for fat. She knew that she was afraid to go away to college. She feared that her mother would become depressed without her. She felt guilty about starting a life of her own and confused about what her parents really wanted her to do about going to college. Tracy did not realize that her overwhelming terror of making a mistake played a major part in her anorexia nervosa.

Family and friends expressed concern about Tracy's weight loss, but she held them off with excuses and with promises to gain. She decided on her own to pursue psychotherapy because of worries about her physical health. After Tracy and I discussed her diagnosis of anorexia nervosa, we agreed to the following treatment plan: a complete medical evaluation by a physician familiar with eating disorders; weight gain at the rate of 1–2 pounds a week; a target weight of 122; weekly "weigh-ins" at the doctor's office (in a hospital gown after voiding, and supervised by the doctor or nurse); and psychotherapy once or twice weekly, depending on her progress.

Tracy took over one and a half years to reach her target weight. She would gain and lose. For a long time, she described her food intake as "huge," when in fact she was eating under 2,000 calories per day (on which she could not gain). Her fatigue and poor concentration, which she correctly understood as the effects of malnutrition, helped motivate her to stop restricting her food.

Psychotherapy centered on three broad topics: her "addiction" to food restriction and how to recover from it, her feelings about her family and about herself as a part of her family, and her body image problems.

Tracy was able to grasp the concept of "addiction to restriction" very easily. She also saw that she would have to learn new coping skills in place of her "addiction." She remained, however, very guarded on the topic of her family. She was able to express some resentment toward her sister, but she just couldn't acknowledge any negative feelings toward her parents. Her body image problems had a lot to do with the rape at age 14. Tracy did come to feel and express her reactions to that trauma, her self-blame, her shame, and last of all, her anger.

Tracy achieved her goal weight and maintained it for over 6 months before ending her psychotherapy. She would return to anorexic ways of thinking when pressured or stressed, but she could resist the temptation to restrict her food. She had also expanded her social network at school, was able to participate in "fun things," share intimate stories with friends, and be silly when she felt like it.

SOURCE: Wagner (1992), pp. 58–59.

Neale, & Kendler, 2000). To summarize, people with anorexia nervosa tend to be intellectually bright and per-fectionistic, overly sensitive, and self-critical, and they may exhibit depression, anxiety, and compulsive behav-iors such as repetitive cleaning rituals (Price Founda-tion Collaborative Group, 2001; Reisch, Thommen, Tschacher, & Hirsbrunner, 2001). Their close relatives also show higher than average rates of these internaliz-ing problems (Lilenfield et al., 1998), which suggests, but does not prove, that anorexia has a genetic basis.

The Course of Anorexia Nervosa

Most anorexics describe experiences that they believe prompted or precipitated their unusual eating behavior. Often the behavior was triggered by some rather com-mon or trivial event that made them feel too heavy or not respected. Sometimes they attribute their problem to a sexual experience or attack. The onset of the disorder is usually quite sudden; victims dramatically reduce their

food intake and begin a rigorous exercise regimen. As the weight loss and compulsive exercise continue, family members or friends notice that the youngster is becom-ing too thin or is beginning to look ill and emaciated. De-spite even strong objections from others, anorexics deny that they are thin and continue their self-destructive be-havior. There is no reasoning with them. Their high ac-tivity level typically continues until they reach such a weakened state that it must be abandoned. They become fatigued and dizzy and may faint when they try to con-tinue exercising. The true anorexic pursues the destruc-tive routine until physically unable to go on.

Physiological changes go far beyond the reduction of body fat and include a wasting of muscle tissue, car-diovascular problems, and alterations of bone marrow, as well as a variety of other health problems associ-ated with starvation (Mehler & Crews, 2001). The physical effects of anorexia-induced starvation are listed in Table 14-2.

Table 14-2 Some Physical Effects of Self-Starvation in Anorexia Nervosa

Cardiac Signs and Symptoms
Heart shrinkage and actual loss of heart tissue.
Very slow heart rate, may lead to marked fatigue.
Cardiac palpitations or arrythmias.
Hypotension (low blood pressure), leading to lightheadedness, dizziness, fainting.
Heart valve clicks, murmurs, may result in chest pain.
Hypothermia, cold extremities, cold intolerance, blue fingers and toes, generally feeling cold compared to peers.
Edema, resulting in swelling of extremities, face, or around eyes.

Gastrointestinal Signs and Symptoms
Gastroparesis (delayed stomach emptying) may result in bloating or nausea.
Constipation may cause abdominal pain.

Dermatological Signs and Symptoms
Dry skin.
Hair loss on head but growth of downy hair on face, neck, arms, legs, and back.
Brittle nails and hair.
Yellowish skin, especially on palms.

Gynecological Signs and Symptoms
Cessation of menstruation.

Skeletal Signs and Symptoms
Osteoporosis contributing to bone loss, fragility, and unexplained fractures.

NOTE: The most prominent signs of anorexia nervosa are severe weight loss and emaciated appearance not due to any other illness. Hyperactivity and excessive exercising are common. Elevated death rate in severe, persistent cases.
SOURCES: American Psychiatric Association (2000); Andersen (1999).

Female patients' menstruation ceases, fails to begin, or becomes infrequent and painful. The body's protective layers of flesh diminish so markedly that the heart becomes small and weak, blood pressure and pulse rate fall, and the woman becomes hypersensitive to the cold. Her flesh is so sparse that she finds it painful to sit on a hard surface such as a wooden chair or in a bathtub. Frequent bruising also occurs as the disorder progresses. Clearly, anorexia nervosa is so dangerous that even seemingly mild cases must be monitored and treated.

Etiology of Anorexia Nervosa

It is difficult to understand how anorexia nervosa can develop. All of their "good," conforming behavior should earn young perfectionists praise and approval and prevent them from developing destructive self-images. Further, why do seemingly trivial occurrences trigger their anorexia? While the events that reportedly precipitate the eating problem vary greatly in magnitude, they often seem too minor to cause a serious disorder (e.g., a joking comment from a classmate about the youngster's weight or habits). Despite much study, the etiology of anorexia nervosa remains unclear. Some writers have attributed the disorder to genetic factors (the significant heritability mentioned previously), hormonal and endocrine problems that affect appetite, or malfunction of the hypothalamus (Brambilla et al., 2001; Corcos et al., 2001; Klump, Miller, Keel, McGue, & Iacono, 2001). Others point to psychological problems as potential causes, including obsessive-compulsive tendencies, depression, and other emotional disturbances that frequently accompany anorexia (Harel, Hallett, Riggs, Vaz, & Kiessling, 2001; Price Foundation Collaborative Group, 2001; Zalsman, Weizman, Carel, & Aizenberg, 2001). Neither genetic nor environmental influences can be ruled out as reasons for the heightened risk for developing anorexia if a family member has the disorder. However, social, cultural, and even economic factors must also be at work to increase the rate of this eating disorder so much and so quickly. Further research is clearly needed to study all possible etiological factors (Dare, Chania, Eisler, Hodes, & Dodge, 2001; Engelsen & Laberg, 2001).

Treatment of Anorexia Nervosa

IN FOCUS 2 ▶ Identify the steps for treating anorexia nervosa.

The treatment process for anorexia nervosa is often long-term and complex because it must focus on both physical and psychological factors. One of the immediate needs is to correct the individual's nutrition problem and achieve medical stabilization before the condition produces irreversible physical damage or becomes fatal. The combination of starvation and purging with laxatives or vomiting seen in the binge-eating/purging type of the disorder is particularly dangerous. Restoring a normal diet can be difficult, since many patients will resist, attempt to exercise surreptitiously, secretly induce vomiting, or even escape from the treatment unit; but appropriate nutrition is essential in order to begin reversing the physical deterioration (Watson, Bowers, & Andersen, 2000).

Many therapeutic procedures have been employed, including hospitalization, individual and group psychotherapy, family psychotherapy, drug treatment, force-feeding, cognitive-behavioral therapy to improve self-image and eating habits, and provision of information regarding the ill effects of restricted eating (Mehler & Crews, 2001; Neiderman, Farley, Richardson, & Lask, 2001; Ruggiero et al., 2001). Treatment must address a variety of factors, since the weight and nutrition problems may be symptoms of other persistent psychological difficulties.

Therapists often focus on the relationships among family members, particularly for youngsters still living at home. Often such treatment is aimed at moderating the family's expectations for conforming, obedience, and striving to achieve, since these children seem to try too hard to meet parental expectations. Therapy approaches may be combinations of the interventions noted above and often include family counseling (Jimerson & Pavelski, 2000; Miller & Pumariega, 2001). Family therapy seems to have more lasting benefits than individual therapy, as judged at a 5-year follow-up (Eisler et al., 1997). Over a 4- to 10-year period and after several years of treatment, about 50% of anorexics recover in weight and menstrual function and most of the remainder are in various stages of recovery (Hsu, 1999).

Most patients do not improve dramatically with medication, although fluoxetine, a selective serotonin reuptake inhibitor (SSRI) used for depression, may help them maintain weight after discharge from the hospital (Kaye, 1999). Fluoxetine has not been found useful earlier, during in-patient treatment (Attia, Haiman, Walsh, & Flater, 1998).

Even with intense therapy regimens, anorexia nervosa is a difficult disorder to treat, because the patient must overcome the delusion about being overweight, strictly follow her therapists' instructions, stop falsifying her actual eating and exercise amounts, and stop purging after eating. To recover, she must eat large amounts of highly nutritious food, initially enough to gain about 2 pounds per week. This is a huge challenge for a food phobic who believes she is hideously fat. However, as patients begin to gain weight, their anxiety and depression also improve (Hsu, 1999). The best prognosis is for those who were ill a shorter time, lost less weight, did not induce vomiting, and had better early adjustment and family functioning (Hsu, 1999). Women who have recovered from this eating disorder may continue to be plagued by perfectionism, exactness, and a sense of loss of control in important areas of their lives (Button & Warren, 2001). Clearly, anorexia nervosa is not a simple disorder. The most effective treatment is individually tailored to address the individual's many problems.

Bulimia Nervosa

IN FOCUS 3 ▶ How are bulimia nervosa and anorexia nervosa different?

Bulimia nervosa is an eating disorder in which there are frequent episodes of uncontrolled binge eating alternating with purging of what has been consumed. During such eating binges, a person may ingest enormous quantities of food in a very short time. Although estimates vary widely, it has been reported that bulimics may consume between 1,200 and 55,000 calories in a single binge, and some individuals binge on a daily basis (Weiss, Katzman, & Wolchik, 1994). These people may not be able to control their binge eating despite the fact that they don't want to do it and typically view it as being abnormal (Hagan, Whitworth, & Moss, 1999; Miller & Pumariega, 2001). Powerful feelings of guilt and self-disgust regarding binge eating may then lead to purging, through vomiting or laxatives, and to periods of fasting. This behavior is also largely out of control. For example, because of increased tolerance, laxative use may reach an extremely high level, perhaps 100 doses daily for some individuals, which causes them to lose normal control of the bowels. The DSM-IV-TR diagnostic criteria for bulimia nervosa are summarized in Table 14-3.

Table 14-3 DSM-IV-TR Diagnostic Criteria for Bulimia Nervosa

A. Recurrent episodes of binge eating. An episode of binge eating is characterized by both of the following:

    (1) eating, in a discrete period of time (e.g., within any 2-hour period), an amount of food that is definitely larger than most people would eat during a similar period of time and under similar circumstances.

    (2) a sense of lack of control over eating during the episode (e.g., a feeling that one cannot stop eating or control what or how much one is eating).

B. Recurrent inappropriate compensatory behavior in order to prevent weight gain, such as self-induced vomiting; misuse of laxatives, diuretics, enemas, or other medications; fasting; or excessive exercise.

C. The binge eating and inappropriate compensatory behaviors both occur, on average, at least twice a week for 3 months.

D. Self-evaluation is unduly influenced by body shape and weight.

E. The disturbance does not occur exclusively during episodes of anorexia nervosa.

Specify type:

Purging Type: During the current episode of bulimia nervosa, the person has regularly engaged in self-induced vomiting or the misuse of laxatives, diuretics, or enemas.

Nonpurging Type: During the current episode of bulimia nervosa, the person has used other inappropriate compensatory behaviors, such as fasting or excessive exercise, but has not regularly engaged in self-induced vomiting or the misuse of laxatives, diuretics, or enemas.

SOURCE: Reprinted with permission from the *Diagnostic and Statistical Manual of Mental Disorders,* 4th ed., Text Revision (2000). Washington, DC: American Psychiatric Association, pp. 549–550.

Bulimia appears to be closely related to anorexia. Symptoms of the two disorders appear similar, but not identical. The DSM-IV-TR outlines distinctions between them that allow for differential diagnosis and classification. Individuals with bulimia are often close to an appropriate weight and are able to maintain that approximate level whereas in the binge-eating/purging type of anorexia nervosa the person is significantly underweight. It is quite possible for a person to be clinically diagnosed as having the binge-eating/purging type of anorexia nervosa at one point and later to be classified as bulimic, but not anorexic, if her weight and menses return to near normal (American Psychiatric Association, 2000). Common to both anorexia nervosa and bulimia is an extreme concern with body weight and overwhelming fear of becoming fat. Individuals with bulimia fluctuate between gaining and losing weight, whereas anorexics are characterized by extreme, life-threatening weight loss.

It is very difficult to pinpoint the prevalence of bulimia because affected individuals are extremely secretive about their bingeing and purging, and their public eating behavior is usually controlled and appropriate. Sometimes their own parents and roommates do not realize what they are doing, except that unusual amounts of food mysteriously disappear from the kitchen, and bulimic individuals may be reduced to stealing from friends and relatives to support expensive binges. The disorder is difficult to detect since there are no obvious physical changes, except for tooth decay, rapid erosion of tooth enamel, and perhaps marks on the hand the person has used to induce vomiting in the early phases of the disorder (see Table 14-4). Bulimics' body weight and condition are typically within the normal range. Like anorexia, bulimia is a disorder that affects many more young females than males. Estimates indicate that about 1–3% of adolescent and young adult females are affected by bulimia (American Psychiatric Association, 2000). Bulimia seems to emerge more frequently among certain populations. For example, for women of college age, the prevalence seems to be considerably higher than for the total population, ranging from nearly 4% to just under 20% (Weiss et al., 1994). Young women with bulimia also report a history of eating problems, especially overeating, as well as other difficulties, including depression (Hunt & Cooper, 2001; Vandereycken, 2001) and obsessive-compulsive behaviors

Table 14-4 Some Physical Problems of Patients with Bulimia Nervosa
Dental and Oral Problems, Mostly Due to Vomiting
Dental caries or cavities
Erosion of tooth enamel
Mouth ulcers
Swollen salivary glands
Periodontal or gum disease
Irritation around the mouth
Increased sensitivity to temperature
Persistent sore throat
The Extremities
Calluses on the back of the hand from induced vomiting
Edema of the hands, feet, or around the eyes
Gastrointestinal Problems
Bloating, pain, cramping from starvation and high-fiber diet
Constipation or diarrhea, mostly from laxatives
Gynecological Problems
Irregular menses
SOURCES: American Psychiatric Association (2000); Andersen (1999).

(Price Foundation Collaborative Group, 2001; Reisch et al., 2001).

Etiology of Bulimia Nervosa

Like other eating disorders, the causes of bulimia are somewhat unclear at this time. People with bulimia seem to be preoccupied with food and have a persistent urge to eat—their lives largely revolve around food and eating. Nearly any incident can trigger an episode of bingeing, rather like the drinking of alcoholics. As noted previously, those with bulimia seem to have more affective disturbance, particularly depression, than most people. They also evidence a higher than normal level of substance abuse, and some report a history of sexual abuse. Similar to anorexia, bulimia probably stems in part from cultural and social pressures to be thin, which may serve as both triggering and long-term causal agents. Clearly, there is a need for additional research on the causal factors contributing to bulimia nervosa. Some individuals (e.g., young females, athletes who must meet weight standards) are more at risk than others, but there is much more to learn regarding causation (Diaz et al., 1999; Raffi, Rodini, Grandi, & Fava, 2000).

Treatment of Bulimia Nervosa

Many different treatments for bulimia have been tried with varying degrees of success. Regardless of other interventions, a medical evaluation of the individual should be undertaken at the outset. A number of medical complications may initially require attention. For example, there may be ruptures in the gastric or esophageal areas due to vomiting; there may be metabolic complications from either the vomiting or the abuse of laxative agents; or there may be musculoskeletal problems that come from strenuous overexercise. Any of these may require medical attention. Serious dental complications include erosion of tooth enamel from highly acidic vomit. Although dental damage is irreversible, further damage can be halted. Medical stabilization is often required prior to addressing the bulimic condition itself and before bulimia becomes a way of life. Those bulimics with the most severe symptoms over a longer period of time have the least positive prognoses and are the most difficult to treat.

Treatment approaches to bulimia have included medication and various combinations of education, counseling, and behavior management. Antidepressants are helpful in reducing binge eating, despite a substantial relapse rate when discontinued (Ferguson & Pigott, 2000; Matsumoto, Miyakawa, Yabana, Iizuka, & Kishimoto, 2001). Fluoxetine or possibly other serotonergic drugs are tried first, and other types of antidepressants may then be tried if necessary to reduce the frequency of bingeing and vomiting (Hudson, Harrison, & Carter, 1999). Various strategies are used in behavioral therapy approaches, but training in self-monitoring is typically a prominent feature, as it is with treatment for anorexia.

A range of cognitive-behavioral therapies, using basic behavioral management principles, have been shown to be quite effective with bulimic patients. These approaches involve interrupting the disordered eating and then examining connections between certain cognitions and eating ("I purge more often when I worry about dating"). Next, the person participates in self-monitoring training and management of self-reinforcement contingencies (e.g., "How can I consistently reward myself royally for normal eating?").

Once some progress has been made, therapy may shift to relapse prevention and the use of multiple interventions such as self-help manuals, development of support groups, and/or family involvement (Mitchell et al., 2001; Raffi et al., 2000). Bulimia is recognized as being very difficult to treat, but "cognitive-behavior therapy is now considered to be the most strongly empirically supported treatment method for bulimia nervosa" (Williamson & Netemeyer, 2000). Interventions include exposure to the irrationally avoided foods through structured meal plans, reassurance, and education, plus prevention of purging through continuous monitoring until the patient improves. Gradually, the patient learns to identify and avoid tempting situations, and she assumes greater control of her own eating. Continued research is important in order to identify and refine effective features of the treatments.

Obesity

IN FOCUS 4 ▶ Define obesity, and tell how many individuals are estimated to be obese.

Obesity is not as easily defined as one might think, primarily because there is no single agreed-upon set of weight guidelines and because popular perceptions of weight norms change greatly over time (Cooper & Burrows, 2001). In general, the condition of **obesity** is characterized by excess body fat and a weight approximately 30% more than is considered normal, based on published expected weights such as the Metropolitan Life Insurance Company tables. The percentage in this definition of obesity was recently increased from 20% to 30%, primarily because so many people exceeded the old level. Evidence suggests that obesity is increasing in the United States and is related to a number of serious health problems as well as psychological and social difficulties (e.g., Bessenoff & Sherman, 2000; Raynor & Epstein, 2001). Estimates suggest that 5–10% of the preschool population is obese, rising to 27% by age 11 and 22% in the teen years. Further, the prevalence of obesity among children has increased substantially in the last 15 years (Jeffery, 2001).

Childhood obesity is a serious health risk because it usually precedes a lifelong battle with obesity. In addition to cardiovascular disease, individuals who are obese may also experience increased risk for hyper-

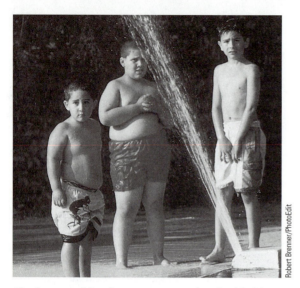

Obesity, a condition that can present serious health risks, is increasing among U.S. children.

and those who become overweight as adults. For example, physiologically, there seem to be two types of obesity: hyperplastic and hypertrophic. *Hyperplastic obesity* occurs when an individual has an abnormally high number of fat cells (nonobese people tend to have about 3 billion such cells; hyperplastic obese individuals may have double that number). *Hypertrophic obesity* occurs when individuals are overweight primarily because of extremely enlarged fat cells rather than because of a larger than normal number of such cells. Obesity that is primarily hyperplastic seems to develop in childhood, while hypertrophic obesity is more an adult disorder. Such causation, however, remains speculative since the distinction regarding onset does not always hold. Biological or physiological explanations feature the inheritance of a tendency toward obesity or slimness. Many times, we hear statements such as "Johnny inherited his fatness from his parents" or "Sally is slender just like her mother." But these remain unsubstantiated popular beliefs, involving oversimplified explanations. One must still overeat considerably in order to become obese.

Many researchers and therapists view learned behavior as an important cause of obesity (Ramirez & Rosen, 2001). There is little question that food consumption in contemporary society serves social as well as physiological purposes, for children and adults. Although eating is a behavior that is under voluntary control, aspects of adult eating appear to occur with little awareness—for example, eating snacks while distracted by a TV program or while driving. A variety of family and social influences may lead to overeating and obesity. Doting parents buy special treats for their kids and are delighted when the children enjoy them, perhaps consuming more than they physiologically need at the moment. Children are frequently admonished to "clean their plate" for one reason or another (e.g., it is socially appropriate, mom may feel hurt, or some convoluted logic regarding "all those starving children" elsewhere). Busy families on the run eat as much as they can as fast as they can in order to keep on schedule. Such practices probably contribute to obesity. Does obesity during childhood destine a person to obesity as an adult?

Research suggests that obesity in youngsters does predict adult obesity. Overweight babies tend to continue to be obese during childhood and adolescence and into adulthood (Benoit, 2000; Jeffery, 2001;

tension, diabetes, sleep problems (notably obstructive sleep apnea), depression, and social maladjustment (Pinhas & Zeitler, 2000). A severely obese person has substantially greater risk of premature death than a person of normal body mass.

Part of the gravity of obesity lies in the fact that it is not easily treated in adults, who typically follow a pattern of dieting and then regaining the lost weight (Devlin, Yanovski, & Wilson, 2000). It is not easy to take weight off, and even more difficult to keep it off. Those who lose substantial amounts of weight must continually battle to maintain their weight loss, and it is much easier to regain than to maintain the weight (Lowe, Foster, Kerzhnerman, Swain, & Wadden, 2001; Nauta, Hospers, Kok, & Jansen, 2000). This difficulty in achieving an acceptable weight once a person is obese makes prevention and early intervention particularly important.

Causes of Obesity

Theories regarding causation of obesity vary and often appear to be in conflict (Bryn, 1999; Dounchis, Hayden, & Wilfley, 2001). One view suggests that obesity is a hereditary or constitutional condition. Support for this perspective is partially derived from cellular differences between obese and nonobese individuals as well as between those who are obese as children

Kurzthaler & Fleishhacker, 2001). There is not a highly optimistic outlook for obese youngsters. The probabilities of continued obesity are compelling. For Scott, being obese at the age of 11 means that he may have to fight obesity all of his life, especially given his mother's eating habits and his own poor food preferences and sedentary life-style.

Being grossly overweight has psychological consequences as well as physical dangers. Contrary to the stereotype of the jolly fat person, obese children and adolescents are unhappy about their weight. They report significantly more negative physical self-perceptions and score lower on general self-worth than nonobese peers (Braet, Mervielde, & Vandereycken, 1997). These negative feelings about themselves begin early in life and probably stem from the rejection they receive from other children. Stigmatization based on weight is most obvious among older children, but is clearly present even in 3-year-olds, who choose nearly everyone else before fat children as playmates (Cramer & Steinwert, 1998). Overweight children themselves expressed even stronger rejection of overweight people than did normal weight children. Obesity predictably leads to rejection by other children and formation of a poor self-image.

Recent literature on obesity and other eating problems illustrates both the importance of research and the need for more sophisticated theoretical perspectives that include multiple and interactive causes (e.g., food addiction, genetic, and environmental causes) (Bryn, 1999; Stein, O'Byrne, Suminski, & Haddock, 1999). It is not clear how a wide variety of factors affect weight and, ultimately, relate to obesity. For example, many people firmly believe that stress-induced eating leads to obesity, but research thus far is not clear on this piece of conventional wisdom (Tanofsky, Wilfley, & Spurrell, 2000; Wolff, Crosby, Roberts, & Wittrock, 2000).

Treatment of Obesity

Weight loss is a difficult process that attracts a great deal of attention in the media. One has only to count the many paid TV advertisements for diet aids and exercise equipment to determine that this is a topic of high interest. Solutions and treatments for being overweight that might seem uncomplicated on the surface, such as dieting and exercise, often fail in the context of chronic obesity (Berg & Rosencrans, 2000; Stein et al., 1999). Although specific strategies for treating obesity are numerous, they can generally be categorized into two broad groups: behavioral therapies and medical treatments.

As a general rule, treatment for obesity must be approached in a systematic fashion based on good research. Current thinking suggests that a multidisciplinary team (perhaps consisting of a physician, nutritionist, psychologist, and exercise therapist) is more effective in addressing the complexities of obesity than a clinician from a single profession who has more limited tools available (Cooper & Fairburn, 2001; Grilo, 2001). Certain characteristics of the person being treated also tend to lead to a greater or lesser probability of successful treatment. For example, eating patterns are quite important. Obese people who can limit themselves to three meals a day as opposed to "grazing" at many times throughout the day tend to respond more favorably to treatment. Also, people who eat all three meals each day seem to experience better success than those who omit a meal, such as breakfast, and then are ravenous and eat too much at night. It is not surprising that people with a history of binge eating are also more difficult to treat (Grilo, 2001). The ability to monitor one's own behavior is important, too. Literature on obesity puts great importance on accurate assessment of amount and type of food and exercise. The necessity for regular monitoring of weight and exercise, which can be burdensome, makes treatment success elusive. Yet if they do not attend to what they eat, obese people find it nearly impossible to change bad eating habits and will not lose weight. The obese boy featured in the chapter opening and his mother would both benefit from information on diet and nutrition; corn dogs, soft drinks, and doughnuts are all high-calorie and unhealthy, and such foods should be eaten sparingly. Unfortunately, kids like Scott encounter temptations to eat foods that are bad for them at schools, recreational facilities, mini-markets, fast-food restaurants, gas stations, shopping malls, and at nearly all times and places throughout their day. Thus, help in detecting and resisting these temptations should be a prominent part of a therapy program.

Pharmacological treatments for obesity are appealing because they appear to offer a simple and rapid solution to a difficult problem. How easy it would be to take a pill that causes you to lose 20 pounds. However, that is not possible, and may never be. Unfortunately, the drugs that suppress appetite often have a number of undesirable or intolerable side effects, patient non-compliance in taking the drugs reduces their effectiveness, and lost weight is rapidly regained once the medication is discontinued (Matsumoto et al., 2001).

A variety of amphetamine-based medications that suppress appetite, increase activity, and heighten mood have been popular in both over-the-counter and prescription forms. The benefits of these drugs may be short-lived. Although psychostimulants may serve to reduce appetite, they may also produce heightened irritability, be addictive, and disrupt sleep. Dexfenfluramine is a medication aimed at increasing secretion of the brain hormone serotonin, which, in turn, reduces the desire for food, particularly carbohydrates. Dexfenfluramine has been used to treat obesity with some degree of success, although weight tends to be regained when patients terminate the medication (Roth, 2000).

People trying to lose weight often take diet drugs in place of, rather than in addition to, increased exercise and continued dieting; so they fail to learn how to control their eating and simply rely on the drugs. At present, the available drugs are probably not used effectively to treat obesity (Bray, 1999).

Surgical interventions have also been used for individuals who suffer from the most severe cases of obesity. Surgical approaches have favored strategies that restrict stomach capacity, either by stapling procedures or by inserting balloon-type devices into the gastric cavity. Both of these procedures are aimed at reducing gastric volume, thereby producing a perception of being full after eating relatively small amounts of food. Complications (e.g., infections, chronic diarrhea, apparatus failures, fatalities associated with major surgery) have plagued both types of treatments, and these approaches should be employed only in the most severe cases when other therapies have been unsuccessful.

Behavioral interventions bring some good news for obese youngsters. A comprehensive review of treatment studies produced this finding: "There is strong evidence for the short- and long-term efficacy of multicomponential behavioral treatment for decreasing weight among children relative to both placebo and education-only treatments" (Jelalian & Saelens, 1999, p. 223). That is, in a number of research studies, multi-faceted behavioral treatment successfully treated obese children. Children are the only age group for whom weight-reduction programs of any type have produced lasting benefits. Why are the behavioral treatments effective?

Behavioral programs tend to focus on managing eating behavior rather than attempting to change personality. While behavioral treatment of obesity does not discount physiological factors, it does focus on those contingencies in the environment that can be manipulated to alter habits related to eating and energy intake and expenditure.

One of the most prominent features of behavioral interventions relates to the development of the obese person's self-monitoring capacity. Obese people frequently do not realize the unsuitability of the foods they consume and how quickly and often they eat. Self-monitoring allows the person to become conscious of behaviors that contribute to undesirable eating, which can then be targeted for modification. In many cases, the individuals being treated keep careful written records of what is eaten, when it was eaten, who was present, and how they felt at the time. Social and environmental circumstances (such as attending parties, feeling disappointment, or viewing TV) can become cues for eating, and also targets for control or change. It is also important to modify the consequences of eating, that is, to provide some type of reward for eating in a manner that promotes weight reduction. Such a process basically involves cognitive-behavioral restructuring that helps the person to lose weight effectively, revise his or her image of self and the environment, and maintain the loss. Maximally effective treatment requires that the specific features of the treatment program be tailored to the individual and his or her environmental context (Grilo, 2001).

Despite the success of behavioral interventions with younger obese clients, maintenance of weight loss continues to be a difficult problem with all weight-reduction programs (Jeffery, 2001). Relapses are the rule rather than the exception for all types of treatment. Relapse prevention is an essential element of any comprehensive treatment program for obesity. Behavioral patterns leading to obesity are not developed overnight, but over a considerable period of time. Further, bad eating habits and little or no exercise become a part of one's life, and it is incredibly difficult to make a change dramatically and permanently.

Continued research on the effective treatment of obesity is essential for promoting a healthy life-style for American youth.

TOILETING PROBLEMS

Most parents at some point express concern regarding their child's toileting behavior, particularly when the youngster is being trained to perform this natural function in a socially appropriate manner. The process of toilet training often generates a certain amount of frustration and stress for parents and children alike. For the most part, problems encountered in toilet training are transient, and appropriate patterns of behavior are developed by the time a child is 2 to 4 years of age. However, for a small percentage of children, this does not occur. Toileting challenges often arise in youngsters with intellectual disabilities or other behavioral disorders (Bainbridge & Myles, 1999; Bruey, 2000; Didden, Skkema, Bosman, Duker, & Curfs, 2001). For such children, toileting remains problematic beyond the normal age at which we expect these behaviors to have been habituated and may continue into and beyond the elementary school years.

It is somewhat surprising that more research has not been undertaken on toileting behaviors. The question of the best time for beginning toilet training has not yet been completely resolved. Obviously, the appropriate age will vary from child to child—a statement that holds true for all behaviors. Around age 2 or 3 seems to be a commonly accepted time for directing serious efforts toward shaping these behaviors, although earlier and later ages have been favored at various times over the last century in the United States (Cummings, 2001). Customary ages for undertaking

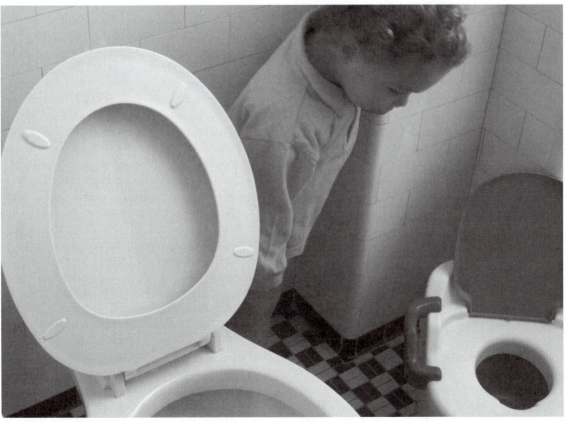

Toilet training can be frustrating for both the child and his or her parents.

Laura Dwight/Corbis

toilet training vary considerably among cultures around the world. Problems with waste elimination should be addressed from a perspective that extends beyond the child to consider the family and cultural context. Such a notion is not unusual in a discussion of habit disorders and has received considerable attention in the literature on toileting problems.

Encopresis

Encopresis is a toileting disorder that involves repeated, unacceptable patterns of fecal expulsion in inappropriate locations (e.g., in clothing or on the floor) by a child who is 4 years of age or older and does not exhibit organic pathology (American Psychiatric Association, 2000). This generic label includes several different types of conditions. On one dimension, encopresis can be viewed in terms of retentive versus nonretentive problems. *Retentive encopresis* is characterized by an excessive retention of fecal material, whereas *nonretentive encopresis* involves uncontrolled expulsion of feces (incontinence) resulting in soiled clothing and bedding. Another dimension relates to whether or not control of fecal expulsion has been established and then ceased (*discontinuous*, or *secondary*, *encopresis*) or has never been reliably established (*continuous*, or *primary*, *encopresis*). It is easy to see how such subcategories represent different disorders, even though the behaviors may appear similar in some cases. These distinctions are very important in trying to establish causation and devise treatment.

Estimates of the prevalence of encopresis vary rather widely, although most figures range between 1% and 3% (Murphy & Carr, 2000). DSM-IV-TR places the prevalence rate at approximately 1% of all 5-year-olds (American Psychiatric Association, 2000). Encopresis occurs more frequently in males than females, and a rather substantial proportion of cases are of the discontinuous type. Although statistics differ depending on the source, over half of all encopretics are children who have established control and then cease to exercise it (Murphy & Carr, 2000).

Obviously, encopresis represents a difficult and frustrating problem for all involved, including the child, parents, and peers. Some difficulties extend far beyond the unpleasant process of cleaning up the mess and the embarrassment of having an accident. In many cases, the negative impact on the child's self-image and sense of personal worth is devastating (Lancioni, O'Reilly, & Basili, 2001). Also, encopresis can generate in caretakers a myriad of negative emotions that can work against treatment.

Treatment of Encopresis

Treatment of encopresis has generally followed one of the three major theoretical perspectives on the problem: medical, psychoanalytic, and behavioral (Christophersen & Mortweet, 2001; Fennig & Fennig, 1999; Smith, Smith, & Lee, 2000). Medical treatment tends to emphasize direct physical control of fecal matter using enemas, laxatives, and stool softeners along with modified diet and sometimes pediatric counseling. In some cases, medication (e.g., imipramine, senokot) has been employed to control bowel actions, although most authorities view encopresis as a combined physiological and behavioral problem and employ combinations of treatment procedures (Christophersen & Mortweet, 2001; Murphy & Carr, 2000). For example, in some cases, effective treatment has required family involvement because of hostility associated with the condition. Multimodal treatments may include behavioral shaping as well as the physical control techniques mentioned above (Fennig & Fennig, 1999; Smith et al, 2000). It is generally thought that clinicians must attend to environmental as well as physical factors in order to effect a cure. The psychoanalytic view of encopresis regards the behavior as a symptom of inner conflicts and tends to employ psychological treatment that emphasizes interpretation of the child's play, acquisition of insight by the older child, and counseling of parents and child. Evidence regarding the success of psychotherapy is very sketchy, primarily because of the absence of adequate research on the approach (Aruffo, Ibarra, & Strupp, 2000).

The primary focus of behavioral treatment is the establishment and maintenance of appropriate toileting behavior through manipulation of environmental consequences. For the continuous encopretic, this involves teaching control skills that presumably have never been learned. For the discontinuous encopretic, it becomes a matter of reestablishing and maintaining such behaviors (Murphy & Carr, 2000). Many procedural variations have been used with impressive success. For the most part, behavioral treatment studies can be grouped into three general categories: (1) those that primarily give positive reinforcement for appropriate control, but no punishment for soiling; (2) those that punish the child who soils; and (3) those that employ a combination of positive reinforcement and punishment. One of the major strengths of behavioral treatments is their provision of specific procedural descriptions for use by clinicians and caretakers. The specificity of behavioral approaches makes evaluation and replication of treatment procedures easier than with treatments based on other theoretical perspectives.

Behavioral treatments of encopresis appear promising. However, since there is great variation in the circumstances surrounding each case, intervention is most likely to be successful when the individual case is precisely evaluated and an individualized treatment program is implemented. Assessment procedures should include complete medical examinations in order to provide comprehensive information regarding the physical status of the child and the family context (Fennig & Fennig, 1999; Smith et al., 2000). Further research that is scientifically sound is badly needed. Not only are investigations of encopresis scarce, relative to research on other disorders, but a substantial portion of the published research lacks important methodological features that would enhance the scientific soundness of the data (Lancioni et al., 2001).

Enuresis

IN FOCUS 5 ▶ What are the prevalence estimates for enuresis, and when is incontinence considered to be a problem in children?

Enuresis is probably more widely recognized as a toileting problem than encopresis. It is certainly a more frequent topic of informal conversation among parents, as well as more frequently examined in the professional literature. There is some good reason for this, since enuresis is more common than encopresis (Christophersen & Mortweet, 2000). DSM-IV-TR cites prevalence figures of 5–10% for children at 5 years of age, 3–5% by age 10, and a lingering 1% for 15-year-olds (American Psychiatric Association, 2000). **Enuresis** is chronic inappropriate wetting by a child who does not have a physical disorder and is old enough to

be toilet-trained. *Nocturnal enuresis* refers to chronic nighttime bed-wetting. *Diurnal enuresis* refers to wetting during the daytime. There is considerable difference of opinion regarding the minimum age at which such behavior should be considered problematic. However, most clinicians view urinary incontinence after about 3 to 5 years of age as a problem.

Although early literature considered encopresis the fecal equivalent of enuresis, there is no solid evidence of a relationship between the two disorders. A child with enuresis may or may not also have encopresis. The major focus of research on enuresis has been on nocturnal occurrences, and the disorder has often been labeled *functional nocturnal enuresis*. Because of this trend in the literature, this section emphasizes the nighttime behavior. This is not meant to suggest that inappropriate urination may not also occur during the day. But in this context, it is interesting to consider the connection between sleep and urinary incontinence.

There are three general classes of theories regarding causation and related treatment of enuresis: medical, psychodynamic (psychoanalytic), and behavioral. Considerable attention has been given to the relationship between enuresis and sleep patterns. It is reasonable to think that enuresis might occur only during deep sleep, when a child is unaware of and does not react to the physiological need to void. Certainly, individual differences could explain why some waken and void themselves in the toilet, and others do not. Some literature relates sleep cycles and sleep abnormalities to enuresis (e.g., Robson & Leung, 2000; Saki & Hebert, 2000). For example, some authorities believe that children with enuresis often have an inadequate release of an antidiuretic hormone during certain sleep stages, which may be accompanied by a deficient muscular inhibition (Murphy & Carr, 2000). These two physiological processes in combination could lead to a lack of control and nighttime wetting. However, further investigation is needed in order to understand the causes of enuresis and its treatment.

The psychodynamic perspective interprets enuresis as a symptom of an inner conflict. This notion is consistent with the fundamental psychoanalytic view of disorders, including encopresis. Effectiveness of psychoanalytic treatment has been poorly documented, and there is little research evidence for a success rate significantly different from that for subjects receiving no treatment.

Medical explanations of enuresis have included developmental or maturational lag, genetic influences, abnormalities of the urinary tract, and a deficit in cortical control (Christophersen & Mortweet, 2001; Stein, Barbaresi, & Benuck, 2001). Obviously, some of these could be interrelated and treatment can be implemented only with some.

A variety of medications have been used over the years to treat enuresis; fluvoxamine is one popular alternative (e.g., Kano & Arisaka, 2000). Use of one family of drugs, the amphetamines, is related to the perspective that views sleep cycles as related to causation. Amphetamines are stimulants and are thought to make it easier for the enuretic to awaken, either by raising the average depth of sleep or by making the individual more easily aroused. This line of reasoning connects enuresis with deficiencies in cortical inhibition and arousal deficits in sleep. Although the logic is reasonable, the evidence does not suggest that stimulants are consistently effective in the treatment of enuresis. Medication has been effective in some cases of enuresis, but the results are not consistent, and there is clear evidence that indicates that other treatments, or certainly combinations of therapies, are preferred (Christophersen & Mortweet, 2001; Horrigan & Barnhill, 2000; Oshlag, 2000).

Behavioral approaches to treating enuresis mainly focus on the environmental contingencies related to urination. Specific treatment procedures have been combined with varying degrees of success. Urine alarms (electric devices that sound a bell or buzzer when urine causes a circuit to close) have been used in mattress pads and in training pants. These devices have been used since the 1930s and remain popular for the treatment of enuresis. Combined with other therapy components, many authorities view urine alarms as a treatment of choice (Alcazar, Rodriguez, & Sanchez, 1999; Murphy & Carr, 2000).

For most cases, combining various procedures seems the most effective approach to treating enuresis (e.g., Alcazar et al., 1999; Murphy & Carr, 2000; Smith et al., 2000). Here again, the treatment program is best determined by a careful analysis of the specific child's characteristics. It should be noted, however, that all treatment approaches suffer from less than complete success and a certain percentage of cases

of enuresis can be expected to relapse and need retreatment.

SLEEP DISORDERS

IN FOCUS 6 ▶ How often do sleep disorders occur in people of different ages?

Many parents voice dissatisfaction or concern about their children's sleep patterns at one time or another. Research suggests that sleep disturbances are relatively common among many different age groups, ranging from children to young adults (Quine, 2001; Smedje, Broman, & Hetta, 2001). Evidence suggests that the overall prevalence of sleep disorders increases with age; they may occur in 30–45% of very young children, and specific difficulties such as insomnia are reported by a similar proportion of adults (American Psychiatric Association, 2000). Different sleep disturbances seem to occur more frequently at different ages. Nightmares, for example, tend to peak in frequency between 3 and 6 years of age, while young adults encounter problems falling asleep and older adults more frequently have difficulty maintaining undisturbed sleep throughout the night. A variety of health-related risks and difficulties can be experienced when sleep is seriously interrupted or when individuals are significantly deprived of sleep (Gelman & King, 2001; Hoban, 2000; Roberts, Roberts, & Chen, 2001). Children's sleep behavior is of considerable concern to parents although, fortunately, a considerable portion of childhood sleep disorders are minor and transient.

Several different stages and states are involved in the normal sleep cycle. It is worthwhile examining these briefly prior to discussing sleeping disorders. Sleep consists of two distinct states: REM sleep is a period during which rapid eye movements occur and an individual dreams; the second state, known as NREM sleep, lacks rapid eye movements and is made up of four distinguishable stages based on brain-wave activity. Stage 1 of NREM sleep represents the transitional period between wakefulness and sleep. Stages 2, 3, and 4 are characterized by differences in amount and type of brain-wave activity and are generally spoken of as increasing in "depth" of sleep. Normal sleep patterns begin with NREM sleep and progress from stage 1 through stage 4 during the first 90 minutes or so of the night. Around this point, the first period of REM sleep occurs and is typically brief, lasting from 5 to 15 minutes. Normal sleep is characterized by repeated cycles of the various stages of NREM sleep and REM sleep. Stage 1 usually accounts for only about 5% of a total night's sleep, stage 2 for about 40–60%, and stages 3 and 4 for the remainder. Most of stage 3 and stage 4 sleep occurs during the first two cycles of NREM sleep. The early portion of a night's sleep rather predictably tends to follow this pattern: awake, stage 1, stage 2, stage 3, stage 4, stage 3, and stage 2. At this point, the first REM period occurs, and then the NREM stages recycle (2, 3, 4, 2), followed by another REM period. Illustrated in Figure 14-1, these sleep cycles and stages are important since certain sleep disturbances tend to occur predominantly during particular sleep states or stages.

In DSM-IV-TR, the American Psychiatric Association classifies sleep disorders into several categories according to causation. We are mainly interested in *primary sleep disorders*, which are those that are not believed to be caused by other mental disorders, a general medical condition, or substance abuse. DSM-IV-TR includes two categories of primary sleep disorders: (1) *dysomnias*, which are sleep disorders related to "excessive sleepiness that is attributable to ongoing sleep deprivation" that may be due to environmental factors such as frequent interruptions of sleep, noise, or light; and (2) *parasomnias*, which are sleep disorders associated with "abnormal behavioral or physiological events occurring

in association with sleep, specific sleep stages, or sleep-wake transitions" (American Psychiatric Association, 2000, pp. 629, 630–631). We will examine selected sleep disorders in both of these categories.

Parasomnias

Parasomnias are sleep disruptions associated with specific parts of the sleep cycle, stages of sleep, or sleep-wake shifts. Parasomnias represent "activation of physiological systems at inappropriate times during the sleep-wake cycle" (American Psychiatric Association, 2000, p. 630). They relate to cognitive processes and often show up on electronic measures of cerebral functioning. Parasomnias may also involve the motor system, as in sleep-walking (Gaylor, Goodlin-Jones, & Anders, 2001). People affected by parasomnias often complain about atypical behaviors *during* sleep rather than incidents of insomnia or unusual sleepiness during the day. People with parasomnias frequently report feeling stressed and often experience co-occurring anxiety and mood disorders (Ohayon, Guilleminault, & Priest, 1999).

Nightmares and Night Terrors

Nightmares and night terrors are sleep disorders in the parasomnia category. There is considerable dreaming during normal sleep, and dream sleep receives continuing attention in the literature (e.g., Kroth, McDavit, Brendlen, Patel, & Zwiener, 2001; Schredl,

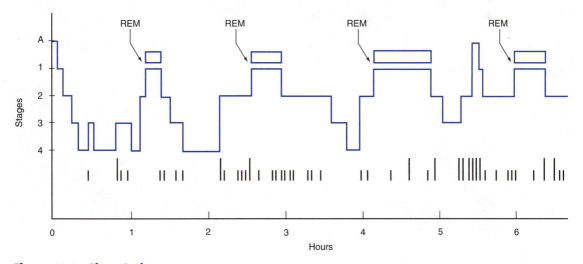

Figure 14-1 Sleep Cycles

2001). As all of us know from experience, dreams can be either pleasant or unpleasant. Most children have occasional bad dreams or nightmares that result in wakefulness and fear. In fact, nighttime fears are present in nearly 75% of normal school children aged 4 to 12 years, and are associated with some of these children's bad dreams and nightmares (Muris, Merckelbach, Gadet, & Moulaert, 2000; Muris, Merckelbach, Ollendick, King, & Bogie, 2001). However, for some children, sleep disturbances are frequent, persistent, and intense, and are then considered serious enough to be considered disorders. This section considers two such sleep disorders: nightmares and night terrors.

Specific research on the prevalence of nightmares and night terrors has been relatively infrequent to date. Prevalence estimates for the two conditions place the frequency of nightmares between 10% and 50% for children 3 to 5 years of age, and that of night terrors between 1% and 6% among children of the same age range (American Psychiatric Association, 2000). Nightmares and night terrors may appear somewhat similar, but only on the surface. As we examine them more closely, distinctions become quite evident.

Nightmares and night terrors tend to happen at different times of night and during different sleep stages. Nightmares generally occur during REM periods, more likely during the latter part of the night when REM sleep periods are longer and dreaming is more intense (American Psychiatric Association, 2000). Dreaming typically occurs during REM sleep, which may suggest that nightmares differ from other dreams mainly in content. Some evidence suggests that nightmares are a more severe expression of the same themes that appear in dreams, such as personal well-being (Zadra & Donderi, 2000). Night terror incidents seem to occur during the first 2 hours of sleep and arise in stage 4 of NREM sleep (Ohayon et al., 1999). This is not a stage during which dreaming normally takes place and is considered to be the stage of deepest sleep. This suggests that night terrors are distinctly different phenomena from ordinary dreams.

There are a number of differences in a child's behavior during nightmares and during night terrors. For example, children experiencing night terrors typically sleep through the episode, even though their be-

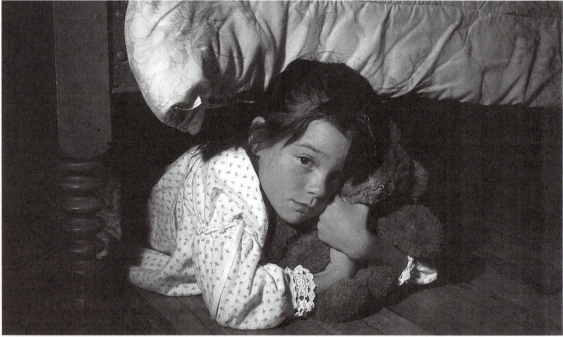

Even though a child's eyes are wide open, she may not remember the episode of night terror when she wakes up.

havior is extremely agitated. Their eyes are often wide open, as though they were staring at something in terror; they make grimaces and exhibit considerable physical movement, sometimes running about the room frantically; they may also shout and scream. Parents often watch such activity helplessly, unable to quiet their children with reassurances or awaken them. Nightmares present a very different picture. Children's movements and verbalization are much more subdued, typically restricted to moaning and slight movements in bed. Beyond this, children having nightmares most often are already awake by the time their parents arrive. From this description, one might conclude that night terrors are merely more fearful episodes of nightmares, perhaps more dramatic in content. Further examination does not support such a deduction.

In most cases, nightmares are followed by a period during which the child is awake, recognizes people and surroundings, can provide a coherent account of what has transpired, and can remember the contents of the dream. Night terrors are followed by instant and peaceful sleep, lack of recognition of people and surroundings, and frequently, complete amnesia regarding both contents and occurrence. Further, children experiencing night terrors often hallucinate; those having nightmares do not. Night terrors may be rather prolonged (15–20 minutes), whereas nightmares tend to be of a much shorter duration (1–2 minutes). At this point, there is little question that nightmares and night terrors are distinctly different phenomena. Either may, however, present a serious difficulty depending on the circumstances and the persistence of the problem. The DSM-IV-TR diagnostic criteria for both nightmares and night terrors are summarized in Table 14-5.

Causes of nightmares and night terrors remain largely unknown at this time, although some theories have proposed a variety of rather elaborate notions, such as sexual impulses that are not understood by

Table 14-5 DSM-IV-TR Diagnostic Criteria for Nightmares (Nightmare Disorder) and Night Terrors (Sleep Terror Disorder)

Nightmare Disorder

A. Repeated awakenings from the major sleep period or naps with detailed recall of extended and extremely frightening dreams, usually involving threats to survival, security, or self-esteem. The awakenings generally occur during the second half of the sleep period.

B. On awakening from the frightening dreams, the person rapidly becomes oriented and alert (in contrast to the confusion and disorientation seen in Sleep Terror Disorder and some forms of epilepsy).

C. The dream experience, or the sleep disturbance resulting from the awakening, causes clinically significant distress or impairment in social, occupational, or other important areas of functioning.

D. The nightmares do not occur exclusively during the course of another mental disorder (e.g., a delirium, Posttraumatic Stress Disorder) and are not due to the direct physiological effects of a substance (e.g., a drug of abuse, a medication) or a general medical condition.

Sleep Terror Disorder

A. Recurrent episodes of abrupt awakening from sleep, usually occurring during the first third of the major sleep period and beginning with a panicky scream.

B. Intense fear and signs of autonomic arousal, such as tachycardia, rapid breathing, and sweating, during each episode.

C. Relative unresponsiveness to efforts of others to comfort the person during the episode.

D. No detailed dream is recalled and there is amnesia for the episode.

E. The episodes cause clinically significant distress or impairment in social, occupational, or other important areas of functioning.

F. The disturbance is not due to the direct physiological effects of a substance (e.g., a drug of abuse, a medication) or a general medical condition.

SOURCE: American Psychiatric Association (2000), pp. 634, 639. Reprinted with permission from the *Diagnostic and Statistical Manual of Mental Disorders*, 4th ed., Text Revision. © 2000 APA.

the individual or experiences in a previous life (da Fonseca, 2000; Koepele & Teixeira, 2000; Koethe & Pietrowsky, 2001). Nightmares and night terrors have also been associated with a variety of other conditions such as bronchial asthma, milk intolerance, night-time feeding, and genetic disposition (Bruni, Verrillo, Miano, & Ottaviano, 2000; Krakow et al., 2000). With both nightmares and night terrors, multiple causes appear to be possible; nearly any event or condition that alters the normal sleep cycle is suspect. Nightmares have been observed as a side effect of the use of certain drugs, although drugs are also employed to treat nightmares. Treatment for both nightmares and night terrors has included the use of a variety of medications, such as prazosin, clonazepam, and fluoxetine (e.g., Brannon, Labbate, & Huber, 2000; Raskind et al., 2000), and psychotherapies, including hypnosis (e.g., Greanleaf, 2000; Howsam, 1999). Treatment results have been rather mixed, although some have claimed that cognitive-behavioral strategies appear to offer a consistently useful treatment approach (Abrahams & Udwin, 2000). The search for effective treatments continues, as illustrated by the procedure outlined in the Research Focus box. Like other therapies, this strategy requires systematic research in order to establish its effectiveness. Past experience with therapies for sleep disorders suggests that the treatment of choice depends to some extent on the individual circumstances of the affected person.

Sleep-Walking Disorder (Somnambulism)

It is estimated that between 1% and 5% of all children have repeated episodes of *somnambulism*, or sleep-walking (American Psychiatric Association, 2000). Somnambulism and night terrors have a number of common features, and it is not unusual to find both problems in the same child. Sleep-walking occurs during NREM sleep in stages 3 and 4. (Children with somnambulism will often start to sleep-walk if they are stood upright during stage 3 or 4 sleep—something that normal children will not do.) Sleep-walkers typically do not remember the incident and are very difficult to awaken. Their eyes are open, and they appear to be walking with a definite purpose, although they show very little emotion. Somnambulism can create serious problems since children can place themselves in danger by walking in unsafe places such as balconies and stairways. Essentially, their senses are not

functioning in a manner that would protect them from falling or other types of accidents.

Somnambulism is most often attributed to some type of emotional stress (e.g., Vgontzas & Kales, 1999). Frequently, some specific accident or other stressful incident is reported to have preceded the sleep-walking (Ohayon et al., 1999). Treatment has followed several approaches with varying degrees of success. A number of different medications have been employed with highly varied results, seeming at times to be almost idiosyncratic (Landry, Warnes, Nielsen, & Montplaisir, 1999). Various therapies have been employed with mixed success, and relapses are relatively common (Stein & Ferber, 2001; Vgontzas & Kales, 1999). The treatment of somnambulism remains largely unexplored relative to treatments for many other childhood disorders.

Dysomnias

Dysomnias are sleep disorders in which the affected individual has significant and chronic difficulty related to the "amount, quality, or timing of sleep" (American Psychiatric Association, 2000, p. 597). Those affected by a dysomnia may experience substantial problems going to sleep or maintaining a sleep state for a sufficient period to be restorative. A dysomnia may also cause individuals to fall asleep at inappropriate times, such as during a conversation or when they are driving an automobile. While the former event may only be embarrassing, the latter circumstance presents some clear dangers to the person involved as well as others. This section focuses on these two types of dysomnias: insomnia and narcolepsy.

Primary Insomnia

Most of us have experienced difficulty falling asleep occasionally, even repeatedly to a point where we are very tired over a period of time. Insomnia as a primary sleep disorder, however, involves a problem in falling asleep that has a duration of at least a month, causes substantial impairment in several areas of functioning, and is not related to substance effects or a general medical condition (American Psychiatric Association, 2000). Primary insomnia seems to begin in the early adult years and is relatively rare during childhood or adolescence. The pattern of insomnia seems to vary, with younger adults experiencing greater difficulty

A Novel Therapy for Night Terror

Dr. Bryan Lask, consulting psychiatrist at the Hospital for Sick Children in London, has reported an effective nondrug treatment for night terrors in children.

Since most such episodes occur within the first hours of sleep, when parents are still awake, Lask suggests that parents note the time they happen for five successive nights. Then he instructs them to wake the child 10–15 minutes before the terror typically occurs, keep the child up for 4 or 5 minutes, and then let the youngster return to sleep.

Lask suggests that parents continue this process until the terrors cease, which is usually within a week of beginning the treatment. If the night terrors recur, which usually happens only once, Lask recommends that the process be repeated.

SOURCE: Condensed from Brody (1996). © 2001 by the New York Times Co. Reprinted by permission.

falling asleep and older individuals more often complaining of problems sleeping through the night. Although prevalence data are incomplete, insomnia seems to vary among populations with physical and mental health problems (e.g., Benca, 2001; Richardson & Roth, 2001). Persistent insomnia seems to increase with age and is more frequent among women. Some prevalence estimates for insomnia are as high as 30–40% of adults, although only 15–25% of those seeking treatment in clinics are identified as having primary insomnia (American Psychiatric Association, 2000; Hajak, 2001; Roberts et al., 2001).

Causes of insomnia are varied, as one would expect. Some evidence suggests that anxiety or worrying is a significant contributor to insomnia (Hajak, 2001; Vgontzas & Kales, 1999). There is also is evidence suggesting that stress, anxiety, and panic attacks are more frequent among individuals with serious insomnia conditions (McKee & Kiffer, 2000; Roberts et al., 2001). General relationships between insomnia and substance abuse (e.g., alcohol, drugs) are also reported in the literature, although such circumstances do not fit the DSM definition of primary insomnia (Brower, Aldrich, Robinson, Zucker, & Greden, 2001; Karam-Hage & Brower, 2000).

Treatments for insomnia have been numerous and have shown highly variable results (Bootzin, 2000). Medication has been widely employed, but with mixed results. Drugs have been used as a means of manipulating the sleep cycle, as sedatives, and as hypnotics (Reite, 2001; Roehrs, Bonahoom, Pedrosi, Rosenthal, & Roth, 2001). Other treatment procedures involving sleep education supplemented with guidance by a therapist have shown promising results. Nonpharmacological treatments have the advantage of avoiding harmful side effects and placing the patient in greater control (McKee & Kiffer, 2000). In most cases, comprehensive behavioral treatment packages have had high success rates and may be tailored more directly to the individual's specific needs (King, Dudley, Melvin, Pallant, & Morawetz, 2001).

Narcolepsy

Narcolepsy is a disorder in which individuals encounter "sleep attacks" at times when they are trying to stay awake (e.g., during the day). Narcolepsy has often been thought of as excessive sleep, but should more correctly be viewed as inappropriate sleep. "Inappropriate" is not meant to suggest a value judgment—narcoleptic incidents can prove physically dangerous and socially embarrassing. They may take place at any time or in any place, when the individuals are walking, standing, driving an automobile, or sitting at the dinner table. Often the episodes are brief, lasting at most about 15 minutes. Patients usually describe the incident in terms of an irresistible urge to sleep. Some are aware that an episode is about to occur, experiencing dream images or hallucinations just before it happens; others experience the episodes without any warning (American Psychiatric Association, 2000). Still others are able to avoid sleep by concentrating intensely on remaining awake.

Estimates regarding the prevalence of narcolepsy vary from 0.02% to 0.16% of the general adult population, or about 10 in 1,000 at the most (American Psychiatric Association, 2000). These figures suggest that there are as many as 250,000 individuals in the United States suffering from narcolepsy. It is unclear how many narcoleptics are children, although the onset of the problem seems to occur predominantly between the ages of 10 and 20.

The cause of narcolepsy has largely eluded researchers to date. One factor that has been identified relates to disturbances of REM sleep. Unlike most people, narcoleptics seem to begin their nocturnal sleep in an REM state. As indicated earlier, in normal people, initial sleep begins with several NREM stages followed later in the cycle by REM sleep. Narcoleptics do, however, seem to have relatively normal *amounts* of REM and NREM sleep during the night.

Treatment of narcolepsy has primarily consisted of drug therapy; benefits have been reported from stimulants such as amphetamines, although some complications and side effects may appear (Scammell et al., 2000; Wisor, Nishino, Sora, Uhl, & Mignot, 2001). Non-pharmacological treatments, such as behavior management and diet alteration, are only recently getting attention in the literature, and considerable research is needed to establish their effectiveness (Fosse, 2000).

SPEECH DISORDERS

IN FOCUS 7 ▶ Identify three types of speech disorders that often present difficulties for children.

Definitions of speech disorders have varied considerably. The definition used here represents a synthesis of several definitions. Defective speech or a **speech disorder** (which are terms often used interchangeably) refers to speech behavior that is sufficiently deviant from normal or accepted speaking patterns that it attracts attention and adversely affects communication for either the speaker or the listener. Like other disorders, speech disorders represent behavior deviations that clearly exceed the normal range of variations.

Prevalence estimates for speaking disabilities in children have varied greatly; consequently, many authors either avoid this topic or are extremely vague. The most frequently quoted figure in the speech pathology literature suggests that about 7–10% of the population is affected (Hardman, Drew, & Egan, 2002). In the 1998–1999 school year, 19% of all children aged 6 to 21 who received services in programs for those with disabilities were classified as having speech or language impairments (U.S. Department of Education, 2000). Speech and language impairments were cited as the second most common disability receiving special services under the Individuals with Disabilities Education Act in 1998–1999 (learning disabilities were first) (U.S. Department of Education, 2000). Both incidence and prevalence vary consistently as a function of age. The incidence of speech disorders is at roughly 12–15% for children in kindergarten through 4th grades, drops to about 4–5% in grades 5 through 8, and remains somewhat constant thereafter, unless therapeutic intervention is undertaken. In some cases, treatment results in improvement; in others, children outgrow a disorder or "self-correct" their problems. Treatment usage varies over time and between types of disorders, and authorities disagree widely on the impact of intervention early in the elementary years (e.g., Johnson & Slomka, 2000; Molfese & Molfese, 2000; Silliman & Diehl, 2002). Once again, we are faced with the reality that prevalence is socially rather than absolutely defined.

Identification and classification approaches to speech disorders have varied depending on etiology and the treatment perspective being employed. This section considers only speech disorders that are related to habit: problems of delayed speech, phonology or articulation, and stuttering. For a more comprehensive examination of speech disorders, you can consult other sources (e.g., Bernstein, 2002). It is important to remember that disorders are deviations from normal that are *significant* or *extreme*. Both children and adults show considerable variation in speaking ability or performance—some people are quite articulate (those "silver-tongued" individuals), whereas others are less facile ("tongue-tied"). The less skilled end of the normal range of speech facility is *not* the focus of the current discussion.

Delayed Speech

Very young children are typically able to communicate to some degree through gestures, noises, squeals, and other means prior to learning to speak

(Bernstein & Levey, 2002; Cheng, 2000). Most such behaviors tend to be dropped as they learn speech. However, some children develop speaking skills much later than is normally expected. In order to examine delayed speech, it is helpful to review the typical development of speech. Table 14-6 summarizes certain landmarks of normal language and speech development in children.

As noted previously, in some cases, maturation serves as a natural cure for certain speech problems. Most young children make a certain number of errors in their speech that do not typically persist. For example, they may delete final consonants ("buy" for *bike*) or unstressed syllables ("nana" for *banana*), and they often substitute certain sounds for others ("tit" for *sit*, "dup" for *soup*). These errors are often considered amusing and cute, and it is not uncommon for parents, siblings, and other individuals to focus attention on them—for example, by imitating the child's pronunciation to others or by speaking in "baby talk" to the child. These behaviors may inadvertently promote speech disorders. Although the precise nature of the impact remains unclear, modeling is thought to influence natural verbal development and is used in interventions (Bernstein & Levey, 2002; Owens, 2002; Weiss, 2002).

Delayed speech represents a failure of speech to develop at the expected age. Some children with delayed speech develop little or no expressive speech

Table 14-6 Normal Language and Prelanguage Development

Age	Behavior
Birth	Crying and making other physiological sounds
1 to 2 months	Cooing as well as crying
3 to 6 months	Babbling as well as cooing
9 to 14 months	Speaking first words as well as babbling
18 to 24 months	Speaking first sentences as well as words
3 to 4 years	Using all basic syntactical structures
4 to 8 years	Articulating correctly all speech sounds in context

SOURCE: Drew & Hardman (2000), p. 204. From *Mental Retardation: A Life Cycle Approach* by Drew & Hardman. Reprinted by permission of Pearson Education, Inc.

beyond vocalizations that are not interpretable as conventional language. Such children may continue to communicate nonverbally through gestures or to use nonspeech vocalizations extensively long after such behavior is typical. Other children with delayed speech can speak a little, but their proficiency is limited for their age and they mainly use nouns without qualifying or auxiliary words.

Etiology of Speech Delays

Delayed speech is a label that is applied to inadequate proficiency that may be caused by any of a number of influences, ranging broadly from heredity to environment. This disorder may stem from experience deprivation, as when a child is raised in an environment that provides little opportunity for learning to speak or in circumstances that actively interfere with mastering speaking skills. Delayed speech may be the result of sensory deprivation from an anatomical defect such as a hearing loss (Hardman et al., 2002; Radziewicz & Antonellis, 2002). Other factors that may contribute to cases of delayed speech include neurological problems (e.g., cerebral palsy), serious emotional disturbances such as childhood schizophrenia and autism, and less severe problems such as negativism (e.g., Chapman, 2000). This discussion focuses on speech delays that may be caused by the establishment of faulty learning, which in turn results from abnormal or unsatisfactory learning circumstances (e.g., experience deprivation, reinforcement contingencies that do not promote speaking) (Bernstein, 2002; Bernstein & Levey, 2002).

The term *negativism* relates to a set of behaviors or conditions that may contribute to delayed speech. When children are developing speech, great pressure is being exerted on them by their parents to learn many other skills as well. During this period, children are expected to learn how to eat properly, to go to bed when it is expected, to control excretory functions, and to perform many other behaviors that characterize adults. These demands exceed some children's tolerance level, and they may be unable to perform as expected by parents and others. Certain children respond negatively to such a situation by refusing to perform—one very effective type of refusal is refusing to talk. It is quite easy for a parent to punish some types of refusal (e.g., refusal to eat or to go to bed), but it is not as simple to handle a refusal to talk. A child cannot easily be forced to talk and may be able to communicate needs quite adequately through gestures. In other circumstances, children are frequently punished for talking because parents view it as inappropriate or inconvenient (e.g., it is too loud or badly timed because the parents are conversing, watching television, or reading). Consequently, it is easy to see how the habit of not speaking may be learned: It is reinforced at times, it is a method of avoiding punishment at other times, and it may be a means of expressing refusal to perform that does not place one in great jeopardy of being punished. If such circumstances persist over a sustained period of time when speech is typically developed, the result may be a child with a significant delay in speech. Not only has the child failed to learn speaking skills, but in some cases he or she has learned *not* to speak (Hardman et al., 2002).

If the child's failure to speak is a form of rebellion, the reward contingencies in the environment must be altered. It must be made more reinforcing to speak than not to do so. Additionally, the child must be taught the skills of speaking that have not yet been learned. It may also be necessary to alter behavior patterns that are only indirectly related to the speech delay, such as those involved in eating and going to bed. Clearly, if the problem persists over a period of years, it becomes increasingly difficult to treat because the delay is more pronounced and the behaviors have become more firmly habituated by continued and increasingly complex reinforcement contingencies.

Another category of causation of delayed speech is experience deprivation, in which environmental circumstances limit the opportunity to learn speaking skills and/or actually interfere with such learning. Environmental contingencies must exist in a configuration that will permit and promote children's learning to speak. This certainly does not mean that the home has to become a contrived miniature language class on a continuing basis. Most households function routinely in a manner that fosters a child's speech acquisition (e.g., encouragement to name objects and reinforcement for response). There are, however, some households that do not promote language acquisition, and significantly delayed child speech may result. In some cases, conversation is unusually infrequent in a child's home. Such circumstances may exist if the parents rarely speak with each other or the child. Conse-

quently, the child does not have much exposure to modeling of speech and perhaps receives little reinforcement for speaking and vocalizing. The basic principles of learning suggest that learning will be retarded in such an environment, and the outcome may well be delayed speech. A family might have additional problems that may contribute to a child's problems in learning to speak. The relationship between the parents may be tense or troubled, which results in a low frequency of verbal communication and also causes anxiety or fear in the child. Perhaps talking that does occur between the parents consists largely of arguing and threatening. This could easily compound the infrequent modeling by adding a component of punishment or aversive stimulation. The child's learning may be further interfered with if speaking is often associated with punishment (e.g., when the father speaks, the mother often shouts obscenities in response).

Other circumstances where there is limited speaking are quite different from those described above, but the net result may be quite similar. For example, a child with normal hearing capacity is born to deaf parents (either one or both). The parents' primary method of communication may be through signing and gestures. There may be little speech learning by a child in this type of environment, or at best, the child's speech proficiency may be significantly delayed. It should be emphasized that the outcomes of such circumstances are extremely variable. One of the authors knows of four brothers with normal hearing who were born to parents who were deaf and had been so from a very early age. The parents used sign language but little or no verbal communication. All of the boys (now adults) learned to speak quite well, and although they experienced some minor problems in school, they have distinguished themselves in a variety of fashions. One holds a Ph.D. degree in special education from a major university. A second has both an M.D. and a Ph.D. (the latter earned at a well-known European university), the third is an able public servant, and the fourth began his rise to the heights of achievement as an inventor and has become a millionaire. Anyone would be fortunate to be so successful, but it is important to remember that this is an exceptional story. An introspective recollection by one of the brothers (in Hardman et al., 2002) suggested a variety of exceptional influences, such as unusually close relationships with their grandparents, that led to a favorable outcome in this particular case. Substantial speech delay is not uncommon in hearing children born into an environment where verbalization is unusually infrequent on account of parental deafness.

Delayed speech caused by experience deprivation may also occur in homes where there is a great deal of verbalization and noise occurring in a very confused and unsystematic fashion. From a learning perspective, such an environment may seriously impede the acquisition of speech at the time when it is normally learned. Learning a complex skill such as speech is a rather delicate process, particularly in its early stages. Stimuli must be presented in an uncomplicated, systematic fashion and without competing or distracting stimuli so that a child can focus on the important features and discriminate those that are central from those that are not important (Nelson, 2002). Additionally, when an appropriate behavior occurs, it needs to be reinforced (and this process must be repeated consistently for learning to progress). A chaotic environment probably will not provide such contingencies and may produce delayed speech.

Children learning to speak will tend to take the route that requires the least effort. Thus, if there is little need to speak, it is unlikely that the child will do so, and in some homes a child has little need to speak. Such conditions are often described in other terms (e.g., the overprotective parent, etc.), but from a learning perspective, there simply may be little need to learn speech. As infants begin to interact with those around them, they communicate in several ways. They may imitate, express pleasure or displeasure, and request with sounds, gestures, facial expressions, and body posture. Reciprocal interactions between parents and infants is very important during this early period, and it is not uncommon to encounter parents who want to satisfy all of their child's needs (Tiegerman-Farber, 2002). Some parents anticipate a child's desires or needs and quickly provide for them by responding to gestures or nonspecific vocalizations. They may rush to feed their children, procure toys for them, and meet a multitude of other needs in response to a mere gesture or cry. By doing this, they may teach (reinforce) such behaviors and delay speech development. It is easy to see how such behaviors, in extreme form, could teach a child to meet needs in a fashion other than speaking. Delayed speech could result from this type of situation.

Treatment of Speech Delays

Speech delay caused by experience deprivation can be treated by using fundamental principles of learning; in theory, this is a simple task, but implementation can be very difficult. Alteration and precise control of stimuli and reinforcement contingencies may be quite complex. Considerable success has been evident in direct teaching interventions that alter the stimulus-reinforcement contingency in order to promote more normal speech development (Robinson & Robb, 2002; Weiss, 2002). Obviously, alternative methods, procedures, and perspectives are useful in order to enhance individualization, and treatment may well involve collaboration between speech clinicians, teachers, and parents (Iacono, Chan, & Waring, 1998; Nelson, 2002). The approach always depends on the specific details of the problem(s) and the viewpoint of the therapist.

Phonological Disorders

Phonological disorders were previously classified as articulation disorders and are the most frequently occurring category of all speech disorders according to DSM-IV-TR (American Psychiatric Association, 2000). These disorders represent the majority of cases encountered by public school speech clinicians, with some prevalence estimates ranging as high as 80% (Cicci, 1998; Hardman et al., 2002). An articulation disorder is basically a disturbance in speech-sound production. In most instances, such problems in children are *functional articulation disorders*; that is, they are not caused by any readily apparent organic defect. In a certain number of cases, articulation difficulties follow a developmental path; as the child grows older, articulation errors often diminish or are eliminated. This has led some public school officials to contend that speech clinicians should not give as much attention as they do to articulation problems, particularly when children are very young. Certainly, there is some logic to such a position in light of the scarcity of fiscal and human resources. However, some articulation errors are not caused solely by immature speech development. Articulation performance is likely to improve with overall development until about the age of 9 or 10. Problems that exist beyond that point are likely to persist unless therapy intervenes; such disorders can become increasingly difficult to remedy if permitted to continue untreated, and individuals may continue to be affected by a disorder for years (Johnson & Slomka, 2000; Molfese & Molfese, 2000).

As with other speech disorders, defective articulation may be caused by a variety of factors. Some cases are due to brain damage or nerve injury (often referred to as *dysartia*); others are caused by physical deformity (such as malformed mouth, jaw, or teeth structures); some are believed to be inherited; and many cases represent learned behaviors (Gibbon, 1999; Hardman et al., 2002; Stimley & Hambrecht, 1999). Those caused by defective learning (functional disorders) constitute a significant problem, since only a small proportion of articulation errors can be attributed to identifiable organic flaws. However, functional articulation disorders also have many causes. The stimulus-reinforcement contingencies that give rise to such problems are as variable as those that promote or permit speech development in general. Perhaps the modeling by parents is inappropriate (e.g., baby talk). Although the influence of baby talk has been questioned, the literature suggests that the nature of parental speech does influence children's linguistic maturity (e.g., Bernstein & Levey, 2002). It may be that household reinforcement for accurate speech production is unsystematic. It is generally less important to pinpoint the causes of functional articulation disorders than to determine the causes of organically based disorders, which may be amenable to surgical correction (Cochrane & Slade, 1999). However, the environmental contingencies cannot be ignored since treatment may need to focus on altering them. The essential task is one of rearranging learning contingencies so that more appropriate speech patterns can be acquired and generalized to diverse environments. A variety of behavior modification procedures have been successful in improving learned articulation problems (Skelton, 1999). Generalization of appropriate learning is obviously important to the child's overall speech performance (Dehaney, 2000; Skelton, 1999), and treatment may, once again, involve collaboration among teachers, parents, and speech therapists (Dettmer, Dyck, & Thurston, 1999; Iacono et al., 1998; Nelson, 2002).

Stuttering

Stuttering is a disorder of fluency and is perhaps the most widely recognized of all speech problems. **Stuttering** is a disturbance in the fluency and rhythm of speech with intermittent blocking, repetition, or prolongation of sounds, syllables, words, or phrases. Nearly all of us at one time or another have known or encountered an individual who stutters, and most of us occasionally exhibit such behaviors ourselves even though we are not stutterers. Furthermore, nearly all young children stutter at times as they develop their speaking abilities. For the most part, these are normal nonfluencies that disappear as the child grows older and progresses in speech development. However, these normal behaviors play a prominent role in certain theories of stuttering.

Many people think of stuttering almost automatically when speech disorders are mentioned. This is not surprising since the interruptions in the flow of speech that characterize stuttering are very evident and easily remembered. Additionally, stuttering makes listeners very uncomfortable. Listeners often try to "help" the stutterer by filling in the relevant words when a block occurs. It is clear that the communication process creates a considerable degree of discomfort for both the stutterer and listener. Despite the fact that stuttering is noticed, it is among the least prevalent of speech disorders (Mansson, 2000; Van Borsel, Verniers, & Bouvry, 1999). Although prevalence statistics are notoriously variable and inaccurate, stuttering consistently appears as a speech disorder that occurs rather infrequently when compared to other problems.

Etiology of Stuttering

The causes of stuttering have been investigated for many years. Many scientists in the past have searched fruitlessly for a single cause. More current thinking has discarded this oversimplified perspective in favor of a view that stuttering may have a variety of causes (Gottwald, 1999; Ludlow, 1999). Theories about the causes of stuttering can basically be divided into three types: those that address it as an emotional or neurotic problem (i.e., wherein stuttering is a behavioral manifestation of some emotional difficulty), those that view it as a constitutional or neurological problem, and those that view it from a learning perspective.

There is decreased interest in attempting to find a constitutional cause of stuttering, although a few studies still appear in the literature. Some investigators have explored neurological dysfunction generally, whereas others have focused more specifically on

Back to the Beginning

Understanding and Treating Eating Disorders

Many disorders have both physiological and psychological sources, symptoms, and consequences. The eating disorders, such as Tina's anorexia nervosa, described at the beginning of this chapter, affect both mind and body. The perfectionism, rejection of help and advice, anxiety, depression, and rigid eating patterns are psychological problems, and the result of severely restricted eating, the starvation syndrome, is a serious physical problem. There are psychological components to Scott's obesity as well. Why would a boy choose food over friends and activities? What would lead him to remain at home while everyone else is playing together and having a good time outside? Why doesn't he do something to lose weight so he won't be teased by the other boys? And why does his family encourage him to eat high-calorie junk food rather than a healthy diet? Here, considerations such as the family's education and income level are important, since better-educated, more advantaged families are usually better informed about nutrition and exercise. Perhaps Scott's mother has never learned what foods to serve her family, or the family's income is low, encouraging them to eat high-carbohydrate meals. Alternatively, his mother could want to keep Scott with her and keeping him fat is an effective way to do so. There are many ways in which psychological and social factors can enter into eating patterns and disorders.

Whatever the psychological basis for Tina's and Scott's unhealthy eating patterns, there are similarities in the treatments they receive. Drugs such as antidepressants can be helpful if teenagers have both eating disorders and depression. However, these drugs are typically not administered for a long period of time, and eating problems may reoccur when the drug is stopped. Cognitive-behavioral therapy is often the treatment of choice, and family therapy is often appropriate, since eating disorders typically involve the entire family. Research indicates that Scott's prognosis is fairly good if he is treated promptly and if he wants to make a change. Tina's is a more difficult case, and she may very well have starved herself into such bad physical condition that she requires hospitalization. With good, individualized treatment involving cognitive-behavioral therapy, family therapy, and perhaps group therapy, she has a reasonable chance of resuming a normal life. However, she may continue to experience compulsive symptoms and mood problems and will certainly have to battle anorexic tendencies in the future.

So we see that physical and mental well-being go hand in hand. Many physical illnesses have psychological contributors, and both medical and psychological treatments are necessary for eating disorders, as well as many other problems that affect children and adolescents.

---

such factors as problems of cerebral dominance or cortical organization. Results have been mixed (Ludlow, 1999). Some evidence has suggested that individuals with fluent speech may have brain organization that differs from those who stutter. There has also been some suggestion that those who stutter use different parts of the brain in information processing. Other researchers have found some support for the notion that problems of cerebral dominance may be present to a greater degree in those who stutter than in those who are fluent. Finally, some have speculated that the separate neural systems controlling various

components of speech production may be out of synchronization in those who stutter (Hardman et al., 2002). Thus, recent research addressing neurological causation of stuttering has shown variable results with rather divergent theoretical outcomes.

Researchers have also explored a variety of other possibilities. Some literature has examined the notion that heredity may play a role in stuttering; this line of thinking is related to observed sex differences in the incidence of the disorder (male stutterers outnumber females about 4 to 1). Some studies have suggested that the hereditary influence exists because of higher incidence of stuttering within certain families, because of disfluency of parents of some stutterers, and because results of twin studies (e.g., Guitar, 1998; Stagg & Burns, 1999). However, it is generally difficult to separate the effects of heredity and environment in speech disorders as well as in other areas (Drew & Hardman, 2000; Yairi, 1999). Often this can be accomplished only by specific genetic analysis (such as in certain types of Down syndrome). Other researchers have explored causal implications of the emotional dimensions of parent-child interactions, although little support has emerged for emotional causation. With regard to emotional causation, it has also been speculated that the stuttering child may experience demands that exceed his or her capacity to respond (e.g., Ratner & Healey, 1999; Whaley & Golden, 2000). Once again, the research has been fragmentary, and substantial support for such a view is lacking.

The learning theory approach to stuttering is not new but has attracted increased attention over the years. Stuttering tends to emerge most often between 3 and 5 years of age (Mansson, 2000). Some have contended that stuttering, in its fully developed form, is a learned and more severe form of the normal nonfluency exhibited in the early years. The hypothesis is that a child may develop stuttering if substantial attention is directed to normal nonfluencies during the early development of speech. Interest in this perspective continues, although it should be noted that it also has its critics (e.g., Max & Caruso, 1998; Ratner, 2000). Even among those who favor the learning theory view of stuttering, there is considerable difference of opinion concerning the functioning and precise form of the learning contingencies. Each case must be examined and treated individually.

Treatment of Stuttering

Treatment of stuttering has been as varied as the theories of its causation. Psychotherapy has met with limited success. Other treatment procedures have focused on the rhythm process of speech, for example, by using a metronome to establish a beat, or have employed relaxation therapy to overcome tenseness (Gilman & Yaruss, 2000). In all cases, results have been mixed. Some success has been evident with play therapy, creative dramatics, parental counseling, and work with teachers and classmates (Howell, Sackin, & Williams, 1999; Kalinowski, Stuart, Wamsley, & Ras-

tatter, 1999). Treatment of stuttering has increasingly included behavioral therapy that attempts to teach the affected individual fluent speaking patterns (Onslow & Packman, 1999). Individualized treatment programs seem to be essential, focusing on the stimulus-reinforcement contingencies in each child's environment. For certain children, it is important to learn to monitor and manage their stuttering, perhaps through speaking more slowly and in a rhythmic fashion. For others, it appears that they must also be aware of physical factors such as breathing. Stuttering is a complex disorder, and its effective treatment may also be rather intricate.

SUMMARY

This chapter has examined a diverse range of disorders that present significant difficulties in a child's development. Many of these create problems that sorely test the resources and patience of families and challenge the knowledge and clinical skill of pediatric psychologists. Parents who seek assistance in solving their children's problems frequently receive conflicting opinions and advice. This further emphasizes the need for systematic and rigorous research that will provide a more solid information base for effective clinical treatment, a fact that is noted repeatedly in this book.

A great deal of public attention has been given to eating problems, including obesity, self-starvation, and binge eating and purging. Although seemingly a simple problem on the surface, obesity is an extremely complex one according to both physiological and psychological research. A variety of treatments have been employed for obesity, but their effectiveness with adults has largely been disappointing. However, with children, behavioral therapy has lasting positive results, suggesting that early intervention is crucial. Anorexia nervosa is a complex eating disorder that is rare but increasing in prevalence. Primarily a problem occurring in adolescent females, anorexia nervosa is a condition of self-inflicted starvation. Health complications can be extremely serious, even resulting in death in a certain percentage of cases, and treatment is quite difficult. Bulimia nervosa, or the binge-purge syndrome, is characterized by episodes of gorging followed by purging via vomiting or laxatives. Like anorexia, bulimia can have serious health consequences. Research and treatment of bulimia are made more difficult because this behavior is denied and kept secret by those affected.

Serious toileting problems include encopresis and enuresis. Toileting problems range from common problems of infancy and childhood to persistent difficulties of the severely mentally ill or people with mental retardation or developmental delays. Encopresis involves problematic patterns of fecal expulsion, whereas enuresis refers to inappropriate wetting. These disorders have been thought to be related to each other although evidence for this view is lacking. Treatment can be very difficult, and relapses are frequent.

Sleep problems are a common difficulty. Researchers have studied the different stages of sleep and related them to sleep disorders, including night terrors, nightmares, and somnambulism. Research seems to indicate that different stages of sleep are associated with these conditions. More research on sleep disorders is clearly needed, since the behaviors can be quite pronounced in some cases and are difficult to treat.

Speech disorders reportedly affect 7–10% of the general population. Stuttering is probably the most widely recognized speech difficulty. However, it is actually found in a much smaller percentage of the population than other types of speech disorders, such as articulation problems. Treatment of speech disorders varies greatly depending on the type of disorder and often the characteristics of the individual case. In some instances, treatment is relatively simple whereas in others it may be complex, lengthy, and of limited effectiveness. Learning-based treatments have been particularly successful in treating certain speech disorders.

INFOTRAC COLLEGE EDITION

For more information, explore this resource at http://www.infotrac-college.com/Wadsworth. Enter the following search terms:

antidepressant medication
cognitive-behavioral therapy
contingency contracting
desensitization
early intervention
modeling
reinforcement
operant learning
problem-solving skills training
primary prevention
family therapy

IN FOCUS ANSWERS

IN FOCUS 1 ▶ Identify four characteristics that are often observed in victims of anorexia nervosa.

- Most often between 14 and 18 years old
- Primarily female
- Often have perfectionist tendencies
- Face a real risk of death

IN FOCUS 2 ▶ Identify the steps for treating anorexia nervosa.

- First, correct the individual's nutrition problem and achieve medical stabilization.
- Restore a normal diet, which can be difficult if patients resist, attempt to exercise surreptitiously, secretly induce vomiting, or even escape from the treatment unit; but appropriate nutrition is essential in order to begin reversing the physical deterioration.
- Treatment must address a variety of factors since the weight and nutrition problems may be symptoms of other persistent psychological difficulties.
- Therapy approaches often include family counseling. Family therapy seems to have more lasting benefits than individual therapy.

IN FOCUS 3 ▶ How are bulimia nervosa and anorexia nervosa different?

- Bulimia nervosa involves frequent episodes of uncontrolled binge eating alternating with purging of what has been consumed. It can co-occur with anorexia nervosa.
- Individuals with bulimia often maintain a weight close to an appropriate level, whereas with anorexia, the person is significantly underweight.
- Individuals with bulimia fluctuate between gaining and losing weight, whereas those with anorexia are characterized by extreme, life-threatening, weight loss.

IN FOCUS 4 ▶ Define obesity, and tell how many individuals are estimated to be obese.

- In general, obese individuals have excess body fat and weigh approximately 30% more than is considered normal, based on published expected weights such as the Metropolitan Life Insurance Company tables.
- Estimates suggest that 5–10% of the preschool population is obese, rising to 27% for ages 6 to 11 and 22% in the teenage years.
- The prevalence of obesity, especially among children, has increased substantially in the last 15 years.

IN FOCUS 5 ▶ What are the prevalence estimates for enuresis, and when is incontinence considered to be a problem in children?

- DSM-IV-TR cites prevalence figures of 5–10% for children at 5 years of age, 3–5% by age 10, and a lingering 1% of 15-year-olds.

- Most clinicians view urinary incontinence after about 3 to 5 years of age as a problem.

IN FOCUS 6 ▶ How often do sleep disorders occur in people of different ages?

- Sleep disorders may occur in 30–45% of very young children.
- Specific sleeping difficulties, such as insomnia, are reported by a similar proportion of adults.

IN FOCUS 7 ▶ Identify three types of speech disorders that often present difficulties for children.

- Delayed speech
- Phonological (articulation) disorders
- Stuttering (fluency disorder)

In the Beginning

Getting Help for Ben

Ben's mother was half expecting the call from his kindergarten teacher. She had seen for herself how Ben tore around the classroom, picking things up and throwing them down, grabbing materials from other children, and not seeming to notice the teacher's instructions to sit down. His behavior was sometimes bad at home, but worse at school, where everything seemed to excite him. He soon became known as one of the most difficult children in his class. Five-year-old Ben was everywhere at once. If he wasn't out of his chair bothering some other child, he was tapping the desk like a drum, looking around the room, whistling, swinging his legs, or doing something else distracting, but rarely attending to his work. He drove everyone wild.

Ben's teacher, Mrs. Johnson, said that many children with problems like Ben's turned out to have attention-deficit/hyperactivity disorder (ADHD) and improved with professional treatment. Ben's mom made an appointment with his pediatrician right away, and they were soon referred to a child and family psychological clinic for assessment. The diagnosis of ADHD was confirmed, and Ben joined a small therapy group of children his age with similar problems.

The therapy consisted of a behavior management program to help the children learn to attend to school tasks for longer periods, to resist impulses to engage in off-task behaviors, to remain seated when appropriate, and to complete their work. If they were following instructions and were on-task when a timer sounded, their therapists and teachers reinforced them by giving them points toward a reward. Later the children would be taught to award points to themselves for appropriate behavior, and finally the program would be gradually removed as they improved. The therapist showed Ben's parents how to set up and administer similar reinforcement programs for him at home. In addition, his pediatrician prescribed a low dosage of a mild stimulant drug, methylphenidate (trade name Ritalin), to help Ben improve his attention to his work and behave less impulsively. Ben's physical reaction to the drug and the dosage level were monitored at regular intervals.

Not all children like Ben with behavior problems receive the best treatment and follow-up, so they fail to improve as much as they could. What is the prognosis for children who receive various types of psychotherapy and medications? Research has provided some answers to this question.

INTRODUCTION

This chapter provides an overview of the different approaches therapists use to treat a wide range of behavior and adjustment problems in infants, children, and adolescents. We describe the various psychotherapies and medications that are used for healing the major types of child psychopathology. Psychotherapies and drug treatments are best viewed as complementary rather than competing ways of helping children. Both drug treatment and psychotherapy are useful under the appropriate circumstances, and they are often used together to address different aspects of a child's problem. For example, a combination of antianxiety medication and behavior therapy reduces children's anxiety; teaching them specific skills to help them cope with stress (Kearney & Silverman, 1998) and giving them a selective serotonin reuptake inhibitor (SSRI) are routinely combined with cognitive-behavioral therapy for the treatment of obsessive-compulsive disorder (March, Franklin, Nelson, & Foa, 2001).

This is not to say that all treatment approaches are equally effective or that they all carry the same level of risk to the child. The chapter points out the better treatments and contrasts them with others that have not withstood research evaluation or are unusually expensive, restrictive, or risky. Although many forms of treatment are sufficiently safe and effective to recommend for use with children, most fall far short of universal effectiveness and complete safety (Werry, 2001). In an era of managed health care, there are demands for greater cost-effectiveness, so the more expensive or lengthy interventions or those that are less effective are quickly winnowed out. This selection process is accomplished largely through rigorous examination of treatment expense and effectiveness. Pursuing this book's theme that research protects children, this chapter examines the research on treatment effectiveness and offers research-based conclusions on treatment choices.

The chapter also stresses the importance of matching the treatment, whether psychological or biological, to the developmental level of the child, emphasizing another theme of this book. Rather than automatically assuming that psychological interventions and drugs developed for adults are safe and effective when administered to children, all interventions should be empirically evaluated for pediatric use. Thus, the theme "development is fundamental" clearly applies to treatment issues, where the child's developmental status is a central consideration. The psychopharmacology section of this chapter considers the ethical use of prescription drugs with children and adolescents. It asks whether many overloaded practitioners follow the guidelines for safe and appropriate use of interventions with children, particularly in view of the widespread and rapidly increasing use of psychiatric drugs originally intended for adults and still untested or insufficiently tested with child patients.

Children have much less freedom of choice than adults do in choosing their medical and psychological treatment. Adults can select the type of treatment they receive, within the limits of their health care plans, but children must follow their parents' wishes regarding their treatment. Younger children, in particular, have very little say in the type and amount of mental health treatment they receive. Treatment alternatives are numerous; over 500 types of psychotherapy are offered to the public (Kazdin, 2000), and new drug treatments for children are being developed constantly. Clinicians need clinical expertise and research knowledge in order to select and deliver the best treatment for an individual child and family. In addition, a child's treatment is often individually tailored and includes techniques from several different treatment approaches. This mixed-method treatment, termed the **eclectic approach**, is used by many clinical practitioners to deal with clients' individual needs (Kazdin, Siegel, & Bass, 1990). Essentially, the clinician picks and chooses from among the different types of therapy to produce a combination of useful intervention techniques for an individual child. For example, a child psychologist first used nonspecific play therapy to gain the confidence of Ann, a 9-year-old girl who was receiving bad grades and complained that she had no friends. Her therapist also gave her parents training in a home-based token reinforcement system to improve her homework and taught Ann how to play with other children and to use self-reinforcement for positive self-talk. These cognitive-behavioral tactics helped her overcome her social isolation, fear of failure, and withdrawal. In virtually all cases, interventions are individually developed to suit the needs of the children being treated. Therapy is definitely not a case of one size fits all, but requires a thorough understanding of each child's unique problems and strengths and of the family and living situation.

However, it may not be necessary to combine therapies in treating a child. A surprising research finding showed that a single form of intervention often proves just as effective as combined approaches (Kazdin, 1996). This research result may indicate that clinicians neglect to apply each treatment fully when several are combined. That is, the intensity of the treatment may suffer when several techniques from behavior therapy, play therapy, special education, and cognitive-behavioral therapy are used with the same child at the same time. Care must be taken to administer each therapy component in full strength for the full time needed in order to ensure that the treatment is fully effective.

The child is not always the only or primary family member who is troubled. Even when the child is initially identified as the client, closer study often reveals that other relatives also have life challenges that may affect the child and require professional attention. It is necessary to understand the child's adjustment difficulties in the context of family relationships, school demands, peer group functioning, and the child's own developmental status. Finally, since appropriate treatment of children requires familiarity with their family and culture, treatment concerns definitely relate to this book's theme that behavior must be understood in context.

DEVELOPMENTAL CONSIDERATIONS

IN FOCUS 1 ▶ Describe some of the most common adjustment problems of infants, elementary school children, and adolescents.

Adults' treatments fit children no better than adult-sized clothing does. In child treatment, many wrong turns and blind alleys have resulted because therapists failed to appreciate youngsters' special, age-related ways of thinking about the world and themselves, their more limited time perspective, their age-related anxieties and fears, and the many other ways in which they differ psychologically from adults. Even today, many types of psychotherapy for children are inadequately adapted forms of adult interventions

intended to provide insight into clients' conflicts and problems. Understanding their own behavior from another person's perspective is a very difficult task for young children, and it is an inappropriate goal for very young therapy clients. Developmental psychology theory and research indicate that there are wider differences in thinking and problem solving between young children and adults than there are between adults from widely dissimilar cultures—for example, impoverished, isolated farmers and middle-class, big-city dwellers. So people who work with troubled youngsters need to become acquainted with the norms of psychological development so that they know what to expect from children of different ages. To appreciate the importance of developmental levels, just ask a preschooler a difficult question, such as what bothers the child and what to do about it. You will feel a real appreciation for the challenges of clinical work with young children, many of whom tend to be shy with unfamiliar adults and may just stop talking at all if they become confused or feel intimidated.

In order to determine the most appropriate type of treatment for a child, a therapist must consider several factors, including the nature, severity, and number of problems, the child's age and cognitive development, and the family composition. The child's developmental level is often related to the child's presenting problem and is thus a major consideration in diagnosis and treatment. The characteristics and adjustment problems typical of children of different ages (described in Chapter 1) guide the choice of treatment, as outlined in Table 15-1.

As the following cases show, each age period has particular features and challenges:

- The youngest children may have difficulty in forming secure attachments with their primary caretakers, so parent training may be necessary. Marti, who is 2 years old, is an example. She resists her mother's attempts to hold her and quiet her and doesn't seem happy when her mom comes home from work. Their interactions are abrupt, tense, and not pleasant for either of them. The mother would benefit from professional help to show her how to be more gentle and loving with Marti and how to calm her when she is irritable and crying. Other infants and toddlers may have developmental delay disorders calling for intensive individual

Table 15-1 Matching Psychosocial Treatments with Children's Developmental Levels	
Child Age Range	**Common Treatment Methods**
Infants and toddlers	Training mother in more sensitive, responsive parenting; therapeutic group care for infants
Preschool children	Parent training in behavior management, play therapy, therapeutic preschool programs
Elementary school	Insight-oriented psychodynamic or client-centered therapy; individual or group behavioral therapy; systems, behavioral, or eclectic family therapy; foster or institutional care
Preadolescents and adolescents	Group psychotherapy of various types, family therapy, individual psychotherapy, foster or institutional care

training in basic skills such as feeding, muscle control, control of tantrums, and following simple instructions.

- When they are in elementary school, children's social adjustment and peer relations become very important. Some children are too shy and awkward to make friends and are bullied; others become the bullies, who must learn to control their aggression. Attention deficit, hyperactivity, and impulsivity are also problems at this age, particularly in classrooms. Many children need to learn to behave appropriately in the controlled setting of the school. Jack, the bully, and Aaron, the victim, are an all-too-typical pair. Jack terrorizes Aaron, takes his things and money, and threatens to beat him up. While one feels powerful and confident, the other becomes powerless and afraid. Both of these boys need the school's intervention and psychological help so that their unhealthy relationship does not continue.

- During their teens, many youngsters have difficulty with schoolwork and reconciling the demands of school, peers, and home. Some become defiant and negative as they attempt to become independent of their parents. Illicit drugs, alcohol, smoking, reckless driving, truancy, sexual experimentation, and thrill seeking of all types are constant temptations for many American teenagers. Adult forms of mood disorders and eating disorders appear at this time, especially in girls. Jeanette is an example. She began to want to stay home a lot rather than go out with her friends, and her weight dropped rapidly; then she started crying at the least little thing. Her self-concept seemed to be at rock-bottom, and she wore long hair and bangs to conceal her face. Try what they might, no one could cheer her up. When she failed to improve

after a month, her parents took her to a mental health clinic for an assessment. She had major depression at the age of 17 years but, fortunately, responded rapidly to treatment and was able to graduate and enter college on schedule.

Motivation Issues

Troubled adults typically go to therapists willingly, seeking relief from their problems. Most want to change their lives and are ready to make a commitment to do so. In contrast, children and adolescents are more likely to blame others for their difficulties, such as teachers, peers, or family members. Adolescents in particular often resist others' explanations of their problems and refuse to take their medication or participate in psychotherapy. A youngster with a tendency to deny problems and assign blame to others is uncooperative and resistant to the idea that he or she must change. Clinical skill of a high order is needed to work with such a therapy client, who comes unwillingly to treatment. It is a good idea to seek help from practitioners who specialize in work with children and adolescents.

Communicating through Play

Therapists who work with children must first win the child's trust through appropriate and interesting activities (Freud, 1945). Play and games are familiar and fun, so therapists who treat young children frequently use such activities as a way of putting children at ease. Play is used at the beginning of treatment even by therapists who later introduce structured behavioral therapy programs with few play-like features. Young children communicate more freely in play than in formal verbal interviews, and play allows them to express

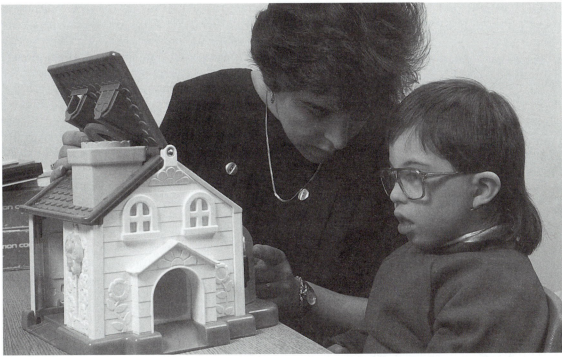

Therapists who work with young children often use play as a way of putting the children at ease so that they can talk more freely about their problems.

their problems and receive help in dealing with them. Guided play activities are a common type of intervention for children (Koocher & D'Angelo, 1992; Leblanc & Ritchie, 2001). Play is particularly useful in the treatment of younger children's fears and anxieties (Russ, 1995). However, dolls can be misused as assessment tools by untrained examiners. Clinicians must be especially cautious in using anatomical dolls in assessing whether children have been sexually abused, as discussed in Chapter 6.

Cultural Diversity

Are cognitive-behavioral interventions as effective with children in Japan or India as they are with children in the United States? There are few published research studies comparing the effects of particular types of therapy with children from different ethnic groups, even groups within the United States. The little research evidence available suggests that similar treatments produce comparable results when used with somewhat different national and ethnic groups

(Christophersen & Mortweet, 2001). However, practitioners should be aware of and sensitive to the child therapy client's cultural context. Ideally, therapists should share the child's ethnicity and cultural background, but that is not often feasible. Practitioners are advised to conduct culturally appropriate assessments of child clients, using language that is familiar to the child. For example, in testing inner-city youth, Black English is preferable to formal, business-style speech, which is foreign to members of the African-American culture (Rodriguez & Walls, 2000). Furthermore, cultures differ in what their members consider to be problem behaviors in children. If children are expected to sleep with their parents or to be very quiet or highly active, these are not problems and do not call for treatment. Surprisingly little is known about the role of cultural issues in assessment and therapy, and a great deal of research is needed in this and other areas of psychology (Hall, 1997). Awareness of and sensitivity to cultural issues is most important for mental health services in a nation rapidly becoming more racially and ethnically diverse.

MAJOR APPROACHES TO PSYCHOLOGICAL TREATMENT

IN FOCUS 2 ▶ Describe the research evidence for the effectiveness of psychodynamic, nondirective play, behavioral, and cognitive-behavioral therapies.

Psychodynamic Therapy

Psychodynamic therapy is based on Freud's psychoanalytic theory and aimed at resolving internal, mental conflict thought to be the cause of the individual's problems. Psychodynamic therapy involves a demanding schedule of sessions three to five times a week, while the more common psychoanalytically oriented therapy features sessions on a reduced schedule of one or two times a week, possibly over a period of 1 or 2 years (Tuma & Russ, 1993). These interventions assume that unconscious inner emotional turmoil, particularly anxiety, lies at the heart of a child's problem. Emotional distress and behavioral disturbances are presumed to stem from mental conflict of which the child is unaware (see Chapter 2). When the child is guided toward understanding the emotional basis of the problem and forms a close alliance with the therapist, the healing process begins.

Although most therapists today are trained in other interventions, the psychodynamic approach to child therapy is still in use. Despite its long history, this approach has attracted little research attention, and so its effectiveness is largely unknown. Traditional child psychotherapy (nonbehavioral, excluding family therapy, and incorporating some psychodynamic elements) was not found to be clearly effective in actual clinical practice (Burns, Hoagwood, & Mrazek, 1999; Weiss, Catron, Harris, & Phung, 1999). Further, based on criteria adapted from the American Psychological Association, psychodynamic therapy was not included in a list of well-established and probably efficacious treatments for conduct disorder (Brestan & Eyberg, 1998). This approach is generally considered to be more appropriate for shyness, anxiety, fear, and social withdrawal than for externalizing, antisocial disorders.

Nondirective Play Therapy

Nondirective play therapy was once among the most frequently used approaches in child treatment. Based on the work of Carl Rogers (1951), this therapy attempts to help the child to accept her own unwelcome impulses and learn to accept more realistic expectations of herself. To do so, the therapist establishes a warm relationship with the child, accepts the child as she is, and encourages the child to express her feelings, whatever they may be (Axline, 1976). This must be a refreshing change for children who are constantly badgered to improve by their parents and teachers. The therapist repeats or reflects the child's expressions without evaluating them, thus encouraging the child to accept herself. It is not clear whether this strategy promotes improvement, since it is not often evaluated in controlled research on therapy outcomes. Nondirective techniques are often used in eclectic out-patient psychotherapy, which is more effective than no therapy (Johnson, Rasbury, & Siegel, 1997) but has limited effectiveness in clinical practice (Burns et al., 1999; Weiss et al., 1999).

Behavioral Therapy

Behavioral therapy typically deals directly with the child's problem behaviors and does not try to provide the child with insight into his own conflicts. For example, in behavioral training, children with autism are taught to attend to and imitate the therapist in speaking words and phrases, children with specific phobias are taught to relax in the presence of the feared stimulus, and socially isolated and awkward children are taught appropriate ways in which to approach and talk with classmates. Behavioral programs are clearly educational, teaching children the skills they need to overcome their difficulties. Skill deficits can arise from various physical and psychological problems, but whatever their cause, a child might profit from well-designed and carefully administered behavioral intervention. Current conditions rather than early childhood experiences, as proposed in the psychodynamic view, are more likely to cause or prolong the child's problems. And the treatment agents are more likely to be parents and teachers who are carefully trained in the procedures than therapists in an office setting.

The first behavioral therapies to be developed were based on Skinner's operant learning principles and featured skill training through the positive reinforcement of desirable behavior. This seemingly simple process can be a very powerful vehicle for improvement, even in children with severe mental retardation and teenagers with extreme eating disorders or conduct disorder. Positive reinforcers are identified through their effects on behavior. Anything that increases the probability that an immediately preceding voluntary behavior will be repeated is termed a *positive reinforcer*. For some children, attention or recognition is a positive reinforcer; others respond to food treats, play opportunities, or TV viewing. The power of Skinner's approach is that reinforcers are individually determined through observing the child's preferences; that is, this approach is tailored to the needs of the individual child. If you see an adult with a clipboard carefully recording the child's behavior or a child making her own behavioral records, it is likely that some operant learning program is in process. Very specific behavioral goals are set by the therapist and adjusted as the child's behavior improves.

Token programs are popular in many child care and treatment settings and for children of different ages and abilities. Children can earn tokens good for a variety of treats and activities by attending to their studies, following the teacher's instructions, doing household chores, or other daily activities. The tokens are positive reinforcers used to reward good behavior in many homes, schools, and treatment settings, much as money is used to sustain adults' job performance.

Undesirable behavior patterns are reduced in a number of ways. In extinction, reinforcement is withheld when the child engages in disruptive behavior, such as tantrums, or refuses to follow instructions. In **time-out from positive reinforcement**, positive reinforcers are withheld very briefly until the child resumes normal behavior. This technique has been embraced by American teachers and parents as an alternative to physical punishment, although many do not understand how to use it correctly.

Some people resist using operant methods, because they see positive reinforcers as bribes for doing what should be done without any special inducement. Unfortunately, the alternatives are often ineffective nagging, criticism, or worse. Like adults, children must be rewarded for their work or they may cease to try. And also like adults, children too frequently receive little or no attention or any other reward for their good behavior. To verify this statement, just observe how seldom adults give children praise and other posi-

tive attention for behaving well at school, church, and home versus how often they reprimand them for behaving badly. Praise is surprisingly rare.

Reinforcement contingency management and other operant techniques have controlled misbehavior and taught adaptive behaviors to many thousands of individual children in therapeutic programs (Weisz, Weiss, Han, Granger, & Morton, 1995). Many demonstrations of the effectiveness of behavioral interventions have used analysis of individual behavior (see Chapter 3) and cannot be compared with group treatment efficacy studies. Nevertheless, the applied behavior analysis studies can provide convincing demonstrations of the potency of behavioral treatment programs with individual children.

All approaches have limitations, and a natural constraint on behavioral treatment is the therapist's inability to control the child's social environment. If the child's reinforcement schedule cannot be precisely controlled, the wrong behaviors will be strengthened, and the amount and timing of positive reinforcers (schedule of reinforcement) will be incorrect, with predictably dismal results. Thus, control of the environment is vital, especially in the early part of the intervention. Also, unless vigorous efforts are made to train children in appropriate behavior wherever they may be, they may behave well only where and when they were trained to do so. Finally, children who have severe disabilities, such as autism and mental retardation, may never graduate from the treatment program. Their behavioral improvement may be so tenuous and dependent on the behavioral skills training that they remain trainees for life.

Cognitive-Behavioral Therapy

To some practitioners, behavioral techniques are too passive; they believe a client should take more personal responsibility for her or his own actions. Actually, behavioral therapy can be used to teach self-control, but a related approach more strongly emphasizes the client's self-direction. Cognitive-behavioral child therapists believe that a child's thoughts, moods, and feelings matter as much and require as much modification as the child's environment. Positive changes in the child's thinking, feeling, and behavior are produced through behavioral techniques such as modeling or imitation and direct training and rehearsal of new routines. Good

Steps in Self-Instruction

1. Pausing to define the problem
2. Considering several alternative solutions
3. Giving self-instructions on how to perform the task
4. Checking one's work and correcting errors calmly
5. Reinforcing oneself for a correct solution

Examples of Self-Instruction

"What does the teacher want me to do?" "I must stop and think before I begin."

"What plans could I try?" "How well would that work?" "What else might work?"

"I have to go slowly and carefully." "Okay, draw the line down, down, good; then to the right . . . Remember, go slowly."

"Have I got it right so far? That's a mistake. I'll just erase it."

"That's OK . . . Even if I make an error, I can go on slowly and carefully."

"Good, I'm doing fine." "I've done a pretty good job." "Good for me!"

Source: Meichenbaum & Goodman (1971).

behavior is reinforced, as it is in behavioral therapy, but cognitive-behavioral therapy aims to integrate cognitive, emotional, behavioral, and social strategies for therapeutic change (Kendall, 1991). Firmly rooted in research, the cognitive-behavioral approach assumes that a person's expectations, assumptions, and evaluations guide behavior, that behavior does not rely on external consequences alone.

Cognitive-behavioral therapy includes various therapeutic techniques. Some cognitive-behavioral interventions focus on appropriate training in problem-solving skills (see Table 15-2), while more complex interventions include many components, such as parenting training, relaxation training (see the Research Focus box), modeling of behavior, and rehearsing of new behavior.

Bandura's *social cognitive approach* (also called *social learning*) stresses that children learn naturally from observations; so providing them with interesting and appropriate models is an effective and noncoercive method of treatment. Skilled models are particularly useful when new behaviors are subtle, complex, and unlikely to be learned in the normal course of

events or when a child is highly anxious. For example, 6-year-old Mark is very frightened of dogs, and dogs are everywhere—in the neighborhood, on the playgrounds, at the lake. Mark needs to overcome his dog phobia so he can lead a normal life. Modeling procedures are particularly useful in the treatment of children's fears and anxieties such as a dog phobia (Bandura, 1969). Mark must build his sense of self-efficacy, his belief in his own ability to handle encounters with dogs, which is a difficult task, since he completely avoids dogs. Guided participation procedures can be used to show Mark fearless models coping calmly with dogs, all types of dogs in many different settings. Then his own therapist pets a dog on a leash in a playpen, a safe-seeming situation. Holding his therapist's hand, Mark manages some brief contact with the friendly dog. Gradually, the therapist demonstrates and then helps Mark to pet, then play with the dog and other dogs of different breeds. Each time Mark masters a new step in the treatment, his self-efficacy rises, which makes his future success with dogs ever more likely.

In the modeling treatment, the child is exposed to the fear stimulus gradually, with no negative consequences, taught skills for dealing with the situation, and helped to increase his self-confidence. Modeling is an effective way to handle many specific fears of childhood (Thorpe & Olson, 1997) and is effectively used in parent training to treat conduct disorder in children (Brestan & Eyberg, 1998; Webster-Stratton, 1996). Modeling procedures are also used as part of cognitive-behavioral therapy for children with obsessive-compulsive disorder, to teach them self-reassuring talk and reduce their anxiety (March et al., 2001).

Kendall's (1991) cognitive-behavioral therapy for anxious children is a good example of a complex intervention. This treatment includes techniques from many different types of behavioral and cognitive approaches. Anxious children are first taught to recognize their anxious feelings and the situations that provoke them. With the therapist, they construct a **fear hierarchy**, or graded sequence of things they fear, beginning with those that cause little fear to those that stimulate paralyzing fright. The children are then trained in progressive muscle relaxation, an activity they pair with imagined encounters with fear-provoking things in their fear hierarchy. This pairing of progressively more fear-provoking scenes with a state of

Research Focus

Progressive Muscle Relaxation

Research has shown that progressive muscle relaxation can be beneficial as part of cognitive-behavioral therapy for children. The therapist uses developmentally appropriate language the child can understand to present these instructions:

Do you know how when you are relaxed, your muscles are relaxed too and feel loose and good? But when you feel nervous or upset, your muscles get really tight. Today, I am going to teach you how to tell whether you are relaxed or tense, and what to do to stop feeling tense. We will practice simple tensing and relaxing first, so you get the idea. Then you can tell all by yourself when you are tense and you can make your muscles relax and feel better. These are very good exercises and they have helped lots of other children learn to relax.

Let's begin by having you test out this couch (or chair). Just get comfortable first. When you are relaxed, you breathe deeply and easily, taking big, slow, deep breaths. Draw a long breath and hold it while I count to 3. Then breathe out slowly until you can't do more. While you exhale, let your jaw and shoulders go loose; just relax. Can you do it? OK, close your eyes, let yourself sink comfortably into the couch (chair). Let's take a slow, deep breath and hold it until you count to 3 silently. Let it out all the way. (Repeat for 2–3 minutes.)

Step 1. Raise your hands above your head, stretch them high and breathe normally (10 seconds). Now drop your hands down.

Step 2. Now hold your arms out and make a really, really tight fist. Pretend you are squeezing a tennis ball as hard as you can. Feel the tension in your hands as you count to 3 slowly. Relax your hands and feel how good it is to be relaxed, all warm and easy.

Step 3. Raise your arms again, and stretch your fingers as wide as you can. Your fingers should be up like you are trying to push against a wall. Stretch those fingers wide, wider. Count to 3. Now drop your hands and feel them relax.

Using the same technique, the therapist teaches the child to tense and relax the different parts of the body from the toes to the facial muscles. When the child is able to do the exercises correctly, the therapist instructs her or him to practice them at home for 10–15 minutes at least twice a day. The exercises can be used whenever the child begins to feel tense. In public places, the child can use the simple breathing exercise and silently think of the word "calm." Audio or video instructions can be used to assist the child's practice, or written instructions may suffice.

SOURCES: Morris & Kratochwill (1983); Schafer (1992).

relaxation is also called *systematic desensitization*, a useful therapy by itself (Johnson et al., 1997). However, it is only one part of Kendall's comprehensive treatment package. Next, the children learn and practice *confident self-talk*, which may boost their morale and help them deal with challenging situations. Previously, they may have been defeated and intimidated, thinking about their own shortcomings, but with instruction in confident self-talk, they can encourage themselves with optimistic thoughts, such as "This isn't too bad. I can do it!" In *problem-solving skills training* (Kazdin et al., 1990), the children learn to recognize and solve problems that impede their progress and are taught behavioral skills for handling the feared situations. After 16 sessions, many participants had progressed from frightened nervous youngsters to much more confident and proficient ones. In one study, 64% of the children who received Kendall's cognitive-behavioral treatment no longer were diagnosed with an anxiety disorder, compared with 5% of those on a waiting list to receive the treatment (Kendall, 1994). Other studies yielded similarly impressive results (Christophersen & Mortweet, 2001).

Evaluation of Cognitive-Behavioral and Behavioral Therapies

Cognitive-behavioral therapies for children are among the more effective types of treatment. Children's fears, anxiety, and phobias have been successfully treated using cognitive-behavioral therapy, modeling, systematic desensitization, and operant training procedures (Burns et al., 1999). None of these therapies is clearly superior to any other, so factors such as convenience, client preference, and expense help determine the choice of intervention. The Society of Clinical Psychology of the American Psychological Association published guidelines for judging the effectiveness of psychotherapies. Using these criteria, cognitive-behavioral therapy was one of only 12 forms of treatment termed "probably efficacious" or better (Brestan & Eyberg, 1998). Many other treatments that were identified as "well-established" or "probably efficacious" included at least some cognitive-behavioral components. In the case of children with anxiety disorders, training parents in behavior management increased treatment effectiveness, especially for younger children (Dadds et al., 1999).

It seems that many types of therapy help children who have behavior disorders. However, most treatment studies are conducted in laboratory settings rather than in mental health clinics, so it remains to be demonstrated that the interventions are effective in everyday use. The long-term potency of behavioral

and cognitive-behavioral interventions is also unproven, but that is true for virtually all types of therapy for children.

FAMILY THERAPIES

IN FOCUS 3 ▶ Describe how a child's problems are viewed in systems-oriented family therapy, behavioral family therapy, and functional family therapy.

Most psychological problems that afflict children develop and are maintained within the family. Family therapy came about as therapists recognized the role played by parents, siblings, and even grandparents in children's disturbances (Everett & Volgy, 1993). One of the more popular types of family treatment is **systems-oriented family therapy**, which treats the entire family group as the client rather than focusing on the child alone. The family system is portrayed as malfunctioning and causing its members to engage in problem behavior. For example, a disobedient and rebellious boy might be expressing family conflict

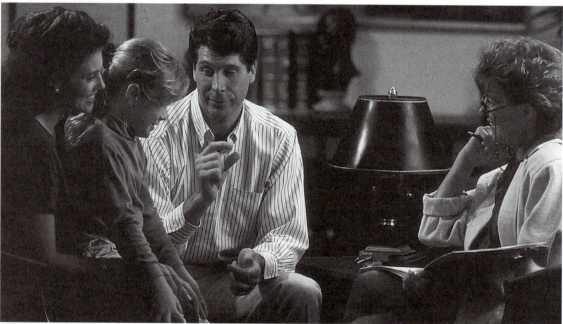

Bruce Ayres/Getty Images

During a family therapy session, a skilled psychotherapist engages the child as well as the parents. The family interaction, rather than the child, is the focus of the therapy.

through his antagonistic behavior, so it would be a mistake to treat him in isolation from the other battling members of his family. According to the family systems view, families naturally target particular members, who are the identified patients, as deviant, and the family's pathology often goes undetected and untreated. Family systems therapy stresses understanding the roles played by every family member, even the youngest and oldest ones. The identified patient's problem probably comes from the family's disturbed interactions. Perhaps the child's deviant behavior serves some function for the family, such as distracting attention from the mother's abuse of prescription drugs or the parents' deteriorating marriage. This functionality of the child's problem behavior may cause the others to unknowingly facilitate the child's behavior, thereby concealing their own problems. The family maintains itself and remains together to fulfill at least some members' needs for security, affection, and support. Dysfunctional families may resist change, including improvement, in order to maintain the shaky balance. The remedy is a treatment that focuses on family interactions rather than on individual behavior.

In systems-oriented family therapy, therapists analyze the verbal and nonverbal messages exchanged in family interactions. Satir (1967) identified *covert family rules* as governing everyone's responding in an unhealthy way. Instead of facing and confronting the unwritten and often unrecognized rules that keep their interactions dysfunctional, family members play by these rules. The therapist must uncover these covert family rules so that they can be altered. One such rule might allow an adolescent daughter to appear helpful when she subtly points out what others are doing wrong, which gets them into trouble, while she appears to be the caring, perfect daughter. Another covert family rule might allow the mother to dominate the others and prevent them from leading lives of their own by being overcome by migraine headaches, asthma attacks, or overwhelming feelings of weakness. Amount and quality of family interaction are analyzed, and families are characterized as *enmeshed* when members continually intrude into one another's affairs. They may demand to be informed concerning the whereabouts and activities of the others, dictating their actions and even how they should feel. *Disengaged* families have the opposite problem: Members

are isolated, offering each other little emotional support. Both enmeshed and disengaged families are dysfunctional, with frustrated and unhappy members. The therapist's response is to point out the covert family rules and explore their consequences, which gives family members the opportunity to develop healthier relationships. Sometimes the therapist labels individuals' behaviors in more positive terms to help the family view them differently. The son they see as selfish and avoidant might be described as becoming more independent and grown-up. The therapist might also "prescribe the symptom" and direct family members to caricature their customary maladaptive behavior and describe it in overexaggerated terms until it becomes so ridiculous that everyone laughs about it. The goal is to help them attain a sense of proportion and develop greater tolerance for each other.

Systems-oriented family therapy can be conducted only when everyone in a family agrees to participate. Fathers are often unavailable or unwilling to attend, which rules out treating the whole family as a system. Another problem is that recognition of the problem interactions by itself may not improve the situation. Family members might need extensive instruction and guided practice in more functional types of interactions. Eclectic (combined) types of family therapies, which include behavioral instruction methods, are sometimes preferable.

Behavioral Family Therapy

Behavioral therapists believe that the behavior of family members is shaped and maintained by everyday consequences. People's maladaptive behavior patterns can best be changed by modifying their environmental contingencies and teaching them new social skills through modeling and positive reinforcement. Members of dysfunctional families commonly communicate unclearly and in coercive ways. They express anger and criticism often, but offer each other little praise or support. Because they are poor at problem-solving, their failures provide many occasions for hostility and mutual recriminations. The therapist attempts to reduce the family members' reliance on coercion and to increase the exchange of positive reinforcers in order to promote improved family relationships (Patterson, Reid, & Dishion, 1975, 1992). In troubled families, positive events are infrequent, and members notice and respond to the others' negative, disruptive actions. Children's aggressive, coercive behaviors are shaped when the other family members give in to them rather than continuing to fight.

In behavioral family therapy, parents are taught to modify their own behavior so that their children are more likely to comply and to reinforce the children generously for good behavior. Family members are trained to detect both positive and coercive exchanges and to systematically increase the rate of positive interactions. **Contingency contracting** is frequently used to ensure that children's desirable behaviors are noted and reinforced by the parents and that the children understand exactly what behaviors are required of them. *Modeling* and *rehearsal* are used to teach family members how to respond to each other more positively.

Some parents find this approach uninviting because it demands so much effort over such a long time period. For example, they might have to make and record daily observations of their and their child's behavior, set goals, and provide reinforcers for behavioral improvement. But it may be worth all the effort. All types of family therapy are beneficial to some degree, but behavioral family therapy has been among the most effective (Burns et al., 1999; Shadish et al., 1993).

Functional Family Therapy

Alexander's functional family therapy (Alexander & Parsons, 1973) is an eclectic approach that combines a systems perspective on the family with behavioral methods such as modeling and contingency contracting to modify specific problem behaviors. Families of adolescent delinquents are a challenging group to treat, in part because a teenager is naturally becoming more independent and more involved with friends and other community influences. Both the adolescent and the family must adapt to their changing relationships. In this approach, the family members are trained to communicate with each other more clearly and accurately, to increase reciprocity rather than having one person dominate, and to explore alternative problem solutions that more closely resemble those of well-functioning families. Functional family therapy has been termed a "well-established" treatment for conduct disorder (Burns et al., 1999).

Parent Training and Foster Parenting

IN FOCUS 4 ▶ Under what conditions is it appropriate to place a child in family foster home care?

Parent training programs are very straightforward and teach parents to use various behavioral techniques appropriate to a child's age and behavioral problems (see the Research Focus box). Using instructional manuals, explanations, and videotaped models, parents are taught to employ techniques such as selectively attending to positive behaviors and ignoring mildly inappropriate behavior to avoid reinforcing it (Webster-Stratton, 1996). Many training programs are designed for parents of antisocial, aggressive children; the parents are trained to use time-out from ongoing positive reinforcement to discourage the children's tantrums and aggressive behavior. The therapists also attempt to improve the parents' attitudes, so they become warmer, more approving, and more loving toward their wayward children. Parents are often taught to use various contingency management techniques, such as using points and tokens with back-up privileges and treats to reinforce appropriate behavior. The family may also require other services such as drug or alcohol abuse treatment groups, social skills training, and other interventions (Patterson, Dishion, & Chamberlain, 1993).

Parent training employing videotaped modeling of good parenting practices is one of the most effective interventions currently available for children between the ages of 3 and 8 years who have oppositional defiant or conduct disorder (Burns et al., 1999). Children older than about 9 are more likely to return to their dysfunctional behaviors after treatment is completed (Patterson & Stoolmiller, 1991). This age difference regarding the effectiveness of parent training may reflect the increasing influence of school and peers; older children may require a different treatment approach.

Adolescents with severe conduct disorders and criminal histories may require foster family treatment or institutional treatment. The best such alternative is family foster home care with psychologically trained, carefully supervised foster parents (Chamberlain & Reid, 1991, 1998). When teenagers have become unmanageable because of substance abuse, defiance of their parents, criminal activity, and chronic truancy, they become candidates for professional foster care. Foster parents in these settings are carefully selected

Don't Just Tell Them What to Do—The Art and Science of Parent Training

Parent training involves much more than simply providing information on how parents should interact with their children. Parent training experts Carolyn Webster-Stratton and Martin Herbert (1993) advise therapists to begin by establishing a supportive, nonjudgmental relationship with the parents, reinforcing and validating their observations, and encouraging them to explore various solutions to the family's problems rather than seeking a "quick fix." Parents of children with conduct disorders frequently feel inadequate as parents and hopeless about their children. Such parents might be taught that they need not be incapacitated by their excessive worry about their situation and instructed to think of reassuring self-statements, for example, that all parents face problems with their children and become discouraged at times, but that the situation will improve if they persevere.

Parents meet in groups with a therapist, are taught general problem-solving skills, and are encouraged to focus on long-term goals of improved child behavior rather than giving in to the insistent demands of a coercive child for the sake of achieving temporary peace in the family. At the same time, they are encouraged to accept the child's limitations and recognize that the child also feels miserable. Webster-Stratton and Herbert (1993) have the following excellent advice for parents who may be inclined to accept defeat too readily:

"Your child needs hundreds of chances to learn from [his] mistakes. His learning more appropriate skills is just like when he was a baby and was learning how to walk. Do you remember how often he tried to get up and fell down? . . . Well this is just the same. It takes lots of small steps and experiments for a child to learn appropriate social skills. And just as you must constantly support the baby who is stumbling, . . . so must you the child who is developing his social skills" (p. 449).

Therapists teach parents in a nondirective fashion through modeling and gently persuading, suggesting, and explaining (e.g., "It is frustrating, but you know it looks like you're doing a nice job of beginning to help him understand the perspective of others in a situation," p. 427). Groups may also view and discuss videotapes of models performing adaptively or incorrectly as parents dealing with children in various common situations, such as handling child disobedience.

Finally, parents in parent training groups are encouraged to continue to meet with each other informally for support after the therapy is concluded. They are encouraged to babysit for each other to provide one another with recreation and some time away from their children.

This program is sensitive to the parents' needs and frustrations as well as to their children's problems. Through a combination of clinical training and experience, plus knowledge derived from therapy research, therapists are offering help to many troubled families.

SOURCES: Webster-Stratton & Herbert (1993, 1994).

graduate students or treatment agency staff members who are trained to provide the adolescents with a structured behavior management program based on social learning principles. Virtually all portions of the day are used for therapeutic and educational programs. Teachers work with the foster parents to specify the closely monitored teen's daily responsibilities at school. A token program reinforces appropriate behavior, with rewards being enjoyable activities such as inviting friends to the house. Undesirable, antisocial friends are declared off-limits, so the teen is shielded from gangs and other negative peer influences. Meanwhile, the youth's real parents receive training in applied behavioral principles so that they can continue the therapeutic program after foster care.

This treatment approach appears to be more effective with chronic juvenile offenders than the more expensive therapeutic group home (Chamberlain & Reid, 1998). Therapeutic group homes are located in the community, and the teens attend the local school. Each home serves 5 to 10 youths and offers various individual and group psychotherapy programs. Family foster home care produced significantly less criminal activity and more successful returns to real families than did group homes. This promising treatment for seriously disturbed adolescents deserves much further study.

DRUG TREATMENTS FOR CHILDHOOD DISORDERS

IN FOCUS 5 ▶ Identify the three types of psychoactive drugs commonly prescribed for children and describe their effectiveness.

Psychoactive drugs (drugs that affect mood, activity level, attention, or thinking) are increasingly used to treat various pediatric psychological disturbances. Medications are prescribed for several reasons:

- To suppress dangerous behaviors, such as self-injurious, suicidal, or violent and aggressive actions
- To suppress intrusive behaviors that interfere with a child's functioning and learning, such as hyperactive, inattentive, or psychotic behaviors
- To enhance positive behavior, such as attentiveness and desirable social interactions (Gadow & Pomeroy, 1993).

Despite widespread enthusiasm for use of psychoactive drugs with children, little research has been directed at testing the safety, efficacy, and long-term effects of drug treatments. Drug research has been concentrated on the adult market. The unfortunate result is that some drugs that have proven effective with adults have been persistently prescribed for children without any research evidence of their effectiveness with younger patients. For example, tricyclic antidepressants, a well-established medication for adult depression, work no better than placebos, or inactive sugar pills, for children with depression. Undeterred, physicians continued to prescribe tricyclic antidepressants for huge numbers of young patients for many years, often at the insistence of parents and teachers. When evaluation research is lacking, practitioners simply do the best they can.

Why is there so little research on medications for children? One reason is the belief that what works for adults should work equally well for children. There is copious evidence that this assumption is false, at least

for some medications. Second, federal regulations governing research with children are highly restrictive, which makes it difficult and expensive to conduct research to assess the effects of drugs, most of which have at least some side effects, sometimes dangerous ones. Since medications developed for adults and approved for the general market can be legally and ethically used to treat children, such use is common. Finally, drug treatment research with children requires a long-term (many-year) follow-up to ensure that the drug treatment benefits continue and that the drug did not adversely affect the child's physical or psychological development. The result of these constraints is that only a very few drugs, such as the central nervous system stimulants, have been adequately investigated and demonstrated to be useful for children with a particular diagnosis, such as attention-deficit/hyperactivity disorder (Jensen et al., 1999; MTA Cooperative Group, 1999a, 1999b [the National Institute of Mental Health–sponsored Multimodal Treatment Study]). Most psychiatric drugs are prescribed for children based on hope rather than proof that they are effective.

This section presents information regarding the leading psychoactive medications for children, the disorders for which they are prescribed, some of the common side effects, and the research verdict on their effectiveness. Guidelines for safe and appropriate use of psychoactive medications with children are also presented, and practitioners and parents should follow these rules as fully as possible for the safety and benefit of the children.

Central Nervous System Psychostimulants

Central nervous system (CNS) psychostimulants (called *stimulants* here) include drugs such as methylphenidate (Ritalin) and dextroamphetamine (Dexedrine). They are among the most frequently prescribed medications for children's psychiatric disorders. These stimulants have been tested repeatedly and found to be effective in reducing the high levels of inattention, impulsivity, and overactivity typical of children with attention-deficit/hyperactivity disorder (MTA Cooperative Group, 1999a). According to various studies, between 70% and 80% of the children who take stimulants improve, while 10% to 30% of children do not benefit from stimulants (Burns et al., 1999). Some children cannot tolerate the side effects, which commonly include insomnia, loss of appetite, stomachaches, headaches, and feelings of jitteriness. These side effects tend to disappear over time in most cases. Stimulants help children with ADHD to attend to and persist in schoolwork. They often become more attentive and efficient and less prone to errors. Moreover, their disruptive and antisocial behavior in the classroom decreases, bringing a welcome decline in their destruction of property, noncompliance, inappropriate bids for attention, and name-calling (Kaplan & Hussain, 1995). Despite their usefulness in the short-term treatment of symptoms of ADHD, stimulants do not produce long-term improvements in peer relationships, school achievement, or academic and social skills (Pelham, Wheeler, & Chronis, 1998). These latter, more complex areas of functioning may require educational and behavioral interventions.

Antidepressant Drugs

Drugs that have been used to treat depression in adults are prescribed for children to treat various conditions, including enuresis, eating disorders, and mood disorders, particularly depression. The two most frequently prescribed antidepressants for children are *tricyclic antidepressants*, such as imipramine (Tofranil) and amitryptiline (Elavil), and the selective serotonin reuptake inhibitors (SSRIs), including fluoxetine and paroxetine. The SSRIs have quickly become the second most commonly prescribed type of psychoactive medication used with children (Jensen et al., 1999). While the tricyclic antidepressants appear to be ineffective in combating childhood depression, the SSRIs proved safe and effective in the first major test of their use to treat this condition (Wagner et al., 1998). Side effects of SSRIs seem to be mostly limited to insomnia, irritability, headache, and gastric upset. However, the long-term safety and effectiveness of the SSRIs have yet to be established.

Antipsychotic (Neuroleptic) Drugs

The antipsychotic (neuroleptic) drugs, such as the phenothiazines, thiaoxanthenes, and haloperidol, were originally developed to control the bizarre, hallucinatory, and occasional violent behavior of adult psychotic patients. These drugs, particularly haloperidol, are sometimes prescribed to decrease violent, agitated behavior in profoundly retarded, brain-injured, or schizo-phrenic children. In particular, antipsychotic drugs are used to reduce assaultiveness, destructiveness, self-injury, and restlessness in children with severe mental retardation and schizophrenia. Although these drugs make the children more tractable, they do nothing to improve their retardation. Typical side effects include sedative action, reduction in alertness, and impairment of thinking and problem-solving skills, at least temporarily. Tardive dyskinesia can occur, with involuntary tongue protrusion, grimacing, drooling, tremor, and stereotyped movements of the head, limbs, and trunk. Although these undesirable effects can be controlled by other medication, they should be avoided wherever possible. Newer atypical neuroleptics, such as clozapine, risperidone, and olanzapine, appear to be more promising, but also have major side effects and are not recommended for routine use at this time (Burns et al., 1999).

Guidelines for Use of Psychoactive Drugs with Children

Psychoactive drug therapy should be considered a moderately restrictive, potentially dangerous treatment that should be used with caution. Such therapy is moderately restrictive because a child cannot choose whether to participate in the treatment. It is potentially dangerous because of the side effects that accompany use of many medications. In most cases, these side effects are minor and dissipate over time, as in the case of the CNS stimulants. But some medications, such as antipsychotics, pose greater risks. Consequently, parents should be advised to inquire about the risks and benefits of any medication their children receive.

Here are some guidelines for children's drug therapy (Murphy, Greenstein, & Pelham, 1993):

1. Drugs should not be the first or only treatment tried. Use less restrictive treatments first.
2. The child should receive a competent medical and psychological exam to establish a diagnosis.
3. The child as well as the parents should consent to the use of drugs. No one should be coerced into taking medications, if at all possible.
4. Drug administration should be conservative, with the smallest dosage possible and for the briefest possible time. Drug-free periods, during which the drug use is discontinued, should be established. A formal treatment plan should include specific, well-

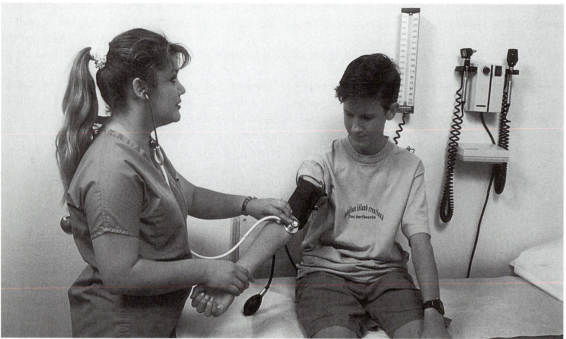

Many psychoactive drugs have side effects, some of which could be dangerous in the absence of regular monitoring and medical supervision.

defined goals, checks for side effects, and follow-up evaluations by qualified professionals.

Use of these guidelines should help ensure that children participate in their own treatment decisions and that they are not exposed to health hazards, or if they are, it is for the shortest possible time. Finally, the guidelines provide for checking up on the child's response to the medication, rather than assuming that the treatment is and continues to be effective. Families need to be well-informed consumers of pharmaceuticals as they are for other items they buy.

PREVENTION AND EARLY INTERVENTION

IN FOCUS 6 ▶ What four types of behavioral problems have been reduced by early intervention programs?

Effective problem prevention greatly benefits children and their families by sparing the children the pain of illness, failure, and rejection. Beyond this, preventing problems before they become established or serious benefits society by reducing the many immediate and long-term social ill effects of mental disorder, including expensive psychiatric treatment and special education services, criminal justice system costs, and tax and welfare costs. Troubled children may become delinquent as adolescents or grow up to become underemployed or unemployed. And, of course, as adults, they are likely to have children who fail to thrive because of their parents' problems. Early intervention, if effective, is unquestionably more humane and cost-effective than trying to remedy a problem that has become serious and costly.

During the past decade, social and behavioral scientists have developed many early intervention programs of increasing potency. Most early intervention efforts are multifaceted, using many different intervention techniques drawn from educational and clinical practice. This section describes only a few of these programs as illustrations of this approach. Like therapy treatments, prevention programs are keyed to the child's developmental level, with programs for infants and toddlers featuring parent education and a stimulating and educational environment. The mother-infant programs typically focus on parent education and aim to improve the cognitive stimulation and quality of emotional care the mother gives her baby. In contrast, programs for adolescents are directed more at them than at their parents and stress their role in dealing with their own problems, often by learning to identify and respond appropriately to problem situations using self-regulation skills.

Early intervention refers to a large set of activities designed to enhance a young child's development. Early intervention programs typically target infants, toddlers, or preschoolers who have special needs or who are at risk for emotional problems and school failure in future years. In most households, no early intervention program is needed to help children to develop normally. Extra guidance is helpful for children raised in extreme poverty and deprivation and those who have developmental disabilities and delays. Intervention should start with a professional assessment of the child's and family's needs and strengths, which serves as a basis for planning an intervention. Typical enrichment services include home visits by child development professionals and provision of high-quality day care programs, which may be followed by special elementary school curricula as the children grow (Ramey & Ramey, 1998). Some early intervention programs are comprehensive and offer such services as health care, education, and job training for unemployed parents. Successful parenting programs feature: (1) parent education, with frequent home visits or practice sessions held elsewhere, (2) interventions that preferably begin before or soon after the baby's birth, and (3) interventions at least 1 year in length (Reichman & McLanahan, 2001).

Over 25 years of research has shown that early intervention programs can produce modest to large beneficial effects on children's cognitive and social development, effects that continue into the elementary school grades (Campbell & Ramey, 1994; Ramey & Ramey, 1996, 1998). Programs that are longer and more intensive produce larger positive effects, and children and parents who participate regularly derive more benefit from the intervention than those who are casually involved. With early intervention, just a little bit of participation does *not* help. Well-designed and carefully administered early intervention programs can be effective, and these programs will become even

more successful as researchers continue to refine them.

One promising nationwide experiment to prevent chronic antisocial behavior and conduct disorder is termed FAST, or Fast Track (Conduct Problems Prevention Research Group, 1999a, 1999b, 2000). The Fast Track program focuses on kindergarten children who have just begun to show disruptive and aggressive behavior and their parents. Program goals are to reduce children's antisocial behavior, teach skills in interpersonal problem-solving and emotional regulation, improve academic skills, particularly the key skill of reading, and generally improve relationships among the children, their parents, and school staff. Employing a research-based, cognitive-behavioral training approach, the Fast Track program provides parent management training, family support services, academic tutoring, and teacher training in the use of classroom interventions. This prevention program has been heavily promoted by the Department of Justice because of its promise. Initial results are encouraging, suggesting that participating children show moderate improvements in the targeted areas of antisocial behavior, school performance, and peer relations and that their parents improve in attitudes and values (Conduct Problems Prevention Research Group, 1999a, 1999b). Nevertheless, much remains to be done to prevent the widespread, serious, and persistent problem of antisocial behavior, and moderate early improvements may not be enough to forestall later problem development. The fundamental individual and social problems that contribute to externalizing disorders, such as poverty, prejudice, crime, and addiction, necessarily remain largely untouched in prevention efforts focused on at-risk families (see Chapter 5 on social conditions and children's problems).

Programs for school-age children are most often conducted in the school and take an educational form. For example, the highly successful Jigsaw Classroom program to combat discrimination of all types brings students of all races, ethnic groups, ability levels, and genders together to do their schoolwork. Small, heterogeneous study groups must work together effectively in order to complete assignments and perform well on exams (Aronson, 2000). Amazingly, this experience leads children to play with those who are different from themselves, reduces their prejudices about other groups, and improves the quality of their school-

Research Focus

Teaching Tolerance in the Jigsaw Classroom

The playground scene was fairly typical for a 3rd-grade class. The popular, aggressive boys collected other boys who were eager to follow their lead, while the shy ones played alone or with just one equally unpopular friend. The girls followed suit, laughing and talking together, except for those who were new to the school, ethnically or racially different, or mainstreamed from special education classes. The ones who were different in some way felt dumb, unattractive, and hopeless about ever being accepted, and some were angry.

Enter social psychologist Dr. Elliott Aronson, with a program to increase every child's acceptance and improve learning at the same time. Aronson's jigsaw classroom, a cooperative learning technique, is in use in hundreds of schools across the United States, and it works. The program uses established principles of social psychology to draw children together to pursue a common goal, so there are no rejected isolates in the class. It is called the jigsaw classroom because, as in a jigsaw puzzle, each piece—each child—is essential for the final product. Having a unique role makes each student essential, which is the key to success.

Here is what the teacher does to create a jigsaw classroom:

- Divide the students into groups of 5 or 6 that are diverse in terms of gender, ethnicity, race, and ability.
- Appoint the most mature student in each group as the leader.
- Divide the day's lesson into 5 or 6 units.
- Give each student the materials to learn only the one segment they are to present.
- Give students time to read over their segment at least twice.
- Form temporary "expert groups" composed of one student from each group assigned to the same segment. These groups discuss the main points of their segment and rehearse their presentations. Students learn to organize and present from each other.
- Have students rejoin their original groups, present their own segments to the group, and answer questions.
- The teacher moves from group to group, observing and intervening if necessary; subtly coaching the leaders by whispering instructions to them.
- Give a quiz on the material at the end of the session so students take the process seriously.

Results include significantly more play contacts across lines of ethnicity, ability, and popularity. Children come to see former outcasts as familiar, useful, and attractive playmates. They value each other as contributors to their shared classroom tasks, and that positive attitude spills over onto the playground. An additional plus is that the children learn the material better than they do in the typical classroom because they play a more active role as learners. The cost? Nothing. The time involved? As little as 1 hour of classroom activity per day. In addition, children's attitudes become less prejudiced. The jigsaw classroom is something any teacher or activity group leader can use to benefit children educationally and socially.

SOURCE: Aronson (2000). See also http://www.jigsaw.org.

work. The jigsaw classroom is an inexpensive, interesting, and successful way to teach academic subjects effectively while reducing students' isolation and rejection of others different from themselves (see the Research Focus box). Perhaps a similar approach would help reduce prejudice toward emotionally and behaviorally disturbed students.

Programs have been developed to reduce depressive symptoms in children and adolescents to prevent them from becoming clinically depressed. The Penn Optimism Program (Gillham, Reivich, Jaycox, & Seligman, 1995) for older school children provides training in relaxation, assertiveness, and active problem-solving, characteristics lacking in mildly depressed people. The children are helped to understand how their negative thinking relates to their mood problems. This cognitive-behavioral program reduced children's depressive symptoms over a 2-year period (Gillham et

Back to the Beginning

Multifaceted Treatment for Ben and His Family

From the wide array of medications available for kids like Ben with ADHD, his pediatrician chose to prescribe Ritalin (methylphenidate). This was a good choice, according to the psychopharmacology research, because the stimulants have been tested in many research studies and were found effective in reducing the symptoms of ADHD. Ben was taken off the medication after 5 months, as soon as his behavior improved and remained controlled. However, Ben had other problems as well. Ben's classroom behavior definitely improved, but his grades remained poor and he still didn't have any friends in his regular classroom. Each of his areas of deficiency must be specifically addressed in a skill-building program. Ben was lucky that his teacher noticed his behavioral problem early, while he was still in kindergarten, and suggested that

his family obtain professional help for him. Research studies suggested that he was given some of the most effective medical and psychological treatments for his condition (American Academy of Pediatrics, 2001; Burns et al., 1999; MTA Cooperative Group, 1999a, 1999b), and he and his parents were trained to manage his treatment themselves rather than continue to rely entirely on professional help. In addition, couples counseling helped Ben's parents to unite and work together to improve the family's relationships. Pills do not cure problems in living and relating to others. Recognizing this fact, his parents sought psychological help for Ben and for themselves. With the best available medical and psychological treatment, Ben and his parents seem to have a brighter future.

---

al., 1995). Another cognitive-behavioral intervention for teens at risk for depression was developed in Oregon by Lewinsohn, Clarke, and their colleagues (Clarke, Hawkins, Murphy, & Sheeber, 1993). In a small group classroom setting, adolescents are taught many skills, including relaxation, stress management, peer relations skills, goal-setting, and monitoring their own moods. Both depression-prone youth and those who were clinically depressed benefited from the program. Participants' depressive symptoms improved significantly and continued to improve over a 2-year period (Clarke, Rohde, Lewinsohn, Hops, & Seeley, 1999). The challenge is to extend this improvement over the longer term.

The transition from adolescence to adulthood is an uncertain time, with many temptations to engage in unhealthy and risky behaviors. The vast majority of young people enter adulthood without major psychological problems. However, it is not enough just to avoid problems in order to live a full and fulfilling life. Teenagers should be helped to become competent, confident, caring, and productive members of their community (Roth & Brooks-Gunn, 2000). Outside of

the classroom, concerned and effective teachers often help at-risk teens cope with their emotional and family problems. Teens with strong emotional attachments to their teachers are less likely to engage in risky behavior, such as using drugs and alcohol, becoming violent, becoming sexually active at an early age, or becoming suicidal (Resnick et al., 1997). Thus, a caring and supportive adult can serve as a guide and mentor for troubled or disadvantaged teens (Dubois, Felner, Meares, & Krier, 1994; Werner & Smith, 1992). Being involved in school-related extracurricular activities also benefits adolescents and reduces their risk-taking behavior and drop-out rates (Cairns & Cairns, 1994). There is a wealth of research information on which to base new prevention and enrichment programs for American youth.

SUMMARY

Selection of an appropriate treatment depends on a child's age, problem type and severity, family relationships, and available treatment resources. In general, younger children are treated through parent training programs, behavioral programs to remedy skills deficits or delays, or play therapy. Older children benefit from parent training in behavior management, skills training, family therapy, and cognitive-behavioral therapy. Insight-oriented psychodynamic therapies remain popular, but have little research support. Behavioral and educational programs attempt to teach the child appropriate social and academic skills, using modeling and reinforcement contingency management. Family therapy is used when the child's problems stem from faulty family communications and maladaptive patterns of interaction at home. Older children and adolescents with conduct disorder may benefit from family foster home care with trained foster parents and detailed daily behavioral programs.

Some types of psychotherapy do benefit children to some extent. Examples of effective or apparently effective psychotherapies include cognitive-behavioral therapy for children's fears and anxieties, family therapy for conduct disorders and delinquency, and videotaped modeling for parent training. The effectiveness of psychotherapy is better established in research settings than in community clinics and hospitals, and long-term outcomes are unstudied in most cases.

Psychoactive drugs are increasingly prescribed for children. Research supports the use of stimulants in the treatment of ADHD, although related problems such as poor school achievement and social relations may require behavioral therapy. The SSRIs have significant promise in the treatment of juvenile depression, but more research is needed. Limitations of using drugs with children include potentially bothersome or dangerous side effects; some children are unable to tolerate some medications. Guidelines for use of medications include trying safer, nondrug interventions first and having minimal dosages and treatment times, a treatment plan, periodic check-ups, and discontinuation of the drug as soon as possible. Developing effective, safe, and practical interventions for children should be a first priority on the nation's health agenda.

INFOTRAC COLLEGE EDITION

For more information, explore this resource at http://www.infotrac-college.com/Wadsworth. Enter the following search terms:

behavior therapy for children
cognitive-behavioral therapy
psychoanalytic/psychodynamic therapy
play therapy
drug therapy for children
ethics and therapy
prevention programs for children

IN FOCUS ANSWERS

IN FOCUS 1 ▶ Describe some of the most common adjustment problems of infants and toddlers, elementary school children, and adolescents.

- Attachment problems or developmental delays in infants and toddlers
- Social adjustment and peer relations problems in elementary school children
- Academic difficulties, mood disorders, substance abuse, eating disorders, and establishing independence in adolescents

IN FOCUS 2 ▶ Describe the research evidence for the effectiveness of psychodynamic, nondirective play, behavioral, and cognitive-behavioral therapies.

- Little research has been done on psychodynamic therapy, so its effectiveness is unknown.
- Probably more effective than no therapy, nondirective play therapy has limited effectiveness in clinic settings.
- Behavioral therapy can teach specific skills, but careful treatment design is needed to produce durable, general effects.
- Cognitive-behavioral therapy treats many of a child's problems at the same time using different techniques. This is effective in controlled laboratory settings, but its utility in actual treatment clinics and in the long term is not established.

IN FOCUS 3 ▶ Describe how a child's problems are viewed in systems-oriented family therapy, behavioral family therapy, and functional family therapy.

- Systems-oriented family therapy views the source of the child's problems as dysfunctional family interactions, not individual psychopathology.
- Behavioral family therapy views the child's problems as coming from inappropriate reinforcement contingencies and lack of social skills.

- Functional family therapy sees both faulty family communications and inappropriate contingencies as creating children's problems.

IN FOCUS 4 ▶ Under what conditions is it appropriate to place a child in family foster home care?

- For teens rather than younger children
- When teens are unmanageable, refuse to obey their parents, are delinquent, and/or abuse drugs
- When their friends are antisocial or gang members

IN FOCUS 5 ▶ Identify the three types of psychoactive drugs commonly prescribed for children and describe their effectiveness.

- Stimulants are used mainly for attention-deficit/hyperactivity disorder. They are effective in treating symptoms, but don't improve social relationships or school achievement in the long term.
- Of antidepressant drugs, the tricyclic antidepressants are ineffective with children, but the SSRIs hold promise of being safe and effective to treat depression and anxiety.

- Antipsychotic drugs, used to control psychotic behavior in adults, are used to reduce assaultiveness, restlessness, and self-injury in severely ill children, but have serious side effects.

IN FOCUS 6 ▶ What four types of behavioral problems have been reduced by early intervention programs?

- Emotional and cognitive problems have been reduced by comprehensive programs for high-risk, disadvantaged infants and preschool children and their parents.
- Conduct disorder and seriously antisocial behavior have been reduced in aggressive kindergarten children by the Fast Track program.
- Prejudice and discrimination have been reduced in school-age children by the Jigsaw Classroom program.
- Depressive symptoms have been reduced in children and adolescents by the Penn Optimism Program.

Glossary

A

Adaptive behavior The ability to respond constructively and independently to demands of the social environment in relation to one's age level and cultural group. Adaptive skill areas specified in the AAMR definition of mental retardation are communication, self-care, home living, social skills, community use, self-direction, health and safety, functional academics, leisure, and work.

Anorexia nervosa A condition of severe weight loss due to self-inflicted starvation accompanied by compulsive exercising and irrational concerns about looking fat.

Antidepressant medications Prescription drugs specifically designed to counteract depressive mood, usually through altering levels of neurotransmitters such as serotonin or dopamine in the brain.

Anxiety Negative mood state marked by bodily tension and apprehension about future dangers or other threatening events.

Articulation disorder A major disturbance in speech-sound production resulting in chronic abnormal vocalization patterns.

Asperger's disorder A pervasive developmental disorder involving severe impairment of social interactions and the development of repetitive patterns of abnormal behaviors, interests, and activities, but without the significant language delays characteristic of autism.

Assessment Process of collecting information on the psychological, physical, and academic achievement and performance of a child, ordinarily through psychological testing, observations, and interviews.

Attachment figure Person to whom the infant forms a significant emotional bond.

Attachment theory View that social relations and self-perceptions are based in early affectional bonds or attachments.

Attention-deficit/hyperactivity disorder (ADHD) Disorder in which a child has primary behavioral difficulties consisting of (1) inability to attend to tasks for extended periods of time, (2) acting before thinking about the consequences (impulsivity), and (3) fidgety or situationally inappropriate excessive motor activity.

Auditory association The act of connecting or relating ideas or information presented verbally, usually as speech.

Auditory blending Combining the parts of a spoken word into an integrated whole, rather than perceiving a series of unconnected syllables.

Auditory discrimination The process of distinguishing between different sounds.

Auditory memory Ability to recognize and recall information conveyed as sounds.

Autism A pervasive developmental disorder that is characterized by an early onset and profound difficulties in relating socially to other people. Often associated with mutism and low IQ.

B

Behavioral genetics The study of possible genetic contributions to observable behavior patterns, especially through comparisons of behavioral similarities between close relations versus nonrelated individuals.

Behavioral observation An assessment technique in which observations of an individual's behavior are recorded using an observation code and the agreement level of the observers (reliability) is analyzed.

Bipolar disorder (formerly *manic depressive disorder*) In general, a mood disorder characterized by shifts between manic episodes of abnormal excitement, hyperactivity, and expansive or irritable mood, episodes of depression, and/or periods of normal mood.

Bulimia nervosa An eating disorder characterized by uncontrolled binge eating followed by purging (vomiting, using laxatives).

C

Capacity (to give consent) A person's mental or emotional ability and legal authority (usually by virtue of age) to give consent to participate in a research project or medical procedure.

Case study In-depth examination of the behavior of an individual or a small social unit such as a family; seeks to determine all of the relevant factors or influences important in the development and current behavior of the person or social unit and often includes a developmental history describing physical, psychological, and social aspects of that development.

Catharsis In psychoanalytic theory, the therapeutic release of pent-up aggressive drive in a socially acceptable manner, such as in pretend attacks with toy weapons.

Central nervous system The brain and the spinal cord.

Cerebral cortex Large forebrain area, divided into left and right hemispheres, active in perceiving, reasoning, creating, planning, and remembering.

Child abuse Actively mistreating a child so as to cause physical, psychological, and/or social or sexual harm. Often combined with neglect.

Child neglect Serious negligence in the care of a child, such as grossly inadequate supervision, health care, nutrition, protection from emotional trauma, or education, or exposure to drug use or delinquency. Often co-occurs with abuse.

Childhood disintegrative disorder A pervasive developmental disorder characterized by significant regression in several areas of functioning following at least 2 years of normal development. Affected areas may include language and communication skills, social skills, motor skills, and bowel or bladder control.

Childhood schizophrenia A childhood psychotic disorder characterized by onset in late childhood and development of thought disorders, hallucinations, delusions, disorganized speech or behavior, movement or motor disturbance such as catatonic-type immobility, and/or unusually flat (expressionless) emotional tone.

Classification Categorization of characteristics or behaviors into groups based on diagnostically relevant sets of criteria, as in identifying the diagnostic characteristics of autistic disorder.

Coercion (coercion hypothesis) An increasingly negative interchange between a child and an adult caretaker or supervisor; characteristic of highly hostile, aggressive children. When the defiant child's antagonistic behavior becomes sufficiently aversive, the adult stops demanding obedience and thus negatively reinforces the behavior.

Cognitive-behavioral therapy (also called *cognitive behavior therapy*) Therapeutic approach that combines systematic control of response consequences, such as provision of positive reinforcement, with training in self-control, including relaxation, confident self-talk, and problem solving.

Cognitive social theory A theory developed by Bandura that stresses the importance of self-regulation and self-efficacy in the origin and maintenance of social behavior.

Cognitive triad In Beck's cognitive theory of depression, the tendency of the depressed person to engage in irrationally negative thoughts about self, the world in general, and the future.

Conduct disorder A persistent social disorder in which the child has primary behavioral difficulties consisting of (1) rule-breaking, (2) aggression, and (3) a disregard for the rights of others. Marked by cruelty and failure to accept blame for misdeeds.

Contingency contracting A behavioral therapy technique in which parents or teachers develop a formal, usually written, agreement with a child to provide specified positive reinforcers in exchange for specific behaviors, such as completing homework, refraining from fighting with siblings, or doing household chores.

Control (experimental control) The concept of holding all variables except the independent variable constant between experimental conditions so that any differences observed in the dependent variable can be attributed to the treatment influence.

Correlation A statistic indicating the strength of association between variables on a scale from 0 (no relationship) to 1 (a perfect relationship).

Cortisol A hormone or corticosteroid secreted by the adrenal glands during stress.

Cross-sectional designs Research designs in which comparisons are made between different groups of participants at different ages.

Cumulative risk model The view that multiple factors (e.g., personality traits, treatment by parents, poverty) accumulate to produce total risk of developing psychopathology.

D

Dependent variable Any behavior or performance that is observed by a researcher to assess the impact of some treatment; sometimes called the *dependent measure*. Often multiple dependent variables are used in studies.

Depression General term for profound, dysphoric feelings, ranging from mild symptoms to a clinical disorder featuring depressed mood. Rare in childhood, depressive mood disorder increases rapidly in prevalence during adolescence.

Descriptive research question Research question that attempts to describe certain naturally occurring groups or situations. No experimental manipulation is involved.

Desensitization (also called *systematic desensitization*) A therapeutic technique based on carefully programmed, increasingly closer or more direct exposure to a feared situation. The actual or imagined stimulus is repeatedly paired with deep muscle relaxation until the fear is overcome.

Developmental psychopathology The interdisciplinary study of the origins, prevention, and treatment of abnormal child behavior, stressing complex interactions and multiple developmental paths. Draws upon developmental psychology and clinical sciences.

Diagnosis Assigning of a categorical label (such as major depressive disorder or conduct disorder) to a group of signs and symptoms exhibited by a person.

***Diagnostic and Statistical Manual of Mental Disorders*, Fourth Edition, Text Revision (DSM-IV-TR)** Published by the American Psychiatric Association, the definitive system of classification used in the United States. Describes many discrete psychological disorders, but also notes physical illnesses, problems in living, and general level of functioning.

Difference research question Research question that compares groups, treatments, or conditions to determine if there is a difference between them.

Discriminative stimulus In operant psychology, any signal that a particular type of response will be followed by reinforcement.

Disorganized/disoriented attachment Pattern of dysfunctional emotional attachment to a caretaker, usually the mother, in which the child appears dazed, unorganized, unfocused, and insecurely attached. Thought to indicate future adjustment problems.

Dopamine A brain neurotransmitter that generally activates other neurotransmitters and is found in excess in some individuals with schizophrenia.

Dyslexia A severe type of learning disability that impairs the ability to read, sometimes totally.

Dysthymic disorder (dysthymia) Mild depression that persists for most of the time for at least 2 years in adults or 1 year in children. Often develops into or is combined with episodes of major depressive disorder.

E

Early intervention Programs to provide special stimulation (e.g., parent training for mothers, educational preschools) for disadvantaged children who are at risk for achievement and adjustment problems.

Echolalia A behavior of some children with mental retardation or autism, in which the individual repeats back (or "parrots") exactly what was said to him or her rather than answering in a socially appropriate manner.

Eclectic treatment Any intervention that combines techniques from several different approaches rather than being limited to a single one. In practice, most psychotherapy is eclectic.

Educational neglect A caretaker's refusal to enroll a child for mandatory schooling, supervise a child's attendance at school, or procure appropriate special education for a child who needs it.

Ego identity A firm, positive sense of the type of person one is. According to Erikson, achieving one's ego identity follows a period of adolescent ego identity crisis.

Ego theory The variety of psychoanalytic theory that stresses ego functions and de-emphasizes instinctual drives.

Elective mutism Selective speaking, limited to certain circumstances but with no physical defect and no deficit in general intellectual ability.

Emotional abuse Attacks on a child's sense of security or self-worth, often accompanied by physical abuse or neglect.

Emotional neglect A caretaker's failure to provide a child with needed psychological care or protection from witnessing chronic or extreme spouse abuse or allowing the child to use drugs or alcohol.

Encopresis Abnormal or unacceptable patterns of fecal expulsion by children beyond the age of toilet training and lacking organic pathology.

Enmeshment In family systems therapy, the failure of family members to respect the autonomy of other members and their inappropriate intrusion into the private affairs of the other members.

Enuresis Elimination disorder involving recurrent bed-wetting or wetting of clothing at least twice a week for 3 months, diagnosed in children over the age of 5 years.

Equifinality A developmental principle stating that a single type of outcome can have many different sources in different children.

Etiology The study of the origins or sources of behavior, especially disturbed behavior.

Experimental matching Assigning of research participants to experimental groups in a way that forces group equivalence on some characteristic(s) thought to be important for the study being conducted (e.g., IQ or reading level).

External validity A measure of the extent to which results of a study generalize to other participants, measures, and settings that were not involved in the research.

Externalizing behavior problems Problems in interpersonal behavior, such as severe aggression and other antisocial behaviors, that are directed externally, toward others and the environment.

Extinction In operant psychology, the cessation of a particular response following withholding of reinforcement.

F

False negative Test result that misidentifies an individual as normal when it should indicate that the person scores in the abnormal range.

False positive Test result that misidentifies an individual as disturbed when it should indicate that the person scores in the normal range.

Family skills-training interventions Programs designed to teach family members particular interaction skills, such as conflict resolution, reinforcing others, and aggression control.

Family therapy Therapeutic approach involving parents and children and aimed at improving family interactions. Includes systems-oriented, behavioral, multidimensional, and multisystemic approaches to treatment.

Fear Feeling of apprehension and alarm about a real or imagined threat.

Fear hierarchy A graded sequence of feared situations listed by a phobic child, beginning with the mildest and ending with the most terrifying scenes. Guided by a therapist, the child then imagines the fears in order, progressing to the more frightening after mastering the less intimidating ones.

Fetal alcohol effects A condition in which the child of a mother who drank heavily while pregnant develops some, but not all, of the signs of fetal alcohol syndrome.

Fetal alcohol syndrome Disorder caused by heavy and prolonged maternal alcohol intake during pregnancy, resulting in damage to the fetus that includes characteristic deformities and mental retardation, with persisting problems throughout life.

Fragile X syndrome A disorder due to a genetic defect on the X chromosome and resulting in mental retardation, unusual physical characteristics, and learning problems.

G

Generalized anxiety disorder Syndrome consisting of incapacitating and unfocused worry, seemingly about nearly everything. Physical symptoms include irritability, tenseness, and restlessness.

Gestational age The age of a developing fetus beginning at the time of fertilization.

Group experimental designs (also *group experimental studies*) Research designs or investigations in which groups of participants are compared to determine the effects of treatments.

H

Haptic perception Relating to the sensation of touch and information received through body movements or position of the body.

Heritability The degree to which a trait is genetically determined and inherited.

Human rights The conditions thought to be necessary for healthy individual development and societal functioning, such as the right to live, access to medical care, free public education, and freedom from slavery, discrimination, and exploitation. Nations differ in their advocacy and respect for these rights for children.

Hyperactivity An excess of activity in inappropriate social circumstances, also referred to as *hyperkinesis*. Often accompanied by attention deficits.

Hypothalamic-pituitary-adrenalcortical axis (HYPAC) Body system involved in responding to stress and regulating emotional responses; consists of the hypothalamus and pituitary gland in the brain and several endocrine glands.

I

Identical twins Twins who developed from the same ovum and so are genetically the same.

Identity crisis Erikson's concept of adolescence as a time of particular stress and strain as the adolescent strives for a clear conception of self (ego identity).

Incidence The rate of occurrence (number of new cases identified) of a disorder during a specified time period (e.g., 1 year).

Independent variable The factor under study that is manipulated by the researcher. Also called *experimental variable*.

Inequality A developmental principle stating that early experiences can have differentially strong effects on later adjustment, depending on their duration, pervasiveness, and potency.

Intelligence tests Standardized tests of mental abilities that compare a child's scores to those of a large group of children of the same age to yield an IQ score.

Intermittent reinforcement Following a particular voluntary behavior by a reinforcing consequence less than 100% of the time.

Internal validity A measure of the degree to which all systematic influences except the independent variable have been controlled or held constant, which allows experimenters to test the effect of the independent variable.

Internalization Totally accepting as one's own the opinions and attitudes and perceptions of oneself held by other significant people.

Internalizing behavior problems Adjustment problems such as anxiety and depression that are directed more inward toward the self than outward toward others.

Interpersonal theory A view influenced by psychoanalysis that holds that a person's early experiences with attachment figures shape perceptions of self and others that are usually strengthened by later relationships.

Introjection In psychodynamic theory, internalized perceptions of parents' reactions to oneself, often originating in childhood. Unrealistic and negative introjections cause persistent psychological distress.

J

Juvenile delinquents Children or adolescents who intentionally break some type of law. Most display some of the same behaviors as children with attention deficits and conduct disorder.

L

Learned helplessness theory Theory developed by Seligman, Abramson, and colleagues that hopelessness or resignation about ever achieving control of one's life lies at the root of depression.

Legal rights Rights guaranteed to children or adults by the U.S. Constitution or by statute or state laws and enforced by the police or courts.

Longitudinal designs Research designs in which a sample of participants is observed repeatedly over an extended period of time to measure change in some factor of interest.

Low birth weight A weight of 2500 grams (5½ pounds) or less at birth; a low-birth-weight baby is considered premature and at risk for higher rates of morbidity and mortality.

M

Major depressive disorder A mental disorder characterized by one or more major depressive episodes, each lasting for at least 2 weeks. Symptoms include depressed mood, loss of interest in usual activities, and additional indicators of depression.

Major depressive episode A pattern of distressing or incapacitating depressive symptoms lasting for at least 2 weeks. Problems include a change in mood and outlook marked by nearly continuous depressed feelings, diminished enjoyment of life, disruptions in eating, sleeping, and activity, fatigue, feelings of guilt, inability to concentrate, and possible suicidal thoughts and impulses.

Mental retardation A fundamental difficulty in learning and performing basic daily life skills, characterized by significantly subaverage intellectual functioning together with limitations in adaptive skills.

Meta-analysis A statistical procedure that allows a researcher to analyze and synthesize the findings of previous empirical studies on a given topic in order to summarize the outcomes of many studies (e.g., how effectively a certain treatment relieves a particular problem).

Minor depression Also called *subclinical depression* because the person feels depressed but fails to show all of the symptoms of a depressive disorder.

Modeling Real-life or symbolic presentation of a specific act or general class of behavior, which provokes imitation or changes the observer's probability of engaging in similar behavior. In therapy, modeling may be used with guided participation to help the child master a feared behavior.

Multifaceted cognitive-behavioral treatments Complex interventions that combine cognitive elements, such as positive self-talk, with skills such as relaxation, and environmental manipulations to reinforce appropriate behavior and discourage inappropriate behavior.

Multifinality A developmental principle stating that similar early experiences can lead to different outcomes for different children.

N

Narcolepsy A sleep disorder involving involuntary and inappropriate sleeping spells.

Negative reinforcement The removal of an unpleasant or noxious stimulus that strengthens a behavior (e.g., when a child's hitting a bully stops the bullying, the hitting is reinforced).

Neglect Failure to provide for the nutrition, shelter, education, or health care of a child.

Neurological dysfunction Presumed malfunctioning of the neurological system. Often the affected individual exhibits behavioral signs of brain injury.

Neuroscience The systematic, scientific study of the relationship between brain and nervous system activity and behavior.

Neurotransmitters Chemicals that cross the gap between neurons to transmit or inhibit nerve impulses. An excess or deficiency of various neurotransmitters is thought to be involved in many different mental disorders.

O

Obesity Condition of being extremely overweight (weighing 30% more than is considered normal), to a degree that it impairs health, normal activity, and social interactions and decreases life expectancy.

Object relations theory (also *interpersonal theory*) A psychodynamic view of interpersonal relationships as being derived from the individual's past experiences with attachment figures such as parents, which become internalized and strengthened by later experiences and then shape perceptions, thoughts, feelings, and behavior.

Observation code The protocol used by observers to record the behavior(s) of a study participant. Contains specific definitions and instructions for accurate observations.

Observational learning Imitation or learning from examples provided by the behavior of others (models).

Obsessive-compulsive disorder An anxiety disorder characterized by persistent, uncontrollable, and intrusive thoughts or impulses accompanied by repetitive rituals aimed at suppressing the unwanted thoughts.

Operant behavior A term from Skinner's psychology for the type of voluntary behavior that operates on or changes the environment in some way and is controlled by its consequences.

Oppositional defiant disorder (ODD) Persistent and severe negativistic behavior with (1) high rates of noncompliance (2) tantrums, and (3) arguing with and resisting adults.

P

Panic Sudden feeling of overwhelming fear and anxiety in the absence of external threat. Physical symptoms may include palpitations, shortness of breath, chest pain, and nausea.

Parsimony Simplicity; a criterion for judging theoretical explanations that specifies that if theories are otherwise equivalent, the less complex one is preferred.

Penetrance The degree to which genes are expressed physically and behaviorally.

Perceptual disorder A deficiency or abnormality in the reception and/or interpretation of sensory stimuli.

Pervasive developmental disorders A general category of disorders, including autism, Rett's disorder, and Asperger's disorder, typically evident in the early years. Characterized by severe and pervasive impairment in several developmental areas, including social interaction and/or communication, or stereotyped behavior, interests, and activities.

Phobia Intense, persistent, irrational fear that interferes with normal activities and causes intense distress.

Phonological disorders Production of speech sounds inappropriate for the speaker's age or dialect.

Physical abuse Physically attacking a child so severely as to produce physical injury. The attack exceeds the cultural and legal standards for appropriate physical discipline.

Physical neglect A caretaker's failure to provide for a child's needs for nourishment, clothing, exercise, or decent housing so as to endanger the child's health.

Placebo In treatment effectiveness research, an inert or inactive procedure used to control for the beneficial effects of participants' positive expectations about the active treatment under investigation.

Polygenic model The view that multiple rather than single gene abnormalities are required for the development of some trait or disorder.

Positive reinforcer Any stimulus, object, or event that follows and increases the rate of a behavior (e.g., when a child receives a compliment on schoolwork and then works more diligently). Often loosely called a *reward*.

Posttraumatic stress disorder (PTSD) An anxiety disorder resulting from experiencing or witnessing an overwhelming, inescapable event, such as a military attack, fire, or earthquake in which the individual persistently re-experiences or morbidly dreads a repetition of the event and experiences high physiological arousal, with insomnia, irritability, and exaggerated startle reactions.

Prevalence The total number of cases of a disorder existing in a population at a particular point in time.

Primary prevention Actions taken before the onset of a condition that prevent the undesirable outcome from occurring (such as preventing maternal drug abuse and thus preventing unborn infants from being damaged).

Problem-solving skills training In cognitive-behavioral therapy, an intervention that teaches impulsive children to slow down, to analyze a problem and what they need to do to solve it, and then to compliment themselves privately as they systematically work on the task.

Psychoactive drugs (substances) Chemical agents that act on the central nervous system, affecting cognition, emotions, or activity level.

Psychoanalytic theory The influential view, developed by Freud, that much of human behavior is motivated by unconscious anxiety, hostility, and sexuality and that personality is formed early in life.

Psychological test Measure of cognitive, emotional, or social functioning through the use of standard test stimuli, observations, scoring, and interpretation.

Punishment An operant psychology term for a stimulus or event that follows and reduces the rate of a particular behavior. Commonly used to describe any painful event used to discipline a child.

Q

Quasi-experimental designs Research designs in which groups that have pre-existing differences (e.g., bright and average groups as measured by IQ) are compared rather than actually manipulating conditions. The pre-existing differences represent the independent variable.

R

Random error Erroneous assessment measure or observation that occurs by chance and in no particular pattern (e.g., the observer's view was temporarily blocked, or someone said something that distracted the observer).

Random sampling Sampling aimed at obtaining a sample of participants that is representative of the population under study; uses a process in which each individual in the population has an equal chance of being selected to participate, often through being chosen by means of a random number table or a computer software program.

Reciprocal gene-environment model The view that genetic make-up influences a person's chances of choosing or creating certain types of environments, which then affect behavior.

Reinforcing consequence (also *reinforcer*) An object, privilege, or event that acts to strengthen an immediately preceding voluntary response (e.g., when a child works harder because the behavior is followed by signs of the teacher's attention and approval).

Relationship research questions Research questions aimed at determining the degree to which two or more measures relate or vary together. Also called *correlational research questions*.

Reliability The agreement level or degree of consistency among observers recording the same behavior type, level, or performance score from simultaneous independent observations.

Research A systematic method of asking questions and obtaining information.

Rett's disorder A pervasive developmental disorder characterized by seemingly normal development through about the first 5 months but a slowing of development thereafter, a loss of purposeful hand movements followed by the development of stereo-typed hand activity, accompanied by serious impairment of language development.

S

School refusal Persistent avoidance or phobia focused on school stemming from family- or school-related factors. Two types are mild acute school refusal, which typically affects younger children, has a sudden onset, and is more easily treated, and severe chronic school refusal, which strikes older children, is associated with other psychological disorders, and is persistent.

Secondary prevention Efforts to remove a problem that already exists or shorten its duration (e.g., controlling the diet of a young child with phenylketonuria, which minimizes the damage to the central nervous system).

Self-efficacy Self-confidence in one's ability to perform adequately in a particular type of task or situation (e.g., academic ability or social skills). High self-efficacy helps people to succeed through persistence and lack of intimidation.

Self-talk (or *positive self-talk*) A technique from cognitive-behavioral therapy in which a child is trained to engage in reassuring self-directed comments, usually subvocally, to improve the child's attitude and likelihood of success at challenging tasks.

Separation anxiety disorder Children's excessive fear that even brief separations from parents and home will seriously harm them or their parents.

Serotonin A neurotransmitter involved in processing information, coordinating movement and general inhibition and restraint, and regulating eating, sexual, and aggressive actions; implicated in some mental disorders.

Sexual abuse Any type of age-inappropriate sexual exploitation of a child by an adult.

Social anxiety disorder (also *social phobia*) Acute and persistent fear of social or performance situations in which one might be publicly embarrassed or humiliated.

Social cognitive theory An approach to the study of behavior that is based on principles of social and cognitive psychology and stresses the effects of modeling and self-determination.

Somnambulism Episodes of walking during sleep as though awake; more commonly known as sleepwalking.

Specific phobia Acute and persistent fear of some particular object or situation.

Speech disorders Speech production that is sufficiently deviant from normal, accepted speaking patterns that it attracts attention, interferes with communication, and adversely impairs communication between the speaker and listener.

Standardized measure A test or procedure that has a set of norms for administration, scoring, and interpretation so that it can be used consistently with different people.

Stimulus overselectivity A perceptual disability in which a child focuses on only part of a stimulus, neglecting other major features.

Structured diagnostic interview A scripted clinical interview consisting of a predetermined set of questions concerning problems and symptoms and used to determine the presence and type of disorder in an individual.

Stuttering A disturbance in the fluency and rhythm of speech, with intermittent blocking, repetition, and prolongation of sounds, syllables, words, or phrases.

Substance abuse Use of a drug or other chemical (often illegally) to the extent that physical or psychological harm results.

Substance dependence Repeated and sustained pattern of self-administration of a drug or other chemical, often producing tolerance, withdrawal, and compulsion to continue usage.

Synapses (also *synaptic clefts*). Spaces between neurons where chemicals (neurotransmitters) are released and move impulses from one neuron to the next.

Systematic error Erroneous assessment measure where the procedure or the person using it is consistently off by a certain degree (e.g., when a coder uses the wrong behavior definition).

Systems-oriented family therapy Approach to treatment that views a child's psychopathology as caused by faulty family interactions rather than the child's weaknesses; teaches family members to detect harmful interactions and replace them with healthy ones.

T

Target behavior In observational studies, particularly applied behavior analysis, the act of central interest; often the behavior to be manipulated or treated (e.g., aggression or in-seat behavior).

Temperament General disposition, including predominant activity level, sociability, and emotionality, which appears in infancy, persists, and may be heritable.

Tertiary prevention Actions that minimize the unfavorable effects of a condition or disorder, thereby improving the person's functioning (e.g., offering specialized training to counteract delayed language skill development).

Time out from positive reinforcement A technique to reduce an unwanted behavior by briefly withholding positive reinforcement that is usually available (e.g., withdrawing all attention from a preschooler for 20 seconds following each tantrum).

Time-series designs Experimental designs in which a researcher manipulates the experimental variable over time and through different phases of treatment conditions (e.g., baseline, treatment, baseline) and records the results. Often used for intensive studies of the behavior of a small number of subjects or single individual.

U

Utility The usefulness or value of a test or procedure in accomplishing a task such as identifying people with a disorder; also the practical usefulness of a psychological theory.

V

Validity Extent to which a test or technique measures what it is intended to measure.

Visual discrimination The process of distinguishing among visually presented stimuli.

Voluntariness A legal term indicating that a person has the mental capacity to consent to participate in a study or treatment.

References

Chapter 1

Aguilar, B., Sroufe, L. A., Egeland, B., & Carlson, E. (2000). Distinguishing the early-onset/persistent and adolescence-onset antisocial behavior types: From birth to 16 years. *Development and Psychopathology, 12,* 109–132.

Allen, J. P., Hauser, S. T., Bell, K. L., & O'Connor, T. G. (1994). Longitudinal assessment of autonomy and relatedness in adolescent-family interactions as predictors of adolescent ego development and self-esteem. *Child Development, 65,* 179–194.

American Psychiatric Association. (2000). *Diagnostic and statistical manual of mental disorders* (4th ed., Text Revision). Washington, DC: Author.

American Psychological Association. (1993). *Violence & youth: Psychology's response. Vol. 1. Summary report of the American Psychological Association Commission on Violence and Youth.* Washington, DC: Author.

Arnett, J. (1995). The young and the reckless: Adolescent reckless behavior. *Current Directions in Psychological Science, 4,* 67–70.

Barrios, B. A., & Dell, S. L. (1998). Fears and anxieties. In E. J. Mash & R. A. Barkley (Eds.), *Treatment of childhood disorders* (2nd ed.) (pp. 249–337). New York: Guilford.

Beidel, D. (1991). Social phobia and overanxious disorder in school-age children. *Journal of the American Academy of Child & Adolescent Psychiatry, 30,* 545–552.

Brown, T. A., & Barlow, D. H. (2001). *Casebook in abnormal psychology.* Belmont, CA: Wadsworth.

Cicchetti, D., & Cohen, D. J. (1995). Perspectives on developmental psychopathology. In D. Cicchetti & D. J. Cohen (Eds.), *Developmental psychopathology: Vol. 1. Theory and methods* (pp. 1–54). New York: Wiley.

Curtiss, S. (1977). *Genie: A psycholinguistic study of a modern-day "wild child."* New York: Academic Press.

Erikson, E. H. (1956). The problems of ego identity. *Journal of the American Psychoanalytic Association, 4,* 56–121.

Geller, B., Reising, D., Leonard, H. L., Riddle, M. A., & Walsh, B. T. (1999). Critical review of tricyclic antidepressant use in children and adolescents. *Journal of the American Academy of Child and Adolescent Psychiatry, 38,* 513–528.

Gilliam, F. D., & Bales, S. N. (2001). Strategic frame analysis: Reframing America's youth. *Social Policy Report: Society for Research in Child Development.* Available: http://www.srcd.org/spr.html

Grotevant, H. D. (1998). Adolescent development in family contexts. In N. Eisenberg (Ed.), *Handbook of child psychology: Vol. 3. Social, emotional, and personality development* (5th ed.) (pp. 1097–1149).

Gullone, E. (1999). The assessment of normal fears in children and adolescents. *Clinical Child and Family Psychology Review, 2,* 91–106.

Ialongo, N., Edelsohn, G., Werthamer-Larsson, L., Crockett, L., & Kellam, S. (1995). The significance of self-reported anxious symptoms in first grade children: Prediction of anxious symptoms and adaptive functioning in fifth grade. *Journal of Child Psychology and Psychiatry, 36,* 427–437.

Keenan, K., & Shaw, D. (1997). Developmental and social influences on young girls' early problem behavior. *Psychological Bulletin, 121,* 95–113.

Lahey, B. B., Schwab-Stone, M., Goodman, S H., Waldman, I. D., Canino, G., Rathouz, P., Miller, T., Dennis, K., Bird, H., & Jensen, P. (2000). Age and gender differences in oppositional behavior and conduct problems: A cross-sectional household study of middle childhood and adolescence. *Journal of Abnormal Psychology, 109,* 488–503.

Lahey, B. B., Waldman, I. D., & McBurnett, K. (1999). The development of antisocial behavior: An integrative causal model. *Journal of Child Psychology and Psychiatry, 40,* 669–682.

Luby, J., & Morgan, K. (1997). Characteristics of an infant/preschool psychiatric clinic sample: Implications for clinical assessment and nosology. *Infant Mental Health Journal, 18*, 209–220.

Meyer, G. J., Finn, S. E., Eyde, L. D., Kay, G. G., Moreland, K. L., Dies, R. R., Eisman, E. J., Kubiszyn, T. W., & Reed, G. M. (2001). Psychological testing and psychological assessment: A review of evidence and issues. *American Psychologist, 56*, 128–165.

Offord, D. R., Boyle, M. H., Szatmari, P., Rae-Grant, N., Links, P., Cadman, D., Byles, J., Crawford, J., Blum, H., Byrne, C., Thomas, H., & Woodward, C. (1987). Ontario Child Health Study: II. Six-month prevalence of disorder and rates of service utilization. *Archives of General Psychiatry, 44*, 832–836.

Panchaud, C., Singh, S., Feivelson, D., & Darroch, J. E. (2000). Sexually transmitted diseases among adolescents in developed countries. *Family Planning Perspectives, 32*, 13–32.

Patterson, G. R., Forgatch, M. S., Yoerger, K. L., & Stoolmiller, M. (1998). Variables that initiate and maintain an early-onset trajectory for juvenile offending. *Development and Psychopathology, 10*, 531–547.

Peterson, A. C. (1993). Creating adolescents: The role of context and process in developmental trajectories. *Journal of Research on Adolescence, 3*, 1–18.

Rovee-Collier, C. (1999). The development of infant memory. *Current Directions in Psychological Science, 8*, 80–85.

Rutter, M., & Sroufe, L. A. (2000). Developmental psychopathology: Concepts and challenges. *Development and Psychopathology, 12*, 265–296.

Rymer, R. (1993). *Genie: An abused child's flight from silence*. New York: Harper Collins.

Shaffer, D., Fisher, P., Duncan, M. K., Davies, M., Piacentini, J., Schwab-Stone, M. E., Lahey, B. B., Bourdon, K., Jensen, P. S., Bird, H. R., Canino, G., & Regier, D. A. (1996). The NIMH Diagnostic Interview Schedule for Children Version 2.3 (DISC-2.3): Description, acceptability, prevalence rates and performance in the MECA study. *Journal of the American Academy of Child and Adolescent Psychiatry, 35*, 865–877.

Silverman, W. K., La Greca, A. M., & Wasserstein, S. (1995). What do children worry about? Worry and its relation to anxiety. *Child Development, 66*, 671–686.

Singh, S., & Darroch, J. E. (2000). Adolescent pregnancy and child bearing: Levels and trends in developed countries. *Family Planning Perspectives, 32*, 14–23.

Smith, J., & Prior, M. (1995). Temperament and stress resilience in school-age children: A within-families study. *Journal of the American Academy of Child and Adolescent Psychiatry, 34*, 168–179.

Tharp, R. G. (1993). Institutional and social context of educational practice and reform. In E. A. Forman, N. Minick, & C. A. Stone (Eds.), *Contexts for learning* (pp. 269–282). New York: Oxford University Press.

Tharp, R. G. (1994). Intergroup differences among Native Americans in socialization and child cognition: An ethnogenetic analysis. In P. M. Greenfield & R. Cocking (Eds.), *Cross-cultural roots of minority child development* (pp. 87–105). Hillsdale, NJ: Erlbaum.

U.S. Department of Education. (2000). *Twenty-second annual report to Congress on the implementation of the Individuals with Disabilities Education Act*. Washington, DC: Author.

U.S. Department of Justice. (2000). *Crime in the United States*. Washington, DC: U.S. Government Printing Office.

U.S. Surgeon General. (2000). *Healthy people*. Washington, DC: U.S. Government Printing Office.

van den Boom, D. C., & Hoeksma, J. B. (1994). The effects of infant irritability on mother-infant interaction: A growth-curve analysis. *Developmental Psychology, 30*, 581–590.

Weems, C. F., Silverman, W. K., & La Greca, A. M. (2000). What do youth referred for anxiety problems worry about? Worry and its relation to anxiety and anxiety disorders in children and adolescents. *Journal of Abnormal Child Psychology, 28*, 63–72.

Werner, E. E., & Smith, R. W. (1992). *Overcoming the odds: High risk children from birth to adulthood*. Ithaca, NY: Cornell University Press.

Youniss, J., & Ruth, A. (2000). *Interim report: Positive indicators of youth development*. Unpublished manuscript, The Catholic University of America, Washington, DC. Cited in F. D. Gilliam & S. N. Bales (2001). Strategic frame analysis: Reframing America's youth. *Social Policy Report*, Vol. 15, Number 3.

Zimmerman, M. A., & Arunkumar, R. (1994). Resiliency research: Implications for schools and policy. *Social Policy Report, 8*, 1–17.

Chapter 2

Ainsworth, M. D. S., Blehar, M., Waters, E., & Wall, S. (1978). *Patterns of attachment*. Hillsdale, NJ: Erlbaum.

Bandura, A. (1995). Exercise of personal and collective efficacy in changing societies. In A. Bandura (Ed.), *Self-efficacy in changing societies* (pp. 1–45). Cambridge, England: Cambridge University Press.

Bandura, A. (1997). *Self-efficacy: The exercise of control*. New York: Freeman.

Bandura, A., Barbaranelli, C., Vittorio, C., & Pastorelli, C. (2001). Self-efficacy beliefs as shapers of children's aspirations and career trajectories. *Child Development*, *72*, 187–206.

Bandura, A., & Walters, R. J. (1963). *Social and personality development*. New York: Holt, Rinehart and Winston.

Benjamin, L. S. (1974). Structural analysis of social behavior (SASB). *Psychological Review*, *81*, 392–425.

Benjamin, L. S. (1993). Every psychopathology is a gift of love. *Psychotherapy Research*, *3*, 1–24.

Benjamin, L. S. (1995). Good defenses make good neighbors. In H. Conte & R. Plutchik (Eds.), *Ego defenses: Theory and measurement* (pp. 53–78). New York: Wiley.

Bowlby, J. (1969). *Attachment and loss. Vol. 1. Attachment*. New York: Basic Books.

Cashdan, S. (1988). *Object relations theory: Using the relationship*. New York: Norton.

Chomsky, N. (1959). Review of *Verbal Behavior* by B. F. Skinner. *Language*, *35*, 26–58.

Cicchetti, D., & Sroufe, L. A. (2000). Editorial: The past as prologue to the future: The times, they've been a changin'. *Development and Psychopathology*, *12*, 255–264.

Cicchetti, D., Toth, S. L., & Lynch, M. (1995). Bowlby's dream comes full circle: The application of attachment theory to risk and psychopathology. In T. Ollendick & R. Prinz (Eds.), *Advances in clinical child psychology*, Vol. 17 (pp. 1–75). New York: Plenum.

Crews, F. (1996). The verdict on Freud. *Psychological Science*, *7*, 63–68.

Erikson, E. H. (1963). *Childhood and society* (2nd ed.). New York: Norton.

Erikson, E. H. (1968). *Identity. Youth and crisis*. New York: Norton.

Fonagy, P., & Target, M. (2000). The place of psychodynamic theory in developmental psychopathology. *Development and Psychopathology*, *12*, 407–425.

Frosh, S. (1997). *For and against psychoanalysis*. London: Routledge.

Hall, C. S. (1954). *A primer of Freudian psychology*. Cleveland: World Publishing.

Hur, Y., Bouchard, T. J., & Eckert, E. (1998). Genetic and environmental influences on self-reported diet: A reared-apart twin study. *Physiology & Behavior*, *64*, 629–636.

Johnson, M. H. (2000). Functional brain development in infants: Elements of an interactive specialization framework. *Child Development*, *71*, 75–81.

Kandel, E. R. (2000). The brain and behavior. In E. R. Kandel, J. H. Schwartz, & T. M. Jessell (Eds.), *Principles of neural science* (4th ed.) (pp. 5–18). New York: McGraw-Hill.

Kelsoe, J. R. (1997). The genetics of bipolar disorder. *Psychiatry Annual*, *27*, 285–292.

Lamb, M. E., Thompson, R. A., Gardner, W., & Charnov, E. L. (1985). *Infant-mother attachment: The origins and significance of individual differences in Strange Situation Behavior*. Hillsdale, NJ: Erlbaum.

Lyons-Ruth, K., Bronfman, E., & Parsons, E. (1999). Maternal disrupted affective communication, maternal frightened or frightening behavior, and disorganized infant attachment strategies. In J. Vondra & D. Barnett (Eds.), *Atypical patterns of infant attachment: Theory, research and current directions. Monographs of the Society for Research in Child Development*, *64* (Serial No. 258), 67–70.

Macmillan, M. (1991). *Freud evaluated: The completed arc. Advances in psychology*. Amsterdam: North-Holland.

McClearn, G. E., Johansson, B., Berg, S., Pedersen, N. L., Ahern, F., Petrill, S. A., & Plomin, R. (1997). Substantial genetic influence on cognitive abilities in twins 80 or more years old. *Science*, *276*, 1560–1563.

McGue, M., & Lykken, D. T. (1992). Genetic influence on risk of divorce. *Psychological Science*, *3*, 368–373.

Mischel, W. (1993). *Introduction to personality* (5th ed.). New York: Holt, Rinehart and Winston.

Newman, D. L., Tellegen, A., & Bouchard, T. J. (1998). Individual differences in adult ego development: Sources of influence in twins reared apart. *Journal of Personality and Social Psychology*, *74*, 985–995.

Owens, G., Crowell, J. A., Pan, H., Treboux, D., et al. (1995). The prototype hypothesis and the origins of attachment working models: Adult relationships with parents and romantic partners. *Monographs of the Society for Research in Child Development*, *60*(2–3), 216–233.

Owens, M. J., Mulcahey, J. J., Stout, S. C., & Plotsky, P. M. (1997). Molecular and neurobiological mechanisms in the treatment of psychiatric disorders. In A. Tasman, J. Kay, & J. A. Lieberman (Eds.), *Psychiatry* (Vol. 1) (pp. 210–257). Philadelphia: W. B. Saunders.

Rapp, B. (Ed.) (2001). *The handbook of cognitive neuropsychology: What deficits reveal about the human mind*. Philadelphia: Psychology Press.

Rende, R., & Plomin, R. (1992). Diathesis-stress models of psychopathology: A quantitative genetic perspective. *Applied & Preventive Psychology*, *1*, 177–182.

Rutter, M., Giller, H., & Hagell, A. (1998). *Antisocial behavior by young people*. New York: Cambridge University Press.

Rutter, M., & Sroufe, L. A. (2000). Developmental psychopathology: Concepts and challenges. *Development and Psychopathology*, *12*, 265–296.

Seifer, R., & Schiller, M. (1995). The role of parenting sensitivity, infant temperament, and dyadic interaction in attachment theory and assessment. In E. Waters, B. Vaughn, G. Posada, & K. Kondo-Ikemura (Eds.), *Caregiving, cultural, and cognitive perspectives on secure-base behavior and working models: New growing points of attachment theory and research. Monographs of the Society for Research in Child Development, 60* (Serial No. 244, Nos. 2–3).

Shoda, Y., Mischel, W., & Wright, J. C. (1994). Intraindividual stability in the organization and patterning of behavior: Incorporating psychological situations into the ideographic analysis of personality. *Journal of Personality & Social Psychology, 67,* 674–687.

Skinner, B. F. (1953). *Science and human behavior.* New York: Macmillan.

Teti, D. M., Gelfand, D. M., Messinger, D. S., & Isabella, R. (1995). Maternal depression and the quality of early attachment: An examination of infants, preschoolers, and their mothers. *Developmental Psychology, 31,* 364–376.

Thompson, R. A. (2000). The legacy of early attachments. *Child Development, 71,* 145–152.

Valenstein, E. S. (1998). *Blaming the brain: The truth about drugs and mental health.* New York: Basic Books.

Yablonsky, L. (1962). *The violent gang.* New York: Crowell-Collier and Macmillan.

Chapter 3

Allen, K. R., & Walker, A. J. (2000). Qualitative research. In C. Hendrick & S. S. Hendrick (Eds.), *Close relationships: A sourcebook* (pp. 19–30). Thousand Oaks, CA: Sage.

Arhar, J. M., Holly, M. L., & Kasten, W. C. (2001). *Action research for teachers: Traveling the yellow brick road.* Upper Saddle River, NJ: Merrill/Prentice Hall.

Babbie, E. (2001). *The practice of social research* (9th ed.). Belmont, CA: Wadsworth/Thomson.

Bersoff, D. N. (1999). *Ethical conflicts in psychology* (2nd ed.). Washington, DC: American Psychological Association.

Brandon, T. (2000). Introduction to the special section on empirical underpinnings of the ethics of alcohol administration in research settings. *Psychology of Addictive Behaviors, 14*(4), 315–318.

Crook, L. S., & Dean, M. C. (1999). Logical fallacies and ethical breaches. *Ethics and Behavior, 9,* 61–68.

Dienstfrey, H. (2000). True or false: The placebo effect as seen in drug studies is definitive proof that the mind can bring about clinically relevant changes in the body: Tabulating the results. *Advances in Mind-Body Medicine, 16*(1), 28–32.

Drew, C. J., & Hardman, M. L. (2000). *Mental retardation: A life cycle approach* (7th ed.). New York: Macmillan.

Drew, C. J., Hardman, M. L., & Hart, A. W. (1996). *Designing and conducting research: Inquiry in education and social science.* Boston: Allyn & Bacon.

Fraenkel, J. R., & Wallen, N. E. (1996). *How to design and evaluate research in education* (3rd ed.). New York: McGraw-Hill.

Freeman, D. (1983). *Margaret Mead and Samoa: The making and unmaking of an anthropological myth.* Cambridge, MA: Harvard University Press.

Freeman, D. (1989). Fa'apua'a Fa'amu and Margaret Mead. *American Anthropologist, 91,* 1017–1022.

Fuller, J. B., & Hester, K. (1999). Comparing the sample-weighted meta-analysis: An applied perspective. *Journal of Management, 25,* 803–828.

Gall, J. P., Gall, M. D., & Borg, W. R. (1998). *Applying educational research: A practical guide* (4th ed.). New York: Longman.

Gay, L., & Airasian, P. (2000). *Educational research: Competencies for analysis and applications* (6th ed.). Columbus, OH: Merrill/Prentice Hall.

Gliner, J. A., & Morgan, G. A. (2000). *Research methods in applied settings: An integrated approach to design and analysis.* Mahwah, NJ: Erlbaum.

Honigmann, J. J. (1963). *Understanding culture.* New York: Harper & Row.

Jones, S. E. (2001). Ethics code draft published for comment. *Monitor on Psychology, 32,* 76.

Karlawish, J. H. T., Hougham, G. W., Stocking, C. B., & Sachs, G. A. (1999). What is the quality of the reporting of research ethics in publications of nursing home research? *Journal of the American Geriatrics Society, 47,* 76–81.

Kavale, K. A., & Forness, S. R. (2000). Policy decisions in special education: The role of meta-analysis. In R. M. Gersten & E. P. Schiller (Eds.), *Contemporary special education research: Syntheses of the knowledge base on critical instructional issues* (pp. 281–326). Mahwah, NJ: Erlbaum.

Kazdin, A. E. (1998). *Methodological issues and strategies in clinical research.* Washington, DC: American Psychological Association.

Kopala, M., & Suzuki, L. A. (1999). *Using qualitative methods in psychology.* Thousand Oaks, CA: Sage.

Loftus, E. F. (1999). Lost in the mall: Misrepresentations and misunderstandings. *Ethics and Behavior, 9,* 51–60.

Luiselli, J. K., & Pine, J. (1999). Social control of childhood stealing in a public school: A case study. *Journal* of *Behavior Therapy and Experimental Psychiatry, 30*, 231–239.

Maxwell, S. E., & Delaney, H. D. (2000). *Designing experiments and analyzing data: A model comparison perspective*. Mahwah, NJ: Erlbaum.

Mead, M. (1928). *Coming of age in Samoa*. New York: Morrow.

Morgan, D. L., & Morgan, R. K. (2001). Single-participant research design: Bringing science to managed care. *American Psychologist, 56*, 119–127.

Oliver, P. J., & Benet-Martinez, V. (2000). Measurement: Reliability, construct validation, and scale construction. In H. T. Reis & C. M. Judd (Eds.), *Handbook of research methods in social and personality psychology* (pp. 339–369). New York: Cambridge University Press.

Posavac, H. D., Sheridan, S. M., & Posavac, S. S. (1999). A cueing procedure to control impulsivity in children with attention deficit hyperactivity disorder. *Behavior Modification, 23*, 234–253.

Powell, S., Calkins, C., Quealy-Berge, D., & Bardos, A. N. (1999). Adolescent day treatment: A school and community based alternative to residential care. *Journal of Developmental and Physical Disabilities, 11*(3), 275–286.

Price, D. D. (2000). True or false: The placebo effect as seen in drug studies is definitive proof that the mind can bring about clinically relevant changes in the body: Do placebo effects in analgesic drug studies demonstrate powerful mind-body interactions? *Advances in Mind-Body Medicine, 16*(1), 21–24.

Richards, S. B., Taylor, R., Ramasamy, R., & Richards, R. Y. (1998). *Single-subject research: Application in education and clinical settings*. Belmont, CA: Wadsworth/Thomson.

Rind, B., Bauserman, R., & Tromovitch, P. (2000). Science versus orthodoxy: Anatomy of the congressional condemnation of a scientific article and reflections on remedies for future ideological attacks. *Applied & Preventive Psychology, 9*, 211–225.

Rind, B., Tromovitch, P., & Bauserman, R. (1998). Meta-analytic examination of assumed properties of child sexual abuse using college samples. *Psychological Bulletin, 124*, 22–53.

Robinson, K. E., & Sheridan, S. M. (2000). Using the mystery motivator to improve child bedtime compliance. *Child & Family Behavior Therapy, 22*, 29–49.

Sales, B. D., & Folkman, S. (2000). *Ethics in research with human participants*. Washington, DC: American Psychological Association.

Schloss, P. J., & Smith, M. A. (1999). *Conducting research*. Upper Saddle River, NJ: Merrill/Prentice-Hall.

Sigafoos, J., & Littlewood, R. (1999). Communication intervention on the playground: A case study on teaching requesting to a young child with autism. *International Journal of Disability, Development, and Education, 46*, 421–429.

Stebbins, R. A. (2001). *Exploratory research in the social sciences*. Thousand Oaks, CA: Sage.

Wallen, N. E., & Fraenkel, J. R. (2000). *Educational research: A guide to the process* (2nd ed.). Mahwah, NJ: Erlbaum.

Willig, C. (2001). *Introducing qualitative research in psychology: Adventures in theory and methods*. Hyattsville, MD: Open University of America Press.

Chapter 4

Ablow, J. C., Measelle, J. R., Kraemer, H. C., Harrington, R., Luby, J., Smider, N., Dierker, L., Clark, V., Dubicka, B., Heffelfinger, A., Essex, M. J., & Kupfer, D. J. (1999). The MacArthur Three-City Outcome Study: Evaluating multi-informant measures of young children's symptomatology. *Journal of the American Academy of Child & Adolescent Psychiatry, 38*, 1580–1590.

Achenbach, T. M. (1991). *Manual for the Child Behavior Checklist/4–18 and 1991 Profile*. Burlington: University of Vermont, Department of Psychiatry.

Achenbach, T. M. (1992). *Manual for the Child Behavior Checklist/2–3 and the 1992 Profile*. Burlington: University of Vermont, Department of Psychiatry.

Ackerman, S. J., Hillsenroth, M. J., Clemence, A. J., Weatherill, R., & Fowler, J. C. (2001). Convergent validity of Rorschach and TAT scales of objective relations. *Journal of Personality Assessment, 77*, 295–306.

Aiken, L. R. (1997). *Psychological testing and assessment* (9th ed.). Needham Heights, MA: Allyn & Bacon.

Akande, A. (1998). Self-monitoring in autistic behavior. *Psychology: A Journal of Human Behavior, 35*, 23–29.

American Psychiatric Association. (2000). *Diagnostic and statistical manual of mental disorders–text revision* (4th ed.). Washington, DC: Author.

American Psychological Association. (1990). *Guidelines for providers of psychological services to ethnic, linguistic, and culturally diverse populations*. Washington, DC: Author.

American Psychological Association. (1999). *Standards for educational and psychological testing*. Washington, DC: Author.

Anastasi, A., & Urbina, S. (1997). *Psychological testing* (7th ed.). New York: MacMillan.

Angold, A., & Costello, E. J. (2000). The Child and Adolescent Psychiatric Assessment (CAPA). *Journal of the*

American Academy of Child & Adolescent Psychiatry, 39, 39–48.

Ardoin, S. P., & Martens, B. K. (2000). Testing the ability of children with attention deficit hyperactivity disorder to accurately report the effects of medication on their behavior. *Journal of Applied Behavior Analysis, 3*, 593–610.

Atlas, R. S., & Pepler, D. J. (1998). Observations of bullying in the classroom. *Journal of Educational Research, 29*, 86–99.

Bardos, A. N. (1993). Human figure drawings: Abusing the abused. *School Psychology Quarterly, 8*, 177–181.

Battle, D. E. (1997). Language and communication disorders in culturally and linguistically diverse children. In D. K. Bernstein & E. Tiegerman-Farber (Eds.), *Language and communication disorders in children* (pp. 382–410). Boston: Allyn & Bacon.

Beutler, L. E., & Malik, M. L. (2002). *Rethinking the DSM: A psychological perspective*. Washington, DC: American Psychological Association.

Binet, A., & Simon, T. (1905). Methodes nouvelles pour le diagnostic du niveau intellectuel des anormaux. *L'Annee Psychologique, 11*, 191–244.

Brems, C. (1998). Cultural issues in psychological assessment: Problems and possible solutions. *Journal of Psychological Practice, 4*, 88–117.

Canino, I., Canino, G., & Arroyo, W. (1998). Cultural considerations for childhood disorders: How much was included in DSM-IV? *Transcultural Psychiatry, 35*, 343–355.

Clare, S. K., Jenson, W. R., Kehle, T. J., & Bray, M. A. (2000). Self-modeling as a treatment for increasing on-task behavior. *Psychology in the Schools, 37*, 517–522.

Cone, J. D. (1999). Introduction to the special section on self-monitoring: A major assessment method in clinical psychology. *Psychological Assessment, 11*, 411–414.

Connors, K. C. (1997). *Connors rating scales revised*. Wilmington, DE: Wide Range.

Davies, S., & Witte, R. (2000). Self-management and peer monitoring within a group contingency to decrease uncontrolled verbalization of children with attention-deficit/hyperactivity disorder. *Psychology in the Schools, 37*, 135–147.

Drasgrow, E., & Yell, M. (2001). Functional behavioral assessments: Legal requirements and challenges. *School Psychology Review, 30*, 239–251.

Drew, C. J., & Hardman, M. L. (2000). *Mental retardation: A life cycle approach* (7th ed.). Columbus, OH: Merrill/Prentice Hall.

Ellingson, S. A., Miltenberger, R. G., Stricker, J., Galensky, T. L., & Garlinghouse, M. (2000). Functional assessment and intervention for challenging behaviors in the classroom. *Journal of Positive Behavior Interventions, 2*, 85–97.

Faust, J., & Ehrich, S. (2001). Children's Apperception Test (C.A.T.). In W. I. Dorfman & M. Hersen (Eds.), *Understanding psychological assessment: Perspectives on individual differences* (pp. 295–312). New York: Kluwer Academic/Plenum.

Follette, W. C. (1996). Introduction to the special section on the development of theoretically coherent alternatives to the *DSM. Journal of Consulting and Clinical Psychology, 64*, 1117–1120.

Foster, S. L., Laverty-Finch, C., Gizzo, D. P., & Osantowski, J. (1999). Practical issues in self-observation. *Psychological Assessment, 11*, 426–438.

Frisby, C. L. (1995). When facts and orthodoxy collide: The Bell Curve and the robustness criterion. *School Psychology Review, 24*, 304–316.

Fu, G. (1999). The development of a Draw-a-Person test in China: The norm from Hongzhu city. *Psychological Science China, 22*, 465–466.

Galton, F. (1869). *Hereditary genius*. London: Macmillan.

Gardner, H. (1983). *Frames of mind: The theory of multiple intelligences*. New York: Basic Books.

Gardner, H. (1998). Are there additional intelligences? The case for naturalist, spiritual, and existential intelligences. In J. Kane (Ed.), *Education, information, and transformation* (pp. 111–131). Englewood Cliffs, NJ: Prentice-Hall.

Gardner, H., Kornhaber, M. L., & Wake, W. K. (1996). *Intelligence: Multiple perspectives*. Ft. Worth, TX: Harcourt Brace College.

Gelfand, D. M., & Hartmann, D. P. (1984). *Child behavior analysis and therapy* (2nd ed.). New York: Pergamon Press.

Gilbert, J. (1978). *Interpreting psychological test data*. New York: Van Nostrand Reinhold.

Gronlund, N. E. (1998). *Assessment of student achievement* (6th ed.). Boston: Allyn & Bacon.

Gronlund, N. E. (2000). *How to write and use instructional objectives* (6th ed.). Columbus, OH: Merrill/Prentice Hall.

Hayes, S. C., Fox, E., Gifford, E. V., Wilson, K. G., Barnes-Holmes, D., & Healy, O. (2001). Derived relational responding as learned behavior. In S. C. Hayes and D. Barnes-Holmes (Eds.), *Relational frame theory: A post-Skinnerian account of human language and cognition* (pp. 21–49). New York: Kluwer Academic/Plenum.

Haynes, S. N. (2001). Clinical applications of analogue behavioral observation: Dimensions of psychometric evaluation. *Psychological Assessment, 13*, 73–85.

Hechtman, L. (2000). Assessment and diagnosis of attention-deficit/hyperactivity disorder. *Child and Adolescent Psychiatric Clinics of North America, 9,* 481–498.

Hernstein, R. J., & Murray, C. (1994). *The bell curve: The reshaping of American life by differences in intelligence.* New York: Free Press.

Holtzman, W. H. (1993). An unjustified, sweeping indictment by Motta et al. of human figure drawings for assessing psychological functioning. *School Psychology Quarterly, 8,* 189–190.

Hopkins, K. D. (1998). *Educational and psychological measurement and evaluation* (8th ed.). Boston: Allyn & Bacon.

Hunsley, J., & DiGiulio, G. (2001). Norms, norming, and clinical assessment. *Clinical Psychology: Science and Practice, 8,* 378–382.

Individuals with Disabilities Education Act Amendments of 1997, 20 U.S.C. § 1400 *et seq.*

Iwata, B. A., Dorsey, M. F., Slifer, K. J., Bauman, K. E., & Richman, G. S. (1994). Toward a functional analysis of self-injury. *Journal of Applied Behavior Analysis, 27,* 197–209.

Janda, L. (1998). *Psychological testing, theory, and applications.* Boston: Allyn & Bacon.

Kamphaus, R. W., Petoskey, M. D., & Rowe, E. W. (2000). Current trends in the psychological testing of children. *Professional Psychology: Research, & Practice, 31,* 155–164.

Klinger, L. G., & Renner, P. (2000). Performance-based measures in autism: Implications for diagnosis, early detection, and identification of cognitive profiles. *Journal of Child Psychology, 29,* 479–492.

Knoff, H. M., Batsche, G. M., & Carlyon, W. (1993). Projective techniques. In T. R. Karotchwill & R. J. Morris (Eds.), *Handbook of psychotherapy with children and adolescents* (pp. 9–37). Boston: Allyn & Bacon.

Koegel, L. K., Koegel, R. L., Hurley, C., & Frea, W. D. (1992). Improving social skills and disruptive behavior in children with autism through self-management. *Journal of Applied Behavior Analysis, 25,* 341–353.

Koppitz, E. M. (1968). *Psychological evaluation of children's Human Figure Drawings.* New York: Grune & Stratton.

Korotitsch, W. J., & Nelson-Gray, R. O. (1999). An overview of self-monitoring research in assessment and treatment. *Psychological Assessment, 11,* 415–425.

Lachar, D., & Gruber, C. P. (1994). *Personality Inventory for Youth manual.* Los Angeles: Western Psychological Services.

Lam, A. L., Cole, C. L., Shapiro, E. S., & Bambara, L. M. (1994). Relative effects of self-monitoring on task behavior, academic accuracy, and disruptive behavior in students with behavior disorders. *School Psychology Review, 23,* 44–58.

Lamison-White, L. (1997). *Poverty in the United States: 1996.* U.S. Bureau of the Census, *Current Population Reports* (Ser. P60–198), U.S. Government Printing Office, Washington, DC.

Larry P. v. Riles, 343 F. Supp. 1306 (D.C.N.D. Cal. 1972), *aff'd,* 502 F. 2d 963 (9th Cir. 1974); *further proceedings,* 495 F. Supp. 926 (D.C.N.D. Cal. 1979), *aff'd,* 502 F. 2d. 693 (9th Cir. 1984).

Lilienfeld, S. O., Wood, J. M., & Garb, H. N. (2001). What's wrong with this picture? *Scientific American, 5,* 81–87.

Mash, E. J., & Terdal, L. G. (1997). *Assessment of childhood disorders* (3rd ed). New York: Guilford.

Mayfield, J. W., & Reynolds, C. R. (1997). Black-white differences in memory test performance among children and adolescents. *Archives of Clinical Neuropsychology, 12,* 111–122.

McComas, J. J., Hoch, H., & Mace, F. C. (2000). Functional analysis. In E. S. Shapiro & T. R. Kratochwill (Eds.), *Conducting school-based assessments of child and adolescent behavior* (pp. 78–120). New York: Guilford.

McConaughy, S. (2000). Self-reports: Theory and practice in interviewing children. In E. S. Shapiro & T. R. Kratochwill (Eds.), *Behavioral Assessment in Schools: Theory, Research, and Clinical Foundations* (2nd ed.) (pp. 173–234). New York: Guilford.

Merrell, K. W. (1999). *Behavioral, social, and emotional assessment of children and adolescents.* Mahwah, NJ: Erlbaum.

Meyer, G., Finn, S. E., Eyde, L. D., Kay, G. G., Moreland, K. L., Dies, R. R., Eisman, E. J., Kubiszyn, T. W., & Reed, G. M. (2001). Psychological testing and psychological assessment: A review of the evidence and issues. *American Psychologist, 56,* 128–165.

Milne, L. C., & Greenway, P. (2001). Free association to Rorschach responses and control of internal states. *Journal of Projective Psychology and Mental Health, 8*(2), 95–106.

Mischel, W. (1993). *Introduction to personality* (5th ed.). New York: Harcourt, Brace, Jovanovich.

Mitsis, E. M., McKay, K. E., Schulz, K. P., Newcorn, J. H., & Halperin, J. M. (2000). Parent-teacher concordance for DSM-IV attention-deficit/hyperactivity disorder in a clinic-referred sample. *Journal of the American Academy of Child & Adolescent Psychiatry, 39,* 308–313.

Murray, H. A. (1943). *Thematic Apperception Test manual.* Cambridge, MA: Harvard University Press.

Naglieri, J. A. (1993). Human figure drawings in perspective. *School Psychology Quarterly, 8,* 170–176.

Nathan, P. E., & Lagenbucher, J. W. (1999). Psychopathology: Description and classification. *Annual Review of Psychology, 50*, 79–107.

Negy, C., Lachar, D., Gruber, C. P., & Garza, N. D. (2001). The Personality Inventory for Youth: Validity and comparability of English and Spanish versions for regular education and juvenile justice samples. *Journal of Personality Assessment, 76*, 250–263.

Nicholls, D., Chater, R., & Lask, B. (2000). Children into DSM don't go: A comparison of classification systems for eating disorders in childhood and early adolescence. *International Journal of Eating Disorders, 28*, 317–324.

Olympia, D. E., Heathfield, L. T., Jenson, W. R., & Clark, E. (2002). Multifaceted functional behavior assessment for students with externalizing behavior disorders. *Psychology in the Schools, 39*(2), 139–155.

O'Neill, R., Horner, R. H., Albin, R. W., Sprague, J. R., Storey, K., & Newton, J. S. (1997). *Functional behavior assessment and program development for problem behavior: A practical handbook* (2nd ed.). Pacific Grove, CA: Brooks/Cole.

Oswald, L., Rhode, G., & Jenson, W. R. (2001). *Classroom observation on a Palm Pilot.* Unpublished manuscript. Salt Lake City: University of Utah.

Paolo, A. M., Ryan, J. J., Ward, L. C., & Hilmer, C. D. (1997). Different WAIS-R short forms and their relation to ethnicity. *Personality and Individual Differences, 21*, 851–856.

Pavuluri, M. N., & Luk, S. (1998). Recognition and classification of psychopathology in preschool children. *Australian & New Zealand Journal of Psychiatry, 32*, 642–649.

Perez, B. (1997). *Sociocultural contexts of language and literacy.* Mahwah, NJ: Erlbaum.

Reavis, K., Jenson, W. R., Morgan, D. P., Likens, M., & Althouse, R. B. (1998). *Functional behavior assessment and interventions program* (*FAIP*). Longmont, CO: Sopris West.

Reeb, R. N. (2000). Classification and diagnosis of psychopathology: Conceptual foundations. *Journal of Psychological Practice, 6*, 3–18.

Reid, J. B. (1978). *A social learning approach to family intervention: Vol. 2. Observation in the home setting.* Eugene, OR: Castalia.

Reid, R. (1995). Assessment of ADHD with culturally different groups: The use of behavior rating scales. *School Psychology Review, 24*, 537–560.

Rorschach, H. (1948). *Psychodiagnostics: A diagnostic test based on perception* (4th ed.). New York: Grune & Stratton.

Rourke, B. P. (1997). Significance of verbal-performance discrepancies for subtypes of children with learning disabilities: Opportunities for the WISC—III. In A. Prifitera & D. H. Saklofske (Eds.), *WISC—III clinical use and interpretation: Scientist-practitioner perspectives* (pp. 139–156). San Diego: Academic.

Saccuzzo, D. P., & Johnson, N. E. (1995). Traditional psychometric tests and proportionate representation: An intervention and program evaluation study. *Psychological Assessment, 7*(2), 183–194.

Sanders, M. (2001). *Observe desktop and palm CD-ROM and instruction manual.* Longmont, CO: Sopris West.

Sattler, J. M. (2001). *Assessment of children: Cognitive applications* (4th ed.). San Diego: Author.

Saunders, C. D., Hall, E. J., Casey, J. E., & Strang, J. D. (2000). Subtypes of psychopathology in children referred for neuropsychological assessment. *Child Neuropsychology, 6*(2), 129–143.

Selznick, L. S., & Savage, R. C. (2000). Using self-monitoring procedures to increase on-task behavior with three adolescent boys with brain injury. *Behavioral Interventions, 15*, 243–260.

Shaffer, D., Fisher, P., Lucas, C. P., Dulcan, M. K., & Schwab-Stone, M. E. (2000). NIMH Diagnostic Interview Schedule for Children Version IV (NIMH DISC-IV): Description, differences from previous versions, and reliability of some common diagnoses. *Journal of the American Academy of Child & Adolescent Psychiatry, 39*, 28–38.

Shapiro, E. S., & Cole, C. L. (1999). Self-monitoring in assessing children's problems. *Psychological Assessment, 11*, 448–457.

Silverstein, M. L. (2001). Clinical identification of compensatory structures on projective tests: A self psychological approach. *Journal of Personality Assessment, 76*, 517–536.

Spearman, C. E. (1927). *The abilities of man.* New York: Macmillan.

Sternberg, R. J. (1997). The triarchic theory of intelligence. In D. P. Flanagan, J. Genshaft, & P. L. Harrison (Eds.), *Contemporary intellectual assessment: Theories, tests, and issues* (pp. 92–104). New York: Guilford.

Szatmari, P. (2000). The classification of autism, Asperger's syndrome, and pervasive developmental disorder. *Canadian Journal of Psychiatry, 45*, 731–738.

Teglasi, H. (2001). *Essentials of TAT and other storytelling techniques assessment.* New York: Wiley.

Valla, J., Bergeron, L., & Smolla, N. (2000). The Dominic-R: A pictorial interview for 6- to 11-year-old children. *Journal of the American Academy of Child & Adolescent Psychiatry, 39*, 85–93.

Van den Broek, A., Golden, C. J., Loonstraa, A., Ghinglia, K., & Goldstein, D. (1998). Short forms of the Wechsler Memory Scale—Revised: Cross-validation and derivation of a two-subtest form. *Psychological Assessment, 10*, 38–40.

Watkins, C. E., Campbell, V. L., Nieberding, R., & Hallmark, R. (1995). Contemporary practice of psychological assessment by clinical psychologists. *Professional Psychology: Research & Practice, 26*, 54–60.

Webster-Stratton, C. L., & Lindsay, D. W. (2000). Social competence and conduct problems in young children: Issues and assessment. *Journal of Clinical Child Psychology, 28*, 25–43.

Wechsler, D. (1958). *The measurement and appraisal of adult intelligence* (4th ed.). Baltimore: Williams & Wilkins.

Wechsler, D. (1991). *WISC-III manual*. San Antonio, TX: Harcourt, Brace, Jovanovich.

Weller, E. B., Weller, R. A., Fristad, M. A., Rooney, M. T., & Schecter, J. (2000). Children's Interview for Psychiatric Syndromes (ChIPS). *Journal of the American Academy of Child & Adolescent Psychiatry, 39*, 76–84.

Westen, D., Feit, A., & Zittel, C. (1999). Focus chapter: Methodological issues in research using projective methods. In P. C. Kendall and J. N. Butcher (Eds.), *Handbook of research methods in clinical psychology* (2nd ed.) (pp. 224–240). New York: Wiley.

Wilson, M. S., & Reschly, D. (1996). Assessment in school psychology training and practice. *School Psychology Review, 25*, 9–23.

World Health Organization. (1992). *International classification of diseases* (10th ed.). Geneva: Author.

Wulfert, E., Greenway, D. E., & Dougher, M. J. (1996). A logical functional analysis of reinforcement-based disorders: Alcoholism and pedophilia. *Journal of Consulting & Clinical Psychology, 64*, 1140–1151.

Chapter 5

American Academy of Child and Adolescent Psychiatry. (1997). Practice parameters for the assessment and treatment of children and adolescents with substance use disorders. *Journal of the American Academy of Child and Adolescent Psychiatry, 36*, 140S-156S.

American Psychiatric Association. (2000). *Diagnostic and Statistical Manual of Mental Disorders* (4th ed., text rev.). Washington, DC: Author.

Azrin, N. H., Acierno, R., Kogan, E., Donahue, B., Besalel, V., & McMahon, P. T. (1996). Follow-up results of supportive versus behavioral therapy for illicit drug abuse. *Behavioral Research & Therapy, 34*, 41–46.

Ballie, R. (2001a, June). Children and parents are having different conversations about substance use. *Monitor on Psychology, 32*(6), 16.

Ballie, R. (2001b, June). Fifty-four percent of youth have tried an illicit drug. *Monitor on Psychology, 32*(6), 17.

Bandura, A. (1969). *Principles of behavior modification*. New York: Holt, Rinehart & Winston.

Barling, J., Rogers, K., & Kelloway, K. (1995). Some effects of teenagers' part-time employment: The quantity and quality of work make the differences. *Journal of Organizational Behavior, 16*, 143–154.

Botsford, C. (2001, May 4). Prescription drug abuse explodes in America. *The NCADI Reporter*. National Clearinghouse for Alcohol and Drug Information. Retrieved May 3, 2002, from the World Wide Web: http://www.health.org/newsroom/rep/168.htm

Briggs, X. S. (1997). Moving up versus moving out: Neighborhood effects in housing mobility programs. *Housing Policy Debate, 8*, 195–234.

Brody, G. H., Ge, X., Conger, R., Gibbons, F. X., McBride, V., Gerrard, M., & Simons, R. L. (2001). The influence of neighborhood disadvantage, collective socialization, and parenting on African American children's affiliation with deviant peers. *Child Development, 72*, 1231–1246.

Carta, J. J., Atwater, J. B., Greenwood, C. R., McConnell, S. R., McEvoy, M. A., & Williams, R. (2001). Effects of cumulative prenatal substance exposure and environmental risks on children's developmental trajectories. *Journal of Community Psychology, 30*, 327–337.

Caspi, A., Moffitt, T., Newman, D., & Silva, P. (1996). Behavioral observations at age 3 years predict adult psychiatric disorders. *Archives of General Psychiatry, 53*, 1033–1039.

Chassin, L., Pitts, S. C., DeLucia, C., & Todd, M. (1999). A longitudinal study of children of alcoholics: Predicting young adult substance use disorders, anxiety, and depression. *Journal of Abnormal Psychology, 108*, 106–119.

Chavkin, W. (2001). Cocaine and pregnancy: Time to look at the evidence. *Journal of the American Medical Association, 285*, 1621–1623.

Children's Defense Fund. (2000). *The state of America's children: Yearbook 2000*. Washington, DC: Author.

Council of Economic Advisors. (2000). *Teens and their parents in the 21st century: An examination of trends in teen behavior and the role of parent involvement*. Washington, DC: Author.

Diamond, G. S., & Liddle, H. A. (1996). Resolving a therapeutic impasse between parents and adolescents in multi-dimensional family therapy. *Journal of Consulting and Clinical Psychology, 64*, 481–488.

Dishion, T. J. (1990). The family ecology of boys' peer relations in middle childhood. *Child Development, 61,* 874–892.

Dishion, T. J., French, D. C., & Patterson, G. R. (1995). The development and ecology of antisocial behavior. In D. Cicchetti & D. J. Cohen (Eds.), *Developmental psychopathology: Vol. 2. Risk, disorder, and adaptation* (pp. 421–471). New York: Wiley.

Ebrahim, S. H., Floyd, R. L., Merritt, R. K., Decoufle, P., & Holtzman, D. (2000). Trends in pregnancy-related smoking rates in the United States, 1987–1996. *Journal of the American Medical Association, 283,* 361–366.

Epstein, J. A., Griffin, K. W., & Botvin, G. J. (2001). Risk taking and refusal assertiveness in a longitudinal model of alcohol use among inner-city adolescents. *Prevention Science, 2,* 193–200.

Foxhall, K. (2001). Adolescents aren't getting the help they need. *Monitor on Psychology, 32,* 56–58.

Franco, P., Chabanski, S., Szliwowski, H., Dramaiz, M., & Kahn, A. (2000). Influence of maternal smoking on autonomic nervous system functioning in healthy infants. *Pediatric Research, 47,* 215–220.

Frank, D. A., Augustyn, M., Grant Knight, W., Pell, T., & Zuckerman, B. (2001). Growth, development, and behavior in early childhood following prenatal cocaine exposure: A systematic review. *Journal of the American Medical Association, 285,* 1613–1625.

Gilvarry, E. (2000). Substance abuse in young people. *Journal of Child Psychology and Psychiatry, 41,* 55–80.

Gold, M. S. (1997). Cocaine (and crack): Clinical aspects. In J. H. Lowinson, P. Ruiz, R. B. Millman, & J. G. Langrod (Eds.), *Substance abuse: A comprehensive textbook* (pp. 181–199). Baltimore: Williams & Wilkins.

Gottfredson, D. C., Gottfredson, G. D., & Hybel, L. G. (1993). Managing adolescent behavior: A multi-year, multi-school study. *American Educational Research Journal, 30,* 179–215.

Grella, C. E., Hser, Y., Joshi, V., & Rounds-Bryant, J. (2001). Drug treatment outcomes for adolescents with comorbid mental and substance use disorders. *Journal of Nervous and Mental Disease, 189,* 384–392.

Henggeler, S. W., Pickrel, S. G., Brondino, M. J., & Crouch, J. L. (1996). Eliminating (almost) treatment dropout of substance abusing or dependent delinquents through home-based multisystemic therapy. *American Journal of Psychiatry, 153,* 427–428.

Hewlett, K. (2001, June 18). Eat dinner with your children. *Monitor on Psychology, 32*(6), 16.

Hofferth, S. L., & Sandberg, J. (1998, November 9). *Changes in American children's time, 1981–1997.*

Bethesda, MD: National Institute of Child Health and Human Development.

Hser, Y., Grella, C. E., Hubbard, R. L., Hsieh, S., Fletcher, B. W., Brown, B. S., & Anglin, D. (2001). An evaluation of drug treatments for adolescents in four U.S. cities. *Archives of General Psychiatry, 58,* 689–695.

Hurt, H., Betancourt, L. M., Brodsky, N. L., & Giannetti, J. M. (2001). A prospective comparison of developmental outcome of children with in utero cocaine exposure and controls using the Battelle Development Inventory. *Journal of Developmental and Behavioral Pediatrics, 22,* 292–296.

Jessor, R., & Jessor, S. L. (1977). *Problem behavior and psychosocial development.* New York: Academic Press.

Kahlenberg, R. (2001). *All together now: Creating middle-class schools through public school choice.* Washington, DC: Brookings Institution Press.

Kilpatrick, D. G., Acierno, R., Saunders, B., Resnick, H. S., Best, C. L., & Schnurr, P. P. (2000). Risk factors for adolescent substance abuse and dependence: Data from a national sample. *Journal of Consulting and Clinical Psychology, 68,* 19–30.

Leshner, A. I. (2001, August). Understanding the risks of prescription drug abuse. *NIDA Notes. Director's Column.* Retrieved May 3, 2002, from the World Wide Web: http://www.nida.nih.gov/NIDA_Notes/NNVol16N3/DirRepVol16N3.html

Liddle, H. A. (1995). Conceptual and clinical dimensions of a multidimensional, multisystems engagement strategy in family-based adolescent treatment. *Psychotherapy: Theory, Research, and Practice, 32,* 39–58.

Ludwig, J., Duncan, G. J., & Hirschfield, P. (1998). *Urban poverty and juvenile crime: Evidence from a randomized housing-mobility experiment.* Unpublished manuscript.

Martin, S. (2001, June). Substance abuse is nation's no. 1 health problem, but there is hope. *Monitor on Psychology, 32,* 10.

Meier, B. (2001, October 28). Overdoses of painkiller are linked to 282 deaths: Federal study details misuse of OxyContin. *New York Times,* p. A-18.

National Clearinghouse for Alcohol and Drug Information. (2001). OxyContin Information. OxyContin: Prescription Drug Abuse-CSAT Advisory. Retrieved October 29, 2001, from the World Wide Web: http://www.health.org/features/oxy/

National Institute for Drug Abuse (NIDA). (1996). *National household survey on drug abuse.* Washington, DC: U.S. Government Printing Office.

National Institute for Drug Abuse (NIDA). (2001, December 19). 2001 Monitoring the Future survey. Retrieved

May 23, 2002, from the World Wide Web: http://www.nida.gov/infofax/hsyouthtrends.html

Ozechowski, T. J., & Liddle, H. A. (2000). Family-based therapy for adolescent drug abuse: Knowns and unknowns. *Clinical Child and Family Psychology Review, 3*, 269–298.

Paltrow, L. M., Cohen, D. S., & Carey, C. A. (2000, October). *Year 2000 overview: Governmental responses to pregnant women who use alcohol or other drugs.* Philadelphia: Women's Law Project, National Advocates for Pregnant Women.

Perry, C. L., Kelder, S. H., & Komro, K. A. (1993). The social world of adolescents: Family, peers, schools, and the community. In S. G. Millstein, A. C. Petersen, & E. O. Nightingale (Eds.), *Promoting the health of adolescents: New directions for the twenty-first century* (pp. 73–96). New York: Oxford.

Portes, A., & Rumbaut, R. G. (2001). *Legacies: The story of the immigrant second generation.* Berkeley: University of California.

Resnick, M. D., Bearman, P. S., Blum, R. W., Bauman, K. E., Harris, K. M., Jones, J., Tabor, J., Beuhring, T., Sieving, R. E., Shew, M., Ireland, M., Bearinger, L. H., & Udry, J. R. (1997). Protecting adolescents from harm: Findings from the National Longitudinal Study on Adolescent Health. *Journal of the American Medical Association, 278*, 823–832.

Roth, J., & Brooks-Gunn, J. (2000). What do adolescents need for healthy development? Implications for youth policy. *Social Policy Report, 14*, 3–19.

Rutter, M. (2000). Psychosocial influences: Critiques, findings, and research needs. *Development and Psychopathology, 12*, 375–405.

Sameroff, A. J., Seifer, R., Barocas, R., Zax, M., & Greenspan, S. (1987). Intelligence quotient scores of 4-year-old children: Social environmental risk factors. *Pediatrics, 79*, 343–350.

Sampson, R. J., & Morenoff, J. (1997). Ecological perspectives on the neighborhood context of urban poverty: Past and present. In J. Brooks-Gunn, G. J. Duncan, & J. L. Aber (Eds.), *Neighborhood poverty: Vol. 2. Policy implications in studying neighborhoods* (pp. 1–22). New York: Sage Foundation.

Santini, J., & Estes, A. (2001, September 2). Speed trap. *The Salt Lake Tribune*, pp. A-1, A-6, A-7.

Sickmund, M., Snyder, H., & Poe-Yamagata, E. (1997). *Juvenile offenders and victims: 1997 update on violence.* Washington, DC: Office of Juvenile Justice and Delinquency Prevention.

Smith, D. (2001). Prevention: Still a young field. *Monitor on Psychology, 3*, 70–72.

Spoth, R. L., Redmond, C., & Shin, C. (2001). Randomized trial of brief family interventions for general populations: Adolescent substance use outcomes 4 years following baseline. *Journal of Consulting and Clinical Psychology, 69*, 627–642.

Steinberg, L. D., Fegley, S., & Dornbusch, S. (1993). Negative impact of part-time work on adolescent adjustment: Evidence from a longitudinal study. *Developmental Psychology, 29*, 171–180.

Walker, A., Rosenberg, M., & Balaban-Gil, K. (1999). Neurodevelopmental and neurobehavioral sequelae of selected substances of abuse and psychiatric medications in utero. *Neurological Disorders: Developmental and Behavioral Sequelae, 8*, 845–867.

Walker, T. (2001, Fall). Class assignment: Can socioeconomic diversity restore the promise of school integration? *Teaching Tolerance, 20*, 34–40.

Weinberg, N., Rahdert, E., Colliver, J. D., & Glantz, M. D. (1998). Adolescent substance abuse: A review of the past 10 years. *Journal of the American Academy of Child and Adolescent Psychiatry, 37*, 252–261.

Werner, E. E., & Smith, R. S. (1992). *Overcoming the odds: High risk children from birth to adulthood.* Ithaca, NY: Cornell.

White, H. R., Loeber, R., Stouthamer-Loeber, M., & Farrington, D. P. (1999). Developmental associations between substance use and violence. *Development and Psychopathology, 11*, 785–803.

Williams, R. J., Chang, S. Y., & Addiction Centre Adolescent Research Group. (2000). A comprehensive and comparative review of adolescent substance abuse treatment outcome. *Clinical Psychology Science and Practice, 7*, 138–166.

Wills, T. A., Sandy, J. M., Yaeger, A., & Shinar, O. (2001). Family risk factors and adolescent substance use: Moderation effects for temperament dimensions. *Developmental Psychology, 37*, 283–297.

Chapter 6

American Medical Association. (1994). Memories of childhood sexual abuse: Report of the Council on Scientific Affairs (CSA 5-A-94). Chicago: Author.

American Psychiatric Association. (1993, December). *Statement on memories of sexual abuse.* Washington, DC: Author.

American Psychological Association. (1994, August). Questions and answers about memories of childhood abuse. Washington, DC: Author.

Bandura, A. (1969). *Principles of behavior modification.* New York: Holt, Rinehart & Winston.

Berliner, L., & Kolko, D. (2000). What works in treatment services for abused children. In M. P. Kluger, G. Alexander, et al. (Eds.), *What works in child welfare* (pp. 97–104). Washington, DC: Child Welfare League of America.

Bernstein, N. (2001, February 2). Plight of 2 boys exposes a long odyssey of abuse. *New York Times*, pp. 1, A19.

Boat, B. W., & Everson, M. D. (1993). The use of anatomical dolls in sexual abuse evaluations: Current research and practice. In G. S. Goodman & B. L. Bottoms (Eds.), *Child victims, child witnesses: Understanding and improving testimony* (pp. 47–70). New York: Guilford.

Bowen, K. (2000). Child abuse and domestic violence in families of children seen for suspected sexual abuse. *Clinical Pediatrics, 39*, 33–40.

Brody, G. H., Xiaojia, G., Rand, C., Gibbons, F. X., Murry, V., Gerrard, M., & Simons, R. L. (2001). The influence of neighborhood disadvantage, collective socialization, and parenting on African American children's affiliation with deviant peers. *Child Development, 72*, 1231–1246.

Brown, J., Cohen, P., Johnson, J. G., & Smailes, E. M. (1999). Childhood abuse and neglect: Specificity and effects on adolescent and young adult depression and suicidality. *Journal of the American Academy of Child & Adolescent Psychiatry, 38*, 1490–1496.

Bruck, M., Ceci, S. J., Francoeur, E., & Barr, R. (1995). "I hardly cried when I got my shot": Influencing children's reports about a visit to their pediatrician. *Child Development, 66*, 193–208.

Caffey, J. (1946). Multiple fractures in the long bones of infants suffering from chronic subdural hematoma. *American Journal of Roentgenology, 56*, 163–173.

Canadian Psychiatric Association. (1996). Position statement: Adult recovered memories of childhood sexual abuse. *Canadian Journal of Psychiatry, 41*, 305–306.

Ceci, S. J., & Bruck, M. (1993, Fall). Child witnesses: Translating research into policy. *Social Policy Report. Society for Research in Child Development, 7*(3).

Ceci, S. J., & Bruck. M. (1995). *Jeopardy in the courtroom: A scientific analysis of children's testimony*. Washington, DC: American Psychological Association.

Cohen, H. (1985). Ending the double standard. Equal rights for children. In A. Cafagna, R. T. Peterson, & C. Staudenbaur (Eds.), *Child nurturance: Philosophy, children, and the family* (Vol.1). New York: Plenum.

Cohen, J. A., & Mannarino, A. P. (1998). Interventions for sexually abused children: Initial treatment findings. *Child Maltreatment, 3*, 17–26.

Cohen, J. A., & Mannarino, A. P. (2000). Predictors of treatment outcome in sexually abused children. *Child Abuse & Neglect, 24*, 983–994.

Coury, D. L. (2000). Recognition of child abuse: Notes from the field. *Archives of Pediatric & Adolescent Medicine, 154*, 178.

Crittenden, P. M. (1988). Maltreated infants: Vulnerability and resilience. *Journal of Child Psychology and Psychiatry, 26*, 85–96.

Davis, M. K., & Gidycz, C. A. (2000). Child sexual abuse prevention programs: A meta-analysis. *Journal of Clinical Child Psychology, 29*, 257–265.

Deater-Deckard, K., & Dodge, K. A. (1997). Externalizing behavior problems and discipline revisited: Nonlinear effects and variation by culture, context, and gender. *Psychological Inquiry, 8*, 161–175.

Deater-Deckard, K., Dodge, K. A., Bates, J. E., & Pettit, G. S. (1996). Physical discipline among African American and European American mothers: Links to children's externalizing behaviors. *Developmental Psychology, 32*, 1065–1072.

Deblinger, E., Lippman, J., & Steer, R. (1996). Sexually abused children suffering post-traumatic stress symptoms: Initial treatment outcome findings. *Child Maltreatment, 1*, 320–321.

DiScala, C., Sege, R., Li, G., & Reece, R. M. (2000). Child abuse and unintentional injuries: A 10-year retrospective. *Archives of Pediatric & Adolescent Medicine, 154*, 16–22.

Doris, J. (1993). *Child witness conference*. Supplemental RFP Children's Justice and Assistance Act funds. Submitted by the Family Life Development Center, Cornell University.

Eckenrode, J., Laird, M., & Doris, J. (1993). School performance and disciplinary problems among abused and neglected children. *Developmental Psychology, 29*, 53–62.

Eckenrode, J., Zielinski, D., Smith, E., Marcynyszyn, L. A., Hanerson, C. R., Kitzman, H., Cole, R., Powers, U., & Olds, D. L. (2001). Child maltreatment and the early onset of problem behaviors: Can a program of nurse home visitation break the link? *Development and Psychopathology, 13*, 873–890.

Finkelhor, D., & Dziuba-Leatherman, J. (1994). Victimization of children. *American Psychologist, 49*, 173–183.

Fleming, J., Mullen, P., & Bammer, G. (1997). A study of potential risk factors for sexual abuse in childhood. *Child Abuse & Neglect, 21*, 49–58.

Foa, E. B., & Riggs, D. S. (1995). Posttraumatic stress disorder following assault: Theoretical considerations and empirical findings. Current Directions in *Psychological Science, 4*, 61–65.

Garfinkel, I., McLanahan, S. S., Meyer, D. R., & Selzer, J. A. (1998). *Fathers under fire*. New York: Russell Sage.

Gelles, R. J. (2000). Treatment resistant families. In R. M. Reece (Ed.), *Treatment of child abuse: Common ground for mental health, medical, and legal practitioners* (pp. 304–312). Baltimore: Johns Hopkins.

Gillham, B., Tanner, G., Cheyne, B., Freeman, I., Rooney, M., & Lambie, A. (1998). Unemployment rates, single parent density, and indices of child poverty: Their relationship to different categories of child abuse and neglect. *Child Abuse & Neglect, 22*, 79–90.

Golden, O. (2000). The federal response to child abuse and neglect. *American Psychologist, 55*, 1050–1057.

Gunnoe, M. L., & Mariner, C. L. (1997). Toward a developmental-contextual model of the effects of parental spanking on children's aggression. *Archives of Pediatrics and Adolescent Medicine, 30*, 4–19.

Hamerman, S., & Ludwig, S. (2000). Emotional abuse and neglect. In R. M. Reece (Ed.), *Treatment of child abuse: Common ground for mental health, medical, and legal practitioners* (pp. 201–210). Baltimore: Johns Hopkins.

Hart, S. N. (1991). From property to person status: Historical perspective on children's rights. *American Psychologist, 46*, 53–39.

Haugaard, J. J. (2000). The challenge of defining child sexual abuse. *American Psychologist, 55*, 1036–1039.

Hempelman, K. A. (2000). *Teen legal rights* (Rev. ed.). Westport, CT: Greenwood.

Holmes, W. C., & Slap, G. B. (1998). Sexual abuse of boys: Definition, correlates, sequelae, and management. *Journal of the American Medical Association, 280*, 1855–1862.

Koocher, G. P., & Keith-Spiegel, P. C. (1990). *Children, ethics, and the law*. Lincoln: University of Nebraska Press.

Kuntz, T. (1997, November 2). Child abuse: A glimpse into a hell for helpless infants. *New York Times*, p. 7.

Lamb, M. E. (1997). Fathers and child development: An introductory overview and guide. In M. E. Lamb (Ed.), *The role of the father in child development* (pp. 1–18). New York: Wiley.

Lamb, M. E., Sternberg. K., & Esplin, P. W. (2000). Effects of age and delay on the amount of information provided by alleged sex abuse victims in investigative interviews. *Child Development, 71*, 1586–1596.

Lamb, M. E., Sternberg, K. J., Orbach, Y., Hershkowitz, I., & Esplin, P. W. (1999). Forensic interviews of children. In A. Memon & R. A. Bull (Eds.), *Handbook of the psychology of interviewing* (pp. 253–277). New York: Wiley.

Lamberg, L. (1999). False memories, lasting scars. *Journal of the American Medical Association, 282*, 192.

Lansdown, G. (2000). Children's rights and domestic violence. *Child Abuse Review, 9*, 416–426.

Larzelere, R. E. (2000). Child outcomes of nonabusive and customary physical punishment by parents: An updated literature review. *Clinical Child and Family Psychology Review, 3*, 199–221.

Levine, M., Anderson, E., Ferretti, L., & Steinberg, K. (1993). Legal and ethical issues affecting clinical child psychology. In T. Ollendick & R. Prinz (Eds.), *Advances in clinical child psychology* (Vol. 15, pp. 81–120). New York: Plenum.

Lief, H. I., & Fetkewicz, J. M. (1999). Casualties of recovered memory therapy: The impact of false allegations of incest on accused fathers. In R. C. Friedman, J. I. Downey, & J. Spurlock (Eds.), *Masculinity and sexuality: Selected topics in the psychology of men. (Review of Psychiatry*, Vol. 18, pp. 145–147). Washington, DC: American Psychiatric Press.

Limber, S. P., & Flekkov, M. G. (1995). The U.N. Convention on the Rights of the Child: Its relevance for social scientists. *Social Policy Report. Society for Research in Child Development, 9*, Whole No. 2.

Lutzker, J. R. (1990). Behavioral treatment of child neglect. *Behavior Modification, 14*, 301–315.

Lyons-Ruth, K., Melnick, S., & Bronfman, E. (In press). Hostile-helpless relational models and disorganized attachment patterns between parents and their young children: Review of research and implications for clinical work. In L. Atkinson & K. Zucker (Eds.), *Clinical applications of attachment*. New York: Guilford.

MacMillan, H. L. (2000). Child maltreatment: What we know in the year 2000. *Canadian Journal of Psychiatry, 45*, 702–709.

Manly, J. T., Kim, J. E., Rogosch, F. A., & Cicchetti, D. (2001). Dimensions of child maltreatment and children's adjustment: Contribution of developmental timing and subtype. *Development and Psychopathology, 13*, 759–782.

Margolin, L. (1990). Fatal child neglect. *Child Welfare, 69*, 309–319.

McLarin, K. J. (1995, July 30). Slaying of Connecticut infant shifts policy on child abuse. *New York Times*, p. Al.

O'Donohue, W. O., & Elliott. A. N. (1991). A model for the clinical assessment of the sexually abused child. *Behavioral Assessment, 13*, 325–340.

Olds, D., Eckenrode, J., Henderson, C. R., Kitzman, H., Powers, J., Cole, R., Sidora, K., Morris, P., & Pettit, L. M. (1997). Long-term effects of home visitation on maternal life course and child abuse and neglect:

Fifteen-year follow-up of a randomized trial. *Journal of the American Medical Association, 278,* 637–643.

Oliver, J. E. (1993). Intergenerational transmission of child abuse: Rates, research, and clinical implications. *American Journal of Psychiatry, 150,* 1315–1324.

Osofsky, J. D., & Fenichel, E. (Eds.). (1994, January). *Caring for infants and toddlers in violent environments: Hurt, healing, and hope. Zero to three* (Vol. 14). Arlington, VA: National Center for Clinical Infant Programs.

Paget, K. D., Philp, I. D., & Abramczvk, L. W. (1993). Recent developments in child neglect. In T. H. Ollendick & R. J. Prinz (Eds.), *Advances in clinical child psychology* (Vol. 15, pp. 121–174). New York: Plenum.

Peterson, U., & Brown, D. (1994). Integrating child injury and abuse-neglect research: Common histories, etiologies, and solutions. *Psychological Bulletin, 116,* 293–315.

Polusny, M. A., & Follette, V. M. (1995). Long-term correlates of child sexual abuse: Theory and review of the empirical literature. *Applied and Preventive Psychology, 4,* 143–166.

Reece, R. M., & Sege, R. (2000). Childhood head injuries: Accidental or inflicted? *Archives of Pediatric & Adolescent Medicine, 154,* 11–15.

Reid, J. B. (1984). Social-interactional patterns in families of abused and nonabused children. In C. Zahn-Waxler, M. Cummings, & M. Radke-Yarrow (Eds.), *Social and biological origins of altruism and aggression.* Cambridge, England: Cambridge University Press.

Riggins v. Nevada. (1992). 112 S. Ct. 1810.

Ryan, K. D., Kilmer, R. P., Cauce, A. M., Watanabe, H., & Hoyt, D. R. (2000). Psychological consequences of child maltreatment in homeless adolescents: Untangling the unique effects of maltreatment and family environment. *Child Abuse & Neglect, 24,* 333–352.

Saywitz, K. J., Mannarino, A. P., Berliner, L., & Cohen, J. A. (2000). Treatment for sexually abused children and adolescents. *American Psychologist, 55,* 1040–1049.

Schumacher, R. B., & Carlson, R. S. (1999). Variables and risk factors associated with child abuse in daycare settings. *Child Abuse & Neglect, 23,* 891–898.

Shonk, S. M., & Cicchetti, D. (2001). Maltreatment, competency deficits, and risk for academic and behavioral maladjustment. *Developmental Psychology, 37,* 1–18.

Southall, D. P., Plunkett, M. C. B., Banks, M. W., Falkov, A. F., & Samuels, M. P. (1997). Covert video recordings of life-threatening child abuse: Lessons for child protection. *Pediatrics, 100,* 735–760.

Stevenson, J. (1999). The treatment of the long-term sequelae of child abuse. *Journal of Child Psychology & Psychiatry & Allied Disciplines, 40,* 89–111.

Stoesz, D., & Karger, H. J. (1996, June). Suffer the children: How government fails its most vulnerable citizens—abused and neglected kids. *The Washington Monthly,* 20–25.

Straus, M. A. (2000). Corporal punishment and primary prevention of physical abuse. *Child Abuse & Neglect, 24,* 1109–1114.

Straus, M. A., & Stewart, J. H. (1999). Corporal punishment by American parents: National data on prevalence, chronicity, severity, and duration, in relation to child and family characteristics. *Clinical Child and Family Psychology Review, 2,* 55–70.

Teitelbaum, L. E., & Ellis, J. W. (1978). The liberty interest of children: Due process rights and their application. *Family Law Quarterly, 12,* 153–202.

Trickett, P. K., & McBride-Chang, C. (1995). The developmental impact of different forms of child abuse and neglect. *Developmental Review, 15,* 311–337.

U.N. Convention on the Rights of the Child. (1991). Unofficial summary of articles. *American Psychologist, 46,* 50–52.

U.S. Department of Health and Human Services. (1989). *Child abuse and neglect: A shared community concern.* Washington, DC: Author.

U.S. Department of Health and Human Services. (2000). *Child maltreatment 1998: Reports from the states to the national child abuse and neglect data system.* Washington, DC: U.S. Government Printing Office.

Walker, N. E., Brooks, C. M., & Wrightsman, L. S. (1999). *Children's rights in the United States: In search of a national policy.* Thousand Oaks, CA: Sage.

Wilcox, B. L., & Naimark, H. (1991). The rights of the child: Progress toward human dignity. *American Psychologist, 46,* 49.

Winick, B. J. (1997). *The right to refuse mental health treatment.* Washington, DC: American Psychological Association.

Yeh, M., & Weisz, J. R. (2001). Why are we here at the clinic? Parent-child (dis)agreement on referral problems at outpatient treatment entry. *Journal of Consulting & Clinical Psychology, 69,* 1018–1025.

Zuravin, S. J. (1989). The ecology of abuse and neglect: Review of the literature and presentation of data. *Violence and Victims, 4,* 101–120.

Chapter 7

Amaya-Jackson, L., & March, J. (1995). Posttraumatic stress disorder. In J. S. March (Ed.), *Anxiety disorders in children and adolescents* (pp. 276–300). New York: Guilford.

American Academy of Child and Adolescent Psychiatry (AACAP). (1998). Summary of the practice parameters for the assessment and treatment of children and adolescents with posttraumatic stress disorder. *Journal of the American Academy of Child and Adolescent Psychiatry, 37*, 997–1001.

American Psychiatric Association. (1994). *Diagnostic and statistical manual of mental disorders* (4th ed. text revision). Washington, DC: Author.

Bandura, A. (1969). *Principles of behavior modification.* New York: Holt, Rinehart and Winston.

Bandura, A. (1986). *Social foundations of thought and action: A social cognitive theory.* Englewood Cliffs, NJ: Prentice-Hall.

Bandura, A., Blanchard, E. B., & Ritter, B. (1969). Relative efficacy of desensitization and modeling approaches for inducing behavioral, affective, and attitudinal changes. *Journal of Personality and Social Psychology, 13*, 173–199.

Barlow, D. H., Chorpita, B. F., & Turovsky, J. (1996). Fear, panic, anxiety, and disorders of emotion. In D. A. Hope (Ed.), *Perspectives on anxiety, panic and fear: The 43rd annual Nebraska Symposium on Motivation* (pp. 251–328). Lincoln: Nebraska University Press.

Barlow, D. H., Gorman, J. M., Shear, K., & Woods, S. W. (2000). Cognitive-behavioral therapy, imipramine, or their combination for panic disorder: A randomized controlled trial. *Journal of the American Medical Association, 283*, 2529–2536.

Barrett, P. M., Duffy, A. L., Dadds, M. R., & Rapee, R. M. (2001). Cognitive-behavioral treatment of anxiety disorders in children: Long-term (6-year) follow-up. *Journal of Consulting and Clinical Psychology, 69*, 135–141.

Bernstein, G. A., Hektner, J. S., Burchardt, C. M., & McMillan, M. H. (2001). Treatment of school refusal: One year follow-up. *Journal of the American Academy of Child and Adolescent Psychiatry, 40*, 206–213.

Berton, M. W., & Stabb, S. D. (1996). Exposure to violence and post-traumatic stress disorder in urban adolescents. *Adolescence, 31*, 489–498.

Breuer, J., & Freud, S. (1957). *Studies on hysteria.* New York: Basic Books. (Original work published 1895.)

Burns, B. J., Hoagwood, K., & Mrazek, P. J. (1999). Effective treatment for mental disorders in children and adolescents. *Clinical Child and Family Psychology Review, 2*, 199–254.

Chorpita, B. F., Albano, A. M., Heimberg, R. G., & Barlow, D. H. (1996). A systematic replication of the prescriptive treatment of school refusal behavior in a single subject. *Journal of Behavior Therapy and Experimental Psychiatry, 27*, 281–290.

Collins, R. L. (1996). For better or worse: The impact of upward social comparison on self-evaluation. *Psychological Bulletin, 119*, 51–69.

Davis, L., & Siegel, L. J. (2000). Posttraumatic stress disorder in children and adolescents: A review and analysis. *Clinical Child and Family Psychology Review, 3*, 135–154.

Eley, T. C., & Stevenson, J. (2000). Specific life events and chronic experiences differentially associated with depression and anxiety in young twins. *Journal of Abnormal Child Psychology, 28*, 383–394.

Elliott, J. G. (1999). School refusal: Issues of conceptualization, assessment, and treatment. *Journal of Child Psychology & Psychiatry, 40*, 1001–1012.

Ficula, T., Gelfand, D. M., Richards, G., & Ulloa, A. (1983, August). *Factors associated with school refusal in adolescents.* Paper presented at the meeting of the American Psychological Association, Anaheim, CA.

Fitzpatrick, C. (1998). Refusal to eat or drink in young children with anxiety disorders. *Clinical Child Psychology & Psychiatry, 3*, 31–37.

Flannery-Schroeder, E. C., & Kendall, P. C. (2000). Group and individual cognitive-behavioral treatments for youth with anxiety disorders: A randomized clinical trial. *Cognitive Therapy & Research, 24*, 251–278.

Fox, N. A., Henderson, H. A., Rubin, K. H., Calkins, S. D., & Schmidt, L. A. (2001). Continuity and discontinuity of behavioral inhibition and exuberance: Psychophysiological and behavioral influences across the first four years of life. *Child Development, 72*, 1–21.

Freud, A. (1977). Fears, anxieties, and phobic phenomena. *The Psychoanalytic Study of the Child, 32*, 85–90.

Freud, S. (1963). Analysis of a phobia in a five-year-old boy. In S. Freud, *The sexual enlightenment of children.* New York: Macmillan. (Original work published in 1909.)

Gullone, E. (1999). The assessment of normal fear in children and adolescents. *Clinical Child and Family Psychology Review, 2,* 91–106.

Heinecke, C. M. (1989). Psychodynamic psychotherapy with children: Current status and guidelines for future research. In B. Lahey & A. Kazdin (Eds.), *Advances in clinical child psychology* (Vol.12, pp. 1–26). New York: Plenum.

Kagan, J., Reznick, M., & Snidman, N. (1987). The physiology and psychology of behavioral inhibition in children. *Child Development, 58*, 1459–1473.

Kaplan, C. A., & Hussain, S. (1995). Use of drugs in child and adolescent psychiatry. *British Journal of Psychiatry, 166*, 291–298.

Kashdan, T. B., & Herbert, J. D. (2001). Social anxiety disorder in childhood and adolescence: Current status and future directions. *Clinical Child and Family Psychology Review, 4,* 37–61.

Kazdin, A. E. (2001). Bridging the enormous gaps of theory with therapy research and practice. *Journal of Clinical Child Psychology, 30,* 59–66.

Kearney, C. A., & Silverman, W. K. (1995). Family environment of youngsters with school refusal behavior: A synopsis with implications for assessment and treatment. *American Journal of Family Therapy, 23,* 59–72.

Kendall, P.C. (1993). Cognitive-behavioral therapies with youth: Guiding theory, current status, and emerging developments. *Journal of Consulting and Clinical Psychology, 61,* 235–247.

Kendall, P. C., Chansky, T. E., Kane, M. T., Kim, R., Kortlander, E., Ronan, K., Sessa, F., & Siqueland, L. (1992). *Anxiety disorders in youth: Cognitive-behavioral interventions.* Needham Heights, MA: Allyn & Bacon.

Kendall, P. C., Flannery-Schroeder, E., Panichelli-Mindel, S. M., Southam-Gerow, M., Henin, A., & Warman, M. (1997). Therapy for youths with anxiety disorders: A second randomized clinical trial. *Journal of Consulting and Clinical Psychology, 65,* 366–380.

Kennedy, W. A. (1965). School phobia: Rapid treatment of fifty cases. *Journal of Abnormal Behavior, 70,* 285–289.

Kessler, R. C., Davis, C. G., & Kendler, K. S. (1997). Childhood adversity and adult psychiatric disorder in the U.S. National Comorbidity Survey. *Psychological Medicine, 27,* 1101–1119.

King, N. J. (1993). Simple and social phobias. In T. Ollendick & R. Prinz (Eds.), *Advances in clinical child psychology* (Vol. 15, pp. 305–341). New York: Plenum.

Last, C. G., Perrin, S., Hersen, M., & Kazdin, A. E. (1996). A prospective study of childhood anxiety disorders. *Journal of the American Academy of Child & Adolescent Psychiatry, 35,* 1502–1510.

Lerner, J., Safren, S. A., Henin, A., Warman, M., Heimberg, R. G., & Kendall, P. C. (1999). Differentiating anxious and depressive self-statements in youth: Factor structure of the Negative Affect Self-Statement Questionnaire among youth referred to an anxiety disorders clinic. *Journal of Clinical Child Psychology, 28,* 82–93.

March, J. S., Frances, A., Kahn, D., & Carpenter, D. (1997). Expert consensus guidelines: Treatment of obsessive-compulsive disorder. *Journal of Clinical Psychiatry, 58* (Suppl. 4), 1–72.

March, J. S., Franklin, M., Nelson, A., & Foa, E. (2001). Cognitive-behavioral psychotherapy for pediatric obsessive-compulsive disorder. *Journal of Clinical Child Psychology, 30,* 8–18.

McCarthy, P. R., & Foa, E. B. (1988). Obsessive-compulsive disorder. In M. Hersen & C. Last (Eds.), *Child behavior therapy casebook* (pp. 55–69). New York: Plenum.

McCloskey, L. A., & Walker, M. (2000). Posttraumatic stress in children exposed to family violence and single-event trauma. *Journal of the American Academy of Child & Adolescent Psychiatry, 39,* 108–115.

McClure, E. B., Brennan, P. A., Hammen, C., & Le Brocque, R. M. (2001). Parental anxiety disorders, child anxiety disorders, and the perceived parent-child relationship in an Australian high-risk sample. *Journal of Abnormal Child Psychology, 29,* 1–10.

McGough, J. J., Speier, P. L., & Cantwell, D. P. (1993). Obsessive-compulsive disorder in childhood and adolescence. *School Psychology Review, 22,* 243–251.

Menzies, R. G., & Clarke, J. C. (1993). A comparison of in vivo and vicarious exposure in the treatment of childhood water phobia. *Behaviour Research and Therapy, 31,* 9–15.

Mitka, M. (2000). Research on children's anxiety needed. *Journal of the American Medical Association, 283,* 1677.

Morris, R. J., & Kratochwill, T. R. (1983). *Treating children's fears and phobias.* New York: Pergamon.

Murphy, D. A., Marelich, W. D., & Hoffman, D. (2000). Assessment of anxiety and depression in young children: Support for two separate constructs. *Journal of Clinical Child Psychology, 29,* 383–391.

Myers, D. G., & Diener, E. (1995). Who is happy? *Psychological Science, 6,* 10–19.

National Institute of Mental Health. (1999). *Facts about social phobia* (No. OM-99 4171, Revised). Bethesda, MD: Author.

Plomin, R., DeFries, J. C., McClearn, G. E., & Rutter, M. (1997). *Behavioral genetics: A primer* (3rd ed.). New York: Freeman.

Rapee, R. M. (1997). Potential role of childrearing practices in the development of anxiety and depression. *Clinical Psychology Review, 17,* 47–67.

Rapoport, J., Inoff-Germain, G., Weissman, M. M., Greenwald, S., Narrow, W. E., Jensen, P. S., Lahey, B. B., & Canino, G. (2000). Childhood obsessive-compulsive disorder in the NIMH MECA study: Parent versus child identification of cases. *Journal of Anxiety Disorders, 14,* 535–548.

Rapoport, J., Swedo, S. E., & Leonard, H. L. (1992). Childhood obsessive compulsive disorder. *Journal of Clinical Psychiatry, 53,* 11–16.

Riddle, M. A., Bernstein, G. A., Cook, E. H., Leonard, H. L., March, J. S., & Swanson, J. M. (1999). Anxiolytics, adrenergic agents, and naltrexone. *Journal of the*

American Academy of Child and Adolescent Psychiatry, 38, 546–556.

Riddle, M. A., Reeve, E. A., Yaryyura-Tobias, J. A., Yang, H. M., Claghorn, J. L., Gathey, G. et al. (2001). Fluvoxamine for children and adolescents with obsessive-compulsive disorder: A randomized, controlled, multicenter trial. *Journal of the American Academy of Child and Adolescent Psychiatry, 40*, 222–229.

Ritter, B. (1968). The group desensitization of children's snake phobias using vicarious and contact desensitization procedures. *Behaviour Research and Therapy, 6*, 1–6.

Rubin, K. H., Nelson, L. J., Hastings, P., & Asendorpf, J. (1999). The transaction between parents' perceptions of their children's shyness and their parenting styles. *International Journal of Behavioral Development, 23*, 937–958.

Russo, M. F., & Beidel, D. C. (1994). Comorbidity of childhood anxiety and externalizing disorders: Prevalence, associated characteristics, and validation issues. *Clinical Psychology Review, 14*, 199–221.

Rutter, M., & Garmezy, N. (1983). Developmental psychopathology. In E. M. Hetherington (Ed.), *Handbook of child psychology* (Vol. IV). New York: Wiley.

Rutter, M., Tizard, J., & Whitmore, K. (Eds.). (1981). *Education, health and behaviour.* Huntington, NY: Krieger.

Schmidt, L. A., Fox, N. A., & Schulkin, J. (1999). Behavioral and psychophysiological correlates of self-presentation in temperamentally shy children. *Developmental Psychobiology, 35*, 119–135.

Schneier, F. R., Johnson, J., Hornig, C. D., Liebowitz, M. R., & Weissman, M. M. (1992). Social phobia: Comorbidity and morbidity in an epidemiologic sample. *Archives of General Psychiatry, 49*, 282–288.

Seligman, M. E. P., & Ollendick, T. H. (1998). Comorbidity of anxiety and depression in children and adolescents: An integrative review. *Clinical Child and Family Psychology Review, 1*, 125.

Silverman, W. K., La Greca, A. M., & Wasserstein, S. (1995). What do children worry about? Worry and its relation to anxiety. *Child Development, 66*, 671–686.

Social phobia, Part II. (1994, November). *The Harvard Mental Health Letter, 11*, 1–3.

Spence, S. H., Donovan, C., & Brechman-Toussaint, M. (1999). Social skills, social outcomes, and cognitive features of childhood social phobia. *Journal of Abnormal Psychology, 108*, 211–221.

Stoppelbein, L., & Greening, L. (2000). Posttraumatic stress symptoms in parentally bereaved children and adolescents. *Journal of the American Academy of Child & Adolescent Psychiatry, 39*, 1112–1119.

Swedo, S. E., Lenanare, M., Rettew, D., Hamburger, S., Bartko, J., & Rapoport, J. (1993). A 2- to 7-year follow-up study of 54 obsessive-compulsive children and adolescents. *Archives of General Psychiatry, 50*, 429–440.

Terr, L. C. (1981). Psychic trauma in children: Observations following the Chowchilla school-bus kidnapping. *American Journal of Psychiatry, 138*, 14–19.

Tremblay, C., Martine, H., & Piche, C. (2000). Type I and type II posttraumatic stress disorder in sexually abused children. *Journal of Child Sexual Abuse, 9*, 65–90.

Twenge, J. M. (2000). The age of anxiety? Birth cohort change in anxiety and neuroticism, 1952–1993. *Journal of Personality and Social Psychology, 79*, 1007–1021.

Vasey, M. W. (1993). Development and cognition in childhood anxiety: The example of worry. In T. Ollendick and R. Prinz (Eds.), *Advances in clinical child psychology* (Vol. 15, pp. 1–40). New York: Plenum.

Vernberg, E. M., La Greca, A. M., Silverman, W. K., & Prinstein, M. J. (1996). Prediction of posttraumatic stress symptoms in children after Hurricane Andrew. *Journal of Abnormal Psychology, 105*, 237–248.

Vila, G., Porche, L. M., & Mouren-Simeoni, M. C. (1999). An 18-month longitudinal study of posttraumatic disorders in children who were taken hostage in their school. *Psychosomatic Medicine, 61*, 746–754.

Walkup, J. T., Labellarte, M. J., Riddle, M. A., Pine, D. S., Greenhill, L., Klein, R., Davies, M., Sweeney, M., Abikoff, H., Hack, S., Klee, B., McCracken, J., Bergman, L., Piacentini, J., March, J., Compton, S., Robinson, J., O'Hara, T., Baker, S., Vitiello, B., Ritz, L., & Roper, M. (2001). Fluvoxamine for the treatment of anxiety disorders in children and adolescents. *New England Journal of Medicine, 344*, 1279–1285.

Wasserstein, S. B., & La Greca, A. M. (1998). Hurricane Andrew: Parent conflict as a moderator of children's adjustment. *Hispanic Journal of Behavioral Sciences, 20*, 212–224.

Weems, C. F., Silverman, W. K., & La Greca, A. M. (2000). What do youth referred for anxiety problems worry about? Worry and its relation to anxiety and anxiety disorders in children and adolescents. *Journal of Abnormal Child Psychology, 28*, 63–72.

Weisenberg, M., Schwarzwald, J., Waysman, M., Solomon, A., & Klingman, A. (1993). Coping of school-age children in the sealed room during Scud missile bombardments and postwar stress reactions. *Journal of Consulting and Clinical Psychology, 61*, 462–467.

Williams, S. L., & Zane, G. (1997). Guided mastery treatment of phobias. *The Clinical Psychologist, 50*(2), 13–15.

Wolpe, J. (1958). *Reciprocal inhibition therapy*. Stanford, CA: Stanford University Press.

Yule, W. (1998). Posttraumatic stress disorder in children and its treatment. In T. W. Miller (Ed.), *Children of trauma: Stressful life events and their effects on children and adolescents* (pp. 219–243). Madison, CT: International Universities Press.

Chapter 8

Abraham, K. (1968). Notes on the psychoanalytical investigation and treatment of manic-depressive insanity and allied conditions. In W. Gaylin (Ed.), *The meaning of despair* (pp. 92–131). New York: Science House.

Abramson, L. Y., Alloy, L. B., & Metalsky, G. I. (1995). Hopelessness depression. In J. N. Buchanan & M. E. P. Seligman (Eds.), *Explanatory style* (pp. 113–134). Hillsdale, NJ: Erlbaum.

Abramson, L. Y., Metalsky, G. I., & Alloy, L. B. (1989). Hopelessness depression: A theory-based subtype of depression. *Psychological Review, 96,* 358–372.

American Psychiatric Association. (2000). *Diagnostic and statistical manual of mental disorders* (4th ed., text revision). Washington, DC: Author.

Andrews, J. A., & Lewinsohn, P. M. (1992). Suicidal attempts among older adolescents: Prevalence and co-occurance with psychiatric disorders. *Journal of the American Academy of Child & Adolescent Psychiatry, 31,* 655–662.

Aseltine, R. H., Gore, S., & Colten, M. E. (1998). The co-occurrence of depression and substance abuse in late adolescence. *Development and Psychopathology, 10,* 549–570.

Bandura, A. (1986). *Social foundations of thought and action: A social cognitive theory*. Englewood Cliffs, NJ: Prentice-Hall.

Beck, A. T. (1967). *Depression: Clinical, experimental, and theoretical aspects*. Philadelphia: University of Pennsylvania Press.

Birmaher, B., Brent, D. A., Kolko, D., Baugher, M., Bridge, J., Holder, D., Iyengar, S., & Ulloa, R. E. (2000). Clinical outcome after short-term psychotherapy for adolescents with major depressive disorder. *Archives of General Psychiatry, 57,* 29–36.

Borowsky, I. W., Resnick, M. D., Ireland, M., & Blum, R. W. (1999). Suicide attempts among American Indian and Alaska Native youth. *Archives of Pediatrics & Adolescent Medicine, 153,* 573–580.

Bowlby, J. (1969/1982). *Attachment and loss. Vol. I: Attachment*. New York: Basic Books.

Brenner, N. D., Hassan, S. S., & Barrios, L. C. (1999). Suicidal ideation among college students in the United States. *Journal of Consulting and Clinical Psychology, 67,* 1004–1008.

Cicchetti, D., Rogosch, F. A., & Toth, S. L. (2000). The efficacy of toddler-parent psychotherapy for fostering cognitive development in offspring of depressed mothers. *Journal of Abnormal Child Psychology, 28,* 135–148.

Cicchetti, D., Toth, S. L., & Lynch, M. (1995). Bowlby's dream comes full circle: The application of attachment theory to risk and psychopathology. In T. Ollendick & R. Prinz (Eds.), *Advances in clinical child psychology* (Vol. 17, pp. 1–76). New York: Plenum.

Clark, R. (1993). Treating the relationships affected by postpartum depression: A group therapy model. *Zero to Three, 13,* 16–23.

Clarke, G., Hops, H., Lewinsohn, P. M., Andrews, J., Seeley, J. R., & Williams, J. (1992). Cognitive-behavioral group treatment of adolescent depression: Prediction of outcome. *Behavior Therapy, 23,* 341–354.

Daley, S. E., Hammen C., & Rao, U. (2000). Predictors of first onset and recurrence of major depression in young women during the 5 years following high school graduation. *Journal of Abnormal Psychology, 109,* 525–533.

D'Augelli, A. R., & Hershberger, S. L. (1993). Lesbian, gay, and bisexual youth in community settings: Personal challenges and mental health problems. *American Journal of Community Psychology, 21,* 421–448.

DiFilippo, J. M., & Overholser, J. C. (2000). Suicidal ideation in adolescent psychiatric inpatients as associated with depression and attachment relationships. *Journal of Clinical Child Psychology, 29,* 155–166.

Emslie, G. J., Rush, A. J., Weinberg, W. A., Kowatch, R. A., Hughes, C. W., Carmody, T., & Rintelmann, J. (1997). A double-blind, randomized, placebo-controlled trial of fluoxetine in children and adolescents with depression. *Archives of General Psychiatry, 54,* 1031–1037.

Ferster, C. B. (1973). A functional analysis of depression. *American Psychologist, 28,* 857–870.

Freud, S. (1965). *Mourning and melancholia* (standard ed.). London: Hogarth Press. (Original work published 1917.)

Garrison, C. Z., Schluchter, M. D., Schoenbach, V. J., & Kaplan, B. K. (1989). Epidemiology of depressive symptoms in young adolescents. *Journal of the American Academy of Child and Adolescent Psychiatry, 28,* 343–351.

Gelfand, D. M., Teti, D. M., Seiner, S. A., & Jameson, P. B. (1996). Helping mothers fight depression: Evaluation of a home-based intervention program for depressed mothers and their infants. *Journal of Clinical Child Psychology, 25,* 406–422.

Gillham, J. E., Reivich, K. J., & Shatte, A. J. (2001). Building optimism and preventing depressive symptoms in children. In E. C. Chang (Ed.), *Optimism and pessimism: Implications for theory, research, and practice* (pp. 301–320). Washington, DC: American Psychological Association.

Gillham, J. E., Shatte, A. J., & Freres, D. R. (2000). Preventing depression: A review of cognitive behavioral and family interventions. *Applied & Preventive Psychology, 9*, 63–88.

Goldsmith, H. H., Buss, K. A., & Lemery, K. S. (1997). Toddler and childhood temperament: Expanded content, stronger genetic evidence, new evidence for the importance of environment. *Developmental Psychology, 33*, 891–905.

Goodman, S. H., & Gotlib, I. H. (1999). Risk for psychopathology in the children of depressed mothers: A developmental model for understanding mechanisms of transmission. *Psychological Review, 106*, 458–490.

Goodman, S. H., & Gotlib, I. H. (Eds.). (2002). Children of depressed parents: Mechanisms of risk and complications for treatment. Washington, DC: *American Psychological Association Press.*

Gotlib, I. H., & Abramson, L. Y. (1999). Attributional theories of emotion. In T. Dalgleish & M. Power (Eds.), *Handbook of cognition and emotion* (pp. 723–740). New York: Wiley.

Gotlib, I. H., & Hammen, C. L. (1992). *Psychological aspects of depression: Toward a cognitive-interpersonal integration.* Chichester, England: Wiley.

Griffith, E. E., & Bell, C. G. (1988). Recent trends in suicide and homicide among Blacks. *Journal of the American Academy of Child & Adolescent Psychiatry, 27*, 349–356.

Gutierrez, P. M., Osman, A., Kopper, A., & Barrios, F. X. (2000). Why young people do not kill themselves: The Reasons for Living Inventory for Adolescents. *Journal of Clinical Child Psychology, 29*, 177–187.

Hamilton, J. D., & Bridge, J. (1999). Outcome at 6 months for 50 adolescents with major depression treated in a HMO. *Journal of the American Academy of Child & Adolescent Psychiatry, 38*, 1340–1346.

Hankin, B. L., Abramson, L., Moffitt, T. E., Silva, P. A., McGee, R., & Andell, K. (1998). Development of depression from preadolescence to young adulthood: Emerging gender differences in a 10-year longitudinal study. *Journal of Abnormal Psychology, 107*, 128–140.

Harrington, R., Rutter, M., & Fombonne, E. (1996). Developmental pathways in depression: Multiple meanings, antecedents, and endpoints. *Development and Psychopathology, 8*, 601–616.

Hawton, K., Haigh, R., Simkin, S., & Fagg, J. (1995). Attempted suicide in Oxford University students, 1976–1990. *Psychological Medicine, 25*, 179–188.

Herzog, D. B., & Rathbun, J. M. (1982). Childhood depression: Developmental considerations. *American Journal of Diseases in Children, 136*, 115–120.

Jameson, P., Gelfand, D. M., Kulcsar, E., & Teti, D. M. (1997). Mother-toddler interaction patterns associated with maternal depression. *Development and Psychopathology, 9*, 537–550.

Jensen, P. S., Bhatara, V. S., Vitiello, B., Hoagwood, K., Feil, M., & Burke, L. B. (1999). Psychoactive medication prescribing practices for U.S. children: Gaps between research and clinical practice. *Journal of the American Academy of Child & Adolescent Psychiatry, 38*, 557–565.

Johnson, V. K., Cowan, P. A., & Cowan, C. P. (1999). Children's classroom behavior: The unique contribution of family organization. *Journal of Family Psychology, 13*, 355–371.

Kessler, R. C., McGonagle, K., Carnelly, K., Nelson, C., Farmer, M. E., & Regier, D. A. (in press). *Comorbidity of mental disorders and substance use disorders: A review of agenda for future research.* Greenwich, CT: JAI Press.

Kessler, R. C., McGonagle, K. A., Zhao, S., Nelson, C., Hughes, M., Eshleman, S., Wittchen, H. U., & Kendler, K. S. (1994). Lifetime and 12-month prevalence of DSM-III-R psychiatric disorders in the United States. *Archives of General Psychiatry, 51*, 8–19.

King, R. A., Pfeffer, C., Gammon, G. D., & Cohen, D. J. (1992). Suicidality of childhood and adolescence. In B. Lahey & A. Kazdin (Eds.), *Advances in clinical child psychology* (Vol. 14, pp. 297–325). New York: Plenum.

Kovacs, M., & Beck, A. T. (1977). An empirical clinical approach toward a definition of childhood depression. In J. Schulterbrandt & A. Raskin (Eds.), *Depression in childhood: Diagnosis, treatment and conceptual model* (pp. 1–25). New York: Raven.

Kovacs, M., Feinberg, T. L., & Crouse-Novak, M. (1984). Depressive disorders in childhood, II: A longitudinal study of the risk for a subsequent major depression. *Archives of General Psychiatry, 41*, 643–649.

Lewinsohn, P. M. (1974). A behavioral approach to depression. In R. Friedman & M. Katz (Eds.), *The psychology of depression: Contemporary theory and research.* Washington, DC: V. H. Winston.

Lewinsohn, P. M., Clarke, G. N., Hops, H., & Andrews, J. (1990). Cognitive-behavioral treatment for depressed adolescents. *Behavior Therapy, 21*, 385–401.

Lewinsohn, P. M., Hops, H., Roberts, R., & Seeley, J. (1993). Adolescent psychopathology: I. Prevalence and incidence of depression and other DSM-III-R disorders in high school students. *Journal of Abnormal Psychology, 102,* 110–120.

Lewinsohn. P. M., & Rohde, P. (1993). The cognitive-behavioral treatment of depression in adolescents: Research and suggestions. *The Clinical Psychologist, 46,* 177–183.

Lewinsohn, P. M., Rohde, P., & Seeley, J. R. (1993). Psychosocial characteristics of adolescents with a history of suicide attempts. *Journal of the American Academy of Child & Adolescent Psychiatry, 32,* 600–668.

Lumsden, W. W. (1980). Intentional self-injury in school age children. *Journal of Adolescence, 3,* 217–228.

Lyons-Ruth, K., Lyubchik, A., Wolfe, R., & Bronfman, E. (2002). Parental depression and child attachment: Hostile and helpless profiles of parent and child behavior among families at risk. In I. H. Gotlib & S. H. Goodman (Eds.), *Children of depressed parents: Mechanisms of risk and implications for treatment* (pp. 89–120). Washington, DC: American Psychological Association Press.

Malcarne, V. L., Hamilton, N. A., Ingram, R. E., & Taylor, L. (2000). Correlates of distress in children at risk for affective disorder: Exploring predictors in the offspring of depressed and nondepressed mothers. *Journal of Affective Disorders, 59,* 243–251.

Malmquist, C. P. (1977). Childhood depression: A clinical and behavioral perspective. In J. Schulterbrandt & A. Raskin (Eds.), *Depression in childhood: Diagnosis, treatment, and conceptual models* (pp. 27–43). Rockville, MD: U.S. Department of Health, Education and Welfare.

Monroe, S. M., Rohde, P., Seeley, J. R., & Lewinsohn, P. M. (1999). Life events and depression in adolescence: Relationship loss as a prospective risk factor in first onset of major depressive disorder. *Journal of Abnormal Psychology, 108,* 606–614.

Murray, C. J. C., & Lopez, A. D. (Eds.). (1996). *Summary: The global burden of disease: A comprehensive assessment of mortality and disability from diseases, injuries, and risk factors in 1990 and projected to 2020.* Cambridge, MA: Harvard University Press.

National Center for Health Statistics. (1995). *Health, United States, 1994.* Hyattsville, MD: Public Health Service.

National Center for Health Statistics. (1999). *Healthy People, 2000: Mental Health and Mental Disorder Progress Review* (ASI, 1999, No. 4148–4). Hyattsville, MD: Public Health Service.

National Institute of Mental Health. (2000). *Suicide facts.* Retrieved June 24, 2001, from the World Wide Web: http://www.nimh.gov/genpop/su_fact.htm

Nolen-Hoeksema, S. (1995). Gender differences in coping with depression across the lifespan. *Depression, 3,* 81–90.

Nolen-Hoeksema, S., Girgus, J. S., & Seligman, M. E. P. (1992). Predictors and consequences of childhood depressive symptoms: A 5-year longitudinal study. *Journal of Abnormal Psychology, 101,* 405–422.

Nottelmann, E. D., & Jensen, P. S. (1995). Comorbidity in children and adolescents: Developmental perspectives. In T. Ollendick & R. Prinz (Eds.), *Advances in clinical child psychology* (Vol. 17, pp. 109–156). New York: Plenum.

Peterson, C. (2000). The future of optimism. *American Psychologist, 55,* 44–55.

Poznanski, E., Mokros, H., Grossman, J., & Freeman, L. (1985). Diagnostic criteria in childhood depression. *American Journal of Psychiatry, 142,* 1168–1173.

Prinstein, M. J., Boergers, J., Spirito, A., Little, T. D., & Grapentine, W. L. (2000). Peer functioning, family dysfunction, and psychological symptoms in a risk factor model for adolescent inpatients' suicidal ideation severity. *Journal of Clinical Child Psychology, 29,* 392–405.

Rapoport, J. L. (2000). Child psychopharmacology comes of age. *Journal of the American Medical Association, 280,* 1785.

Regier, D. A., Narrow, W. E., & Rae, D. S. (1993). The de facto mental and addictive disorders service system. Epidemiologic catchment area prospective 1-year prevalence rates of disorders and services. *Archives of General Psychiatry, 50,* 85–94.

Regier, D. A., Rae, D. S., Narrow, W. E., et al. (1998). Prevalence of anxiety disorders and their comorbidity with mood and addictive disorders. *British Journal of Psychiatry Supplement, 34,* 24–28.

Reifman, A., & Windle, M. (1995). Adolescent suicidal behaviors as a function of depression, hopelessness, alcohol use, and social support: A longitudinal investigation. *American Journal of Community Psychology, 23,* 329–354.

Remafedi, G., French, S., Story, M., Resnick, M. D., & Blum, R. (1998). The relationship between suicide risk and sexual orientation: Results of a population-based study. *American Journal of Public Health, 88,* 57–60.

Reynolds, W. (1994). Depression in adolescents. In T. Ollendick & R. Prinz (Eds.), *Advances in clinical child psychology* (Vol. 16, pp. 261–316). New York: Plenum.

Rogan, M. (2001, March 4). Please take our children away. *New York Times Magazine*, pp. 40–45.

Rotheram-Borus, M. J., Piacentini, J., Cantwell, C., Belin, T. R., & Song, J. (2000). The 18-month impact of an emergency room intervention for adolescent female suicide attempters. *Journal of Consulting and Clinical Psychology, 68*, 1081–1093.

Russ, S. W. (1995). Play psychotherapy research: State of the science. In T. Ollendick & R. Prinz (Eds.), *Advances in clinical child psychology* (Vol. 17, pp. 365–391). New York: Plenum.

Safren, S. A., & Heimberg, R. G. (1999). Depression, hopelessness, suicidality, and related factors in sexual minority and heterosexual adolescents. *Journal of Consulting and Clinical Psychology, 67*, 859–866.

Seligman, M. E. P., & Csikszentmihalyi, C. (2000). Positive psychology: An introduction. *American Psychologist, 55*, 5–14.

Seppa, N. (1997, June). Internalizing disorders overlooked in schools. *APA Monitor*, p. 30.

Sheeber, L., Davis, B., & Hops, H. (2002). Gender specific vulnerability to depression in children of depressed mothers. In I. H. Gotlib & S. H. Goodman (Eds.), *Children of depressed parents: Mechanisms of risk and implications for treatment*. Washington, DC: American Psychological Association Press.

Spirito, A., Brown, L., Overholser, J., & Fritz, G. (1989). Attempted suicide in adolescence: A review and critique of the literature. *Clinical Psychology Review, 9*, 335–363.

Stark, K., Humphrey, L., Laurent, J., Livingston, R., & Christopher, J. (1993). Cognitive, behavioral, and family factors in the differentiation of depressive and anxiety disorders during childhood. *Journal of Consulting and Clinical Psychology, 61*, 878–886.

Stice, E., Hayward, C., Cameron, R. P., Killen, J. D., & Taylor, C. B. (2000). Body image and eating disturbances predict onset of depression among female adolescents: A longitudinal study. *Journal of Abnormal Psychology, 109*, 438–444.

Stoelb, M., & Chirboga, J. (1998). A process for assessing adolescent risk for suicide. *Journal of Adolescence, 21*, 359–370.

Summerville, M. G., Kaslow, N. J., & Doepke, K. J. (1996). Psychopathology and cognitive and family functioning in suicidal African-American adolescents. *Current Directions in Psychological Science, 5*, 7–11.

Teti, D. M., & Gelfand, D. M. (1991). Behavioral competence among mothers of infants in the first year: The mediational role of maternal self-efficacy. *Child Development, 62*, 918–929.

Teti, D. M., Gelfand, D. M., Messinger, D. S., & Isabella, R. (1995). Maternal depression and the quality of early attachment: An examination of infants, preschoolers, and their mothers. *Developmental Psychology, 31*, 364–376.

Tsuang, M. T., & Faraone, S. V. (1990). *The genetics of mood disorders*. Baltimore: Johns Hopkins.

U.S. Surgeon General. (2001). *Mental health: A report of the Surgeon General—Chapter 2*. Retrieved January 10, 2001, from the World Wide Web: http://www.surgeongeneral.gov/Library/MentalHealth/chapter2/sec2_l.html

Weinberg, M. K., & Tronick, E. Z. (1998). The impact of maternal psychiatric illness on infant development. *Journal of Clinical Psychiatry, 59*, 53–61.

Weissman, M. M., Wolk, S., Goldstein, R., Moreau, D., Adams, P., Greenwald, S., Klier, C. M., Ryan, N. D., Dahl, R., & Wickramaratne, P. (1999). Depressed adolescents grown up. *Journal of the American Medical Association, 281*, 1707–1713.

Weisz, J. R. (1986). Understanding the developing understanding of control. In M. Perlmutter (Ed.), *Cognitive perspectives on children's social and behavioral development: The Minnesota Symposia on Child Psychology* (Vol. 18, pp. 219–285). Hillsdale, NJ: Erlbaum.

Weisz, J. R., Southam-Gerow, M. A., & McCarty, C. A. (2001). Control-related beliefs and depressive symptoms in clinic-referred children and adolescents: Developmental differences and model specificity. *Journal of Abnormal Psychology, 110*, 97–109.

Wilson, G. T. (1991). Comment: Suicidal behavior-clinical considerations and risk factors. *Journal of Consulting and Clinical Psychology, 59*, 869–873.

Woolston, J. L. (1999). Combined pharmacotherapy: Pitfalls of treatment. *Journal of the American Academy of Child & Adolescent Psychiatry, 38*, 1455–1457.

Wright, C., George, T. P., Burke, R., Gelfand, D. M., & Teti, D. M. (2000). Early maternal depression and children's adjustment to school. *Child Study Journal, 30*, 153–168.

Younggren, J. N. (2001). *Legal and ethical risks and risk management in professional psychological practice. Sequence II: Risk management in specific high risk areas*. APA Insurance Trust and Utah Psychological Association, Salt Lake City, January 26.

Chapter 9

Abikoff, H. (2001). Tailored psychosocial treatments for ADHD: The search for a good fit. *Journal of Clinical Child Psychology, 30*, 122–125.

Albaret, J. M., Soppelsa, R., & Marquet-Doleac, J. (2000). Interest in the matching figures test in the diagnosis of the impulsiveness component in attention deficit hyperactivity disorder: A comparative study. *Approche Neuropsychologique de Apprentissages chez l'Enfant, 12*(3), 98–102.

American Psychiatric Association. (2000). *Diagnostic and statistical manual of mental disorders* (4th ed., text revision). Washington, DC: Author.

Antrop, I., Roeyers, H., Van Oost, P., & Buysse, A. (2000). Stimulation seeking and hyperactivity in children with ADHD. *Journal of Child Psychology and Psychiatry and Allied Disciplines, 41*, 225–231.

Ardoin, S. P., & Martens, B. K. (2000). Testing the ability of children with attention deficit hyperactivity disorder to accurately report the effects of medication on their behavior. *Journal of Applied Behavior Analysis, 33*, 593–610.

Aro, T., Ahonen, T., Tolvanen, A., Lyytinen, H., & Todd-de-Barra, H. (1999). Contribution of ADHD characteristics to the academic treatment outcome of children with learning difficulties. *Developmental Neuropsychology, 15*(2), 291–305.

Auerbach, J. G., Benjamin, J., Faroy, M., Gellar, V., & Ebstein, R. (2001). DRD4 related to infant attention and information processing: A developmental link to ADHD? *Psychiatric Genetics, 11*, 31–35.

Austin, K. M. (1999). Adult attention deficit hyperactivity disorder: Personality characteristics and comorbidity. *Dissertation Abstracts International: Section B: The Sciences and Engineering, 59*(7-B), 3751.

Ayers, T., Sellers, T., Schneider, D., Gottschling, H., & Soucar, E. (2001). Problems with Danforth's early diagnosis and observational bias in behavior management. *Child and Family Behavior Therapy, 23*, 57–59.

Barkley, R. A. (1998). *Attention-deficit hyperactivity disorder: A handbook for diagnosis and treatment.* New York: Guilford.

Battle, E. S., & Lacey, B. (1972). A context for hyperactivity in children, over time. *Child Development, 43*, 757–773.

Beck, C., Silverstone, P., Glor, K., & Dunn, J. (1999). Psychostimulant prescriptions by psychiatrists higher than expected: A self-report survey. *Canadian Journal of Psychiatry, 44*, 680–684.

Bender, W. N. (1998). *Learning disabilities: Characteristics, identification, and teaching strategies* (3rd ed.). Boston: Allyn and Bacon.

Benedetto-Nasho, E., & Tannock, R. (1999). Math computation, error patterns and stimulant effects in children with attention deficit hyperactivity disorder. *Journal of Attention Disorders, 3*(3), 121–134.

Bhaumik, S., Branford, D., Naik, B. I., & Biswas, A. B. (2000). A retrospective audit of selective serotonin reuptake inhibitors (fluoxetine and paroxetine) for the treatment of depressive episodes in adults with learning disabilities. *British Journal of Developmental Disabilities, 46*(91, Pt. 2), 131–139.

Breggin, P. R. (1999a). Psychostimulants in the treatment of children diagnosed with ADHD: Risks and mechanisms of action. *International Journal of Risk and Safety in Medicine, 12*, 3–35.

Breggin, P. R. (1999b). Psychostimulants in the treatment of children diagnosed with ADHD: Part II—Adverse effects on brain and behavior. *Ethical Human Sciences and Services, 1*, 213–242.

Brockel, B. J., & Cory-Slechta, D. A. (1998). Lead, attention, and impulsive behavior: Changes in a fixed-ratio waiting-for-reward paradigm. *Pharmacology, Biochemistry and Behavior, 60*, 545–552.

Buckingham, D. (1999). Psychopharmacology of children and adolescents. In J. M. Herrera and W. B. Lawson (Eds.), *Cross-cultural psychiatry* (pp. 373–381). Chichester, England: Wiley.

Casey, B. J. (2001). Disruption of inhibitory control in developmental disorders: A mechanistic model of implicated frontostriatal circuitry. In J. L. McClelland and R. S. Siegler (Eds.), *Mechanisms of cognitive development: Behavioral and neural perspectives. Carnegie Mellon Symposium on Cognition* (pp. 327–349). Mahwah, NJ: Erlbaum.

Castellanos, F. X. (2001). Neuroimaging studies of ADHD. In M. V. Solanto and A. F. Arnsten (Eds.), *Stimulant drugs and ADHD: Basic and clinical neuroscience* (pp. 243–258). New York: Oxford.

Cherland, E., & Fitzpatrick, R. (1999). Psychotic side effects of psychostimulants: A 5-year review. *Canadian Journal of Psychiatry, 44*, 811–813.

Colledge, E., & Blair, R. J. R. (2001). The relationship in children between the inattention and impulsivity component of attention deficit and hyperactivity disorder and psychopathic tendencies. *Personality and Individual Differences, 30*, 1175–1187.

Connors, C. K. (2000). Attention-deficit/hyperactivity disorder-historical development and overview. *Journal of Attention Disorders, 3*(4), 173–191.

Cook, E. J., Jr. (1999). Genetics of attention-deficit hyperactivity disorder. *Mental Retardation and Developmental Disabilities Research Reviews, 5*(3), 191–198.

Crystal, D. S., Ostrander, R., Chen, R., & August, G. J. (2001). Multimethod assessment of psychopathology among DSM-IV subtypes of children with attention-deficit/hyperactivity disorder: Self-, parent, and teacher reports. *Journal of Abnormal Child Psychology, 29,* 189–205.

Cunningham, C. E. (1999). In the wake of the MTA: Charting a new course for the study and treatment of children with attention-deficit hyperactivity disorder. *Canadian Journal of Psychiatry, 44,* 999–1006.

Dane, A. V., Schachar, R. J., & Tannock, R. (2000). Does actigraphy differentiate ADHD subtypes in a clinical research setting? *Journal of the American Academy of Child and Adolescent Psychiatry, 39,* 752–760.

Danforth, J. S. (1999). The outcome of parent training using the Behavior Management Flow Chart with a mother and her twin boys with oppositional defiant disorder and attention-deficit hyperactivity disorder. *Child and Family Behavior Therapy, 21,* 59–80.

Danforth, J. S. (2001). Comments on parent training research. A reply to Ayers et al. *Child and Family Behavior Therapy, 23,* 61–63.

Davies, S., & Witte, R. (2000). Self-management and peer-monitoring within a group contingency to decrease uncontrolled verbalizations of children with attention-deficit/hyperactivity disorder. *Psychology in the Schools, 37,* 135–147.

Dinn, W. M., Robbins, N. C., & Harris, C. L. (2001). Adult attention-deficit/hyperactivity disorder: Neuropsychological correlates and clinical presentation. *Brain and Cognition, 46*(1–2), 114–121.

Drew, C. J., & Hardman, M. L. (2000). *Mental retardation: A life cycle approach* (7th ed.). Columbus, OH: Merrill.

Driskill, J. D. (2000). Structured child and parent groups with ADHD children: Evaluation of varying levels of parent involvement. *Dissertation Abstracts International: Section B: The Sciences and Engineering, 60*(9-B), 4884.

DuPaul, G. J., & Eckert, T. L. (1997). The effects of school-based interventions for attention deficit hyperactivity disorder: A meta-analysis. *School Psychology Review, 26,* 5–27.

DuPaul, G. J., & Eckert, T. L. (1998). Academic interventions for students with attention-deficit/hyperactivity disorder: A review of the literature. *Reading and Writing Quarterly: Overcoming Learning Difficulties, 14,* 59–82.

Eaves, L., Rutter, M., Silberg, J. L., Shillady, L., Maes, H., & Pickles, A. (2000). Genetic and environmental causes of covariation in interview assessments of disruptive behavior and adolescent twins. *Behavior Genetics, 30,* 321–334.

Elia, J., Ambrosini, P. J., & Rapoport, J. L. (1999). Drug therapy: Treatment of attention-deficit/hyperactivity disorder. *New England Journal of Medicine, 340*(10), 780–788.

Entwistle, P. C. (2000). Assessment of attention in children with attention deficit hyperactivity problems in primary care settings. *Journal of Clinical Psychology in Medical Settings, 7,* 159–166.

Ervin, R. A., Kern, L., Clarke, S., DuPaul, G. J., Dunlap, G., & Friman, P. C. (2000). Evaluating assessment-based intervention strategies for students with ADHD and comorbid disorders within the natural classroom context. *Behavioral Disorders, 25,* 344–358.

Eshleman, A. S. (1999). Relationship between perinatal complications and attention deficit hyperactivity disorder and other behavioral characteristics. *Dissertation Abstracts International: Section A: Humanities and Social Sciences, 59*(10-A), 3836.

Evans, S. W., Pelham, W. E., Smith, B. H., Bukstein, O., Gnagy, E. M., Greiner, A. R., Altenderfer, L., & Baron-Myak, C. (2001). Dose-response effects of methylphenidate on ecologically valid measures of academic performance and classroom behavior in adolescents with ADHD. *Experimental and Clinical Psychopharmacology, 9,* 163–175.

Faraone, S. V., Biederman, J., & Monuteaux, M. C. (2001). Attention deficit hyperactivity disorder with bipolar disorder in girls: Further evidence for a familial subtype? *Journal of Affective Disorders, 64,* 19–26.

Faraone, S. V., Biederman, J., Weiffenbach, B., Keith, T., Chu, M. P., Weaver, A., Spencer, T. J., Wilens, T. E., Frazier, J., Cleves, M., & Sakai, J. (1999). Dopamine D-sub-4 gene 7-repeat allele and attention deficit hyperactivity disorder. *American Journal of Psychiatry, 156,* 768–770.

Faraone, S. V., Doyle, A. E., Mick, E., & Biederman, J. (2001). Meta-analysis of the association between the 7-repeat allele of the dopamine D-sub-4 receptor gene and attention deficit hyperactivity disorder. *American Journal of Psychiatry, 158,* 1052–1057.

Feingold, B. F. (1975). Hyperkinesis and learning disabilities linked to artificial food flavors and colors. *American Journal of Nursing, 75,* 797–803.

Fleck, S. G. (1998). Executive functions in ADHD adults. *Dissertation Abstracts International: Section B: The Sciences and Engineering, 58*(11-B), 6232.

Folstrom-Bergeron, B. M. (1998). Metamemory knowledge and application in children with attention deficit hyperactivity disorder: A developmental perspective. *Dissertation Abstracts International: Section B: The Sciences and Engineering, 58*(10-B), 5670.

Forbes, G. B. (2001). A comparison of the Conners' Parent & Teacher Rating Scales, the ADD-H Comprehensive Teacher's Rating Scale, and the Child Behavior Checklist in the clinical diagnosis of ADHD. *Journal of Attention Disorders, 5,* 25–40.

Goldstein, S. (1999). Attention-deficit hyperactivity disorder. In S. Goldstein and C. R. Reynolds (Eds.), *Handbook of neurodevelopmental and genetic disorders in children* (pp. 154–184). New York: Guilford.

Gordon, M. (1979). The assessment of impulsivity and mediating behaviors in hyperactive and nonhyperactive boys. *Journal of Abnormal Child Psychology, 7,* 317–326.

Greene, R. W., & Ablon, J. S. (2001). What does the MTA study tell us about effective psychosocial treatment for ADHD? *Journal of Clinical Child Psychology, 30,* 114–121.

Greenhill, L. L. (2001). Clinical effects of stimulant medication in ADHD. In M. V. Solanto and A. F. T. Arnsten (Eds.), *Stimulant drugs and ADHD: Basic and clinical neuroscience* (pp. 31–71). New York: Oxford.

Hankin, C. S., Wright, A., & Gephart, H. (2001). The burden of attention-deficit/hyperactivity disorder. *Drug Benefit Trends, 13*(4), 7BH-13BH.

Hardman, M. L., Drew, C. J., & Egan, M. W. (2002). *Human exceptionality: Society, school, and family* (7th ed.). Newton, MA: Allyn & Bacon.

Harwood, T. M., & Beutler, L. E. (2001). Commentary on Greene and Ablon: What does the MTA study tell us about effective psychosocial treatment for ADHD? *Journal of Clinical Child Psychology, 30,* 141–143.

Henker, B., & Whalen, C. K. (1999). The child with attention-deficit/hyperactivity disorder in school and peer settings. In H. C. Quay & A. E. Hogan (Eds.), *Handbook of disruptive behavior disorders* (pp. 157–178). New York: Kluwer Academic/Plenum.

Hoza, B. (2001). Psychosocial treatment issues in the MTA: A reply to Greene and Ablon. *Journal of Clinical Psychology, 30,* 126–130.

Jensen, P. S., Hinshaw, S. P., Swanson, J. M., Greenhill, L. L., Conners, C. K., Arnold, L. E., Abikoff, H. B., Elliott, G., Hechtman, L., Hoza, B., March, J. S., Newcorn, J. H., Severe, J. B., Vitiello, B., Wells, K., & Wigal, T. (2001). Findings from the NIMH multimodal treatment study of ADHD (MTA): Implications and applications for primary care providers. *Journal of Developmental and Behavioral Pediatrics, 22,* 60–73.

Jensen, P. S., Kettle, L., Roper, M. T., Sloan, M. T., Dulcan, M. K., Hoven, C., Bird, H. R., Bauermeister, J. J., & Payne, J. D. (1999). Are stimulants overprescribed? Treatment of ADHD in four U.S. communities. *Journal of the American Academy of Child and Adolescent Psychiatry, 38,* 797–804.

Johnson, R. C., & Rosen, L. A. (2000). Sports behavior of ADHD children. *Journal of Attention Disorders, 4*(3), 150–160.

Johnson-Cramer, N. L. (1999). Assessment of school-aged children with comorbidity of attention deficit hyperactivity disorder and low birth weight classification. *Dissertation Abstracts International: Section A: Humanities and Social Sciences, 59*(7-A), 2344.

Johnston, C., Fine, S., Weiss, M., Weiss, J., Weiss, G., & Freeman, W. S. (2000). Effects of stimulant medication treatment on mother's and children's attributions for the behavior of children with attention deficit hyperactivity disorder. *Journal of Abnormal Child Psychology, 28,* 371–382.

Jones, M. L. (2001). The effect of pharmacotherapy on parenting stress in mothers of children with attention-deficit hyperactivity disorder. *Dissertation Abstracts International: Section B: The Sciences and Engineering, 61*(8-B), 0419.

Kagan, J. (1966). Reflection impulsivity: The generality and dynamics of conceptual tempo. *Journal of Abnormal Psychology, 71,* 17–24.

Kollins, S. H., MacDonald, E. K., & Rush, C. R. (2001). Assessing the abuse potential of methylphenidate in nonhuman and human subjects: A review. *Pharmacology, Biochemistry and Behavior, 68,* 611–627.

Konrad, K., Gauggel, S., Manz, A., & Schoell, M. (2000). Inhibitory control in children with traumatic brain injury (TBI) and children with attention deficit/hyperactivity disorder (ADHD). *Brain Injury, 14,* 859–875.

Levy, F., Barr, C., & Sunahara, G. (1998). Directions of aetiologic research on attention deficit hyperactivity disorder. *Australian & New Zealand Journal of Psychiatry, 32,* 97–103.

Lochman, J. E., & Szczepanski, R. G. (1999). Externalizing conditions. In V. L. Schwean & D. H. Saklofske (Eds.), *Handbook of psychosocial characteristics of exceptional children* (pp. 219–246). New York: Kluwer Academic/Plenum.

Luk, E. S. L., Staiger, P. K., Wong, L., & Mathai, J. (1999). Children who are cruel to animals: A revisit. *Australian and New Zealand Journal of Psychiatry, 33,* 29–36.

Mancini, C., Van Ameringen, M., Oakman, J. M., & Figueirdo, D. (1999). Childhood attention deficit/hyperactivity disorder in adults with anxiety disorders. *Psychological Medicine, 29,* 515–525.

Merrell, K. W. (1999). *Behavioral, social, and emotional assessment of children and adolescents.* Mahwah, NJ: Erlbaum.

Molina, B. S. G., Smith, B. H., & Pelham, W. E. (2001). Factor structure and criterion validity of secondary school teacher ratings of ADHD and ODD. *Journal of Abnormal Child Psychology, 29,* 71–82.

Moore, J., & Fombonne, E. (1999). Psychopathology in adopted and nonadopted children: A clinical sample. *American Journal of Orthopsychiatry, 69,* 403–409.

Morris, M. M. (2001). Parental stress and marital satisfaction in families of children with attention deficit/hyperactivity disorder. *Dissertation Abstracts International: Section A: Humanities and Social Sciences, 61*(7-A), 2607.

Mulsow, M. H., O'Neal, K. K., & Murray, V. M. (2001). Adult attention deficit hyperactivity disorder, the family, and child maltreatment. *Trauma, Violence and Abuse, 2,* 36–50.

Nadder, T. S., Silberg, J. L., Rutter, M., Maes, H., & Eaves, L. J. (2001). Comparison of multiple measures of ADHD symptomatology: A multivariate genetic analysis. *Journal of Child Psychology and Psychiatry and Allied Disciplines, 42,* 475–486.

National Institute of Mental Health. (2000). *Attention deficit hyperactivity disorder (ADHD)-questions and answers.* Retrieved May 20, 2002 from the World Wide Web: www.nimh.nih.gov/publicat/adhdqu.cfm

National Institute of Mental Health. (2001). *Attention deficit hyperactivity disorder.* Retrieved May 20, 2002 from the World Wide Web: www.nimh.nih.gov/publicat/adhd.cfm

National Institutes of Health. (1998, November 16–18). Diagnosis and treatment of attention deficit hyperactivity disorder. *NIH Consensus Statement Online, 16*(2), 1–37.

Nolan, M., & Carr, A. (2000). Attention deficit hyperactivity disorder. In A. Carr (Ed.), *What works with children and adolescents? A critical review of psychological interventions with children, adolescents and their families* (pp. 65–101). Florence, KY: Taylor & Francis/Routledge.

Ohan, J. L., & Johnston, C. (1999). Attributions in adolescents medicated for attention-deficit/hyperactivity disorder. *Journal of Attention Disorders, 3,* 49–60.

Padolsky, I. P. (2001). The efficacy of EEG neurofeedback in the treatment of ADHD children: A case study analysis. *Dissertation Abstracts International: Section B: The Sciences and Engineering, 61*(12-B), 6716.

Pisecco, S., Baker, D. B., Silva, P. A., & Brooke, M. (2001). Boys with reading disabilities and/or ADHD: Distinctions in early childhood. *Journal of Learning Disabilities, 43*(2), 98–106.

Power, T. J., Karustis, J. L., & Habboushe, D. F. (2001). *Homework success for children with ADHD: A family-school intervention program.* New York: The Guilford.

Pozzi, M. E. (2000). Ritalin for whom? Understanding the need for Ritalin in psychodynamic counselling with families of under-5s. *Journal of Child Psychotherapy, 26,* 25–43.

Putnam, S. C. (2001). *Nature's Ritalin for the marathon mind: Nurturing your ADHD child with exercise.* Hinesburg, VT: Upper Access.

Raggio, D. J. (1999). Use of the School Performance Rating Scale with children treated for attention deficit hyperactivity disorder. *Perceptual and Motor Skills, 88*(3, Pt.1), 957–960.

Ralph, N. B., Oman, D., & Forney, W. (2001). Treatment outcomes with low income children and adolescents with attention deficit. *Children and Youth Services Review, 23,* 145–167.

Rapport, M. D. (2001). Attention-deficit/hyperactivity disorder. In M. Hersen and V. B. Van Hasselt (Eds.), *Advanced abnormal psychology* (2nd ed.), (pp. 191–208). New York: Kluwer Academic/Plenum.

Reddy, L. A., Spencer, P., Hall, T. M., & Rubel, E. (2001). Use of developmentally appropriate games in a child group training program for young children with attention-deficit/hyperactivity disorder. In A. A. Drewes and L. J. Carey (Eds.), *School-based play therapy* (pp. 256–274). New York: Wiley.

Rhee, S. H. (2000). A genetic epidemiological study of sex differences in ADHD. *Dissertation Abstracts International: Section B: The Sciences and Engineering, 60*(11-B), 5788.

Rhee, S. H., Waldman, I. D., Hay, D. A., & Levy, F. (1999). Sex differences in genetic and environmental influences on DSM-III-R attention-deficit/hyperactivity disorder. *Journal of Abnormal Psychology, 108,* 24–41.

Ross, R. G., & Campagnon, N. (2001). Diagnosis and treatment of psychiatric disorders in children with a schizophrenic parent. *Schizophrenia Research, 50*(1–2), 121–129.

Sagvolden, T. (1999). Attention deficit/hyperactivity disorder. *European Psychologist, 4*(2), 109–114.

Sakelaris, T. L. (1999). Effects of a self-managed study skills intervention on homework and academic performance of middle school students with attention deficit hyperactivity disorder (ADHD). *Dissertation Abstracts International: Section A: Humanities and Social Sciences, 60*(2-A), 0337.

Shaver, S. M. (1999). The relationship among teaching practices, attitudes about ADHD, and medical and special education referral by teachers. *Dissertation Abstracts International: Section A: Humanities and Social Sciences, 59*(8-A), 2854.

Shimabukuro, S. M., Prater, M. A., Jenkins, A., & Edelen-Smith, P. (1999). The effects of self-monitoring of academic performance on students with learning disabilities and ADD/ADHD. *Education and Treatment of Children, 22,* 397–414.

Silver, L. B. (1999). *Attention-deficit/hyperactivity disorders: A clinical guide to diagnosis and treatment for health and mental health professionals* (2nd ed.). Washington, DC: American Psychiatric Press.

Smith, C. M. (2001). The use of pictorial cues and parent education to increase on-task behavior, compliance, and task completion for children with attention deficit hyperactivity disorder. *Dissertation Abstracts International: Section B: The Sciences and Engineering, 61*(7-B), 3826.

Smith, C. R. (1998). *Learning disabilities: The interaction of learner, task, and setting* (4th ed.). Boston: Allyn & Bacon.

Snider, V. E., Frankenberger, W., & Aspenson, M. R. (2000). The relationship between learning disabilities and attention deficit hyperactivity disorder: A national survey. *Developmental Disabilities Bulletin, 28,* 18–38.

Solanto, M. V. (2001). Attention-deficit/hyperactivity disorders: Clinical features. In M. V. Solanto and A. F. T. Arnsten (Eds.), *Stimulant drugs and ADHD: Basic and clinical neuroscience* (pp. 3–30). New York: Oxford.

Solanto, M. V., Abikoff, H., Sonuga-Barke, E., Schachar, R., Logan, G. D., Wigal, T., Hechtman, L., Hinshaw, S., & Turkel, E. (2001). The ecological validity of delay aversion and response inhibition as measures of impulsivity in AD/HD: A supplement to the NIMH multimodal treatment study of AD/HD. *Journal of Abnormal Child Psychology, 29,* 215–228.

Sonuga-Barke, E. J. S., Daley, D., Thompson, M., Laver-Bradbury, C., & Weeks, A. (2001). Parent-based therapies for preschool attention-deficit/hyperactivity disorder: A randomized controlled trial with a community sample. *Journal of the American Academy of Child and Adolescent Psychiatry, 40,* 402–408.

Speltz, M. L., DeKlyen, M., Calderon, R., Greenberg, M. T., & Fisher, P. A. (1999). Neuropsychological characteristics and test behaviors of boys with early onset conduct problems. *Journal of Abnormal Psychology, 108,* 315–325.

Stahl, N. D., & Clarizio, H. F. (1999). Conduct disorder and comorbidity. *Psychology in the Schools, 36,* 41–50.

Steele, J. L. B. (2000). Exploring the relationship between diet and attention deficit/hyperactivity disorder: The structure of nutritional intake of children with AD/HD as compared to normal controls. *Dissertation Abstracts International: Section A: Humanities and Social Sciences, 61* (1-A), 87.

Stein, M. A., Fischer, M., & Szumowski, E. (1999). Evaluation of adults for ADHD. *Journal of the American Academy of Child and Adolescent Psychiatry, 38,* 940–941.

Stewart, G. A., Steffler, D. J., Lemoine, D. E., & Leps, J. D. (2001). Do quantitative EEG measures differentiate hyperactivity in attention deficit/hyperactivity disorder? *Child Study Journal, 31*(2) 103–121.

Strecker, E. (1929). Behavior problems in encephalitis. *Archives of Neurology and Psychiatry, 21,* 137–144.

Strecker, E., & Ebaugh, F. (1924). Neuropsychiatric sequelae of cerebral trauma in children. *Archives of Neurology and Psychiatry, 12,* 443–453.

Teeter, P. A., & Semrud-Clikeman, M. (1997). *Child neuropsychology: Assessment and interventions for neurodevelopmental disorders.* Boston: Allyn & Bacon.

Tramo, M. J. (1999). Metamemory knowledge and applications in children with attention deficit hyperactivity disorder: A developmental perspective. *Dissertation Abstracts International: Section B: The Sciences and Engineering, 59*(10-B), 5670.

Trawick-Smith, J. (2000). *Early childhood development: A multicultural perspective* (2nd ed.). Columbus, OH: Merrill/Prentice Hall.

Tripp, G., Luk, S. L., Schaughency, E. A., & Singh, R. (1999). DSM-IV and ICD-10: A comparison of the correlates of ADHD and hyperkinetic disorder. *Journal of the American Academy of Child and Adolescent Psychiatry, 38*(2), 156–164.

U.S. Department of Education, Office of Special Education Programs. (2000). *Twenty-first annual report to Congress on the implementation of the Individuals with Disabilities Education Act.* Washington, DC: Author.

Vance, A. L. A., Luk, E. S. L., Costin, J., Tonge, B. J., & Pantelis, C. (1999). Attention deficit hyperactivity disorder: Anxiety phenomena in children treated with psychostimulant medication for 6 months or more. *Australian and New Zealand Journal of Psychiatry, 33*(3), 399–406.

Venn, J. J. (2000). *Assessing students with special needs* (2nd ed.). Columbus, OH: Merrill/Prentice Hall.

Voeller, K. S. (2001). Attention-deficit/hyperactivity disorder as a frontal-subcortical disorder. In D. G. Lichter and J. L. Cummings (Eds.), *Frontal-subcortical circuits in psychiatric and neurological disorders* (pp. 334–371). New York: Guilford.

Weller, E., Rowan, A., Weller, R., & Elia, J. (1999). Aggressive behavior associated with attention-deficit/hyperactivity disorder, conduct disorder, and developmental disabilities. *Journal of Clinical Psychiatry Monograph Series, 17*(2), 2–7.

Wells, K. C. (2001). Comprehensive versus matched psychosocial treatment in the MTA study: Conceptual and empirical issues. *Journal of Clinical Child Psychology, 30*, 131–135.

Wells, K. C., Epstein, J. N., Hinshaw, S. P., Conners, C. K., Klaric, J., Abikoff, H. B., Abramowitz, A., Arnold, L. E., Elliott, G., Greenhill, L. L., Hechtman, L., Hoza, B., Jensen, P. S., March, J. S., Pelham, W., Jr., Pfiffner, L., Severe, J., Swanson, J. M., Vitiello, B., & Benedetto, W. T. (2000). Parenting and family stress treatment outcomes in attention deficit hyperactivity disorder (ADHD): An empirical analysis of the MTA study. *Journal of Abnormal Child Psychology, 28*, 543–553.

Wendt, M. S. (2000). The effect of an activity program designed with intense physical exercise on the behavior of attention deficit hyperactivity disorder (ADHD) children. *Dissertation Abstracts International: Section A: Humanities and Social Sciences, 61*(2-A), 500.

Whalen, C. K. (2001). ADHD treatment in the 21st century: Pushing the envelope. *Journal of Clinical Child Psychology, 30*, 136–140.

Willcutt, E. G., & Pennington, B. F. (2000). Comorbidity of reading disability and attention-deficit/hyperactivity disorder: Differences by gender and subtype. *Journal of Learning Disabilities, 33*, 179–191.

Wood, J. W. (1997). Attention deficit disorders. In J. W. Wood and A. M. Lazarri (Eds.), *Exceeding the boundaries: Understanding exceptional lives* (pp. 161–194). Ft. Worth, TX: Harcourt.

Ylvisaker, M., & DeBonis, D. (2000). Executive function impairment in adolescence: TBI and ADHD. *Topics in Language Disorders, 20*(2), 29–57.

Zentall, S. S., Moon, S. M., Hall, A. M., & Grskovic, J. A. (2001). Learning and motivational characteristics of boys with AD/HD and/or giftedness. *Exceptional Children, 67*, 499–519.

Zillessen, K. E., Scheuerpflug, P., Fallgatter, A. J., Strik, W. K., & Warnke, A. (2001). Changes of the brain electrical fields during the continuous performance test in attention-deficit hyperactivity disorder boys depending on methylphenidate medication. *Clinical Neurophysiology, 112*, 1166–1173.

Chapter 10

Alterson, C. J. (2000). High-probability command sequence versus noncontingent reinforcement in the treatment of escape-maintained problem behavior. *Dissertation Abstracts International: Section B: The Sciences and Engineering, 60*(8-B), 4199.

Anderson, D. R., Bryant, J., Wilder, A., Santomero, A., Williams, M., & Crawley, A. M. (2000). Researching Blue's Clues: Viewing behavior and impact. *Media Psychology, 2*, 179–194.

American Academy of Pediatrics, Committee on Public Education. (1999). Policy statement: Media education (RE9911). *Pediatrics, 104*, 341–343.

American Psychiatric Association. (2000). *Diagnostic and statistical manual of mental disorders* (4th ed., text revision). Washington DC: Author.

Angold, A., & Costello, E. J. (2001). The epidemiology of disorders of conduct: Nosological issues and comorbidity. In J. Hill and B. Maughan (Eds.), *Conduct disorders in childhood and adolescence. Cambridge child and adolescent psychiatry* (pp. 126–168). New York: Cambridge University Press.

Annambhotla, K. (2000). Social information processing and emotion in hypermasculine men after rejection by a woman. *Dissertation Abstracts International: Section B: The Sciences and Engineering, 61*(6-B), 3268.

Antrop, I., Roeyers, H., Van Oost, P., & Buysse, A. (2000). Stimulation seeking and hyperactivity in children with ADHD. *Journal of Child Psychology and Psychiatry and Allied Disciplines, 41*, 225–231.

Arnold, A. P. (1996). Genetically triggered sexual differentiation of brain and behavior. *Hormones and Behavior, 30*, 495–505.

Ashford, J. B., Sales, B. D., & LeCroy, C. W. (2001). Aftercare and recidivism prevention. In J. B. Ashford and B. D. Sales (Eds.), *Treating adult and juvenile offenders with special needs* (pp. 373–400). Washington, DC: American Psychological Association.

Atkins, M. S., & McKay, M. M. (2001). Conduct disorder. In M. Hersen and V. B. Van Hasselt (Eds.), *Advanced abnormal psychology* (2nd ed.) (pp. 209–222). New York: Kluwer Academic/Plenum.

Atkins, M. S., Osborne, M. L., Bennett, D. S., Hess, L. E., & Halperin, J. M. (2001). Children's competitive peer aggression during reward and punishment. *Aggressive Behavior, 27*, 1–13.

Auerbach, J. G., Benjamin, J., Faroy, M., Gellar, V., & Ebstein, R. (2001). DRD4 related to infant attention and information processing: A developmental link to ADHD? *Psychiatric Genetics, 11*, 31–35.

August, G. J., Realmuto, G. M., Hektner, J. M., & Bloomquist, M. L. (2001). An integrated components preventive intervention for aggressive elementary school children: The Early Risers program. *Journal of Consulting and Clinical Psychology, 69*, 614–626.

Barkley, R. A. (1998). *Attention-deficit hyperactivity disorder: A handbook for diagnosis and treatment*. New York: Guilford.

Barratt, E. S., Felthous, A., Kent, T., Liebman, M. J., & Coates, D. D. (2000). Criterion measures of aggression-impulsive versus premeditated aggression. In D. H. Fiesbein (Ed.), *The science, treatment, and prevention of antisocial behaviors: Application to the criminal justice system* (pp. 4–2 to 4–15). Kingston, NJ: Civic Research Institute.

Barrera, M., Jr., Biglan, A., Ary, D., & Li, F. (2001). Replication of a problem behavior model with American Indian, Hispanic, and Caucasian youth. *Journal of Early Adolescence, 21*, 133–157.

Bateson, P., & Martin, P. (2000). *Design for a life: How biology and psychology shape human behavior.* New York: Touchstone Books/Simon and Schuster.

Benda, B. B., Flynn-Corwyn, R., & Toombs, N. J. (2001). Recidivism among adolescent serious offenders: Prediction of entry into the correctional system for adults. *Criminal Justice and Behavior, 28*, 588–613.

Bettner, B. L., & Lew, A. (2000). Talking to parents about hitting. *Journal of Individual Psychology, 56*, 110–114.

Bodtker, A. (2001). Conflict education and special-needs students, part two: Improving conflict competence and emotional competence. *Mediation Quarterly, 18*, 377–395.

Braga, A. A., Kennedy, D. M., Waring, E. J., & Piehl, A. M. (2001). Problem-oriented policing, deterrence, and youth violence: An evaluation of Boston's Operation Ceasefire. *Journal of Research in Crime and Delinquency, 38*, 195–225.

Brestan, E. V., & Eyberg, S. M. (1998). Effective psychological treatments of conduct-disordered children and adolescents: 29 years, 82 studies, and 5,272 kids. *Journal of Clinical Child Psychology, 27*, 180–189.

Bushman, B. J., Baumeister, R. F., & Phillips, C. M. (2001). Do people aggress to improve their mood? Catharsis beliefs, affect regulation opportunity, and aggressive responding. *Journal of Personality and Social Psychology, 81*, 17–32.

Cantor, J., Bushman, B. J., Huesmann, L. R., Groebel, J., Malamuth, N. M., Impett, E. A., Donnerstein, E., & Smith, S. (2001). Some hazards of television viewing: Fears, aggression, and sexual attitudes. In D. G. Singer and J. L. Singer (Eds.), *Handbook of children and the media* (pp. 207–307). Thousand Oaks, CA: Sage.

Cantor, J., & Mares, M. L. (2001). Effects of television on child and family emotional well-being. In J. Bryant and J. A. Bryant (Eds.), *Television and the American family* (2nd ed.) (pp. 317–332). Mahwah, NJ: Erlbaum.

Cavell, T. A. (2001). Updating our approach to parent training. I: The case against targeting noncompliance. *Clinical Psychology: Science and Practice, 8*, 299–318.

Centers for Disease Control. (2000). *National vital statistics reports, 48*(11).

Centers for Disease Control. (2001). Surveillance for fatal and nonfatal firearm-related injuries-United States, 1993–1998. *MMWR, 50*(SS-2): 1–34.

Cherulnik, P. D. (2001). *Methods for behavioral research: A systematic approach.* Thousand Oaks, CA: Sage.

Christenson, S. L., & Sheridan, S. M. (2001). *Schools and families: Creating essential connections for learning.* New York: Guilford.

Collins, W. A., Maccoby, E. E., Steinberg, L., & Hetherington, E. M. (2000). Contemporary research on parenting: The case for nature and nurture. *American Psychologist, 55*, 218–232.

Conduct Problems Prevention Research Group. (2000). Merging universal and indicated prevention programs: The Fast Track model. *Addictive Behaviors, 25*, 913–927.

Costello, E. J., & Angold, A. (2001). Bad behaviour: An historical perspective on disorders of conduct. In J. Hill and B. Maughan (Eds.), *Conduct disorders in childhood and adolescence. Cambridge child and adolescent psychiatry* (pp. 1–31). New York: Cambridge University Press.

Cottle, C. C., Lee, R. J., & Heilbrun, K. (2001). The prediction of criminal recidivism in juveniles: A meta-analysis. *Criminal Justice and Behavior, 28*, 367–394.

Cottle, T. J. (2001). *At peril: Stories of injustice.* Amherst: University of Massachusetts Press.

Cowart, L. U. (2000). The efficacy of a school-home note in reducing disruptive classroom behavior: The differential effects of selecting social and academic targets. *Dissertation Abstracts International: Section B: The Sciences and Engineering, 60*(9-B), 4869.

Crespi, T. D., & Giuliano, A. J. (2001). Juvenile delinquency and adolescent violence: Focus for family therapy and consultation in independent practice. *Journal of Psychotherapy in Independent Practice, 2*(2), 83–95.

Crystal, D. S., Ostrander, R., Chen, R. S., & August, G. J. (2001). Multimethod assessment of psychopathology among DSM-IV subtypes of children with attention-deficit/hyperactivity disorder: Self-, parent, and teacher reports. *Journal of Abnormal Child Psychology, 29*(3), 189–205.

Cullen, F. T., & Gendreau, P. (2001). From nothing works to what works: Changing professional ideology in the 21st century. *Prison Journal, 81*, 313–338.

Cunningham, C. E. (1996). Improving availability, utilization, and cost efficacy of parent training programs for children with substance abuse and delinquency. In R. D. Peters and R. J. McMahon (Eds.), *Preventing childhood disorders, substance abuse, and delinquency* (pp. 144–160). Thousand Oaks, CA: Sage.

Curtner-Smith, M. E. (2000). Mechanisms by which family processes contribute to school-age boys' bullying. *Child Study Journal, 30*, 169–186.

Dahlberg, L. L., & Potter, L. B. (2001). Youth violence: Developmental pathways and prevention challenges. *American Journal of Preventive Medicine, 20* (Suppl. 1), 3–14.

Dane, A. V., Schachar, R. J., & Tannock, R. (2000). Does actigraphy differentiate ADHD subtypes in a clinical research setting? *Journal of the American Academy of Child and Adolescent Psychiatry, 39,* 752–760.

Danforth, J. S. (1999). The outcome of parent training using the Behavior Management Flow Chart with a mother and her twin boys with oppositional defiant disorder and attention-deficit hyperactivity disorder. *Child and Family Behavior Therapy, 21,* 59–80.

Danforth, S., & Boyle, J. R. (2000). *Cases in behavior management.* Columbus, OH: Merrill/Prentice Hall.

Darley, J. M., Carlsmith, K. M., & Robinson, P. H. (2000). Incapacitation and just desserts as motives for punishment. *Law and Human Behavior, 24,* 659–683.

de Brito-Orsini, C. M. (2000). Freud and the "sandman." *Percurso: Revista de Psicanalise, 13*(25)[2], 53–58.

Denham, S. A., Workman, E., Cole, P. M., Weissbrod, C., Kendziora, K. T., & Zahn-Waxler, C. (2000). Prediction of externalizing behavior problems from early to middle childhood: The role of parental socialization and emotion expression. *Developmental Psychopathology, 12,* 23–45.

Donovan, W. L., Leavitt, L. A., & Walsh, R. O. (2000). Maternal illusory control predicts socialization strategies and toddler compliance. *Developmental Psychology, 36,* 402–411.

Drabick, D. A. G., Strassberg, Z., & Kees, M. R. (2001). Measuring qualitative aspects of preschool boys' noncompliance: The response style questionnaire (RSQ). *Journal of Abnormal Child Psychology, 29,* 129–139.

Dumas, J. E., Prinz, R. J., Smith, E. P., & Laughlin, J. (1999). The Early Alliance prevention trial: An integrated set of interventions to promote competence and reduce risk for conduct disorder, substance abuse, and school failure. *Clinical Child and Family Psychology Review, 2,* 37–53.

Eaves, L., Rutter, M., Silberg, J. L., Shillady, L., Maes, H., & Pickles, A. (2000). Genetic and environmental causes of covariation in interview assessments of disruptive behavior and adolescent twins. *Behavior Genetics, 30,* 321–334.

Eisenberg, N., Fabes, R. A., Murphy, B. C., Shepard, S., Gutherie, I. K., Mazsk, P., Poulin, R., & Jones S. (1999). Prediction of elementary school children's socially appropriate and problem behavior from anger reactions at age 4–6 years. *Journal of Applied Developmental Psychology, 20,* 119–142.

Esbensen, F. A., Deschenes, E. P., & Winfree, L. T., Jr. (1999). Differences between gang girls and gang boys: Results from a multisite survey. *Youth and Society, 31,* 27–53.

Escamilla, A. G. (2001). Effects of self-instructional cognitive-behavioral techniques on anger management in juveniles. *Dissertation Abstracts International: Section A: Humanities and Social Sciences, 61*(8-A), 3117.

Farrington, D. P., Petrosino, A., & Welsh, B. C. (2001). Systematic reviews and cost-benefit analyses of correctional interventions. *Prison Journal, 81,* 339–359.

Feinberg, M., & Hetherington, E. M. (2001). Differential parenting as a within-family variable. *Journal of Family Psychology, 15,* 22–37.

Feinberg, M., Neiderhiser, J., Howe, G., & Hetherington, E. M. (2001). Adolescent, parent, and observer perceptions of parenting: Genetic and environmental influences on shared and distinct perceptions. *Child Development, 72,* 1266–1284.

Fisch, S., Truglio, R. T., & Cole, C. F. (1999). The impact of Sesame Street on preschool children: A review and synthesis of 30 years' research. *Media Psychology, 1,* 165–190.

Fombonne, E., Wostear, G., Cooper, V., Harrington, R., & Rutter, M. (2001a). The Maudsley long-term follow-up of children and adolescent depression: 1. Psychiatric outcomes in adulthood. *British Journal of Psychiatry, 179,* 210–217.

Fombonne, E., Wostear, G., Cooper, V., Harrington, R., & Rutter, M. (2001b). The Maudsley long-term follow-up of children and adolescent depression: 2. Suicidality, criminality and social dysfunction in adulthood. *British Journal of Psychiatry, 179,* 218–223.

Forbes, G. B., & Adams-Curtis, L. E. (2001). Experiences with sexual coercion in college males and females: Role of family conflict, sexist attitudes, acceptance of rape myths, self-esteem, and the Big Five personality factors. *Journal of Interpersonal Violence, 16,* 865–889.

Friedlander, K. (2001). Latent delinquency and ego development. In J. R. Meloy (Ed.), *The mark of Cain: Psychoanalytic insight and the psychopath* (pp. 79–90). Hillsdale, NJ: Analytic Press.

Goldsmith, H. (2001). The interaction of management and treatment in a residential youth corrections/ treatment setting. *Residential Treatment for Children and Youth, 18*(4), 23–32.

Goldsmith, H. H., Aksan, N., Essex, M., & Vandell, D. L. (2001). Temperament and socioemotional adjustment to kindergarten: A multi-informant perspective. In T. D. Wachs and G. A Kohnstamm (Eds.), *Temperament in context* (pp. 103–138). Mahwah, NJ: Erlbaum.

Goldstein, A. P. (1999). Aggression reduction strategies: Effective and ineffective. *School Psychology Quarterly, 14,* 40–58.

Gonzalez, A., Greenwood, G., & WenHsu, J. (2001). Undergraduate students' goal orientations and their relationship to perceived parenting styles. *College Student Journal, 35,* 182–192.

Green, S. (2001). Systemic vs. individualistic approaches to bullying. *Journal of the American Medical Association, 286,* 787.

Grier, L. K. (2000). Identity diffusion and development among African Americans: Implications for crime and corrections. In N. J. Pallone (Ed.), *Race, ethnicity, sexual orientation, violent crime: The realities and the myths* (pp. 81–94). Binghamton, NY: Haworth.

Guidubaldi, J., & Duckworth, J. (2001). Divorce and children's cognitive ability. In E. L. Grigorenko and R. J. Sternberg (Eds.), *Family environment and intellectual functioning: A life-span perspective* (pp. 97–118). Mahwah, NJ: Erlbaum.

Gumpel, T. P., & David, S. (2000). Exploring the efficacy of self-regulatory training as a possible alternative to social skills training. *Behavior Disorders, 25,* 131–141.

Gupta, V. B., Nwosa, N. M., Nadel, T. A., & Inamdar, S. (2001). Externalizing behaviors and television viewing in children of low-income minority parents. *Clinical Pediatrics, 40,* 337–341.

Hardman, M. L., Drew, C. J., & Egan, M. W. (2002). *Human exceptionality: Society, school, and family* (7th ed.). Boston: Allyn & Bacon.

Harris, G. T., Rice, M. E., & Lalumeire, M. (2001). Criminal violence: The roles of psychopathy, neurodevelopmental insults, and antisocial parenting. *Criminal Justice and Behavior, 28,* 402–426.

Hetherington, E. M. (1999a). Should we stay together for the sake of the children? In E. M. Hetherington (Ed.), *Coping with divorce, single parenting, and remarriage: A risk and resiliency perspective* (pp. 93–116). Mahwah, NJ: Erlbaum.

Hetherington, E. M. (1999b). Social capital and the development of youth from nondivorced, divorced, and remarried families. In W. A. Collins and B. Laursen (Eds.), *Relationships as developmental contexts. The Minnesota symposia on child psychology, Vol. 30* (pp. 177–209). Mahwah, NJ: Erlbaum.

Hill, J., & Maughan, B. (2001). *Conduct disorders in childhood and adolescence. Cambridge child and adolescent psychiatry.* New York: Cambridge University Press.

Hoffner, C., Plotkin, R. S., Buchanan, M., Anderson, J. D., Kamigaki, S. K., Hubbs, L. A., Kowalszyk, L., Silberg, K., & Pastorek, A. (2001). The third-person effect in perceptions of the influence of television violence. *Journal of Communication, 51,* 283–299.

Hogben, M., Byrne, D., Hamburger, M. E., & Osland, J. (2001). Legitimized aggression and sexual coercion: Individual differences in cultural spillover. *Aggressive Behavior, 27,* 26–43.

Horgan, J. (1993). Eugenics revisited. *Scientific American, 268*(6), 122–128, 130–131.

Huesman, L. R., & Miller, L. S. (1994). Longterm effects of repeated exposure to media violence in childhood. In L. R. Huesman (Ed.), *Aggressive behavior: Current perspectives* (pp. 153–180). New York: Plenum.

Hunt, G. P., & Laidler, K. J. (2001). Alcohol and violence in the lives of gang members. *Alcohol Research and Health, 25,* 66–71.

Ison, M. S. (2001). Training in social skills: An alternative for handling disruptive child behavior. *Psychological Reports, 88,* 903–911.

Johnson, J. K. (2001). Sibling, peer, and personality influences on substance use: A multivariate genetic analysis. *Dissertation Abstracts International: Section B: The Sciences and Engineering, 61*(8-B), 4408.

Joseph, J. (2001). Is crime in the genes? A critical review of twin and adoption studies of criminality and antisocial behavior. *Journal of Mind and Behavior, 22,* 179–218.

Kazdin, A. E. (1985). *Treatment of antisocial behavior in children and adolescents.* Homewood, IL: Dorsey.

Kazdin, A. E. (2001). Treatment of conduct disorders. In J. Hill and B. Maughan (Eds.), *Conduct disorders in childhood and adolescence. Cambridge child and adolescent psychiatry* (pp. 408–448). New York: Cambridge University Press.

Kellner, M. H., & Bry, B. H. (1999). The effects of anger management groups in a day school for emotionally disturbed adolescents. *Adolescence, 34,* 645–651.

Kennedy, R. W. (2001). *The encouraging parent: How to stop yelling at your kids and start teaching them confidence, self-discipline, and joy.* New York: Three Rivers.

Kinder, M. (1999). *Kids' media culture.* Durham, NC: Duke University Press.

Kipps, V. D. (2000). The integration of object relations family therapy and cognitive behavior therapy: The development of a treatment protocol for increasing anger control in male adolescents with externalizing behavior difficulties. *Dissertation Abstracts International: Section B: The Sciences and Engineering, 61*(3-B), 1639.

Klorman, R. (2000). Psychophysiological research on childhood psychopathology. In M. Hersen and R. T. Ammerman (Eds.), *Advanced abnormal child psychology* (2nd ed.) (pp. 57–80). Mahwah, NJ: Erlbaum.

Kochanska, G., Coy, K. C., & Murray, K. T. (2001). The development of self-regulation in the first four years of life. *Child Development, 72*, 1091–1111.

Koles, M., & Jenson, W. R. (1985). A comprehensive treatment approach for chronic firesetting in a boy. *Journal of Behavior Therapy and Experimental Psychiatry, 16*, 81–86.

Kolko, D. J., Day, B. T., Bridge, J. A., & Kazdin, A. E. (2001). Two-year prediction of children's firesetting in clinically referred and nonreferred samples. *Journal of Child Psychology and Psychiatry and Allied Disciplines, 42*, 371–380.

Kozioff, M. A., LaNunziata, L., Cowardin, J., & Bessellieu, F. B. (2000). Direct instruction: Its contributions to high school achievement. *High School Journal, 84*, 54–71.

Krcmar, M., & Cooke, M. C. (2001). Children's moral reasoning and their perceptions of television violence. *Journal of Communication, 51*, 300–316.

Kunitz, S. J., Gabriel, K. R., Levy, J. E., Henderson, E., Lampert, K., McCloskey, J., Quintero, G., Russell, S., & Vince, A. (1999). Alcohol dependence and conduct disorder among Navajo Indians. *Journal of Studies on Alcohol, 60*, 159–167.

Lacayo, R. (2000). Are you man enough? *Time, 155*(16), 58–63.

Ladouceur, R., Gosselin, P., Laberge, M., & Blaszczynski, A. (2001). Dropouts in clinical research: Do results reported reflect clinical reality? *Behavior Therapist, 24*(2), 44–46.

Lamb, M. E. (1999). *Parenting and child development in "nontraditional" families*. Mahwah, NJ: Erlbaum.

Landy, S., & Menna, R. (2001). Play between aggressive young children and their mothers. *Clinical Child Psychology and Psychiatry, 6*, 223–240.

Lee, D. L. (1999). The effects of stimulation on the operant responses of children with attention-deficit/hyperactivity disorder. *Dissertation Abstracts International: Section A: Humanities and Social Sciences, 60*(3-A), 0703.

Lemmey, D., McFarlane, J., Wilson, P., & Malecha, A. (2001). Intimate partner violence: Mothers' perspectives of effects on their children. *American Journal of Maternal/Child Nursing, 26*(2), 98–103.

Levine, S. (1999). Youth in terroristic groups, gangs, and cults: The allure, the animus, and the alienation. *Psychiatric Annals, 29*, 342–349.

Levitt, S. D., & Lochner, L. (2001). The determinants of juvenile crime. In J. Gruber (Ed.), *Risky behavior among youths: An economic analysis* (pp. 327–373). Chicago: University of Chicago Press.

Loeber, R., & Coie, J. (2001). Continuities and discontinuities of development, with particular emphasis on emotional and cognitive components of disruptive behaviour. In J. Hill and B. Maughan (Eds.), *Conduct disorders in childhood and adolescence. Cambridge child and adolescent psychiatry* (pp. 379–407). New York: Cambridge University Press.

Loeber, R., Farrington, D. P., Stouthamer-Loeber, M., Moffit, T. E., & Caspi, A. (2001). The development of male offending: Key findings from the first decade of the Pittsburgh Youth Study. In R. Bull (Ed.), *Children and the law: The essential readings in developmental psychology* (pp. 336–378). Malden, MA: Blackwell.

Loeber, R., Green, S. M., Lahey, B. B., & Kalb, L. (2000). Physical fighting in childhood as a risk factor for later mental health problems. *Journal of the American Academy of Child and Adolescent Psychiatry, 39*, 421–428.

Lynn, R. (2001). *Eugenics: A reassessment*. Westport, CT: Praeger/Greenwood.

Lyons, J. S., Baerger, D. R., Quigly, P., Erlich, J., & Griffin, E. (2001). Mental health service needs of juvenile offenders: A comparison of detention, incarceration, and treatment settings. *Children's Services: Social Policy, Research, and Practice, 4*(2), 69–85.

MacDonald, A. W., III, Pogue-Geile, M. F., Debski, T. T., & Manuck, S. (2001). Genetic and environmental influences on schizotypy: A community-based twin study. *Schizophrenia Bulletin, 27*, 47–48.

Mahony, D. L. (1999). Children witnessing domestic violence: A developmental approach. *Clinical Excellence for Nurse Practitioners, 3*, 362–369.

Marmorstein, N. R., & Iacono, W. G. (2001). An investigation of female adolescent twins with both major depression and conduct disorder. *Journal of the American Academy of Child and Adolescent Psychiatry, 40*, 299–306.

Martinez, C. R., Jr., & Forgatch, M. S. (2001). Preventing problems with boys' noncompliance: Effects of a parent training intervention for divorcing mothers. *Journal of Consulting and Clinical Psychology, 69*, 416–428.

Matsumoto, D. (2001). *The handbook of culture and psychology*. London: Oxford University Press.

McBurnett, K., Lahey, B. B., Rathouz, P. J., & Loeber, R. (2000). Low salivary cortisol and persistent aggression in boys referred for disruptive behavior. *Archives of General Psychiatry, 57*, 38–43.

McCloskey, L. A., & Stuewig, J. (2001). The quality of peer relationships among children exposed to family violence. *Development and Psychopathology, 13*, 83–96.

McConnell, M. J. (2000). The effects of family type on the developmental trajectories of internalizing and externalizing behaviors in children and adolescents. *Dissertation Abstracts International: Section B: The Sciences and Engineering, 60*(12-B), 6374.

McCoy, A. R., & Reynolds, A. J. (1999). Grade retention and school performance: An extended investigation. *Journal of School Psychology, 37*, 273–298.

McCurdy, M., Skinner, C. H., Grantham, K., Watson, T. S., & Hindman, P. M. (2001). Increasing on-task behavior in an elementary student during mathematics seatwork by interspersing additional brief problems. *School Psychology Review, 30*, 23–32.

McDonald, R., Jouriles, E. N., Norwood, W., Ware, H. S., & Ezell, E. (2000). Husbands' marital violence and the adjustment problems of clinic-referred children. *Behavior Therapy, 31*, 649–665.

McDonnell, J., Thorson, N., Allen, C., & Mathot-Buckner, C. (2000). The effects of partner learning during spelling for students with severe disabilities and their peers. *Journal of Behavioral Education, 10*(2–3), 107–121.

McNeely, R. L., Cook, P. W., & Torres, J. B. (2001). Is domestic violence a gender issue, or a human issue? *Journal of Human Behavior in the Social Environment, 4*, 227–251.

Meloy, J. R. (2001). *The mark of Cain: Psychoanalytic insight and the psychopath*. Hillsdale, NJ: Analytic Press.

Modestin, J., Matutat, B., & Wuermle, O. (2001). Antecedents of opioid dependence and personality disorder: Attention-deficit/hyperactivity disorder and conduct disorder. *European Archives of Psychiatry and Clinical Neuroscience, 251*, 42–47.

Munneke, D. M. (2001). A preliminary investigation of the acceptability and effectiveness of a computer-based adjunct to therapist-delivered parent training for child noncompliance. *Dissertation Abstracts International: Section B: The Sciences and Engineering, 61*(8-B), 4419.

Murray, J. P. (1995). Children and television violence. *Kansas Journal of Law and Public Policy, 4*, 7–14.

Murray, J. P., & Lonnborg, B. (1995). *Children and television: Using TV sensibly*. Manhattan, KS: Cooperative Extension Service.

Nadder, T. S., Silberg, J. L., Rutter, M., Maes, H., & Eaves, L. J. (2001). Comparison of multiple measures of ADHD symptomatology: A multivariate genetic analysis. *Journal of Child Psychology and Psychiatry and Allied Disciplines, 42*, 475–486.

Nansel, T. R., Overpeck, M., Pilla, R. S., Ruan, W. J., Simmons-Morton, B., & Scheidt, P. (2001). Bullying behaviors among U.S. youth: Prevalence and association with psychosocial adjustment. *Journal of the American Medical Association, 285*, 2094–2100.

Nelson, J. R., Johnson, A., & Marchand-Martella, N. (1996). Effects of direct instruction, cooperative learning, and independent learning practices on the classroom behavior of students with behavioral disorders: A comparative analysis. *Journal of Emotional and Behavioral Disorders, 4*, 53–62.

Nichols-Anderson, C. L. (2001). The effects of parental practices and acculturation upon sexual risk taking among Latino adolescents. *Dissertation Abstracts International: Section B: The Sciences and Engineering, 61*(9-B), 4998.

Nielsen Media Research (2000). *2000 report on television*. New York: Author.

Norris, A. K. (2000). An examinaton of the role of anger in the relationship between hypermasculinity and sexual aggression. *Dissertation Abstracts International: Section B: The Sciences and Engineering, 60*(11-B), 5785.

Norris, J., George, W. H., Davis, K. C., Martell, J., & Leonesio, R. J. (1999). Alcohol and hypermasculinity as determinants of men's empathetic responses to violent pornography. *Journal of Interpersonal Violence, 14*, 683–700.

O'Connor, B. P., & Dyce, J. A. (2001)). Personality disorders. In M. Hersen and V. B. Van Hasselt (Eds.), *Advanced abnormal psychology* (2nd ed.) (pp. 399–417). New York: Kluwer Academic/Plenum.

O'Koon, J. H. (2001). Co-occurrence of conduct problems and depressive symptoms among urban adolescents: Reported rates, effects on functioning, and pathways of risk. *Dissertation Abstracts International, 61*(7-B), 3855.

Patterson, G. R., Dishion, T. J., & Yoerger, K. (2000). Adolescent growth in new forms of problem behavior: Macro- and micro-peer dynamics. *Prevention Science, 1*, 3–13.

Patterson, G. R., & Forgatch, M. S. (2001). Therapist behavior as a determinant for client noncompliance: A paradox for the behavior modifier. In C. E. Hill (Ed.), *Helping skills: The empirical foundation* (pp. 271–283). Washington, DC: American Psychological Association.

Pearce, J. C. (2000). The effect of cognitive-behavioral group counseling on adolescent depression, academic performance, and self-esteem. *Dissertation Abstracts International: Section B: The Sciences and Engineering, 61*(3-B), 1648.

Pettit, G. S., Polaha, J. A., & Mize, J. (2001). Perceptual and attributional processes in aggression and conduct problems. In J. Hill and B. Maughan (Eds.), *Conduct disorders in childhood and adolescence. Cambridge child and adolescent psychiatry* (pp. 292–319). New York: Cambridge University Press.

Poulin, F., & Boivin, M. (2000). The role of proactive and reactive aggression in the formation and development of boys' friendships. *Developmental Psychology, 36*, 233–240.

Preski, S., & Shelton, D. (2001). The role of contextual, child and parent factors in predicting criminal outcomes in adolescence. *Issues in Mental Health Nursing, 22,* 197–205.

Regehr, C., Edward, M., & Bradford, J. (2000). Research ethics and forensic patients. *Canadian Journal of Psychiatry, 45,* 892–898.

Rhee, S. H. (2000). A genetic epidemiological study of sex differences in ADHD. *Dissertation Abstracts International: Section B: The Sciences and Engineering, 60* (11-B), 5788.

Ridenour, T. A. (2000). Genetic epidemiology of antisocial behavior. In D. H. Fishbein (Ed.), *The science, treatment, and prevention of antisocial behaviors: Application to the criminal justice system* (pp. 7–1 to 7–24). Kingston, NJ: Civic Research Institute.

Riedel, M. (2000). Homicide. In V. B. Van Hasselt and M. Hersen (Eds.), *Aggression and violence: An introductory text* (pp. 214–236). Needham Heights, MA: Allyn & Bacon.

Robins, L. N. (1999). A 70-year history of conduct disorder: Variations in definition, prevalence, and correlates. In P. Cohen and C. Slomkowski (Eds.), *Historical and geographical influences on psychopathology* (pp. 37–56). Mahwah, NJ: Erlbaum.

Rodemaker, J. E. (2000). Emotion recognition and social competence in children with and without conduct disorders. *Dissertation Abstracts International: Section B: The Sciences and Engineering, 60*(9-B), 4907.

Russo, D. C., Cataldo, M. F., & Cushing, P. J. (1981). Compliance training and behavioral covariation in the treatment of multiple behavior problems. *Journal of Applied Behavior Analysis, 14,* 209–222.

Sanders, M. R., Montgomery, D. T., & Brechman-Toussaint, M. L. (2000). The mass media and the prevention of child behavior problems: The evaluation of a television series to promote positive outcome for parents and their children. *Journal of Child Psychology and Psychiatry and Allied Disciplines, 41,* 939–948.

Sarat, A. (1999). Remorse, responsibility, and criminal punishment: An analysis of popular culture. In S. A. Bandes (Ed.), *The passions of law: Critical America* (pp. 168–190). New York: New York University Press.

Scharrer, E. (2001). Men, muscles, and machismo: The relationship between television violence exposure and aggression and hostility in the presence of hypermasculinity. *Media Psychology, 3*(2), 159–188.

Schmeck, K., & Poustka, F. (2001). Temperament and disruptive behavior disorders. *Psychopathology, 34,* 159–163.

Schubiner, H., Tzelepis, A., Milberger, S., Lockhart, N., Kruger, M., Kelly, B. J., & Schoener, E. P. (2000). Prevalence of attention-deficit/hyperactivity disorder and conduct disorder among substance abusers. *Journal of Clinical Psychiatry, 61,* 244–251.

Serdahl, E. (2000). The influence of parent-teacher relationships on the adjustment of aggressive children: An ecosystemic perspective on the home-school mesosystem. *Dissertation Abstracts International: Section A: Humanities and Social Sciences, 61*(4-A), 1296.

Seroczynski, A. D., Bergeman, C. S., & Coccaro, E. F. (1999). Etiology of the impulsivity/aggression relationship: Genes or environment? *Psychiatry Research, 86,* 41–57.

Short, J. F., Jr. (2001). Youth collectivities and adolescent violence. In S. O. White (Ed.), *Handbook of youth and justice. The Plenum series in crime and justice* (pp. 237–264). New York: Kluwer Academic/Plenum.

Sigurdsson, J. F., Gudjonsson, G. H., & Peersen, M. (2001). Differences in the cognitive ability and personality of desisters and re-offenders: A prospective study among young offenders. *Psychology, Crime and Law, 7,* 33–43.

Simic, M., & Fombonne, E. (2001). Depressive conduct disorder: Symptom patterns and correlates in referred children and adolescents. *Journal of Affective Disorders, 62* (3), 175–185.

Sims, B. (2001). Domestic violence. In H. M. Rebach and J. G. Bruhn (Eds.), *Handbook of clinical sociology* (2nd ed.) (pp. 313–326). Dordrech, Netherlands: Kluwer Academic/Plenum.

Spillane-Grieco, E. (2000). From parent verbal abuse to teenage physical aggression? *Child and Adolescent Social Work Journal, 17,* 411–430.

Stifter, C. A., Spinrad, T. L., & Braungart-Rieker, J. M. (1999). Toward a developmental model of child compliance: The role of emotion regulation in infancy. *Child Development, 70,* 21–32.

Stormshak, E. A., Bierman, K. L., McMahon, R. J., & Legua, L. J. (2000). Parenting practices and child disruptive behavior problems in early elementary school. *Journal of Clinical Child Psychology, 29,* 17–29.

Sullivan, M. L. (2001). Hyperghettos and hypermasculinity: The phenomonology of exclusion. In A. Booth and A. C. Crouter (Eds.), *Does it take a village? Community effects on children, adolescents, and families* (pp. 95–101). Mahwah, NJ: Erlbaum.

Summers, D. R. (2000). Conduct-disordered youth: A comparative study of personality traits, relationships, and moral development. *Dissertation Abstracts International: Section B: The Sciences and Engineering, 60*(9-B), 4870.

Taylor, E. R., Kelly, J., Valescu, S., Reynolds, G. S., Sherman, J., & German, V. (2001). Is stealing a gateway crime? *Community Mental Health Journal, 37*, 347–358.

Tedeschi, J. T. (2001). Social power, influence, and aggression. In J. P. Forgas and K. D. Williams (Eds.), *Social influence: Direct and indirect processes. The Sydney symposium of social psychology* (pp. 109–126). Philadelphia: Psychology/Taylor & Francis.

Tremblay, R. E., LeMarquand, D., & Vitaro, F. (1999). The prevention of oppositional defiant disorder and conduct disorder. In H. C. Quay and A. E. Hogan (Eds.), *Handbook of disruptive behavior disorders* (pp. 525–555). New York: Kluwer Academic/Plenum.

U.S. Department of Justice, Bureau of Justice Statistics. (2001). *Homicide trends in the U.S.: Age trends.* Retrieved May 22, 2002, from the World Wide Web: www.ojp.usdoj.gov/bjs/homicide/teens/htm

U.S. Department of Justice, Office of Justice Programs. (1998). *Violence by intimates: Analysis of data on crimes by current or former spouses, boyfriends, and girlfriends* (NCJ-167237). Washington, DC: Author.

Verona, E., & Patrick, C. J. (2000). Suicide risk in externalizing syndromes: Temperamental and neurobiological underpinnings. In T. E. Joiner and D. M. Rudd (Eds.), *Suicide science: Expanding the boundaries* (pp. 137–173). Norwell, MA: Kluwer Academic.

Vitaro, F. (1998). The interdependence between developmental research and the prevention of adjustment problems in youth. *Revue Canadienne de Psycho Education, 27*, 231–251.

Vitaro, F., Brendgen, M., & Tremblay, R. E. (2001). Preventative intervention: Assessing its effects on the trajectories of delinquency and testing for mediational processes. *Applied Developmental Science, 5*, 201–213.

Wakschlag, L. S., Gordon, R. A., Lahey, B. B., Loeber, R., Green, S. M., & Leventhal, B. L. (2000). Maternal age at first birth and boys' risk for conduct disorder. *Journal of Research on Adolescence, 10*, 417–441.

Wann, D. L., Carlson, J. D., Holland, L. C., Jacob, B. E., Owens, D. A., & Wells, D. D. (1999). Beliefs in symbolic catharsis: The importance of involvement with aggressive sports. *Social Behavior and Personality, 27*, 155–164.

Weiner, B. (2001). Responsibility for social transgressions: An attributional analysis. In B. F. Malle and L. J. Moses (Eds.), *Intentions and intentionality: Foundations of social cognition* (pp. 331–344). Cambridge, MA: MIT Press.

Weist, M. D., & Cooley-Quille, M. (2001). Advancing efforts to address youth violence involvement. *Journal of Clinical Child Psychology, 30*, 147–151.

Weisz, J. R., Weiss, B., Han, S. S., Granger, D. A., & Morton, T. (1995). Effects of psychotherapy with children and adolescents revisited: A meta-analysis of treatment outcome studies. *Psychological Bulletin, 117*, 450–468.

Welte, J. W., Zhang, L., & Wieczorek, W. F. (2001). The effects of substance use on specific types of criminal offending in young men. *Journal of Research in Crime and Delinquency, 38*, 416–438.

Willcutt, E. G., & Pennington, B. F. (2000). Comorbidity of reading disability and attention-deficit/hyperactivity disorder: Differences by gender and subtype. *Journal of Learning Disabilities, 33*, 179–191.

Wong, S. E. (1999). Treatment of antisocial behavior in adolescent inpatients: Behavioral changes and client satisfaction. *Research on Social Work Practice, 9*, 25–44.

Yanof, J. (1999). Eric's analysis. In A. A. Rothstein and J. Glenn (Eds.), *Learning disabilities and psychic conflict: A psychoanalytic casebook* (pp. 277–303). Madison, CT: International Universities.

Ziegler, D. (2001). To hold, or not to hold . . . Is that the right question? *Residential Treatment for Children and Youth, 18* (4), 33–45.

Chapter 11

Alarcon, M., Knopik, V. S., & DeFries, J. C. (2000). Covariation of mathematics achievement and general cognitive ability in twins. *Journal of School Psychology, 38*, 63–77.

Allen, D. (2000). Recent research on physical aggression in persons with intellectual disability: An overview. *Journal of Intellectual and Developmental Disability, 25*, 41–57.

American Psychiatric Association. (2000). *Diagnostic and statistical manual of mental disorders* (4th ed., text revision). Washington, DC: Author.

Aro, T., Ahonen, T., Tolvanen, A., Lyytinen, H., & Todd-de-Barra, H. (1999). Contribution of ADHD characteristics to the academic treatment outcome of children with learning difficulties. *Developmental Neuropsychology, 15*(2), 291–305.

Badian, N. A. (1999). Reading disability defined as a discrepancy between listening and reading comprehension: A longitudinal study of stability, gender differences, and prevalence. *Journal of Learning Disabilities, 32*(2), 138–148.

Barkley, R. A. (1998). *Attention-deficit hyperactivity disorder: A handbook for diagnosis and treatment.* New York: Guilford.

Barra, H. (1999). Contribution of ADHD characteristics to the academic treatment outcome of children with learning difficulties. *Developmental Neuropsychology, 15*(2), 291–305.

Bender, W. N. (1998). *Learning disabilities: Characteristics, identification, and teaching strategies* (3rd ed.). Boston: Allyn and Bacon.

Bhaumik, S., Brandford, D., Naik, B. I., & Biswas, A. B. (2000). A retrospective audit of selective serotonin reuptake inhibitors (fluoxetine and paroxetine) for the treatment of depressive episodes in adults with learning disabilities. *British Journal of Developmental Disabilities, 46*(91, Pt. 2), 131–139.

Blanchett, W. J. (2000). Sexual risk behaviors of young adults with LD and the need for HIV/AIDS education. *Remedial and Special Education, 21,* 336–345.

Bocian, K. M., Beebe, M. E., MacMillan, D. L., & Gresham, F. M. (1999). Competing paradigms in learning disabilities classification by schools and the variations in the meaning of discrepant achievement. *Learning Disabilities Research and Practice, 14,* 1–14.

Boden, C., & Brodeur, D. A. (1999). Visual processing of verbal and nonverbal stimuli in adolescents with reading disabilities. *Journal of Learning Disabilities, 32*(1), 58–71.

Boucher, C. R. (1999). *Students in discord: Adolescents with emotional and behavioral disorders.* Westport, CT: Greenwood.

Brown, D. S. (2000). *Learning a living: A guide to planning your career and finding a job for people with learning disabilities, attention deficit disorder, and dyslexia.* Bethesda, MD: Woodbine House.

Bryant, D. P., Bryant, B. R., & Hammill, D. D. (2000). Characteristic behaviors of students with LD who have teacher-identified math weaknesses. *Journal of Learning Disabilities, 33*(2), 168–177.

Cambridge, P., & Mellan, B. (2000). Reconstructing the sexuality of men with learning disabilities: Empirical evidence and theoretical interpretations of need. *Disability and Society, 15,* 293–311.

Codina, G. E., Yin, Z., Katims, D. S., & Zapata, J. T. (1998). Marijuana use and academic achievement among Mexican American school-age students: Underlying psychosocial and behavioral characteristics. *Journal of Child and Adolescent Substance Abuse, 7*(3), 79–96.

Connors, C. K. (2000). Attention-deficit/hyperactivity disorder-historical development and overview. *Journal of Attention Disorders, 3*(4), 173–191.

Cordell, A. S. (1999). Self-esteem in children. In J. C. Carlock (Ed.), *Enhancing self-esteem* (3rd ed.) (pp. 287–376). Philadelphia: Accelerated Development.

Culbertson, J. L. (1998). Learning disabilities. In T. H. Ollendick & M. Hersen (Eds.), *Handbook of child psychopathology* (3rd ed.) (pp. 117–156). New York: Plenum.

D'Amato, R. C., Dean, R. S., & Rhodes, R. L. (1998). Subtyping children's learning disabilities with neuropsychological, intellectual, and achievement measures. *International Journal of Neuroscience, 96,* 107–125.

Dole, S. (2000). The implications of the risk and resilience literature for gifted students with learning disabilities. *Roeper Review, 23*(2), 91–96.

Drew, C. J., & Hardman, M. L. (2000). *Mental retardation: A life cycle approach* (7th ed.). Columbus, OH: Merrill/Prentice Hall.

Drew, C. J., Hardman, M. L., & Hart, A. W. (1996). *Designing and conducting research: Inquiry in education and social science.* Boston: Allyn & Bacon.

Elia, J., Ambrosini, P. J., & Rapoport, J. L. (1999). Drug therapy: Treatment of attention-deficit-hyperactivity disorder. *New England Journal of Medicine, 340*(10), 780–788.

Escera, C., Alho, K., Schroeger, E., & Winkler, I. (2000). Involuntary attention and distractibility as evaluated with event-related brain potentials. *Audiology and Neuro-Otology, 5*(3–4), 151–166.

Ferretti, R. P., MacArthur, C. A., & Dowdy, N. S. (2000). The effects of an elaborated goal on the persuasive writing of students with learning disabilities and their normally achieving peers. *Journal of Educational Psychology, 92,* 694–702.

Gardill, M. C., & Jitendra, A. K. (1999). Advanced story map instruction: Effects on the reading comprehension of students with learning disabilities. *Journal of Special Education, 33,* 2–17.

Gersten, R., & Baker, S. (1998). Real world use of scientific concepts: Integrating situated cognition with explicit instruction. *Exceptional Children, 65,* 23–35.

Goldstein, K. (1936). The modifications of behavior consequent to cerebral lesions. *Psychiatric Quarterly, 10,* 586–610.

Goldstein, K. (1939). *The organism.* New York: American Book.

Gomez, R., & Condon, M. (1999). Central auditory processing ability in children with ADHD with and without learning disabilities. *Journal of Learning Disabilities, 32*(2), 150–158.

Gordon, M., & Keiser, S. (1998). *Accommodations in higher education under the Americans with Disabilities Act (ADA): A no-nonsense guide for clinicians, educators, administrators, and lawyers.* New York: Guilford.

Gralton, E., James, A., & Crocombe, J. (2000). The diagnosis of schizophrenia in the borderline learning-disabled forensic population: Six case reports. *Journal of Forensic Psychiatry, 11*, 185–197.

Hadley, R. L. (1998). The Americans with Disabilities Act of 1990: Faculty and student perceptions of reasonable accommodations versus competency in graduate psychology programs. *Dissertation Abstracts International: Section B: The Sciences and Engineering, 28*(11-B), 6235.

Hagborg, W. J. (1999). Scholastic competence subgroups among high school students with learning disabilities. *Learning Disability Quarterly, 22*, 3–10.

Halfon, N., & Newcheck, P. W. (1999). Prevalence and impact of parent-reported disabling mental health conditions among U.S. children. *Journal of the American Academy of Child and Adolescent Psychiatry, 38*, 600–609.

Hardman, M. L., Drew, C. J., & Egan, M. W. (2002). *Human exceptionality: Society, school, and family* (7th ed.). Newton, MA: Allyn & Bacon.

Hazell, P. L., Carr, V. J., Lewin, T. J., Dewis, S. A. M., Heathcote, D. M., & Brucki, B. M. (1999). Effortful and automatic information processing in boys with ADHD and specific learning disorders. *Journal of Child Psychology and Psychiatry and Allied Disciplines, 40*(2), 275–286.

Heath, N. L., & Ross, S. (2000). Prevalence and expression of depressive symptomatology in students with and without learning disabilities. *Learning Disability Quarterly, 23*, 2436.

Hollins, S., Perez, W., Abdelnoor, A., & Webb, B. (1999). *Falling in love*. London: Gaskell/St. George's Hospital Medical School.

Humphreys, G. W., & Riddoch, M. J. (1999). Impaired development of semantic memory: Separating semantic from structural knowledge and diagnosing a role for action in establishing stored memories for objects. *Neurocase, 5*(6), 519–532.

Jenkins, Y. M. (1999). *Diversity in college settings: Directives for helping professionals*. New York: Routledge.

Jitendra, A. K., Hoppes, M. K., & Xin, Y. P., (2000). Enhancing main idea comprehension for students with learning problems: The role of summarization strategy and self-monitoring instruction. *Journal of Special Education, 34*(3), 127–139.

Johnson, B. D., Altmaier, E. M., & Richman, L. C. (1999). Attention deficits and reading disabilities: Are immediate memory defects additive? *Developmental Neuropsychology, 15*(2), 213–226.

Johnson, E. O., & Breslau, N. (2000). Increased risk of learning disabilities in low birth weight boys at age 11 years. *Biological Psychiatry, 47*(6), 490–500.

Jordan, N. C., & Hanich, L. B. (2000). Mathematical thinking in second-grade children with different forms of LD. *Journal of Learning Disabilities, 33*(6), 567–578.

Kamann, M. P., & Wong, B. Y. L. (1993). Inducing adaptive coping self-statements in children with learning disabilities through self-instruction training. *Journal of Learning Disabilities, 26*, 630–638.

Kaplan, B. J., Wilson, B. N., Dewey, D., & Crawford, S. G. (1998). DCD may not be a discrete disorder. *Human Movement Science, 17*(4–5), 471–490.

Kauffman, J. M., Hallahan, D. P., & Lloyd, J. W. (1998). Politics, science and the future of learning disabilities. *Learning Disability Quarterly, 21*, 276–280.

Kavale, K. A., & Forness, S. R. (2000). Auditory and visual perception processes and reading ability: A quantitative reanalysis and historical reinterpretation. *Learning Disability Quarterly, 23*, 253–270.

Kehrer, C. A., Sanchez, P. N., Habif, U., Rosenbaum, J. G., & Towness, B. D. (2000). Effects of a significant-other observer on neuropsychological test performance. *Clinical Neuropsychologist, 14*, 67–71.

Kirk, S. A. (1963). Behavioral diagnosis and remediation of learning disabilities. *Proceedings: Conference on Exploration into the Problems of the Perceptually Handicapped Child. First Annual Meeting* (Vol. 1). Chicago.

Kovner, R., Budman, C., Frank, Y., Sison, C., Lesser, M., & Halprin, J. (1999). Neuropsychological testing in adult attention deficit hyperactivity disorder: A pilot study. *International Journal of Neuroscience, 97*, 277.

Kraus, N., & Cheour, M. (2000). Speech sound representation in the brain. *Audiology and Neuro-Otology, 5*(3–4), 140–150.

Krueger, R. F. (2000). Phenotypic, genetic, and nonshared environmental parallels in the structure of personality: A view from the Multidimensional Personality Questionnaire. *Journal of Personality and Social Psychology, 79*, 1057–1067.

Larsen-Miller, L. (1994). *An investigation to determine the effects of a video-mediated metacognitive reading comprehension strategy in a complimentary environment*. Unpublished master's thesis, University of Utah.

Lefrancois, G. R. (1999). *The lifespan* (6th ed.). Belmont, CA: Wadsworth.

Livingston, R. B., Gray, R. M., Haak, R. A., & Jennings, E. (2000). Factor structure of the Reitan-Indiana Neuropsychological Battery for Children. *Assessment, 7*, 189–199.

Lorsbach, T. C. (2000). Source monitoring as a framework for conceptualizing the nature of memory difficulties in children with learning disabilities. In K. P. Roberts and M. Blades (Eds.), *Children's source monitoring* (pp. 115–145). Mahwah, NJ: Erlbaum.

Mangina, C. A., Beuzeron-Mangina, J. H., & Grizenko, N. (2000). Event-related brain potentials, bilateral electrodermal activity and Mangina-Test performance in learning disabled/ADHD pre-adolescents with severe behavioral disorders as compared to age-matched normal controls. *International Journal of Psychophysiology, 37*, 71–85.

Mastropieri, M. A., Sweda, J., & Scruggs, T. E. (2000). Putting mnemonic strategies to work in an inclusive classroom. *Learning Disabilities Research and Practice, 15*(2), 69–74.

McLean, J. F., & Hitch, G. J. (1999). Working memory impairments in children with specific arithmetic learning difficulties. *Journal of Experimental Child Psychology, 74*, 240–260.

Meyer, M. S. (2000). The ability-achievement discrepancy: Does it contribute to an understanding of learning disabilities? *Educational Psychology Review, 12*(3), 315–337.

Moss, S., Emerson, E., Kiernan, C., Turner, S., Hatton, C., & Alborz, A. (2000). Psychiatric symptoms in adults with learning disability and challenging behavior. *British Journal of Psychiatry, 177*, 452–456.

Most, T., & Greenbank, A. (2000). Auditory, visual, and auditory-visual perception of emotions by adolescents with and without learning disabilities and their relationship to social skills. *Learning Disabilities Research and Practice, 15*(4), 171–178.

Murray, C., Goldstein, D. E., Nourse, S., & Edgar, E. (2000). The postsecondary school attendance and completion rates of high school graduates with learning disabilities. *Learning Disabilities Research and Practice, 15*(3), 119–127.

Naglieri, J. A. (1999). How valid is the PASS theory and CAS? *School Psychology Review, 28*, 145–162.

Naglieri, J. A., & Johnson, D. (2000). Effectiveness of a cognitive strategy intervention in improving arithmetic computation based on the PASS theory. *Journal of Learning Disabilities, 33*(6), 591–597.

Nicholls, M. E. R., Schier, M., Stough, C. K. K., & Box, A. (1999). Psychophysical and electrophysiologic support for a left hemisphere temporal processing advantage. *Neuropsychiatry, Neuropsychology, and Behavioral Neurology, 12*, 11–16.

Olivier, C., Hecker, L., Klucken, J., & Westby, C. (2000). Language: The embedded curriculum in postsecondary education. *Topics in Lanuguage Disorders, 21*(1), 15–29.

Palladino, P., Poli, P., Masi, G., & Marcheschi, M. (2000). The relation between metacognition and depressive symptoms in preadolescents with learning disabilities: Data in support of Borkowski's model. *Learning Disabilities Research and Practice, 15*(3), 142–148.

Persinger, M. A., & Tiller, S. G. (1999). Personality not intelligence or educational achievement differentiates university students who access special needs for "learning disabilities." *Social Behavior and Personality, 27*, 1–10.

Pineda, D., Ardila, A., & Roselli, M. (1999). Neuropsychological and behavioral assessment of ADHD in seven- to twelve-year-old children: A discriminant analysis. *Journal of Learning Disabilities, 32*, 159–173.

Prior, M., Smart, D., Sanson, A., & Oberklaid, F. (1999). Relationships between learning difficulties and psychological problems in preadolescent children from a longitudinal sample. *Journal of the American Academy of Child and Adolescent Psychiatry, 38*(4), 429–436.

Rankin-Erickson, J. L., & Pressley, M. (2000). A survey of instructional practices of special education teachers nominated as effective teachers of literacy. *Learning Disabilities Research and Practice, 15*(4), 206–225.

Renninger, K. A. (2000). Individual interest and its implications for understanding intrinsic motivation. In C. Sansome & J. M. Harackiewicz (Eds.), *Intrinsic and extrinsic motivation: The search for optimal motivation and performance* (pp. 373–404). San Diego: Academic.

Rojewski, J. W. (1999). Occupational and educational aspirations and attainment of young adults with and without LD 2 years after high school completion. *Journal of Learning Disabilities, 32*, 533–552.

Rose, S. A., Feldman, J. F., Jankowski, J. J., & Futterweit, L. R. (1999). Visual and auditory temporal processing, cross-modal transfer, and reading. *Journal of Learning Disabilities, 32*(3), 256–266.

Rothenberger, A., Banaschewski, T., Heinrich, H., Moll, G. H., Schmidt, M. H., & van-t-Klooster, B. (2000). Comorbidity in ADHD children: Effects of coexisting conduct disorder or tic disorder on event-related brain potential in an auditory selective-attention task. *European Archives of Psychiatry and Clinical Neuroscience, 250*(2), 101–110.

Samango-Sprouse, C. (1999). Frontal lobe development in childhood. In B. L. Miller & J. L. Cummings (Eds.), *The human frontal lobes: Functions and disorders* (pp. 584–603). New York: Guilford.

Schallert, T., Bland, S. T., Leasure, J. L., Tillerson, J., Gonzales, R., Williams, L., Arronowski, J., & Grotta, J. (2000). Motor rehabilitation, use-related neural events, and reorganization of the brain after injury. In H. S. Levin & J. Grafman (Eds.), *Cerebral reorganization of function after brain damage* (pp. 145–167). New York: Oxford University Press.

Shamir, E., Rotenberg, V. S., Laudon, M., Zisapel, N., & Elizur, A. (2000). First-night effect of melatonin treatment in patients with chronic schizophrenia. *Journal of Clinical Psychopharmacology, 20,* 691–694.

Shapiro, E. S., & Kratochwill, T. R. (2000). *Behavioral assessment in schools: Theory, research, and clinical foundations* (2nd ed.). New York: Guilford.

Silliman, E. R., Jimerson, T. L., & Wilkinson, L. C. (2000). A dynamic systems approach to writing assessment in students with language learning problems. *Topics in Language Disorders, 20*(4), 45–64.

Silver, L. B. (1999). *Attention-deficit/hyperactivity disorders: A clinical guide to diagnosis and treatment for health and mental health professionals* (2nd ed.). Washington, DC: American Psychiatric Press.

Simner, M. L., & Eidlitz, M. R. (2000). Towards an empirical definition of developmental dysgraphia: Preliminary findings. *Canadian Journal of School Psychology, 16,* 103–110.

Smith, C. R. (1998). *Learning disabilities: The interaction of learner, task, and setting* (4th ed.). Boston: Allyn and Bacon.

Snider, V. E., Frankenberger, W., & Aspenson, M. R. (2000). The relationship between learning disabilities and attention deficit hyperactivity disorder: A national survey. *Developmental Disabilities Bulletin, 28*(1), 18–38.

Speltz, M. L., DeKlyen, M., Calderon, R., Greenberg, M. T., & Fisher, P. A. (1999). Neuropsychological characteristics and test behaviors of boys with early onset conduct problems. *Journal of Abnormal Psychology, 108,* 315–325.

Swanson, H. L. (1999). Reading comprehension and working memory in learning-disabled readers: Is the phonological loop more important than the executive system? *Journal of Experimental Child Psychology, 72,* 1–31.

Swanson, H. L. (2000a). Are working memory deficits in readers with learning disabilities hard to change? *Journal of Learning Disabilities, 33*(6), 551–566.

Swanson, H. L. (2000b). What instruction works for students with learning disabilities? Summarizing the results from a meta-analysis of intervention studies. In R. Gersten, E. P. Schiller, & S. Vaughn (Eds.), *Contemporary special education research: Syntheses of the knowledge base on critical instructional issues* (pp. 1–30). Mahwah, NJ: Erlbaum.

Swanson, H. L., & Sachse, L. C. (2000). A meta-analysis of single-subject-design intervention research for students with LD. *Journal of Learning Disabilities, 33*(2), 114–136.

Taylor, H. G., Anselmo, M., Foreman, A. L., Schatschneider, C., & Angelopoulos, J. (2000). Utility of kindergarten teacher judgments in identifying early learning problems. *Journal of Learning Disabilities, 33*(2), 200–210.

Tirosh, E. & Cohen, A. (1998). Language deficit with attention-deficit disorder: A prevalent comorbidity. *Journal of Child Neurology, 13*(10), 493–497.

U.S. Department of Education. (1999). *To assure the free appropriate public education of all children with disabilities: Twenty-first annual report to Congress on the implementation of the Individuals with Disabilities Education Act.* Washington, DC: U.S. Government Printing Office.

U.S. Department of Education. (2000). *Twenty-second annual report to Congress on the implementation of the Individuals with Disabilities Education Act.* Washington, DC: Author.

Vadasy, P. F., Jenkins, J. R., & Pool, K. (2000). Effects of tutoring in phonological and early reading skills on students at risk for reading disabilities. *Journal of Learning Disabilities, 33*(6), 579–590.

van Strien, J. W. (1999). Verbal learning in boys with P-type dyslexia, L-type dyslexia, and boys without learning disabilities: Differences in learning curves and in serial position curves. *Child Neuropsychology, 5*(3), 145–153.

Wanzek, J., Dickson, S., Bursuck, W. D., & White, J. M. (2000). Teaching phonological awareness to students at risk for reading failure: An analysis of four instructional programs. *Learning Disabilities Research and Practice, 15*(4), 226–239.

Ward, M. C., & Bernstein, D. J. (1998). Promoting academic performance among students with special needs. *Ethics and Behavior, 8*(3), 276–281.

Warner-Rogers, J., Taylor, A., Taylor E., & Sandberg, S. (2000). Inattentive behavior in childhood: Epidemiology and implications for development. *Journal of Learning Disabilities, 33*(6), 520–536.

Watson, A. L., Franklin, M. E., Ingram, M. A., & Eilenberg, L. B. (1998). Alcohol and other drug abuse among persons with disabilities. *Journal of Applied Rehabilitation Counseling, 29*(2), 22–29.

Weiler, M. D., Harris, N. S., Naomi, S., Marcus, D. J., Bellinger, D., Kosslyn, S. M., & Waber, D. P. (2000). Speed of information processing in children referred for learning problems: Performance on a visual filtering test. *Journal of Learning Disabilities, 33*(6), 538–550.

Welch, M., Brownell, K., & Sheridan, S. M. (1999). What's the score and game plan on teaming in schools? A review of the literature on team teaching and school-based problem solving teams. *Remedial and Special Education, 20*(1), 36–49.

Welch, M., & Sheridan, S. M. (1995). *Educational partnerships: An ecological approach to serving students at risk*. San Francisco: Harcourt Brace Jovanovich.

Werner, H., & Strauss, A. A. (1939). Types of visuo-motor activity in their relation to low and high performance ages. *Proceedings of the American Association on Mental Deficiency, 44*, 163–168.

Werner, H., & Strauss, A. A. (1941). Pathology of figure-background relation in the child. *Journal of Abnormal and Social Psychology, 36*, 236–248.

Willcutt, E. G., & Pennington, B. F. (2000). Comorbidity of reading disability and attention-deficit/hyperactivity disorder: Differences by gender and subtype. *Journal of Learning Disabilities, 33*(2), 179–191.

Willcutt, E. G., Pennington, B. F., & DeFries, J. C. (2000). Etiology of inattention and hyperactivity/impulsivity in a community sample of twins with learning difficulties. *Journal of Abnormal Child Psychology, 28*, 149–159.

Wong, B. Y. L. (1999). Metacognition in writing. In R. Gallimore, L. P. Bernheimer, D. L. MacMillan, D. L. Speece, & S. Vaughn (Eds.), *Developmental perspectives on children with high-incidence disabilities* (pp. 183–198). Mahwah, NJ: Erlbaum.

Wong, B. Y. L. (2000). Writing strategies instruction for expository essays for adolescents with and without learning disabilities. *Topics in Language Disorders, 20*(4), 29–44.

Wren, C., & Einhorn, J. (2000). *Hanging by a twig: Understanding and counseling adults with learning disabilities and ADD*. New York: Norton.

Yanez, G., Harmony, T., Bernal, J., Rodriguez, M., Marosi, E., & Fernandez, T. (2000). Presentation of a neuropsychological battery for the evaluation of children with learning disorders in reading: Study of a normal population. *Revista Latina de Pensamiento y Lenguaje, 8*(1), 87–107.

Chapter 12

Adnams, C. M., Kodituwakku, P. W., Hay, A., Molteno, C. D., Viljoen, D., & May, P. A. (2001). Patterns of cognitive-motor development in children with fetal alcohol syndrome from a community in South Africa. *Alcoholism: Clinical and Experimental Research, 25*, 557–562.

American Association on Mental Retardation. (1992). *Mental retardation: Definition, classification, and systems of supports* (9th ed.). Washington, DC: Author.

American Psychiatric Association. (2000). *Diagnostic and statistical manual of mental disorders* (4th ed., text revision). Washington, DC: Author.

Bailey, D. B., Jr., Hatton, D. D., Mesibov, G., Ament, N., & Skinner, M. (2000). Early development, temperament, and functional impairment in autism and fragile X syndrome. *Journal of Autism and Developmental Disorders, 30*, 49–59.

Balboni, G., Pedrabissi, L., Molteni, M., & Villa, S. (2001). Discriminant validity of the Vineland Scales: Score profiles of individuals with mental retardation and a specific disorder. *American Journal on Mental Retardation, 106*, 162–172.

Bell, D. M., & Espie, C. A. (2000). Age recognition in adults with intellectual disabilities: A literature review and an exploratory study. *Journal of Applied Research in Intellectual Disabilities, 13*(3), 132–158.

Berk, L. E. (1998). *Development through the lifespan*. Boston: Allyn & Bacon.

Bochner, S., Outhred, L., & Pieterse, M. (2001). A study of functional literacy skills in young adults with Down Syndrome. *International Journal of Disability, Development and Education, 48*, 67–90.

Bosner, S. M., & Belfiore, P. J. (2001). Strategies and considerations for teaching an adolescent with Down Syndrome and Type I diabetes to self-administer insulin. *Education and Training in Mental Retardation and Developmental Disabilities, 36*, 94–102.

Brock, S. R. (2000). An investigation of the long-term neuropsychological outcome of prenatal teratogenic exposure: Fetal alcohol syndrome and maternal PKU syndrome. *Dissertation Abstracts International: Section B: The Sciences and Engineering, 60*(7-B), 3591.

Browder, D. M. (2001). *Curriculum and assessment for students with moderate and severe disabilities*. New York: Guilford.

Campbell, F. A., Pungello, E. P., Miller-Johnson, S., Burchinal, M., & Ramey, C. T. (2001). The development of cognitive and academic abilities: Growth curves from an early childhood educational experiment. *Developmental Psychology, 37*, 231–242.

Chinn, P. L. (1979). *Child health maintenance: Concepts in family-centered care* (2nd ed., p. 109). St. Louis: C. V. Mosby.

Clifft, M. A. (1986). Writing about psychiatric patients: Guidelines for disguising case material. *Bulletin of the Menninger Clinic, 50*, 511–524.

Cornish, K. M., Munir, F., & Cross, G. (2001). Differential impact of the FMR-1 full mutation on memory and attention functioning: A neuropsychological perspective. *Journal of Cognitive Neuroscience, 13*(1), 144–150.

Dickinson, H. (2000). Idiocy in nineteenth-century fiction compared with medical perspectives of the time. *History of Psychiatry, 11*(43, Pt. 3), 291–309.

Dion, E., Prevost, M. J., Carriere, S., Babin, C., & Gois-neau, J. (2001). Phenylalanine restricted diet treatment of the aggressive behaviours of a person with mental retardation. *British Journal of Developmental Disabilities, 47*(92, Pt. 1), 21–29.

Dorland, N. W. (1974). *Dorland's illustrated medical dictionary* (25th ed.). Philadelphia: Saunders.

Drake, E. R., Engler-Todd, L., O'Connor, A. M., Surh, L. C., & Hunter, A. (1999). Development and evaluation of a decision aid about prenatal testing for women of advanced maternal age. *Journal of Genetic Counseling, 8*, 217–233.

Drew, C. J., & Hardman, M. L. (2000). *Mental retardation: A life cycle approach* (7th ed.). New York: MacMillan.

Dykens, E. M., & Hodapp, R. M. (2001). Research in mental retardation: Toward an etiologic approach. *Journal of Child Psychology and Psychiatry and Allied Disciplines, 42*, 49–71.

Dykens, E. M., Hodapp, R. M., & Finucane, B. M. (2000). *Genetics and mental retardation syndromes: A new look at behavior and interventions*. Baltimore: Brookes.

Espy, K. A., Francis, D. J., & Riese, M. L. (2000). Prenatal cocaine exposure and prematurity: Neurodevelopmental growth. *Journal of Developmental and Behavioral Pediatrics, 21*, 262–270.

Felce, D., Lowe, K., Perry, J., Hones, E., Baxter, H., & Bowley, C. (1999). The quality of residential and day services for adults with intellectual disabilities in eight local authorities in England: Objective data gained in support of a social services inspectorate inspection. *Journal of Applied Research in Intellectual Disabilities, 12*(4), 273–293.

Flynn, J. R. (2000). The hidden history of IQ and special education: Can the problems be solved? *Psychology, Public Policy, and Law, 6*(1), 191–198.

Golbeck, S. L. (2001). *Psychological perspectives on early childhood education: Reframing dilemmas in research and practice*. Mahwah, NJ: Erlbaum.

Guralnick, M. J. (2000). *Interdisciplinary clinical assessment of young children with developmental disabilities*. Baltimore: Brookes.

Hall, S., & Oliver, C. (2000). An alternative approach to the sequential analysis of behavioral interactions. In T. Thompson & D. Felce (Eds.), *Behavioral observation: Technology and applications in developmental disabilities* (pp. 335–348). Baltimore: Brookes.

Hardman, M. L., Drew, C. J., & Egan, M. W. (2002). *Human exceptionality: Society, school, and family* (7th ed.). Boston: Allyn & Bacon. *Jackson v. Indiana*. 406 U. S. 715 (1972).

Joyce, T., Ditchfield, H., & Harris, P. (2001). Challenging behaviour in community services. *Journal of Intellectual Disability Research, 45*(2), 130–138.

Kasari, C., & Freeman, S. F. N. (2001). Task-related social behavior in children with Down syndrome. *American Journal on Mental Retardation, 106*, 253–264.

Kau, A. S. M., Reider, E. E., Payne, L., Meyer, W. A., & Freund, L. (2000). Early behavior signs of psychiatric phenotypes in fragile × syndrome. *American Journal on Mental Retardation, 105*, 266–299.

Keith, K. D., & Schalock, R. L. (2000). *Cross-cultural perspectives on quality of life*. Washington, DC: American Association on Mental Retardation.

Keogh, B. K., Garnier, H. E., Bernheimer, L. P., & Gallimore, R. (2000). Models of child-family interactions for children with developmental delays: Child-driven or transactional? *American Journal on Mental Retardation, 105*, 32–46.

Kessler, D. B., & Dawson, P. (1999). *Failure to thrive and pediatric undernutrition: A transdisciplinary approach*. Baltimore: Brookes.

Klinger, L. G., & Dawson, G. (2001). Prototype formation in autism. *Development and Psychopathology, 13*, 111–124.

Kumin, L., & Adams, J. (2000). Developmental apraxia of speech and intelligibility in children with Down syndrome. *Down Syndrome Quarterly, 5*(3), 1–7.

Lacerda, F., von Hofsten, C., & Heimann, M. (2001). *Emerging cognitive abilities in early infancy*. Mahwah, NJ: Erlbaum.

Larson, S. A., Lakin, K. C., Anderson, L., Nohoon, K., Lee, J. H., & Anderson, D. (2001). Prevalence of mental retardation and developmental disabilities: Estimates from the 1994/1995 National Health Interview Survey Disability Supplements. *American Journal on Mental Retardation, 106*, 231–252.

Luckasson, R., & Reeve, A. (2001). Naming, defining, and classifying in mental retardation. *Mental Retardation, 39*, 47–52.

Mank, D., O'Neill, C. T., & Jensen, R. (1998). Quality in supported employment: A new demonstration of the capabilities of people with severe disabilities. *Journal of Vocational Rehabilitation, 11*, 83–95.

McWilliam, P. J. (2000). *Lives in progress: Case stories in early intervention*. Baltimore: Brookes.

Menkes, J. H., Hurst, P. L., & Craig, J. M. (1954). A new syndrome: Progressive familial infantile cerebral dysfunction associated with an unusual urinary substance. *Pediatrics, 14*, 462–467.

Mervis, C. B., Klein-Tasman, B. P., & Mastin, M. E. (2001). Adaptive behavior of 4- through 8-year-old children with Williams syndrome. *American Journal on Mental Retardation, 106*, 82–93.

Miller-Loncar, C. L., Winter, J. M., & Whitman, T. L. (2001). Mental retardation. In M. Hersen & V. B. Van Hasselt (Eds.). *Advanced abnormal psychology* (2nd ed.) (pp. 147–163). New York: Kluwer Academic/Plenum.

Minde, K. (2000). Prematurity and serious medical conditions in infancy: Implications for development, behavior, and intervention. In C. H. Zeanah, Jr. (Ed.), *Handbook of infant mental health* (2nd ed.) (pp. 176–194). New York: Guilford.

Nadeau, L., Boivin, M., Tessier, R., Lefebvre, F., & Robaey, P. (2001). Mediators of behavioural problems in 7-year-old children born after 24 to 28 weeks of gestation. *Journal of Developmental and Behavioral Pediatrics, 22*, 1–10.

National Information Center for Children and Youth with Disabilities. (2001). *General information about Down syndrome* (Fact Sheet No. 4). Washington, DC: Author. Retrieved June 12, 2002 from the World Wide Web: http://www.nichcy.org/pubs/factshe/fs4txt.htm

Nickel, R. E., & Desch, L. W. (2000). *The physician's guide to caring for children with disabilities and chronic conditions*. Baltimore: Brookes.

O'Brien, G. V. (1999). Protecting the social body: Use of the organism metaphor in fighting the "menace of the feebleminded." *Mental Retardation, 37*(3), 188–200.

Oswald, D. P., Coutinho, M. J., Best, A. M., & Nguyen, N. (2001). Impact of sociodemographic characteristics on the identification rates of minority students as having mental retardation. *Mental Retardation, 39*, 351–367.

Picard, E. M., Del-Dotto, J. E., & Breslau, N. (2000). Prematurity and low birthweight. In K. O. Yeates & M. D. Ris (Eds.), *Pediatric neuropsychology: Research, theory, and practice* (pp. 237–251). New York: Guilford.

Roberts, J. E., Mirrett, P., & Burchinal, M. (2001). Receptive and expressive communication development of young males with Fragile X Syndrome. *American Journal on Mental Retardation, 106*, 216–230.

Romski, M. A., Sevcik, R. A., & Wilkinson, K. M. (1994). Peer-directed communicative interactions of augmented language learners with mental retardation. *American Journal on Mental Retardation, 98*, 527–538.

Schonfeld, A. M., Mattson, S. N., Lang, A., Delis, D. C., & Riley, E. P. (2001). Verbal and nonverbal fluency in children with heavy prenatal alcohol exposure. *Journal of Studies on Alcohol, 62*, 239–246.

Schwartz, C., & Armony-Sivan, R. (2001). Students' attitudes to the inclusion of people with disabilities in the community. *Disability and Society, 16*, 401–413.

Shapiro, J., et al. (1993). Separate but equal. *U.S. News & World Report*, December 13.

Slininger, D., Sherrill, C., & Jankowski, C. M. (2000). Children's attitudes toward peers with severe disabilities: Revisiting contact theory. *Adapted Physical Activity Quarterly, 17*, 176–196.

Smith, D. W., & Wilson, A. A. (1973). *The child with Down syndrome (mongolism)*. Philadelphia: Saunders.

Smith, T., Groen, A. D., & Wynn, J. W. (2000). Randomized trial for intensive early intervention for children with pervasive developmental disorder. *American Journal of Mental Retardation, 105*, 269–285.

The Arc (2000). *An introduction to genetics and mental retardation*. Silver Springs, MD: Author. Retrieved June 12, 2002 from the World Wide Web: http://TheArc.org/depts/gbr01.html

U.S. Department of Education. (2000). To assure the free appropriate public education of all children with disabilities. *Twenty-second annual report to Congress on the implementation of the Individuals with Disabilities Education Act*. Washington, DC: U. S. Government Printing Office.

Wakschlag, L. S., Gordon, R. A., Lahey, B. B., Loeber, R., Green, S. M., & Leventhal, B. L. (2000). Maternal age at first birth and boys' risk for conduct disorder. *Journal of Research on Adolescence, 10*, 417–441.

White, D. A., Nortz, M. J., Mandernach, T., Huntington, K., & Steiner, R. D. (2001). Deficits in memory strategy use related to prefrontal dysfunction during early development: Evidence from children with phenylketonuria. *Neuropsychology, 15*, 221–229.

Widaman, K. F. (1999). The process of analyses of data: Benefits and costs associated with collaborative studies. *Mental Retardation and Developmental Disabilities Research Reviews, 5*(2), 155–161.

Yoder, P. J., & Warren, S. F. (2001). Intentional communication elicits language-facilitating maternal responses in dyads with children who have developmental disabilities. *American Journal on Mental Retardation, 106*, 327–335.

York, A., von Fraunhofer, N., Turk, J., & Sedgwick, P. (1999). Fragile-x syndrome, Down's syndrome, and autism: Awareness and knowledge amongst special educators. *Journal of Intellectual Disability Research, 43*, 314–324.

Chapter 13

Abraham, K. (1955). *Selected papers on psychoanalysis*. New York: Basic Books.

Allison, D. B., & Casey, D. E. (2001). Antipsychotic-induced weight gain: A review of the literature. *Journal of Clinical Psychiatry, 62* (Suppl. 7), 22–31.

Aman, M. G., Arnold, L. E., & Armstrong, S. C. (1999). Review of serotonergic agents and perseverative behavior in patients with developmental disabilities. *Mental Retardation and Developmental Disabilities Research Reviews, 5*(4), 279–289.

American Psychiatric Association. (2000). *Diagnostic and statistical manual of mental disorders* (4th ed., text revision). Washington, DC: Author.

Auranen, M., Vanhala, R., Levander, M., Varilo, T., Hietala, M., Riikonen, R., Peltonen, L., Jaervelae, I., & Vosman, M. (2001). MECP2 gene analysis in classical Rett syndrome and patients with Rett-like features. *Neurology, 56,* 611–617.

Ayers, T., Sellers, T., Schneider, D., Gottschling, H., & Soucar, E. (2001). Danforth's comments on parent training research: A rejoinder. *Child and Family Behavior Therapy, 23*(2), 65–66.

Bagalkote, H., Pang, D., & Jones, P. B. (2001). Maternal influenza and schizophrenia in the offspring. *International Journal of Mental Health, 29*(4), 3–21.

Bailey, D. B., Jr., Hatton, D. D., Skinner, M., & Mesibov, G. (2001). Autistic behavior, FMR1 protein, and developmental trajectories in young males with Fragile X syndrome. *Journal of Autism and Developmental Disorders, 31,* 165–174.

Baker, M. J. (2000). Incorporating the thematic ritualistic behaviors of children with autism into games: Increasing social play interactions with siblings. *Journal of Positive Behavior Interventions, 2*(2), 66–84.

Balla, A., Koneru, R., Smiley, J., Sershen, H., & Javitt, D. C. (2001). Continuous phencyclidine treatment induces schizophrenia-like hyperreactivity of striatal dopamine release. *Neuropsychopharmacology, 25,* 157–164.

Barry, L. M., & Singer, G. H. S. (2001). A family in crisis: Replacing the aggressive behavior of a child with autism toward an infant sibling. *Journal of Positive Behavior Interventions, 3,* 28–38.

Bauminger, N., & Yirmiya, N. (2001). The functioning and well-being of siblings of children with autism: Behavioral-genetic and familial contributions. In J. A. Burack and T. Charman (Eds.), *The development of autism: Perspectives from theory and research* (pp. 61–80). Mahwah, NJ: Erlbaum.

Bettelheim, B. (1967). *The empty fortress.* New York: Free Press.

Biklen, D. (1990). Communication unbound: Autism and praxis. *Harvard Educational Review, 60,* 291–314.

Biklen, D. (1992). Typing to talk: Facilitated communication. *American Journal of Speech-Language Pathology, 1*(2), 15–17.

Bishop, D. V. M. (2000). What's so special about Asperger syndrome? The need for further exploration of the borderlands of autism. In A. Klin, F. R. Volkmar, & S. S. Sparrow (Eds.), *Asperger syndrome* (pp. 254–277). New York: Guilford.

Botting, N., & Conti-Ramsden, G. (1999). Pragmatic language impairment without autism: The children in question. *Autism, 3*(4), 371–396.

Broderick, A. A., & Kasa-Hendrickson, C. (2001). "SAY JUST ONE WORD AT FIRST": The emergence of reliable speech in a student labeled with autism. *Journal of the Association for Persons with Severe Handicaps, 26,* 13–24.

Brown, A. S., Cohen, P., Harkavy-Friedman, J., Babulas, V., Malaspina, D., Gorman, J. M., & Susser, E. S. (2001). Prenatal rubella, premorbid abnormalities, and adult schizophrenia. *Biological Psychiatry, 49,* 473–486.

Brushwick, N. L. (2001). Social learning and the etiology of autism. *New Ideas in Psychology, 19,* 49–75.

Cardno, A. G., Sham, P. C., Murray, R. M., & McGuffin, P. (2001). Twin study of symptom dimensions in psychoses. *British Journal of Psychiatry, 179,* 39–45.

Carrington, S., & Graham, L. (2001). Perceptions of school by two teenage boys with Asperger syndrome and their mothers: A qualitative study. *Autism, 5,* 37–48.

Clarke, D. J. (2001). Treatment of schizophrenia. In A. Dosen and K. Day (Eds.), *Treating mental illness and behavior disorders in children and adults with mental retardation* (pp. 183–200). Washington, DC: American Psychiatric Press.

Consenza, A., Bruni, G., & Muratori, F. (2001). VEOS in a six year old girl: Premorbid state, onset, course and therapy. *Psychiatry: Interpersonal and Biological Processes, 63,* 385–398.

Constantino J. N., & Todd, R. D. (2000). Genetic structure of reciprocal social behavior. *American Journal of Psychiatry, 157,* 2043–2044.

Conti-Ramsden, G., Botting, N., Simkin, Z., & Knox, E. (2001). Follow-up of children attending infant language units: Outcomes at 11 years of age. *International Journal of Language and Communication Disorders, 36,* 207–219.

Cormier, S., & Cormier, B. (1998). *Interviewing strategies for helpers: Fundamental skills and cognitive behavioral interventions* (4th ed.). Pacific Grove, CA: Brooks/Cole.

Dales, L., Hammer, S. J., & Smith, N. J. (2001). Time trends in autism and in MMR immunization coverage in California. *Journal of the American Medical Association, 285,* 1183–1185.

Demeter, K. (2000). Assessing the developmental level in Rett syndrome: An alternative approach? *European Child and Adolescent Psychiatry, 9*, 227–233.

Dennis, M., Lazenby, A. L., & Lockyer, L. (2001). Inferential language in high-function children with autism. *Journal of Autism and Developmental Disorders, 31*, 47–54.

Dennis, M., Lockyer, L., Lazenby, A. L., Donnelly, R. E., Wilkinson, M., & Schoonheyt, W. (1999). Intelligence patterns among children with high-functioning autism, phenylketonuria, and childhood head injury. *Journal of Autism and Developmental Disorders, 29*, 5–17.

Depatie, L., & Lal, S. (2001). Apomorphine and the dopamine hypothesis of schizophrenia: A dilemma? *Journal of Psychiatry and Neuroscience, 26*, 203–220.

Dewey, J. T. (1999). Child characteristics affecting stress reactions in parents of children with autism. *Dissertation Abstracts International Section A: Humanities and Social Sciences, 60*(2-A), 0388.

Dissanayke, C., & Sigman, M. (2001). Attachment and emotional responsiveness in children with autism. In L. M. Glidden (Ed.), *International review of research in mental retardation: Autism* (Vol. 23) (pp. 239–266). San Diego, CA: Academic.

Dominigue, B., Cuttler, B., & McTarnaghan, J. (2000). The experience of autism in the lives of families. In A. M. Wetherby and B. M. Prizant (Eds.), *Autism spectrum disorders: A transactional developmental perspective* (Vol. 9) (pp. 369–393). Baltimore: Brookes.

Drew, C. J., & Hardman, M. L. (2000). *Mental retardation: A life cycle approach* (7th ed.). Columbus, OH: Merrill.

Dunn, D. W., & McDougle, C. J. (2001). Childhood-onset schizophrenia. In A. Breier & P. V. Tran (Eds.), *Current issues in the psychopharmacology of schizophrenia* (pp. 375–388). Philadelphia: Lippincott Williams & Wilkins.

Eliez, S., & Reiss, A. L. (2000). MRI neuroimaging of childhood psychiatric disorders: A selective review. *Journal of Child Psychology and Psychiatry and Allied Disciplines, 41*, 679–694.

Erlandson, A., Hallberg, B., Hagberg, B., Wahlstroem, J., & Matinsson, T. (2001). MECP2 mutation screening in Swedish classical Rett syndrome females. *European Child and Adolescent Psychiatry, 10*(2), 117–121.

Evans, I. M., & Meyer, L. H. (2001). Having friends and Rett syndrome: How social relationships create meaningful contexts for limited skills. *Disability and Rehabilitation: An International Multidisciplinary Journal, 23*(3–4), 167–176.

Evans, J. D., Negron, A. E., Palmer, B. W., Paulsen, J. S., Heaton, R. K., & Jeste, D. V. (1999). Cognitive deficits and psychopathology in institutionalized versus community-dwelling elderly schizophrenia patients. *Journal of Geriatric Psychiatry and Neurology, 12*, 11–15.

Fatemi, S. H., Cuadra, A., El Fakahany, E. E., Sidwell, R. W., & Thuras, P. (2000). Prenatal viral infection causes alterations in nNOS expression in developing mouse brains. *NeuroReport, 11*, 1493–1496.

Fein, D. (2001). The primacy of social and language deficits in autism. *Japanese Journal of Special Education, 38*(6), 1–16.

Folstein, S. E., Santangelo, S. L., Gilman, S. E., Piven, J., Landa, R., Lainhart, J., Hein, J., & Wzorek, M. (1999). Predictors of cognitive test patterns in autism families. *Journal of Child Psychology and Psychiatry and Allied Disciplines, 40*, 1117–1128.

Fombonne, E., Simmons, H., Ford, T., Meltzer, H., & Goodman, R. (2001). Prevalence of pervasive developmental disorders in the British Nationwide Survey of Child Mental Health. *Journal of the American Academy of Child and Adolescent Psychiatry, 40*, 820–827.

Frea, W. D., & Vittimberga, G. L. (2000). Behavioral intervention for children with autism. In J. Austin and J. E. Carr (Eds.), *Handbook of applied behavior analysis* (pp. 247–273). Reno, NV: Context Press.

Freedman, R. I., & Boyer, N. C. (2000). The power to choose: Supports for families caring for individuals with developmental disabilities. *Health and Social Work, 25*, 59–68.

Friedman, J. I., Harvey, P. D., Coleman, T., Moriarty, P. J., Bowie, C., Parrella, M., White, L., Adler, D., & Davis, K. L. (2001). Six-year follow-up study of cognitive and functional status across the lifespan in schizophrenia: A comparison with Alzheimer's disease and normal aging. *American Journal of Psychiatry, 158*, 1441–1448.

Glidden, L. M. (2001). *International review of research in mental retardation: Autism* (Vol. 23). San Diego, CA: Academic.

Goldstein, M. J. (1999). Psychosocial treatments for individuals with schizophrenia and related disorders. In N. E. Miller and K. M. Magruder (Eds.), *Cost-effectiveness of psychotherapy: A guide for practitioners, researchers, and policymakers* (pp. 235–247). New York: Oxford University Press.

Green, M. F. (2001). *Schizophrenia revealed: From neurons to social interactions.* New York: Norton.

Gresham, F. M., Beebe-Frankenberger, M. E., & MacMillan, D. L. (1999). A selective review of treatments for children with autism: Description and methodological considerations. *School Psychology Review, 28*, 559–575.

Hardan, A. Y., Minshew, N. J., Harenski, K., & Keshavan, M. S. (2001). Posterior fossa magnetic resonance imaging in autism. *Journal of the American Academy of Child and Adolescent Psychiatry, 40,* 666–672.

Hardman, M. L., Drew, C. J., & Egan, M. W. (2002). *Human exceptionality: Society, school, and family* (7th ed.). Boston: Allyn & Bacon.

Hatton, D. D., & Bailey, D. B., Jr. (2001). Fragile X syndrome and autism. In E. Schopler and N. Yirmiya (Eds.), *The research basis for autism intervention* (pp. 75–89). New York: Kluwer Academic/Plenum.

Heaton, P., Pring, L., & Hermelin, B. (1999). A pseudo-savant: A case of exceptional musical splinter skills. *Neurocase, 5,* 503–509.

Hecimovic, A., Powell, T. H., & Christensen, L. (1999). Supporting families in meeting their needs. In D. B. Zager (Ed.), *Autism: Identification, education, and treatment* (2nd ed.) (pp. 261–299). Mahwah, NJ: Erlbaum.

Henderson, L. A., Yu, P. L., Frysinger, R. C., Galons, J. P., Bandler, R., & Harper, R. M. (2002). Neural responses to intravenous serotonin revealed by functional magnetic resonance imaging. *Journal of Applied Physiology, 92,* 331–342.

Hendry, C. N. (2000). Childhood disintegrative disorder: Should it be considered a distinct diagnosis? *Clinical Psychology Review, 20,* 77–90.

Herken, H., & Erdal, M. E. (2001). Catechol-O-methyltransferase gene polymorphism in schizophrenia: Evidence for association between symptomology and prognosis. *Psychiatric Genetics, 11*(2), 105–109.

Hermelin, B., Pring, L., Buhler, M., Wolff, S., & Heaton, P. (1999). A visually impaired savant artist: Interacting perceptual and memory representations. *Journal of Child Psychology and Psychiatry and Allied Disciplines, 40,* 1129–1139.

Howlin, P. (2000). Outcome in adult life for more able individuals with autism or Asperger syndrome. *Autism, 4,* 63–68.

Huebner, R. A., & Emery, L. J. (1998). Social psychological analysis of facilitated communication: Implications for education. *Mental Retardation, 36,* 259–268.

Ivey, A. E., & Ivey, M. B. (1999). *Intentional interviewing and counseling: Facilitating client development in a multicultural society* (4th ed.). Pacific Grove, CA: Brooks/Cole.

Jacobsen, K., Viken, A., & Von Tetzchner, S. (2001). Rett syndrome and ageing: A case study. *Disability and Rehabilitation: An International Multidisciplinary Journal, 23*(3–4), 160–166.

Jolliffe, T., & Baron-Cohen, S. (2001). A test of central coherence theory: Can adults with high-functioning autism or Asperger syndrome integrate objects in context? *Visual Cognition, 8,* 67–101.

Karmali, I. A. L. (2000). Reducing palilalia and echolalia by teaching the tact operant to young children with autism. *Dissertation Abstracts International: Section B: The Sciences and Engineering, 61*(6-B), 3265.

Karp, B. I., Garvey, M., Jacobsen, L. K., Frazier, J. A., Hamburger, S. D., Bedwell, J. S., & Rapoport, J. L. (2001). Abnormal neurologic maturation in adolescents with early-onset schizophrenia. *American Journal of Psychiatry, 158,* 118–122.

Kauffman, J. (2001). *Characteristics of emotional and behavioral disorders of children and youth* (7th ed.). Columbus, OH: Merrill/Prentice Hall.

Kielinen, M., Linna, S. L., & Moilanen, I. (2000). Autism in northern Finland. *European Child and Adolescent Psychiatry, 9*(3), 162–167.

Kim, J. A., Szatmari, P., Bryson, S. E., Streiner, D. L., & Wilson, F. J. (2000). The prevalence of anxiety and mood problems among children with autism and Asperger syndrome. *Autism, 4*(2), 117–132.

Kjelgaard, M. M., & Tager-Flusberg, W. (2001). An investigation of language impairment in autism: Implications for genetic subgroups. *Language and Cognitive Processes, 16,* 287–308.

Klauber, T. (1999). Warren: From passive and sensuous compliance to a more lively independence: Limited therapeutic objectives with a verbal adolescent. In A. Alvarez & S. Reid (Eds.), *Autism and personality: Findings from the Tavistock Autism Workshop* (pp. 213–227). Florence, KY: Taylor & Francis/Routledge.

Klin, A., Volkmar, F. R., & Sparrow, S. S. (2000). *Asperger syndrome.* New York: Guilford.

Kodama, S., Fukuzako, H., Fukuzako, T., Kiura, T., Nozoe, S., Hashiguchi, T., Yamada, K., Takenouchi, K., Takigawa, M., Nakabeppu, Y., & Nakajo, M. (2001). Aberrant brain activation following motor skill learning in schizophrenic patients as shown by functional magnetic resonance imaging. *Psychological Medicine, 31,* 1079–1088.

Koning, C., & Magill-Evans, J. (2001). Social and language skills in adolescent boys with Asperger syndrome. *Autism, 5,* 23–36.

Koppenhaver, D. A., Erickson, K. A., Harris, B., McLellan, J., Skotko, B. G., & Newton, R. A. (2001). Storybook-based communication intervention for girls with Rett syndrome and their mothers. *Disability and Rehabilitation: An International Multidisciplinary Journal, 23*(3–4), 149–159.

Lenior, M. E., Dingemans, P. M. A. J., Linszen, D. H., de-Haan, L., & Schene, A. H. (2001). Social functioning and the course of early-onset schizophrenia: Five-year follow-up of a psychosocial intervention. *British Journal of Psychiatry, 179*, 53–58.

Liss, M., Harel, B., Fein, D., Allen, D., Dunn, M., Feinstein, C., Morris, R., Waterhouse, L., & Rapin, I. (2001). Predictors and correlates of adaptive functioning in children with developmental disorders. *Journal of Autism and Developmental Disorders, 31*, 219–230.

Magnusson, P., & Saemundsen, E. (2001). Prevalence of autism in Iceland. *Journal of Autism and Developmental Disorders, 31*, 153–163.

Malhotra, S., & Gupta, N. (1999). Childhood disintegrative disorder. *Journal of Autism and Developmental Disorders, 29*, 491–498.

Manning, J. T., Baron-Cohen, S., Wheelwright, S., & Sanders, G. (2001). The 2nd to 4th digit ratio and autism. *Developmental Medicine and Child Neurology, 43*(3), 160–164.

Mastropieri, M. A., & Scruggs, T. E. (2000). The inclusive classroom: Strategies for effective instruction. Upper Saddle River, NJ: Prentice-Hall.

Matthews, B., Shute, R., & Rees, R. (2001). An analysis of stimulus overselectivity in adults with autism. *Journal of Intellectual and Developmental Disability, 26*(2), 161–176.

Mayes, S. D., Calhoun, S. L., & Crites, D. L. (2001). Does DSM-IV Asperger's disorder exist? *Journal of Abnormal Child Psychology, 29*, 263–271.

McDowell, J. E., & Clementz, B. A. (2001). Behavioral and brain imaging studies of saccadic performance in schizophrenia. *Biological Psychology, 57*(1–3), 5–22.

McIntosh, H. (1999). Two autism studies fuel hope—and skepticism. *Monitor on Psychology, 30*(8), 28.

McKerchar, T. L., Kahng, S. W., Casioppo, E., & Wilson, D. (2001). Functional analysis of self-injury maintained by automatic reinforcement: Exposing masked social functions. *Behavioral Interventions, 16*, 59–63.

Moes, D. R., & Frea, W. D. (2000). Using family context to inform intervention planning for the treatment of a child with autism. *Journal of Positive Behavior Interventions, 2*(1), 40–46.

Moldavsky, M., Lev, D., & Lerman-Sagie, T. (2001). Behavioral phenotypes of genetic syndromes: A reference guide for psychiatrists. *Journal of the American Academy of Child and Adolescent Psychiatry, 40*, 749–761.

Mount, R. H., Hastings, R. P., Reilly, S., Cass, H., & Charman, T. (2001). Behavioural and emotional features in Rett Syndrome. *Disability and Rehabilitation: An International Multidisciplinary Journal, 23*(3–4), 129–138.

Moxon, L., & Gates, D. (2001). Children with autism: Supporting the transition to adulthood. *Educational and Child Psychology, 18*(2), 28–40.

Munk-Jorgensen, P., & Ewald, H. (2001). Epidemiology in neurobiological research: Exemplified by the influenza-schizophrenia theory. *British Journal of Psychiatry, 178*(Suppl. 40), s30–s32.

Nally, B., Houlton, B., & Ralph, S. (2000). Researches in brief: The management of television and video by parents of children with autism. *Autism, 4*, 331–337.

Nesbitt, S. (2000). An evaluation of multi-agency service provision for children with autistic spectrum disorders. *British Journal of Developmental Disabilities, 46*(90, Pt. 1), 43–50.

Nunneley, S. A., Martin, C. C., Slauson, J. W., Hearon, C. M., Nickerson, L. D. H., & Mason, P. A. (2002). Changes in regional cerebral metabolism during systemic hyperthermia in humans. *Journal of Applied Physiology, 92*, 846–851.

Oezcankaya, R., Mumcu, N., & Istanbullu, O. (2000). Herpes simplex and cytomegalovirus antibody levels in schizophrenic patients: A controlled study. *Klinik Psikofarmakoloji Buelteni, 10*, 201–204.

Ozonoff, S., Dawson, G., and McPartland, J. (2002). *A parent's guide to Asperger syndrome and high-functioning autism: How to meet the challenges and help your child thrive.* New York: Guilford.

Ozonoff, S., & Griffith, E. M. (2000). Neuropsychological function and the external validity of Asperger syndrome. In A. Klin, F. R. Volkmar, & S. S. Sparrow (Eds.), *Asperger syndrome* (pp. 72–96). New York: Guilford.

Parisse, C. (1999). Cognition and language acquisition in normal and autistic children. *Journal of Neurolinguistics, 12*(3–4), 247–269.

Patterson, A., & Rafferty, A. (2001). Making it to work: Towards employment for the young adult with autism. *International Journal of Language and Communication Disorders, 36*(Suppl.), 475–480.

Pilowsky, T., Yirmiya, N., Arbelle, S., & Mozes, T. (2000). Theory of mind abilities of children with schizophrenia, children with autism, and normally developing children. *Schizophrenia Research, 42*, 145–155.

Piven, J., & Palmer, P. (1999). Psychiatric disorder and the broad autism phenotype: Evidence from a family study of multiple-incidence autism families. *American Journal of Psychiatry, 156*, 557–563.

Posey, D. J., & McDougle, C. J. (2000). The pharmacotherapy of target symptoms associated with autistic disorder and other pervasive developmental disorders. *Harvard Review of Psychiatry, 8*(2), 45–63.

Purcell, A. E., Rocco, M. M., Lenhart, J. A., Hyder, K., Zimmerman, A. W., & Pevsner, J. (2001). Assessment of neural cell adhesion molecule (NCAM) in autistic serum and postmortem brain. *Journal of Autism and Developmental Disorders, 31,* 183–194.

Randall, P., & Parker, J. (1999). *Supporting the families of children with autism.* Chichester, England: Wiley.

Ratey, J. J., Dymek, M. P., Fein, D., Joy, S., Green, L. A., & Waterhouse, L. (2000). Neurodevelopmental disorders. In B. S. Fogel & R. B. Schiffer, (Eds.), *Synopsis of neuropsychiatry* (pp. 245–271). Philadelphia: Lippincott-Raven.

Remington, G., Sloman, L., Konstantareas, M., Parker, K., & Gow, R. (2001). Clomipramine versus haloperidol in the treatment of autistic disorder: A double-blind, placebo-controlled, crossover study. *Journal of Clinical Psychopharmacology, 21,* 440–444.

Rinehart, N. J., Bradshaw, J. L., Brereton, A. V., & Tonge, B. J. (2001). Movement preparation in high-functioning autism and Asperger disorder: A serial choice reaction time task involving motor reprogramming. *Journal of Autism and Developmental Disorders, 31,* 79–88.

Roane, H. S., Piazza, C. C., Sgro, G. M., Volkert, V. M., & Anderson, C. M. (2001). Analysis of aberrant behaviour associated with Rett syndrome. *Disability and Rehabilitation: An International Multidisciplinary Journal, 23*(3–4), 139–148.

Roberts, J. E., Mirrett, P., & Burchinal, M. (2001). Receptive and expressive communication development of young males with Fragile X syndrome. *American Journal on Mental Retardation, 106,* 216–230.

Rode, M. (1999). Echo or answer? The move towards ordinary speech in three children with autistic spectrum disorder. In A. Alvarez & S. Reid (Eds.), *Autism and personality: Findings from the Tavistock Autism Workshop* (pp. 79–92). New York: Routledge.

Romera, M. I., & Gurpegui, M. (2001). Visuo-perceptual processing in patients with schizophrenia treated with typical or atypical antipsychotics. *Acta Espanolas de Psiquiatria, 29,* 19–24.

Rungreangkulkij, S. (2001). Experience of Thai families of a person with schizophrenia: Family stress and adaptation. *Dissertation Abstracts International: Section B: The Sciences and Engineering, 61*(8-B), 4080.

Rutter, M. (2000). Genetic studies of autism: From the 1970s into the millenium. *Journal of Abnormal Child Psychology, 28,* 3–14.

Sabaratnam, M. (2000). Pathological and neuropathological findings in two males with fragile-X syndrome. *Journal of Intellectual Disability Research, 44,* 81–85.

Sacks, O. (1993, December 27/1994, January 3). A neurologist's notebook: An anthropologist on Mars. *The New Yorker,* 106–125.

Safran, S. P. (2001). Asperger syndrome: The emerging challenge to special education. *Exceptional Children, 67,* 151–160.

Satoi, M., Matsuishi, T., Yamada, S., Yamashita, Y., Ohtaki, E., Mori, K., Riikonen, R., Kato, H., & Percy, A. K. (2000). Decreased cerebrospinal fluid levels of beta-phenylethylamine in patients with Rett syndrome. *Annals of Neurology, 47,* 801–803.

Schreibman, L. (2000). Intensive behavioral/psychoeducational treatments for autism: Research needs and future directions. *Journal of Autism and Developmental Disorders, 30,* 373–378.

Sheppard, S. (2000). Autism outreach services—influencing inclusive practice? *Educational and Child Psychology, 17*(4), 17–28.

Shu, B. C., Lung, F. W., Tien, A. Y., & Chen, B. C. (2001). Executive function deficits in non-retarded autistic children. *Autism, 5,* 165–174.

Siff, K. (2001). *Finding Jake: A mother's story.* Retrieved June 20, 2002 from the World Wide Web: http://more.abcnews.go.com/sections/nightline/dailynews/nl_010309_autism_jake1.html

Sperry, V. W. (2001). *Fragile success: Ten autistic children, childhood to adulthood* (2nd ed.). Baltimore: Brookes.

Stodgell, C. J., Ingram, J. L., & Hyman, S. L. (2001). The role of candidate genes in unraveling the genetics of autism. In L. M. Glidden (Ed.), *International review of research in mental retardation: Autism* (Vol. 23). San Diego, CA: Academic.

Sturmey, P., & James, V. (2001). Administrative prevalence of autism in the Texas school system. *Journal of the American Academy of Child and Adolescent Psychiatry, 40,* 621.

Sudhalter, V., & Belser, R. C. (2001). Conversational characteristics of children with Fragile X syndrome: Tangential language. *American Journal on Mental Retardation, 106,* 389–400.

Symon, J. B. (2001). Parent education for autism: Issues in providing services at a glance. *Journal of Positive Behavior Interventions, 3*(3), 160–174.

Szatmari, P. (2000). The classification of autism, Asperger's syndrome, and pervasive developmental disorder. *Canadian Journal of Psychiatry, 45,* 731–738.

Tjus, T., Heimann, M., & Nelson, K. E. (2001). Interaction patterns between children and their teachers when using a specific multimedia and communication strategy: Observations from children with autism and mixed intellectual disabilities. *Autism, 5,* 175–187.

Umansky, R., Watson, J. S., Hoffbuhr, K., Painter, K. M., Devaney, J., & Hoffman, E. (2001). Social facilitation of object-oriented hand use in a Rett syndrome variant girl: Implications for partial preservation of an hypothesized specialized cerebral network. *Journal of Developmental and Behavioral Pediatrics, 22*, 119–122.

U.S. Department of Education. (1991, August 19). Notice of proposed rulemaking. *Federal Register, 56*(160), 41271.

Volkmar, F. R. (2000). Childhood schizophrenia: Developmental aspects. In H. Remschmidt (Ed.), *Schizophrenia in children and adolescents. Cambridge child and adolescent psychiatry* (pp. 60–81). New York: Cambridge University Press.

Volkmar, F. R., & Klin, A. (2001). Asperger's disorder and higher functioning autism: Same or different? In L. M. Glidden (Ed.), *International review of research in mental retardation: Autism* (Vol. 23) (pp. 83–110). San Diego, CA: Academic.

Walton, J. A. (2000). Schizophrenia and life in the world of others. *Canadian Journal of Nursing Research, 32*(3), 69–78.

Ward, M. J., & Meyer, R. N. (1999). Self-determination for people with developmental disabilities and autism: Two self-advocates' perspectives. *Focus on Autism and Other Developmental Disabilities, 14*(3), 133–139.

Wassink, T. H., Piven, J., & Patil, S. R. (2001). Chromosomal abnormalities in a clinic sample of individuals with autistic disorder. *Psychiatric Genetics, 11*(2), 57–63.

Weimer, A. K., Schatz, A. M., Lincoln, A., Ballantyne, A. O., & Trauner, D. A. (2001). "Motor" impairment in Asperger syndrome: Evidence for a deficit in proprioception. *Journal of Developmental and Behavioral Pediatrics, 22*(2), 92–101.

Weiskop, S., Matthews, J., & Richdale, A. (2001). Treatment of sleep problems in a 5-year-old boy with autism using behavioural principles. *Autism, 5*, 209–221.

Weiss, M. J., & Harris, S. L. (2001). *Reaching out, joining in: Teaching social skills to young children with autism.* Bethesda, MD: Woodbine House.

Wheatcraft, T. K., & Bracken, B. A. (1999). Early identification and intervention of psychosocial and behavioral effects of exceptionality. In V. L. Schwean and D. H. Saklofske (Eds.), *Handbook of psychosocial characteristics of exceptional children* (pp. 543–562). New York: Kluwer Academic/Plenum.

Williams, D. (1992). *Nobody nowhere: The extraordinary autobiography of an autistic.* New York: Avon.

Willick, M. S. (2001). Psychoanalysis and schizophrenia: A cautionary tale. *Journal of the American Psychoanalytic Association, 49*, 27–56.

Wing, L. (1981). Asperger's syndrome: A clinical account. *Psychological Medicine, 11*, 115–129.

Wing, L., & Shah, A. (2000). Catatonia in autistic spectrum disorders. *British Journal of Psychiatry, 176*, 357–362.

Witte-Bakken, J. K. (1998). The effects of feedback on the validity of facilitated communication. *Dissertation Abstracts International: Section B: The Sciences and Engineering, 58*(9-B), 5148.

Wolery, M. (2000). The environment as a source of variability: Implications for research with individuals who have autism. *Journal of Autism and Developmental Disorders, 30*, 379–381.

Wootton, A. J. (1999). An investigation of delayed echoing in a child with autism. *First Language, 19*(57, Pt. 3), 359–381.

Ziedonis, D. M., & Stern, R. (2001). Dual recovery therapy for schizophrenia and substance abuse. *Psychiatric Annals, 31*, 255–264.

Zwaigenbaum, L., Szatmari, P., Mahoney, W., Bryson, S., Bartolucci, G., & MacLean, J. (2000). High functioning autism and childhood disintegrative disorder in half brothers. *Journal of Autism and Developmental Disorders, 30*(2), 121–126.

Chapter 14

Abrahams, S., & Udwin, O. (2000). Treatment of post-traumatic stress disorder in an eleven-year-old boy using imaginal and in vivo exposure. *Clinical Child Psychology and Psychiatry, 5*, 387–401.

Alcazar, A. I. R., Rodriguez, J. O., & Sanchez, M. J. (1999). Meta-analysis of behavioural interventions of enuresis in Spain. *Anales de Psicologia, 15*, 157–167.

American Psychiatric Association. (2000). *Diagnostic and statistical manual of mental disorders* (4th ed., text revision). Washington, DC: Author.

Andersen, A. E. (1999). The diagnosis and treatment of eating disorders in primary care medicine. In P. S. Mehler & A. E. Andersen (Eds.), *Eating disorders: A guide to medical care and complications* (pp. 1–26). Baltimore: Johns Hopkins University Press.

Aruffo, R. N., Ibarra, S., & Strupp, K. R. (2000). Encopresis and anal masturbation. *Journal of the American Psychoanalytic Association, 48*, 1327–1354.

Attia, E., Haiman, C., Walsh, B., & Flater, S. R. (1998). Does fluoxetine augment the inpatient treatment of anorexia nervosa? *American Journal of Psychiatry, 255*, 548–551.

Bainbridge, N., & Myles, B. S. (1999). The use of priming to induce toilet training to a child with autism. *Focus on Autism and Other Developmental Disabilities, 14*, 106–109.

Benca, R. M. (2001). Consequences of insomnia and its therapies. *Journal of Clinical Psychiatry, 62* (Supplement 10), 33–38.

Benoit, D. (2000). Regulation and its disorders. In C. Violato & E. Oddone-Paolucci (Eds.), *The changing family and child development* (pp. 149–161). Calgary, Canada: International Congress on the Changing Family and Child Development.

Berg, F. M., & Rosencrans, K. (2000). *Women afraid to eat: Breaking free in today's weight-obsessed world.* Hettinger, ND: Healthy Weight Network.

Bernstein, D. K. (2002). The nature of language and its disorders. In D. K. Bernstein and E. Tiegerman-Farber (Eds.), *Language and communication disorders in children* (5th ed.) (pp. 2–26). Needham Heights, MA: Allyn & Bacon.

Bernstein, D. K., & Levey, S. (2002). Language development: A review. In D. K. Bernstein and E. Tiegerman-Farber (Eds.), *Language and communication disorders in children* (5th ed.) (pp. 27–94). Needham Heights, MA: Allyn & Bacon.

Bessenoff, G. R., & Sherman, J. W. (2000). Automatic and controlled components of prejudice toward fat people: Evaluation versus stereotype activation. *Social Cognition, 18,* 329–353.

Bootzin, R. R. (2000). Cognitive-behavioral treatment of insomnia: Knitting up the ravell'd sleeve of care. In D. T. Kenny & J. G. Carlson (Eds.), *Stress and health: Research and clinical applications* (pp. 243–266). Amsterdam, Netherlands: Harwood Academic Publishers.

Braet, C., Mervielde, I., & Vandereycken, W. (1997). Psychological aspects of childhood obesity: A controlled study in a clinical and nonclinical sample. *Journal of Pediatric Psychology, 22,* 59–71.

Brambilla, F., Bellodi, L., Arancio, C., Limonta, D., Ferrari, E., & Solerte, B. (2001). Neurotransmitter and hormonal background of hostility in anorexia nervosa. *Neuropsychobiology, 43,* 225–232.

Brannon, N., Labbate, L., & Huber, M. (2000). Gabapentin treatment for posttraumatic stress disorder. *Canadian Journal of Psychiatry, 45,* 84.

Bray, G. S. (1999). Pharmacologic therapy of obesity. In D. J. Goldstein (Ed.), *The management of eating disorders and obesity* (pp. 213–248). Totowa, NJ: Humana Press.

Brody, J. E. (1996, January 17). Personal health. *The New York Times,* p. B8.

Brower, K. J., Aldrich, M. S., Robinson, E. A. R., Zucker, R. A., & Greden, J. F. (2001). Insomnia, self-medication, and relapse to alcoholism. *American Journal of Psychiatry, 158,* 399–404.

Bruey, C. T. (2000). Daily life with your child. In M. D. Powers (Ed.), *Children with autism: A parents' guide* (2nd ed.) (pp. 91–118). Bethesda, MD: Woodbine House.

Brumberg, J. J. (2000). *Fasting girls: The history of anorexia nervosa.* New York: Vintage Books.

Bruni, O., Verrillo, E., Miano, S., & Ottaviano, S. (2000). Clinical and historical predictors of sleep disturbances in school-age children. *Sleep and Hypnosis, 2*(4), 147–151.

Bryn, A. S. (1999). Fat, loathing and public health: The complicity of science in a culture of disordered eating. *Culture, Medicine and Psychiatry, 23,* 245–268.

Bulik, C. M., & Sullivan, P. F. (1997). Predictors of the development of bulimia nervosa in women with anorexia nervosa. *Journal of Nervous and Mental Disease, 185,* 704–707.

Button, E. J., & Warren, R. L. (2001). Living with anorexia nervosa: The experience of a cohort of sufferers from anorexia nervosa 7.5 years after initial presentation to a specialized eating disorders service. *European Eating Disorders Review, 9*(2), 74–96.

Chapman, R. S. (2000). Children's language learning: An interactionist perspective. *Journal of Child Psychology and Psychiatry and Allied Disciplines, 41,* 33–54.

Cheng, L. R. L. (2000). Children of yesterday, today and tomorrow: Global implications for child language. *Folia Phoniatrica et Logopaedica, 52*(1–3), 39–47.

Christophersen, E. R., & Mortweet, S. L. (2001). *Treatments that work with children: Empirically supported strategies for managing childhood problems.* Washington, DC: American Psychological Association.

Cicci, R. (1998). Speech and language evaluation. In H. S. Ghuman and R. M. Sarles (Eds.), *Handbook of child and adolescent outpatient, day treatment, and community psychiatry* (pp. 107–114). Philadelphia: Brunner/Mazel.

Cochrane, V. M., & Slade, P. (1999). Appraisal and coping in adults with cleft lip: Associations with well-being and social anxiety. *British Journal of Medical Psychology, 72*(4), 485–503.

Cooper, M., & Burrows, A. (2001). Underlying assumptions and core beliefs related to eating disorders in the mothers of overweight girls. *Behavioural and Cognitive Psychotherapy, 29*(2), 143–149.

Cooper, Z., & Fairburn, C. G. (2001). A new cognitive behavioural approach to the treatment of obesity. *Behaviour Research and Therapy, 39,* 499–511.

Corcos, M., Guilbaud, O., Chaouat, G., Cayol, V., Speranza, M., Chambry, J., Paterniti, S., Moussa, M., Flament, M., & Jeammet, P. (2001). Cytokines and anorexia nervosa. *Psychosomatic Medicine, 63*, 502–504.

Cramer, P., & Steinwert, T. (1998). Thin is good, fat is bad: How early does it begin? *Journal of Applied Developmental Psychology, 19*, 429–451.

Cummings, L. L. (2001). Parent training: A program for parents of two- and three-year-olds. *Dissertation Abstracts International, Section A: Humanities and Social Sciences, 61*(7-A), 4209.

da Fonseca, F. L. (2000). Aesthetic censorship in Maria's dream. *Percurso: Revista de Psicanalise, 13*(25), 59–67.

Dare, C., Chania, E., Eisler, I., Hodes, M., & Dodge, E. (2001). The Eating Disorder Inventory as an instrument to explore change in adolescents in family therapy for anorexia nervosa. *European Eating Disorders Review, 8*(5), 369–383.

Dehaney, R. (2000). Literacy hour and the literal thinker: The inclusion of children with semantic-pragmatic language difficulties in the literacy hour. *Support for Learning, 15*, 35–40.

de Jonge, P. V. H., & van Furth, E. F. (1999). Eating disorders in models: Fiction or fact? *European Eating Disorders Review, 7*, 235–238.

Dettmer, P., Dyck, N., & Thurston, L. P. (1999). *Consultation, collaboration, and teamwork for students with special needs* (3rd ed.). Boston: Allyn & Bacon.

Devlin, M. J., Yanovski, S. Z., & Wilson, G. T. (2000). Obesity: What mental health professionals need to know. *American Journal of Psychiatry, 157*, 854–866.

Diaz, J. M. M., Gasga, L. M., Rodriguez, E. M., Rayon, G. L. A., Aguilar, X. L., & Fernandez, M. R. (1999). Risk factors in eating disorders. *Revista Mexicana de Psicologia, 16*, 37–46.

Didden, R., Skkema, S. P. E., Bosman, I. T. M., Duker, P. C., & Curfs, L. M. G. (2001). Use of a modified Azrin-Foxx toilet training procedure with individuals with Angelman Syndrome. *Journal of Applied Research in Intellectual Disabilities, 14*, 64–70.

Dounchis, J. Z., Hayden, H. A., Wilfley, D. E. (2001). Obesity, body image, and eating disorders in ethnically diverse children and adolescents. In J. K. Thompson & L. Smolak (Eds.), *Body image, eating disorders, and obesity in youth: Assessment, prevention, and treatment* (pp. 67–98). Washington, DC: American Psychological Association.

Drew, C. J., & Hardman, M. L. (2000). *Mental retardation: A life cycle approach* (7th ed.). Columbus, OH: Merrill/Prentice-Hall.

Eisler, I., Dare, C., Russell, G. F. M., Szmukler, G., Le Grange, D., & Dodge, E. (1997). Family and individual therapy in anorexia nervosa: A 5-year follow-up. *Archives of General Psychiatry, 54,* 1025–1030.

Engelsen, B. K., & Laberg, J. C. (2001). A comparison of three questionnaires (EAT-12, EDI, and EDE-Q) for assessment of eating problems in healthy female adolescents. *Nordic Journal of Psychiatry, 55*(2), 129–135.

Fennig, S., & Fennig, S. (1999). Management of encopresis in early adolescence in a medical-psychiatric unit. *General Hospital Psychiatry, 21*, 360–367.

Ferguson, C. P., & Pigott, T. A. (2000). Anorexia and bulimia: Neurobiology and pharmacotherapy. *Behavior Therapy, 31*, 237–263.

Fosse, R. (2000). REM mentation in narcoleptics and normals: Reply to Tore Nielsen. *Consciousness and Cognition: An International Journal, 9*, 514–515.

Gaylor, E. E., Goodlin-Jones, B. L., & Anders, T. F. (2001). Classification of young children's sleep problems: A pilot study. *Journal of the American Academy of Child and Adolescent Psychiatry, 40*, 61–67.

Gelman, V. S., & King, N. J. (2001). Wellbeing of mothers with children exhibiting sleep disturbance. *Australian Journal of Psychology, 53*, 18–22.

Gibbon, F. E. (1999). Undifferentiated lingual gestures in children with articulation/phonological disorders. *Journal of Speech, Language, and Hearing Research, 42*, 382–397.

Gilman, M., & Yaruss, J. S. (2000). Stuttering and relaxation: Applications for somatic education in stuttering treatment. *Journal of Fluency Disorders, 25*, 59–76.

Gottwald, S. R. (1999). Family communication patterns and stuttering development: An analysis of the research literature. In N. B. Ratner and C. E. Healey (Eds.), *Stuttering research and practice: Bridging the gap* (pp. 175–191). Mahwah, NJ: Erlbaum.

Greanleaf, E. (2000). *The problem of evil.* Phoenix, AZ: Xeig, Tucker.

Grilo, C. M. (2001). Pharmacological and psychological treatments of obesity and binge eating disorder. In M. T. Sammons & N. B. Schmidt (Eds.), *Combined treatment for mental disorders: A guide to psychological and pharmacological interventions* (pp. 239–269). Washington, DC: American Psychological Association.

Guitar, B. (1998). *Stuttering: An integrated approach to its nature and treatment* (2nd ed.). Baltimore, MD: Williams & Wilkins.

Hagan, M. M., Whitworth, R. H., & Moss, D. E. (1999). Semistarvation-associated eating behaviors among college binge eaters: A preliminary description and assessment scale. *Behavioral Medicine, 25*(3), 125–132.

Hajak, G. (2001). Epidemiology of severe insomnia and its consequences in Germany. *European Archives of Psychiatry and Clinical Neuroscience, 251*(2), 49–56.

Halmi, K. A., Sunday, S. R., Strober, M., Kaplan, A., Woodside, D. B., Fichter, M., Treasure, J., Berrettini, W. H., & Kaye, W. H. (2000). Perfectionism in anorexia nervosa: Variation by clinical subtype, obsessionality, and pathological eating behavior. *American Journal of Psychiatry, 157,* 1799–1805.

Hardman, M. L., Drew, C. J., & Egan, M. W. (2002). *Human exceptionality: Society, school, and family* (7th ed.). Boston: Allyn & Bacon.

Harel, Z., Hallett, J., Riggs, S., Vaz, R., & Kiessling, L. (2001). Antibodies against human putamen in adolescents with anorexia nervosa. *International Journal of Eating Disorders, 29,* 463–469.

Hoban, T. F. (2000). Sleepiness in children with neurodevelopmental disorders: Epidemiology and management. *CNS-Drugs, 14,* 11–22.

Horrigan, J. P., & Barnhill, L. J. (2000). "Fluvoxamine and enuresis": Comment. *Journal of the American Academy of Child and Adolescent Psychiatry, 39,* 1465–1466.

Howell, P., Sackin, S., & Williams, R. (1999). Differential effects of frequency-shifted feedback between child and adult stutterers. *Journal of Fluency Disorders, 24*(2), 127–136.

Howsam, D.G. (1999). Hypnosis in the treatment of insomnia, nightmares and nightterrors. *Australian Journal of Clinical and Experimental Hypnosis, 27,* 32–39.

Hsu, L. K. G. (1999). Treatment of anorexia nervosa. In D. J. Goldstein (Ed.), *The management of eating disorders and obesity* (pp. 59–70). Totowa, NJ: Humana Press.

Hudson, J. I., Harrison, G. P., & Carter, W. P. (1999). Pharmacologic therapy of bulimia nervosa. In D. J. Goldstein (Ed.), *The management of eating disorders and obesity* (pp. 19–45). Totowa, NJ: Humana Press.

Hunt, J., & Cooper, M. (2001). Selective memory bias in women with bulimia nervosa and women with depression. *Behavioural and Cognitive Psychotherapy, 29,* 93–102.

Iacono, T. A., Chan, J. B., & Waring, R. E. (1998). Efficacy of a parent-implemented early language intervention based on collaborative consultation. *International Journal of Language and Communication Disorders, 33,* 281–303.

Jeffery, R. W. (2001). Public health strategies for obesity treatment and prevention. *American Journal of Health Behavior, 25,* 252–259.

Jelalian, E., & Saelens, B. E. (1999). Empirically supported treatments in pediatric psychology: Pediatric obesity. *Journal of Pediatric Psychology, 24,* 223–248.

Jimerson, S. R., & Pavelski, R. (2000). The school psychologist's primer on anorexia nervosa: A review of research regarding epidemiology, etiology, assessment, and treatment. *California School Psychologist, 5,* 65–77.

Johnson, C. R., & Slomka, G. (2000). Learning, motor, and communication disorders. In M. Hersen & R. T. Ammerman (Eds.), *Advanced abnormal child psychology* (2nd ed.) (pp. 371–385). Mahwah, NJ: Erlbaum.

Kalinowski, J., Stuart, A., Wamsley, L., & Rastatter, M. P. (1999). Effects of monitoring condition and frequency-altered feedback on stuttering frequency. *Journal of Speech, Language, and Hearing Research, 42,* 1347–1354.

Kano, K., & Arisaka, O. (2000). Fluvoxamine and enuresis. *Journal of the American Academy of Child and Adolescent Psychiatry, 39,* 1464–1465.

Karam-Hage, M. & Brower, K. J. (2000). Gabapentin treatment for insomnia associated with alcohol dependence. *American Journal of Psychiatry, 157,* 151.

Kaye, W. H. (1999). Pharmacologic therapy for anorexia nervosa. In D. J. Goldstein (Ed.), *The management of eating disorders and obesity* (pp. 71–79). Totowa, NJ: Humana Press.

Kepele, K. C., & Teixeira, M. A. (2000). Annihilation anxiety: A metapsychological exploration of D. W. Winnicott's *The Piggle. Psychoanalysis and Psychotherapy, 17,* 229–256.

King, N. J., Dudley, A., Melvin, G., Pallant, J., & Morawetz, D. (2001). Empirically supported treatments for insomnia. *Scandinavian Journal of Behaviour Therapy, 30,* 23–32.

Klump, K. L., Miller, K. B., Keel, P. K., McGue, M., & Iacono, W. G. (2001). Genetic and environmental influences on anorexia nervosa syndromes in a population-based twin sample. *Psychological Medicine, 31,* 737–740.

Koethe, M., & Pietrowsky, R. (2001). Behavioral effects of nightmares and their correlations to personality patterns. *Dreaming: Journal of the Association for the Study of Dreams, 11,* 43–52.

Krakow, B., Lowry, C., Germain, A., Gaddy, L., Hollifield, M., Koss, M., Tandberg, D., Johnston, L., & Melendrez, D. (2000). A retrospective study on improvements in nightmares and post-traumatic stress disorder following treatment for co-morbid sleep-disordered breathing. *Journal of Psychosomatic Research, 49,* 291–298.

Kroth, J., McDavit, J., Brendlen, C., Patel, A., & Zwiener, L. (2001). Risk-taking, death anxiety, and dreaming. *Psychological Reports, 88,* 514–516.

Kurzthaler, I., & Fleischhacker, W. W. (2001). The clinical implications of weight gain in schizophrenia. *Journal of Clinical Psychiatry, 62*(Suppl. 7), 32–37.

Lai, K. Y. C. (2000). Anorexia nervosa in Chinese adolescents—Does culture make a difference? *Journal of Adolescence, 23*, 561–568.

Lancioni, G. E., O'Reilly, M. F., & Basili, G. (2001). Treating encopresis in people with disabilities: A literature review. *Journal of Applied Research in Intellectual Disabilities, 14*, 47–63.

Landry, P., Warnes, H., Nielsen, T., & Montplaisir, J. (1999). Somnambulistic-like behaviour in patients attending a lithium clinic. *International Clinical Psychopharmacology, 14*, 173–175.

Levenkron, S. (2000). *Anatomy of anorexia*. New York: W.W. Norton.

Lilenfield, L. R., Kaye, W. H., Greeno, C. G., Merikangas, K. R., Plotnicov, K., Pollice, C., Rao, R., Strober, M., Bulik, C. M., & Nagy, L. (1998). A controlled family study of anorexia nervosa and bulimia nervosa: Psychiatric disorders in first-degree relatives and effects of proband comorbidity. *Archives of General Psychiatry, 55*, 603–610.

Lowe, M. R., Foster, G. D., Kerzhnerman, I., Swain, R. M., & Wadden, T. A. (2001). Restrictive dieting vs. "undieting": Effects on eating regulation in obese clinic attenders. *Addictive Behaviors, 26*, 253–266.

Ludlow, C. L. (1999). A conceptual framework for investigating the neurobiology of stuttering. In N. B. Ratner and C. E. Healey (Eds.), *Stuttering research and practice: Bridging the gap* (pp. 63–84). Mahwah, NJ: Erlbaum.

Mansson, H. (2000). Childhood stuttering: Incidence and development. *Journal of Fluency Disorders, 25*, 47–57.

Matsumoto, T., Miyakawa, T., Yabana, T., Iizuka, H., & Kishimoto, H. (2001). A clinical study of comorbid eating disorders in female methamphetamine abusers: Second report. *Seishin Igaku Clinical Psychiatry, 43*, 57–64.

Max, L., & Caruso, A. J. (1998). Adaptation of stuttering frequency during repeated readings: Associated changes in acoustic parameters of perceptually fluent speech. *Journal of Speech, Language, and Hearing Research, 41*, 1265–1281.

McKee, M. G., & Kiffer, J. F. (2000). Biofeedback and stress. In D. T. Kenny & J. G. Carlson (Eds.), *Stress and health: Research and clinical applications* (pp. 163–178), Amsterdam, Netherlands: Harwood Academic Publishers.

Mehler, P. S., & Crews, C. K. (2001). Refeeding the patient with anorexia nervosa. *Eating Disorders: The Journal of Treatment and Prevention, 9*(2), 167–171.

Miller, M. N., & Pumariega, A. J. (2001). Eating disorders: Bulimia and anorexia nervosa. In V. H. Booney & A. Pumariega (Eds.), *Clinical assessment of child and adolescent behavior* (pp. 234–268). New York: John Wiley & Sons.

Mitchell, J. E., Fletcher, L., Hanson, K., Mussell, M. P., Seim, H., Crosby, R., & AlBanna, M. (2001). The relative efficacy of fluoxetine and manual-based self-help in the treatment of outpatients with bulimia nervosa. *Journal of Clinical Psychopharmacology, 21*, 298–304.

Molfese, D. L., & Molfese, V. J. (2000). The continuum of language development during infancy and early childhood. In C. Rovee-Collier & L. P. Lipsitt (Eds.), *Progress in infancy research* (Vol. 1, pp. 251–287). Mahwah, NJ: Erlbaum.

Muris, P., Merckelbach, H., Gadet, B., & Moulaert, V. (2000). Fears, worries, and scary dreams in 4- to 12-year-old children: Their content, developmental pattern, and origins. *Journal of Clinical Child Psychology, 29*, 43–52.

Muris, P., Merckelbach, H., Ollendick, T. H., King, N. J., & Bogie, N. (2001). Children's nighttime fears: Parent-child ratings of frequency, content, origins, coping behaviors and severity. *Behaviour Research and Therapy, 39*, 13–28.

Murphy, E., & Carr, A. (2000). Enuresis and encopresis. In A. Carr. (Ed.), *What works with children and adolescents?: A critical review of psychological interventions with children, adolescents and their families* (pp. 49–64). Florence, KY: Taylor & Francise/Routledge.

Nauta, H., Hospers, H., Kok, G., & Jansen, A. (2000). A comparison between a cognitive and a behavioral treatment for obese binge eaters and obese non-binge eaters. *Behavior Therapy, 31*, 441–461.

Neiderman, M., Farley, A., Richardson, J., & Lask, B. (2001). Nasogastric feeding in children and adolescents with eating disorders: Toward good practice. *International Journal of Eating Disorders, 29*, 441–448.

Nelson, N. W. (2002). Language intervention in school settings. In D. K. Bernstein and E. Tiegerman-Farber (Eds.), *Language and communication disorders in children* (5th ed.) (pp. 315–353). Needham Heights, MA: Allyn & Bacon.

Neumaerker, K. J., Bettle, N., Neumaerker, U., & Bettle, O. (2000). Age- and gender-related psychological characteristics of adolescent ballet dancers. *Psychopathology, 33*(3), 137–142.

Ohayon, M. M., Guilleminault, C., & Priest, R. G. (1999). Night terrors, sleep-walking, and confusional arousal in the general population: Their frequency and relationship to other sleep and mental disorders. *Journal of Clinical Psychiatry, 60*, 268–276.

Onslow, M., & Packman, A. (1999). The Lidcombe Program of early stuttering intervention. In N. B. Ratner and C. E. Healey (Eds.), *Stuttering research and prac-*

tice: Bridging the gap (pp. 193–209). Mahwah, NJ: Erlbaum.

Oshlag, R. S. (2000). The development and testing of "dry nights" A cognitive-behavioral treatment of nocturnal enuresis. *Dissertation Abstracts International, Section A: Humanities and Social Sciences, 61*(1-A), 84.

Owens, R. E., Jr. (2002). Mental retardation: Difference and delay. In D. K. Bernstein and E. Tiegerman-Farber (Eds.), *Language and communication disorders in children* (5th ed.) (pp. 436–509). Needham Heights, MA: Allyn & Bacon.

Pinhas, H. O. & Zeitler, P. (2000). "Who is the wise man?—the one who foresees consequences": Childhood obesity, new associated comorbidity and prevention. *Preventive Medicine: An International Journal Devoted to Practice and Theory, 31*, 702–705.

Price Foundation Collaborative Group, (2001). Deriving behavioural phenotypes in an international, multicentre study of eating disorders. *Psychological Medicine, 31*, 635–645.

Quine, L. (2001). Sleep problems in primary school children: Comparison between mainstream and special school children. *Child: Care, Health and Development, 27*, 201–221.

Radziewicz, C., & Antonellis, S. (2002). Considerations and implications for habilitation of hearing impaired children. In D. K. Bernstein and E. Tiegerman-Farber (Eds.), *Language and communication disorders in children* (5th ed.) (pp. 565–598). Needham Heights, MA: Allyn & Bacon.

Raffi, A. R., Rodini, M., Grandi, S., & Fava, G. A. (2000). The prodromal phase of bulimia nervosa. *Rivista di Psichiatria, 35*, 270–275.

Ramirez, E. M., & Rosen, J. C. (2001). A comparison of weight control and weight control plus body image therapy for obese men and women. *Journal of Consulting and Clinical Psychology, 69*, 440–446.

Raskind, M. A., Dobie, D. J., Kanter, E. D., Petrie, E. C., Thompson, C. E., & Peskind, E. R. (2000). The alphasub-1-adrenergic antagonist prazosin ameliorates combat trauma nightmares in veterans with posttraumatic stress disorder: A report of 4 cases. *Journal of Clinical Psychiatry, 61*(2) 129–133.

Ratner, N. B., & Healey, C. E. (1999). *Stuttering research and practice: Bridging the gap.* Mahwah, NJ: Erlbaum.

Raynor, H. A., & Epstein, L. H. (2001). Dietary variety, energy regulation, and obesity. *Psychological Bulletin, 127*, 325–341.

Reisch, T., Thommen, M., Tschacher, W., & Hirsbrunner, H. P. (2001). Outcomes of a cognitive-behavioral day treatment program for a heterogeneous patient group. *Psychiatric Services, 52*, 970–972.

Reite, M. (2001). Treatment of insomnia. In A. F. Schatzberg & C. B. Nemeroff (Eds.), *Essentials of clinical psychopharmacology* (pp. 681–714). Washington, DC: American Psychiatric Association.

Richardson, G. S., & Roth, T. (2001). Future directions in the management of insomnia. *Journal of Clinical Psychiatry, 62* (Suppl. 10), 39–45.

Roberts, R. E., Roberts, C. R., & Chen, I. G. (2001). Functioning of adolescents with symptoms of disturbed sleep. *Journal of Youth and Adolescence, 30*, 1–18.

Robinson, N. B., & Robb, M. P. (2002). Early communication assessment and intervention: A dynamic process. In D. K. Bernstein and E. Tiegerman-Farber (Eds.), *Language and communication disorders in children* (5th ed.) (pp. 155–196). Needham Heights, MA: Allyn & Bacon.

Robson, W. L. M., & Leung, A. K. C. (2000). Secondary nocturnal enuresis. *Clinical Pediatrics, 39*, 379–385.

Roehrs, T., Bonahoom, A., Pedrosi, B., Rosenthal, L., & Roth, T. (2001). Treatment regimen and hypnotic self-administration. *Psychopharmacology, 155*, 11–17.

Roth, J. D. (2000). Combined drug treatment for obesity. *Dissertation Abstracts International: Section B: The Sciences and Engineering, 60*(9-B), 4940.

Ruggiero, G. M., Laini, V., Mauri, M. C., Ferrari, V. M. S., Clemente, A., Lugo, F., Mantero, M., Redaelli, G., Zappulli, D., & Cavagnini, F., (2001). A single blind comparison of amisulpride, fluoxetine and clomipramine in the treatment of restricting anorectics. *Progress in Neuro-Psychopharmacology and Biological Psychiatry, 25*, 1049–1059.

Saki, J., & Hebert, F. (2000). Secondary enuresis associated with obstructive sleep apnea. *Journal of the American Academy of Child and Adolescent Psychiatry, 38*, 140–141.

Scammell, T. E., Estabrooke, I. V., McCarthy, M. T., Chemelli, R. M., Yanagisawa, M., Miller, M. S., & Saper, C. B. (2000). Hypothalamic arousal regions are activated during modafinil-induced wakefulness. *Journal of Neuroscience, 20*, 8620–8628.

Schredl, M. (2001). Dreams of singles: Effects of waking-life social contacts on dream content. *Personality and Individual Differences, 31*, 269–275.

Silliman, E. R., & Diehl, S. F. (2002). Assessing children with language learning disabilities. In D. K. Bernstein and E. Tiegerman-Farber (Eds.), *Language and communication disorders in children* (5th ed.) (pp. 181–255). Needham Heights, MA: Allyn & Bacon.

Skelton, S. L. (1999). A comparison of concurrent and hierarchial task sequencing in single-phoneme phonological treatment and generalization. *Dissertation*

Abstracts International: Section B: The Sciences and Engineering, 59(7-B), 3393.

Smedje, H., Broman, J. E., & Hetta, J. (2001). Associations between disturbed sleep and behavioural difficulties in 635 children aged 6 to 8 years: A study based on parents' perceptions. *European Child and Adolescent Psychiatry, 10,* 1–9.

Smith, L., Smith, P., & Lee, S. K. Y. (2000). Behavioural treatment of urinary incontinence and encopresis in children with learning disabilities. *Developmental Medicine and Child Neurology, 42,* 276–279.

Stagg, V., & Burns, M. S. (1999). Specific developmental disorders. In R. T. Ammerman & M. Hersen (Eds.), *Handbook of prescriptive treatments for children and adolescents* (2nd ed.) (pp. 48–62). Boston: Allyn & Bacon.

Stein, M. T., Barbaresi, W. J., & Benuck, I. (2001). An opportunity for office-based research. *Journal of Developmental and Behavioral Pediatrics, 22,* 35–39.

Stein, M. T., & Ferber, R. (2001). Recent onset of sleepwalking in early adolescence. *Journal of Developmental and Behavioral Pediatrics, 22*(Suppl. 2), S33–S35.

Stein, R. J., O'Byrne, K. K., Suminski, R. R., & Haddock, C. K. (1999). Etiology and treatment of obesity in adults and children: Implications for the addiction model. *Drugs and Society, 15*(1–2), 103–121.

Steinhausen, H. C., & Verhulst, F. (1999). *Risks and outcomes in developmental psychopathology.* New York: Oxford University Press.

Stimley, M. A., & Hambrecht, G. (1999). Comparisons of children's single-word articulation proficiency, single-word speech intelligibility, and conversational speech intelligibility. *Journal of Speech Language Pathology and Audiology, 23,* 19–23.

Sullivan, P. F. (1995). Mortality in anorexia nervosa. *American Journal of Psychiatry, 152,* 1073–1074.

Tanofsky, K. M., Wilfley, D. E., & Spurrell, E. (2000). Impact of interpersonal and ego-related stress on restrained eaters. *International Journal of Eating Disorders, 27,* 411–418.

Thomsen, S. R., McCoy, J. K., & Williams, M. (2001). Internalizing the impossible: Anorexic outpatients' experiences with women's beauty and fashion magazines. *Eating Disorders: The Journal of Treatment and Prevention, 9,* 49–64.

Tiegerman-Farber, E. (2002). Interactive teaming: The changing role of the speech/language pathologist. In D. K. Bernstein and E. Tiegerman-Farber (Eds.), *Language and communication disorders in children* (5th ed.) (pp. 96–125). Needham Heights, MA: Allyn & Bacon

U.S. Department of Education, Office of Special Education Programs (2000). *Twenty-second Annual Report to Congress on the Implementation of the Individuals with Disabilities Education Act.* Washington, DC: Author.

Van Borsel, J., Verniers, I., & Bouvry, S. (1999). Public awareness of stuttering. *Folia Phoniatrica et Logopaedica, 51,*(3), 124–132.

Vandereycken, W. (2001). Overeating and overweight: A neglected or disguised disorder? *European Eating Disorders Review, 9,* 141–143.

Vgontzas, A. N., & Kales, A. (1999). Sleep and its disorders. *Annual Review of Medicine, 50,* 387–400.

Wade, T. D., Bulik, C. M., Neale, M., & Kendler, K. S. (2000). Anorexia nervosa and major depression: Shared genetic and environmental risk factors. *American Journal of Psychiatry, 157,* 469–471.

Wagner, S. (1992). Eating disorder treatment stories: Four cases. In R. Lemberg (Ed.), *Controlling eating disorders with facts, advice, and resources* (pp. 58–64). Phoenix, AZ: Oryx Press.

Watson, T. L., Bowers, W. A., & Andersen, A. E. (2000). Involuntary treatment of eating disorders. *American Journal of Psychiatry, 157,* 1806–1810.

Weiss, A. L. (2002). Planning language intervention for young children. In D. K. Bernstein and E. Tiegerman-Farber (Eds.), *Language and communication disorders in children* (5th ed.) (pp. 256–314). Needham Heights, MA: Allyn & Bacon.

Weiss, L., Katzman, M., & Wolchik, S. (1994). Bulimia nervosa: Definition, diagnostic criteria, and associated psychological problems. In L. A. Alexander-Mott & D. B. Lumsden (Eds.), *Understanding eating disorders: Anorexia nervosa, bulimia nervosa, and obesity* (pp. 161–180). Washington, DC: Taylor & Francis.

Westen, D., & Harnden-Fischer, J. (2001). Personality profiles in eating disorders: Rethinking the distinction between Axis I and Axis II. *American Journal of Psychiatry, 158,* 547–562.

Whaley, B. B., & Golden, M. A. (2000). Communicating with persons who stutter: Perceptions and strategies. In D. O. Braithwaite and T. L. Thompson (Eds.), *Handbook of communication and people with disabilities: Research and application* (pp. 423–438). Mahwah, NJ: Erlbaum.

Williamson, D. A., & Netemeyer, S. B. (2000). Cognitive-behavior therapy. In K. J. Miller & J. S. Mizes (Eds.), *Comparative treatments for eating disorders* (pp. 61–81). New York: Springer.

Wisor, J. P., Nishino, S., Sora, I., Uhl, G. H., & Mignot, E. (2001). Dopaminergic role in stimulant-induced wakefulness. *Journal of Neuroscience, 21,* 1787–1794.

Wolff, G. E., Crosby, R. D., Roberts, J. A., & Wittrock, D. A. (2000). Differences in daily stress, mood, coping, and eating behavior in binge eating and nonbinge eating. *Addictive Behaviors, 25,* 205–216.

Yairi, E. (1999). Epidemiologic factors and stuttering research. In N. B. Ratner and C. E. Healey (Eds.), *Stuttering research and practice: Bridging the gap* (pp. 45–53). Mahwah, NJ: Erlbaum.

Zadra, A., & Donderi, D. C. (2000). Nightmares and bad dreams: Their prevalence and relationship to well-being. *Journal of Abnormal Psychology, 109,* 273–281.

Zalsman, G., Weizman, A., Carel, C. A., & Aizenberg, D. (2001). Geriatric Depression Scale (GDS-15): A sensitive and convenient instrument for measuring depression in young anorexic patients. *Journal of Nervous and Mental Disease, 189,* 338–339.

Chapter 15

Alexander, J. F., & Parsons, B. V. (1973). Short-term behavioral intervention with delinquent families: Impact on family process and recidivism. *Journal of Abnormal Psychology, 81,* 219–225.

American Academy of Pediatrics. (2001, October). Guidelines for treatment of attention-deficit/hyperactivity disorder. *Pediatrics.* Accessed Oct. 15, 2001, from the World Wide Web: http://www.aap.org/advocacy/releases/octadhd.htm

Aronson, E. (2000). *Nobody left to hate: Teaching compassion after Columbine.* New York: Worth Publishers.

Axline, V. M. (1976). Play therapy procedures and results. In C. Shaefer (Ed.), *The therapeutic use of child's play.* New York: Jason Aronson.

Bandura, A. (1969). *Principles of behavior modification.* New York: Holt, Rinehart & Winston.

Brestan, E. V., & Eyberg, S. M. (1998). Effective psychosocial treatments of conduct-disordered children and adolescents: 29 years, 82 studies, and 5,272 kids. *Journal of Clinical Child Psychology, 27,* 180–189.

Burns, B. J., Hoagwood, K., & Mrazek, P. J. (1999). Effective treatment for mental disorders in children and adolescents. *Clinical Child and Family Psychology Review, 2,* 199–254.

Cairns, R. B., & Cairns, B. D. (1994). *Lifelines and risks: Pathways of youth in our time.* New York: Cambridge University Press.

Campbell, F. A., & Ramey, C. T. (1994). Effects of early intervention on intellectual and academic achievement: A follow-up study of children from low-income families. *Child Development, 65,* 684–698.

Chamberlain, P., & Reid, J. B. (1991). Using a specialized foster care community treatment model for children and adolescents leaving the state mental hospital. *Journal of Community Psychology, 19,* 266–276.

Chamberlain, P., & Reid, J. B. (1998). Comparison of two community alternatives to incarceration for chronic juvenile offenders. *Journal of Consulting and Clinical Psychology, 66,* 624–633.

Christophersen, E. R., & Mortweet, S. L. (2001). *Treatments that work with children: Empirically supported strategies for managing childhood problems.* Washington, DC: American Psychological Association.

Clarke, G. N., Hawkins, W., Murphy, M., & Sheeber, L. (1993). School-based primary prevention of depressive symptomatology in adolescents: Findings from two studies. *Journal of Adolescent Research, 8,* 183–204.

Clarke, G. N., Rohde, P., Lewinsohn, P. M., Hops, H., & Seeley, J. R. (1999). Cognitive-behavioral treatment of adolescent depression: Efficacy of acute group treatment and booster sessions. *Journal of the American Academy of Child and Adolescent Psychiatry, 38,* 272–279.

Conduct Problems Prevention Research Group. (1999a). Initial impact of the Fast Track prevention trial for conduct problems: I. The high-risk sample. *Journal of Consulting and Clinical Psychology, 67,* 631–647.

Conduct Problems Prevention Research Group. (1999b). Initial impact of the Fast Track prevention trial for conduct problems: II. Classroom effects. *Journal of Consulting and Clinical Psychology, 67,* 648–657.

Conduct Problems Prevention Research Group. (2000). Merging universal and indicated prevention programs: The Fast Track model. *Addictive Behaviors, 25,* 913–927.

Dadds, M. R., Holland, D. E., Laurens, K. R., Mullins, M., Barrett, P. M., & Spence, S. H. (1999). Early intervention and prevention of anxiety disorders in children: Results at a 2-year follow-up. *Journal of Consulting and Clinical Psychology, 67,* 145–150.

DuBois, D. L., Felner, R. D., Meares, H., & Krier, M. (1994). Prospective investigation of the effects of socioeconomic disadvantage, life stress, and social support on early adolescent adjustment. *Journal of Abnormal Psychology, 103,* 511–522.

Everett, C. A., & Volgy, S. S. (1993). Treating the child in systemic family therapy. In T. Kratochwill & R. Morris (Eds.), *Handbook of psychotherapy with children and adolescents* (pp. 247–257). Boston: Allyn & Bacon.

Freud, A. (1945). *The psychoanalytic study of the child: Vol. 1. Indications for child analysis.* New York: International Universities Press.

Gadow, K. D., & Pomeroy, J. C. (1993). Pediatric psychopharmacotherapy: A clinical perspective. In T. Kratochwill & R. Morris (Eds.), *Handbook of psychotherapy with children and adolescents* (pp. 356–402). Needham Heights, MA: Allyn & Bacon.

Gillham, J. E., Reivich, K. J., Jaycox, L. H., & Seligman, M. E. P. (1995). Preventing depressive symptoms in schoolchildren: Two year follow-up. *Psychological Science, 6*, 343–351.

Hall, C. C. (1997). Cultural malpractice: The growing obsolescence of psychology with the changing U.S. population. *American Psychologist, 52*, 642–651.

Jensen, P. S., Bhatara, V. S., Vitiello, B., Hoagwood, K., Feil, M., & Burke, L. B. (1999). Psychoactive medication prescribing practices for U.S. children: Gaps between research and clinical practice. *Journal of the American Academy of Child and Adolescent Psychiatry, 38*, 557–565.

Johnson, J. H., Rasbury, W. C., & Siegel, L. J. (1997). *Approaches to child treatment: Introduction to theory, research, and practice*. Boston: Allyn & Bacon.

Kaplan, C. A., & Hussain, S. (1995). Use of drugs in child and adolescent psychiatry. *British Journal of Psychiatry, 166*, 291–298.

Kazdin, A. E. (1996). Combined and multimodal treatments in child and adolescent psychotherapy: Issues, challenges, and research directions. *Clinical Psychology Science and Practice, 3*, 69–100.

Kazdin, A. E. (2000). *Psychotherapy for children and adolescents: Directions for research and practice*. New York: Oxford University Press.

Kazdin, A. E., Siegel, T. C., & Bass, D. (1990). Drawing upon clinical practice to inform research on child and adolescent psychotherapy. *Professional Psychology: Research and Practice, 21*, 189–190.

Kearney, C. A., & Silverman, W. K. (1998). A critical review of pharmacotherapy for youth with anxiety disorders: Things are not as they seem. *Journal of Anxiety Disorders, 12*, 83–102.

Kendall, P. C. (1991). *Child and adolescent therapy: Cognitive-behavioral procedures*. New York: Guilford.

Kendall, P. C. (1994). Treating anxiety disorders in children: Results of a randomized clinical trial. *Journal of Consulting and Clinical Psychology, 62*, 100–110.

Koocher, G., & D'Angelo, E. J. (1992). Evolution of practice in child psychotherapy. In I. Freedheim (Ed.), *History of psychotherapy* (pp. 457–492). Washington, DC: American Psychological Association.

Leblanc, M., & Ritchie, M. (2001). A meta-analysis of play therapy outcomes. *Counselling Psychology Quarterly, 14*, 149–163.

March, J. S., Franklin, M., Nelson, A., & Foa, E. (2001). Cognitive-behavioral psychotherapy for pediatric obsessive-compulsive disorder. *Journal of Clinical Child Psychology, 30*, 8–18.

Meichenbaum, D., & Goodman, J. (1971). Training impulsive children to talk to themselves: A means of developing self-control. *Journal of Abnormal Psychology, 77*, 115–126.

Morris, R. J., & Kratochwill, T. R. (1983). *Treating children's fears and phobias: A behavioral approach*. New York: Pergamon Press.

MTA Cooperative Group. (1999a). A 14-month randomized clinical trial of treatment strategies for attention-deficit/hyperactivity disorder. *Archives of General Psychiatry, 56*, 1073–1086.

MTA Cooperative Group. (1999b). Moderators and mediators of treatment response for children with attention-deficit/hyperactivity disorder. *Archives of General Psychiatry, 56*, 1088–1095.

Murphy, D. A., Greenstein, J. J., & Pelham, W. E. (1993). Pharmacological treatment. In V. B. Van Hasselt & M. Hersen (Eds.), *Handbook of behavior therapy and pharmacotherapy for children* (pp. 333–378). Boston: Allyn & Bacon.

Patterson, G. R., Dishion, T. J., & Chamberlain, P. (1993). Outcomes and methodological issues related to treatment of antisocial children. In T. R. Giles (Ed.), *Handbook of effecive psychotherapy* (pp. 43–88). New York: Plenum.

Patterson, G. R., Reid, J. B., & Dishion, T. J. (1975). *A social learning approach: I. Families with aggressive children*. Eugene, OR: Castalia.

Patterson, G. R., Reid, J. B., & Dishion, T. J. (1992). *Antisocial boys*. Eugene, OR: Castalia.

Patterson, G. R., & Stoolmiller, M. (1991). Replications of a dual failure model for boys' depressed mood. *Journal of Consulting and Clinical Psychology, 59*, 491–498.

Pelham, W. E., Wheeler, T., & Chronis, A. (1998). Empirically supported psychosocial treatments for attention-deficit hyperactivity disorder. *Journal of Clinical Child Psychology, 27*, 190–205.

Ramey, C. T., & Ramey, S. L. (1996). Early intervention: Optimizing development for children with disabilities and risk conditions. In M. Wolraich (Ed.), *Disorders of development and learning: A practical guide to assessment and management* (2nd ed.) (pp. 141–158). Philadelphia: Mosby.

Ramey. C. T., & Ramey, S. L. (1998). Early intervention and early experience. *American Psychologist, 53*, 109–120.

Reichman, N. E., & McLanahan, S. S. (2001). Self-sufficiency programs and parenting interventions: Lessons from New Chance and the Teenage Parent Demonstration. *Social Policy Report, 15*, 1–14.

Resnick, M. D., Bearman, P. S., Blum, R. W., Bauman, K. E., Harris, K. M., Jones, J., Tabor, J., Beuhring, T., Sieving, R. E., Shew, M., Ireland, M., Bearinger, L. H., & Udry, J. R. (1997). Protecting adolescents from harm: Findings from the National Longitudinal Study on Adolescent Health. *Journal of the American Medical Association, 278,* 823–832.

Rodriguez, R. R., & Walls, N. E. (2000). Culturally educated questioning: Toward a skills-based approach in multicultural counselor training. *Applied & Preventive Psychology, 9,* 89–99.

Rogers, C. T. (1951). *Client-centered therapy: Its current practice, implications, and theory.* Boston: Houghton Mifflin.

Roth, J., & Brooks-Gunn, J. (2000). What do adolescents need for healthy development? Implications for youth policy. *Social Policy Report, 14,* 1–20.

Russ, S. W. (1995). Play psychotherapy research: State the science. In T. Ollendick & R. Prinz (Eds.), *Advances in clinical child psychology,* Vol. 17 (pp. 365–392). New York: Plenum Press.

Satir, V. (1967). *Conjoint family therapy: A guide.* Palo Alto, CA: Science and Behavior Books.

Schafer, W. (1992). *Stress management for wellness.* Fort Worth: Holt, Rinehart & Winston.

Shadish, W. R., Montgomery, L. M., Wilson, P., Wilson, M. R., Bright, I., & Okwumabua, T. (1993). Effects of family and marital psychotherapies: A meta-analysis. *Journal of Consulting and Clinical Psychology, 61,* 992–1002.

Thorpe, G. L., & Olson, S. L. (1997). *Behavior therapy: Concepts, procedures, and applications* (2nd ed). Boston: Allyn & Bacon.

Tuma, J., & Russ, S. W. (1993). Psychoanalytic psychotherapy with children. In T. Kratochwill & R. Morris (Eds.), *Handbook of psychotherapy with childen and adolescents* (pp. 131–161). Boston: Allyn & Bacon.

Wagner, K. D., Birmaher, B., Carlson, G., Clarke, G., Emslie, G., Geller, B., Keller, M. R., Klein, R., Kutcher, S., Papatheodorou, G., Ryan, N., Strober, M., & Weller, E. (1998). *Safety of paroxetine and imipramine in the treatment of adolescent depression.* Paper presented at the 38th annual Meeting of the NIMH New Clinical Drug Evaluation Unit, Boca Raton, FL, June 10–13.

Webster-Stratton, C. (1996). Early intervention with videotape modeling: Programs for families of children with oppositional defiant disorder or conduct disorder. In E. D. Hibbs & P. S. Jensen (Eds.), *Psychosocial treatment research of child and adolescent disorders: Empirically based strategies for clinical practice* (pp. 435–474). Washington, DC: American Psychological Association.

Webster-Stratton, C., & Herbert, M. (1993). "What really happens in parent training?" *Behavior Modification, 17,* 407–456.

Webster-Stratton, C., & Herbert, M. (1994). *Troubled families—problem children: A collaborative approach to working with families.* Chichester, England: Wiley.

Weiss, B., Catron, T., Harris, V., & Phung, T. M. (1999). The effectiveness of traditional child psychotherapy. *Journal of Consulting and Clinical Psychology, 67,* 82–94.

Weisz, J. R., Weiss, B., Han, S. S., Granger, D. A., & Morton, T. (1995). Effects of psychotherapy with children and adolescents revisited: A meta-analysis of treatment outcome studies. *Psychological Bulletin, 117,* 450–468.

Werry, J. S. (2001). Pharmacological treatments of autism, attention-deficit/hyperactivity disorder, oppositional defiant disorder, and depression in children and youth—Commentary. *Journal of Clinical Child Psychology, 30,* 110–113.

Werner, E. E., & Smith, R. S. (1992). *Overcoming the odds: High risk children from birth to adulthood.* Ithaca, NY: Cornell University Press.

Name Index

Bruni, G., 308
Bruni, O., 332
Brushwick, N. L., 303
Bry, B. H., 230
Bryant, B. R., 243
Bryant, D. P., 243
Bryn, A. S., 322, 323
Bryson, S. E., 294
Buckingham, D., 210
Buhler, M., 292
Bulik, C. M., 314, 315
Burchardt, C. M., 163, 164
Burchinal, M., 270, 279, 305
Burke, R., 182
Burns, B. J., 169, 348, 352, 354, 356, 357, 361
Burns, M. S., 340
Burrows, A., 321
Bursuck, W. D., 243
Bushman, B. J., 230
Buss, K. A., 183
Button, E. J., 319
Buysse, A., 204, 226
Byrne, D., 222

C

Caffey, J., 124
Cairns, B. D., 361
Cairns, R. B., 361
Calderon, R., 200, 243
Calhoun, S. L., 289
Calkins, C., 60
Calkins, S. D., 165
Cambridge, P., 255
Cameron, R. P., 181
Campbell, F. A., 279, 359
Campbell, V. L., 88
Canadian Psychiatric Association, 134
Canino, G., 99
Canino, I., 99
Cantor, J., 229
Cantwell, C., 192
Cantwell, D. P., 172
Cardno, A. G., 305
Carel, C. A., 318
Carey, C. A., 116
Carlsmith, K. M., 234
Carlson, E., 16
Carlson, R. S., 132
Carlyon, W., 88
Carpenter, D., 171
Carr, A., 211, 326, 327, 328
Carriere, S., 270
Carrington, S., 294
Carta, J. J., 113
Carter, W. P., 321

Caruso, A. J., 340
Casey, B. J., 206
Casey, D. E., 307
Casey, J. E., 91
Cashdan, S., 37
Casioppo, E., 291
Caspi, A., 109, 218
Cass, H., 295
Castellanos, F. X., 206
Cataldo, M. F., 224
Catron, T., 348
Cauce, A. M., 126
Caudra, A., 304
Cavell, T. A., 227
Ceci, S. J., 135, 137, 138
Centers for Disease Control, 232
Chabanski, S., 114
Chamberlain, P., 354, 355
Champagnon, N., 207
Chan, J. B., 337
Chang, S. Y., 121
Chania, E., 318
Chapman, R. S., 335
Charman, T., 295
Charnov, E. L., 37
Chassin, L., 109
Chater, R., 99
Chavkin, W., 116
Chen, B. C., 291
Chen, I. G., 328
Chen. R., 204
Chen, R. S., 217
Cheng, L. R. L., 335
Cheour, M., 245
Cherland, E., 207
Cherulnik, P. D., 218
Children's Defense Fund, 107
Chinn, P. L., 274
Chirboga, J., 194
Chomsky, N., 42
Chorpita, B. F., 158, 162
Christensen, L., 291
Christenson, S. L., 230
Christopher, J., 184
Christophersen, E. R., 326, 327, 328, 347, 351
Chronis, A., 357
Cicchetti, D., 37, 39, 141, 142, 144, 184, 189
Cicci, R., 337
Clare, S. K., 96
Clarizio, H. F., 205
Clark, E., 95
Clark, R., 189
Clarke, D. J., 306, 307
Clarke, G. N., 187, 361
Clarke, J. C., 167

Clemence, A. J., 88
Clementz, B. A., 304
Clifft, M. A., 261
Coates, D. D., 218
Coccaro, E. F., 227
Cochrane, V. M., 338
Codina, G. E., 254
Cohen, A., 241
Cohen, D. J., 192
Cohen, D. S., 116
Cohen, H., 147, 150
Cohen, P., 142
Coie, J., 218, 220, 232, 234
Cole, C. F., 229
Cole, C. L., 96
Colledge, E., 200
Collins, R. L., 155
Collins, W. A., 227
Colliver, J. D., 108
Colten, M. E., 179
Condon, M., 249
Conduct Problems Prevention Research Group, 230, 359
Cone, J. D., 95, 96
Connors, C. K., 210, 255
Connors, K. C., 94
Consenza, A., 308
Constantino, J. N., 305
Conti-Ramsden, N., 292, 300
Cook, E. J., Jr., 208
Cook, P. W., 228
Cooke, M. C., 229
Cooley-Quille, M., 232
Cooper, M., 320, 321
Cooper, V., 221
Cooper, Z., 323
Corcos, M., 318
Cordell, A. S., 250
Cormier, B., 306
Cormier, S., 306
Cornish, K. M., 270
Cory-Slechta, D. A., 208
Costello, E. J., 98, 219, 220
Costin, J., 207
Cottle, C. C., 230
Cottle, T. J., 220
Council of Economic Advisors, 111
Coury, D. L., 135
Coutinho, M. J., 276
Cowan, C. P., 182
Cowan, P. A., 182
Cowardin, J., 231
Cowart, L. U., 223
Coy, K. C., 223
Craig, J. M., 271
Cramer, P., 323
Crawford, S. G., 240

Emery, L. J., 306
Emslie, G. J., 187
Engelsen, B. K., 318
Engler-Todd, L., 271
Entwistle, P. C., 202
Epstein, J. A., 108
Epstein, L. H., 321
Erdal, M. E., 303, 305
Erikson, E. H., 14, 35
Erlandson, A., 295
Erlich, J., 234
Ervin, R. A., 211
Esbensen, F. A., 233
Escamillo, A. G., 230
Escera, C., 250
Eshleman, A. S., 208
Espie, C. A., 263
Esplin, P. W., 134, 139
Espy, K. A., 273
Essex, M., 225
Estes, A., 116
Evans, I. M., 295
Evans, J. D., 308
Evans, S. W., 210
Everett, C. A., 352
Everson, M. D., 136, 138
Ewald, H., 303, 304
Eyberg, S. M., 229, 348, 350, 352
Ezell, E., 227

F

Fagg, J., 191
Fairburn, C. G., 323
Falkov, A. F., 136
Fallgatter, A. J., 200
Faraone, S. V., 186, 206, 207, 209
Farley, A., 318
Faroy, M., 226
Farrington, D. P., 111, 218, 234
Fatemi, S. H., 304
Faust, J., 89
Fava, G. A., 321
Fegley, S., 107
Fein, D., 303
Feinberg, M., 227
Feinberg, T. L., 188
Feingold, B. F., 208
Feisher, P. A., 200
Feit, A., 88
Feivelson, D., 14
Felce, D., 283
Feldman, J. F., 248
Felner, R. D., 361
Felthous, A., 218
Fenichel, E., 142, 143, 144
Fennig, S., 326, 327

Ferber, R., 332
Ferguson, C. P., 321
Ferretti, L., 148
Ferretti, R. P., 244
Ferster, C. B., 185
Fetkewicz, J. M., 134
Ficula, T., 162, 163
Figueirdo, D., 200
Finkelhor, D., 131, 132, 135
Finucane, B. M., 270
Fisch, S., 229
Fischer, M., 202
Fisher, P. A., 243
Fisher, P., 98
Fitzpatrick, C., 158
Fitzpatrick, R., 207
Flannery-Schroeder, E. C., 169
Flater, S. R., 319
Fleck, S. G., 202
Fleishhacker, W. W., 323
Flekkov, M. G., 147
Flemming, J., 130, 135
Floyd, R. D., 114
Flynn, J. R., 263
Flynn-Corwyn, R., 234
Foa, E., 171, 344
Foa, E. B., 146, 171
Folkman, S., 72
Follette, V. M., 142
Follette, W. C., 99
Folstein, S. E., 290
Folstrom-Bergeron, B. M., 211
Fombonne, E., 179, 202, 221, 295
Fonagy, P., 34
Forbes, G. B., 205, 222
Ford, T., 295
Foreman, A. L., 243
Forgatch, M. S., 12, 223
Forness, S. R., 67, 248
Forney, W., 200
Fosse, R., 334
Foster, G. D., 322
Foster, S. L., 95
Fowler, J. C., 88
Fox, N. A., 165
Foxhall, K., 108, 116
Fraenkel, J. R., 55, 65
Frances, A., 171
Francis, D. J., 273
Franco, P., 114
Francoeur, E., 138
Frank, D. A., 116
Frankenberger, W., 205, 241
Franklin, M., 171, 344
Franklin, M. E., 255
Frea, W. D., 96, 306, 307, 308
Freedman, R. I., 291

Freeman, D., 56
Freeman, L., 181
Freeman, S. F. N., 270
French, D. C., 108
French, S., 193
Freres, D. R., 190
Freud, A., 33, 164, 346
Freud, S., 33, 164, 171, 184
Freund, L., 270
Friedlander, K., 229
Friedman, J. I., 308
Frisby, C. L., 83
Fristad, M. A., 98
Fritz, G., 194
Frosh, S., 34
Fu, G., 89
Fuller, J. B., 67
Futterweit, L. R., 248

G

Gadet, B., 330
Gadow, K. D., 356
Gall, J. P., 54
Gall, M. D., 54
Gallimore, R., 276
Galton, F., 86
Gammon, G. D., 192
Garb, H. N., 88
Gardill, M. C., 243, 257
Gardner, H., 87, 88
Gardner, W., 37
Garfinkel, I., 130
Garmezy, N., 162
Garnier, H. E., 276
Garrison, C. Z., 179
Garza, N. D., 91
Gates, D., 308
Gauggel, S., 206
Gay, L., 65
Gaylor, E. E., 329
Gelfand, D. M., 37, 100, 103, 143, 162, 163, 182, 184, 189
Gellar, V., 200, 226
Geller, B., 8
Gelles, R. J., 145
Gelman, V. S., 328
Gendreau, P., 234
George, T. P., 182
George, W. H., 226
Gephart, H., 209
Gerpegui, M., 307
Gersten, R., 250
Ghinglia, K., 86
Giannetti, J. M., 116
Gibbon, F. E., 338
Gidycz, C. A., 145

Hebert, F., 327
Hechtman, L., 96
Hecimovic, A., 291
Hecker, L., 257
Heilbrun, K., 230
Heimann, M., 276, 290
Heimberg, R. G., 162, 193
Heinecke, C. M., 166
Hektner, J. M., 230
Hektner, J. S., 163, 164
Hempelman, K. A., 124
Henderson, H. A., 165
Henderson, L. A., 304
Hendry, C. N., 295, 296
Henggeler, S. W., 121
Henker, B., 205
Herbert, J. D., 161
Herbert, M., 355
Herken, H., 303
Hermelin, B., 292
Hernstein, R. J., 83
Hersen, M., 166
Hershberger, S. L., 193
Hershkowitz, I., 139
Herzog, D. B., 181
Hess, L. E., 227
Hester, K., 67
Hetherington, E. M., 227
Hetta, J., 328
Hewlett, K., 110
Hill, J., 218, 221
Hillsenroth, M. J., 88
Hilmer, C. D., 88
Hindman, P. M., 223
Hirsbrunner, H. P., 317
Hirschfield, P., 112
Hitch, G. J., 250
Hoagwood, K., 169, 348
Hoban, T. F., 328
Hoch, H., 100
Hodapp, R. M., 268, 270
Hodes, M., 318
Hoeksma, J. B., 20
Hofferth, S. L., 111
Hoffman, D., 158
Hoffner, C., 229
Hogben, M., 222
Hollins, S., 256
Holly, M. L., 75
Holmes, W. C., 133, 135
Holtzman, D., 114
Holtzman, W. H., 90
Honigmann, J. J., 56
Hopkins, K. D., 87, 94
Hoppes, M. K., 244
Hops, H., 181, 185, 187, 361
Horgan, J., 226
Hornig, C. D., 161

Horrigan, J. P., 328
Hospers, H., 322
Hougham, G. W., 74
Houlton, B., 302
Howe, G., 227
Howell, P., 340
Howlin, P., 308
Howsam, D. G., 332
Hoyt, D. R., 126
Hoza, B., 210
Hser, Y., 108, 119
Hsu, L. K. G., 318, 319
Huber, M., 332
Hudson J. I., 321
Huebner, R. A., 306
Huesman, L. R., 228
Humphrey, L., 184
Humphreys, G. W., 248
Hunsley, J., 89
Hunt, G. P., 233
Hunt, J., 320
Hunter, A., 271
Huntington, K., 270
Hur, Y., 27
Hurley, C., 96
Hurst, P. L., 271
Hurt, H., 116
Hussain, S., 169, 172, 357
Hybel, L. G., 112
Hyman, S. L., 305

I

Iacono, T. A., 337, 338
Iacono, W. G., 221, 318
Ialongo, N., 12
Ibarra, S., 326
Iizuka, H., 321
Inamdar, S., 216
Individuals with Disabilities Act
   (IDEA), 79, 100
Ingram, J. L., 305
Ingram, M. A., 255
Ingram, R. E., 188
Ireland, M., 193
Isabella, R., 37, 184
Ison, M. S., 230
Istanbullu, O., 304
Ivey, A. E., 306
Ivey, M. B., 306
Iwata, B. A., 100

J

Jackson v. Indiana, 282
Jacobsen, K., 295
James, A., 250

James, V., 297, 298
Jameson, P., 182, 189
Janda, L., 94
Jankowski, C. M., 281
Jankowski, J. J., 248
Jansen, A., 322
Javitt, D. C., 305
Jaycox, L. H., 360
Jeffery, R. W., 321, 322, 324
Jelalian, E., 324
Jenkens, Y. M., 250, 254
Jenkins, A., 210
Jenkins, J. R., 245
Jennings, E., 252
Jensen, P. S., 181, 187, 207, 209, 356, 357
Jensen, R., 281
Jenson, W. R., 95, 96, 99, 222
Jessor, R., 106
Jessor, S. L., 106
Jimerson, S. R., 315, 318
Jitendra, A. K., 243, 244, 257
Johnson, A., 231
Johnson, B. D., 241, 243
Johnson, C. R., 334, 338
Johnson, D., 245, 250, 257
Johnson, E. O., 253
Johnson, J., 161
Johnson, J. G., 142
Johnson, J. H., 348, 351
Johnson, J. K., 226
Johnson, M. H., 31
Johnson, N. E., 87
Johnson, R. C., 204
Johnson, V. K., 182
Johnson-Cramer, N. L., 208
Johnston, C., 209
Jolliffe, T., 294
Jones, M. L., 209
Jones, P. B., 304
Jones, S. E., 71
Jordan, N. C., 245
Joseph, J., 227
Joshi, V., 108
Jouriles, E. N., 227
Joyce, T., 283

K

Kagan, J., 202
Kahlenberg, R., 113
Kahn, A., 114
Kahn, D., 171
Kahng, S. W., 291
Kalb, L., 225
Kales, A., 332
Kalinowski, J., 340
Kamann, M. P., 247

Mehler, P. S., 317, 318
Meichenbaum, D., 350
Meier, B., 117
Mellan, B., 255
Melnick, S., 141
Meloy, J. R., 229
Meltzer, H., 295
Menkes, J. H., 271
Menna, R., 217, 218
Menzies, R. G., 167
Merckelbach, H., 330
Merrell, K. W., 79, 204
Merritt, R. K., 114
Mervielde, I., 323
Mervis, C. B., 263
Mesibov, G., 270, 305
Messinger, D. S., 37, 184
Metalsky, G. I., 184
Meyer, D. R., 130
Meyer, G., 83
Meyer, G. J., 17, 18
Meyer, L. H., 295
Meyer, M. S., 243
Meyer, R. N., 290
Meyer, W. A., 270
Miano, S., 332
Mick, E., 207
Mignot, E., 334
Miller, L. S., 228
Miller, K. B., 318
Miller, M. N., 318, 319
Miller-Johnson, S., 279
Miller-Loncar, C. L., 265
Milne, L. C., 88
Minde, K., 273, 275
Minshew, N. J., 304
Mirrett, P., 270, 305
Mischel, W., 42, 45, 85
Mitchell, J. E., 321
Mitka, M., 153
Mitsis, E. M., 99
Miyakawa, T., 321
Mize, J., 219
Modestin, J., 223
Moes, D. R., 307
Moffitt, T., 109
Moffitt, T. E., 218
Moilanen, I., 290
Mokros, H., 181
Moldavsky, M., 295
Molfese, D. L., 334, 338
Molfese, V. J., 334, 338
Molina, B. S. G., 202
Molteni, M., 263
Monroe, S. M., 183, 185, 193
Montgomery, D. T., 228
Montplaisir, J., 332

Monuteaux, M. C., 207
Moon, S. M., 210
Moore, J., 202
Morawetz, D., 333
Morenoff, J., 108
Morgan, D. L., 63
Morgan, D. P., 99
Morgan, G. A., 55
Morgan, K., 12
Morgan, R. K., 63
Morris, M. M., 209
Morris, R. J., 167, 351
Morton, T., 230, 349
Mortweet, S. L., 326, 327, 328, 347, 351
Moss, D. E., 319
Moss, S., 241, 257
Most, T., 249
Moulaert, V., 330
Mount, R. H., 295
Mouren-Simeoni, M. C., 159
Moxon, L., 308
Mozes, T., 296
Mrazek, P. J., 169, 348
MTA Cooperative Group, 356, 361
Mulcahey, J. J., 30
Mullen, P., 130
Mulsow, M. H., 209
Mumcu, N., 304
Munir, F., 270
Munk-Jorgensen, P., 303, 304
Munneke, D. M., 223
Muratori, F., 308
Muris, P., 330
Murphy, D. A., 158, 357
Murphy, E., 326, 327, 328
Murphy, M., 361
Murray, C., 83, 258
Murray, C. J. C., 179
Murray, H. A., 90
Murray, J. P., 229
Murray, K. T., 223
Murray, R. M., 305
Murray, V. M., 209
Myers, D. G., 155
Myles, B. S., 325

N

Nadder, T. S., 208, 227
Nadeau, L., 275
Nadel, N. M., 216
Naglieri, J. A., 90, 241, 245, 250, 257
Naik, B. I., 210, 255
Naimark, H., 147
Nally, B., 302
Nansel, T. R., 231
Narrow, W. E., 178

Nathan, P. E., 99
National Center for Health Statistics, 190, 191
National Clearinghouse for Alcohol and Drug Information, 117
National Information Center for Children and Youth with Disabilities, 269
National Institute of Mental Health (NIMH), 161, 191, 208, 209
National Institute on Drug Abuse (NIDA), 103, 108, 114
National Institutes of Health (NIH), 199, 210, 211
Nauta, H., 322
Neale, M., 317
Negy, C., 91
Neiderhiser, J., 227
Neiderman, M., 318
Nelson, A., 171, 344
Nelson, J. R., 231
Nelson, K. E., 290
Nelson, L. J., 165
Nelson, N. W., 337, 338
Nelson-Gray, R. O., 96
Nesbitt, S., 289
Netemeyer, S. B., 321
Neumaerker, K. J., 314
Neumaerker, U., 314
Newcheck, P. W., 240
Newcorn, J. H., 99
Newman, D. L., 27, 109
Nguyen, N., 276
Nicholls, D., 99
Nicholls, M. E. R., 245, 252
Nichols-Anderson, C. L., 227
Nickel, R. E., 278
Nieberding, R., 88
Nielsen Media Research, 228
Nielson, T., 332
Nishino, S., 334
Nolan, M., 211
Nolen-Hoeksema, S., 181, 185
Norris, A. K., 226
Norris, J., 226
Nortz, M. J., 270
Norwood, W., 227
Nottelmann, E. D., 181
Nourse, S., 258
Nunneley, S. A., 304
Nwosa, N. M., 216

O

Oakman, J. M., 200
Oberklaid, F., 250
O'Brien, G. V., 262

O'Byrne, K. K., 323
O'Connor, A. M., 271
O'Connor, B. P., 226
O'Connor, T. G., 14
O'Donohue, W. O., 139
Oezcankaya, R., 304
Offord, D. R., 17
Ohan, J. L., 209
Ohayon, M. M., 329, 330, 332
O'Koon, J. H., 221
Olds, D., 144
Oliver, C., 270
Oliver, J. E., 129
Oliver, P. J., 56
Olivier, C., 257
Ollendick, T. H., 158, 330
Olson, S. L., 350
Olympia, D. E., 95
Oman, D., 200
O'Neal, K. K., 209
O'Neill, C. T., 281
O'Neill, R., 99, 100
Onslow, M., 340
Orbach, Y., 139
O'Reilly, M. F., 326
Osantowski, J., 95
Osborne, M. L., 227
Oshlag, R. S., 328
Osland, J., 222
Osman, A., 194
Osofsky, J. D., 142, 143, 144
Ostrander, R., 204, 217
Oswald, D. P., 276
Oswald, L., 95
Ottaviano, S., 332
Outhred, L., 270
Overholser, J. C., 191, 194
Owens, G., 36, 37
Owens, M. J., 30
Owens, R. E., Jr., 335
Ozechowski, T. J., 119, 120
Ozonoff, S., 290, 292, 294

P

Packman, A., 340
Paget, K. D., 140, 144
Palladino, P., 250, 254
Pallant, J., 333
Palmer, P., 303
Paltrow, L. M., 116
Panchaud, C., 14
Pang, D., 304
Pantelis, C., 207
Paolo, A. M., 88
Parisse, C., 292, 300
Parker, J., 291

Parker, K., 307
Parsons, B. V., 354
Parsons, E., 37
Pastorelli, C., 44
Patel, A., 329
Patil, S. R., 303
Patrick, C. J., 216
Patterson, A., 290, 298
Patterson, G. R., 12, 108, 223, 232, 353, 354
Pavelski, R., 315, 318
Pavuluri, M. N., 99
Payne, L., 270
Pearce, J. C., 221, 234
Pedrabissi, L., 263
Pedrosi, B., 333
Peersen, M., 230
Pelham, W. E., 202, 357
Pell, T., 116
Pennington, B. F., 208, 227, 243, 253
Pepler, D. J., 94
Perez, B., 87
Perez, W., 256
Perrin, S., 166
Perry, C. L., 112
Persinger, M. A., 250
Peterson, A. C., 17
Peterson, C., 190
Peterson, U., 130, 144
Petoskey, M. D., 88
Petrosino, A., 234
Pettit, G. S., 129, 219
Pfeffer, C., 192
Phillips, C. M., 230
Philp, I. D., 140
Phung, T. M., 348
Piacentini, J., 192
Piazza, C. C., 295
Picard, E. M., 271, 275
Piche, C., 159
Pickrel, S. G., 121
Piehl, A. M., 234
Pieterse, M., 270
Pietrowsky, R., 330
Pigott, T. A., 321
Pilowsky, T., 296
Pine, J., 58, 59, 60
Pineda, D., 241
Pinhas, H. O., 322
Pisecco, S., 206
Pitts, S. C., 109
Piven, J., 303
Plomin, R., 28, 165
Plotsky, P. M., 30
Plunkett, M. C. B., 136
Podolsky, I. P., 205

Poe-Yamagata, E., 111
Pogue-Geile, M. F., 226
Polaha, J. A., 219
Poli, P., 250
Polusny, M. A., 142
Pomeroy, J. C., 356
Pool, K., 245
Porche, L. M., 159
Portes, A., 108, 109, 113
Posavac, H. D., 51, 53
Posavac, S. S., 51, 53
Posey, D. J., 307
Potter, L. B., 218
Poulin, F., 222
Poustka, F., 227
Powell, S., 60
Powell, T. H., 291
Power, T. J., 211
Poznanski, E., 181
Pozzi, M. E., 205
Prater, M. A., 210
Preski, S., 220, 221, 234
Pressley, M., 244
Prevost, M. J., 270
Price, D. D., 69
Price Foundation Collaborative Group, 317, 318, 320
Priest, R. G., 329
Pring, L., 292
Prinstein, M. J., 160, 194
Prinz, R. J., 220
Prior, M., 20, 250
Pumariega, A. J., 318, 319
Pungello, E. P., 279
Purcell, A. E., 304
Putnam, S. C., 207

Q

Quealy-Berge, D., 60
Quigly, P., 234
Quine, L., 328

R

Radziewicz, C., 335
Rae, D. S., 178
Rafferty, A., 290, 298
Raffi, A. R., 321
Raggio, D. J., 206
Rahdert, E., 108
Ralph, N. B., 200
Ralph, S., 302
Ramasamy, R., 63
Ramey, C. T., 279, 359
Ramey, S. L., 359
Ramirez, E. M., 322

Subject Index

Anafranil, 187, 307
Anal stage, Freud's, 33
Anatomically correct dolls, 136–138, 347
Anencephaly, 273
Anger control training, 230
Anorexia nervosa, 17, 313, 314–319
   case studies on, 312, 316, 340
   diagnostic criteria for, 315
   and personality traits, 315
   treatment of, 318–319
Anoxia, 275
Antecedents, 95, 99
Antidepressants, 8, 169, 186–187, 318–319, 321, 356, 357
Antipsychotic drugs, 307, 357
Antisocial behavior, 16–17, 28, 222–223, 226–229. *See also* Antisocial personality disorder; Conduct disorder; Oppositional defiant disorder
Antisocial personality disorder, 231–232
   diagnostic criteria for, 231
Anxiety, 12, 13, 21
   in adolescents, 154–156
   case studies on, 1, 21, 163
   cognitive-behavioral therapy for, 350–351
   definition of, 153
   and depression, 158
   divorce and, 155–156
   math, 241, 245, 246–247, 251–252
   separation, 78, 101, 157–158
   social, 1, 21, 161
Anxiety disorders, 115. *See also specific disorders*
   causes of, 164–165
Anxious children, 153
Applied behavior analysis (ABA), 256–257, 288, 307, 309
Appropriateness (of behaviors)
   age-, 11–15
   cultural, 10
Arithmetic subtest, of WISC-III, 87
Arousal, 45
Articulation disorders. *See* Phonological disorders
Asperger's disorder, 292–294
   diagnostic criteria for, 293
Assessment, 79–82, 94–96. *See also specific techniques*
   case study on, 294
   of child sexual abuse, 135–139
   collection procedures used in, 79
   and research, 84
Association, auditory, 249
Association techniques, 88
Attachment figure, 36–37
Attachment relationship, 20
Attachment theory, 20, 34, 36–37, 183, 184
Attention, selective, 250
Attention deficit disorder (ADD), 204–205
Attention-deficit/hyperactivity disorder (ADHD), 13, 16, 199–200
   case studies on, 59–60, 198, 212, 343, 361
   causes of, 206–209

characteristics of, 200–206
diagnostic criteria for, 201
DSM-IV-TR definition of, 201
and Feingold Diet, 208
and learning disabilities, 241, 243
possible causes of, 206–209
research on, 51, 53
and substance use, 117, 119
treatment of, 209–213, 343, 357. *See also* Ritalin
Attention problems, of children with learning disabilities, 250
Attitudes, set of, 19–20
Atypical autism, 292
Auditory association, 249
Auditory blending, 249
Auditory discrimination, 248–249
Auditory memory, 249
Auditory perception, 248–249
Augmented language, system of, 280
Autism, 289–292, 293
   atypical, 292
   case studies on, 288, 291, 301, 309
   causes of, 303–305
   and childhood schizophrenia, 296–303
   diagnostic criteria for, 293
   and language, 300, 308
   and mental retardation, 267
   social development of children with, 298–300
   treatment of, 305–308
Autism spectrum disorders, 289–290
Autobiographical memory, 8
Autonomic nervous system, 29
Average score, 84

B

Baby talk, 335, 338
Barbiturates, 117
Basal ganglia, and obsessive-compulsive disorder, 171
Beck's cognitive theory of depression, 183, 184
Bed-wetting, 327
Behavior(s)
   abnormal, 10, 12, 24–32. *See also specific types*
   adaptive, 264, 265
   age-appropriate, 11–15
   antisocial, 16–17, 28, 222–223
   depressive, 181
   externalizing, 216–217
   and gender, 16–18
   mediating, 202
   observation of, 94–96
   operant, 40–42
   rating scales for, 91–94
   Skinner's superstitious, 43
   stereotypic, 291, 301–302, 306
   roots of, 7
   target, 95

Behavior management, 80, 99–100, 210–213, 235, 246–247, 256–257, 288, 309, 343
Behavior rating scales, 91–94
Behavioral family therapy, 353–354
Behavioral genetics, 26–27
Behavioral observation, 95–96
Behavioral therapy, 348–349, 351–352, 353–354. *See also* Cognitive-behavioral therapy
Bell Curve, The, 83
Benzodiazepines, 117, 161, 169
Berkeley Puppet Interview, 97
Bias, 60, 87
Binge eating, 313, 314, 319–320, 323
Binge-eating/purging type of anorexia nervosa, 314, 315
Biology, and behavior, 3, 6–7, 24–32, 106, 165, 185–186
Bipolar disorder, 26, 177–178
Birth, precipitous, 275
Birth trauma, 273–274
Birth weight, 114, 275–276
Blending, auditory, 249
Block design subtest, of WISC-III, 87
Blood, Rh incompatibility of, 272, 278
Bonding, infant-caregiver, 36
Borderline personality disorder, 192
Brain
    and ADHD, 200, 206–207
    and autism, 304
    damage to, 206, 253
    functions and structure of, 29–32
    and childhood schozophrenia, 304
Brain-behavior link, 25, 29, 30–32, 186
Brain scans, 304
Breech presentation, 274
Broad-spectrum factors, 91
Bulimia nervosa, 17, 313, 319–321
    causes of, 320–321
    diagnostic criteria for, 319
    treatment of, 321
Bullying, case study on, 7

C

California Psychological Inventory, 91
CAPA, 98
Capacity, in consent, 72–73, 74
Caretaker interview, 100
Carolina Abecedarian Project, 279
Case studies, 57–60, 67
    on attention-deficit/hyperactivity disorder, 59–60, 198, 212, 343, 361
    on African Americans in special education, 282
    on aggression, 7
    on alcoholism and abuse, 125
    on anorexia nervosa, 312, 316, 340
    on anxiety, 1, 21, 163
    on Asperger's disorder, 294
    on autism, 288, 291, 301, 309

on child abuse, 6, 123, 125, 128, 134, 136, 137, 149
on childhood obesity, 312, 340
on chronic fire-setting, 222
on conduct disorder, 175, 195, 215, 221, 222, 235
on depression, 175, 195
on disordered behavior, 23, 45
on eating problems, 175, 195, 312, 340
on false memories and sexual abuse, 134
on gang membership, 109
on illicit drug use, 103, 120
on learning disabilities, 23, 238, 259
on math anxiety, 251–252
on mental retardation, 261, 282, 284–285, 295
on meth moms and abuse, 116
on neglect, 6, 123
on phonological coding problems, 198, 212
on physical abuse, 6, 123, 136, 149
on posttraumatic stress disorder, 152, 160, 172
on reading problems, 48, 75
on Rett's disorder, 295
on schoolbus kidnapping, 152, 172
on selective mutism, 78, 101
Case studies, (*cont.*)
    on separation anxiety, 78, 101
    on sexual abuse, 123, 134, 149
    on skill development, 284–285, 295
    on sleeping problems, 175, 195
    on socioeconomic integration in schools, 113
    on stealing, 59–60
    on stress, 152, 155–156, 160, 163, 172
    on using Ritalin, 343, 361
    on using anatomically correct dolls, 137
    on using applied behavior analysis, 288, 309
CAT, 89
Categorical Educational Classification System, 80
Catharsis, 229–230
CBCL, 84, 91–93
CBM, 246–247
CBT, 21, 144, 146
CCC model, 185
Central nervous system (CNS), 29, 30
    psychostimulants, 356
Cerebellum. 31
Cerebral cortex, 30–31
Child abuse, 18, 50, 133–134. *See also* Neglect
    assessment of, 135–139
    causes of, 127–132
    characteristics of victims of, 131–132
    definition of, 126
    effects of, 141–142
    mandatory reporting of, 124–125
    prevention of, 142–144
    research on, 51
    treatment of, 145–146
    types of, 126
Child and Adolescent Psychiatric Assessment (CAPA), 98
Child & Family WebGuide, 20

Cueing procedure, 53
Cultural appropriateness, of behavior, 10
Cultural factors, 6
    in academic achievement, 13–14
    and appropriateness of behaviors, 10
    and behavior checklists, 94
    and intelligence tests, 87
    and physical punishment, 127, 129
    in suicide, 192–193
    in therapy, 347
Culturally pervasive experiences, 6
Cumulative risk model, 113

D

D.A.R.E., 118, 156
Day care centers, and child abuse, 133
Deafness, of parents, 336–337
Decade for a Culture of Nonviolence, 148
Deception, in research, 73–74
Defective speech, 334–339
Defects, clinical, 273
Deinstitutionalization, 283
Delayed echolalia, 300
Delayed speech, 334–337
Delinquency, juvenile, 43, 230–236
Deoxyribonucleic acid (DNA), 24, 25. *See also* Genetics
Dependence, substance, 104, 105
    Freud's explanation of, 33
Dependent variable, 60
Depression
    and anxiety, 158
    and autism, 303
    case study on, 1, 175, 195
    diagnostic criteria for, 177
    double, 178
    and gender, 17, 181–182
    and heredity, 185–186
    minor, 178
    postpartum, 189
    prevalence of, 179–180
    symptoms of, 177
    theories of, 183–185
    treatment of, 8, 119, 186–189
Deprivation of experiences, and delayed speech, 336–337
Descriptive research questions, 52, 58
Desensitization
    in vivo, 167
    systematic, 167, 351
Desensitization therapies, 167, 351
Designs, experimental, 61–65
Desipramine, 186
Development, 7–9, 11–15, 61
    and environment, 3–6, 24
    fetal, and mental retardation, 268–277
    of language, 334–335
    and learning disabilities, 252

psychosexual personality, 33–34
    and therapy, 345–347
Developmental disorders, pervasive, 289–290. *See also
    specific disorders*
Developmental psychopathology, 39–40
Deviation, standard, 84
Dexedrine, 117, 255, 356
Dexfenfluramine, 324
Dextroamphetamine, 356
*Diagnostic and Statistical Manual of Mental
    Disorders*, 4th ed., Text Revision (DSM-IV-TR), 9, 80,
    99
Diagnostic criteria, 9–10
    for anorexia nervosa, 315
    for antisocial personality disorder, 231
    for Asperger's disorder, 293
    for attention-deficit/hyperactivity disorder, 201
    for autism, 293
    for bulimia nervosa, 319
    for conduct disorder, 219
    for depression, 177
    for learning disorders, 242
    for mental retardation, 267
    for nightmare disorder, 331
    for night terrors, 331
    for oppositional defiant disorder, 218
    for schizophrenia, 297
    for substance abuse, 104
    for substance dependence, 105
Diagnostic Interview Schedule for Children (DISC-IV), 98
Diagnostic interviews, 98
Diagnostic process, 79–80, 98. *See also* Assessment;
    Classification
    for mental retardation, 265–266
Diencephalon, 31
Diet, and ADHD, 208
Dieting, 313, 314, 322, 323
Difference research questions, 52, 58, 59
Differential reinforcement, 203
Digit span subtest, of WISC-III, 87
Dimensions, of AAMR diagnostic-classification process,
    265–266
Dining together, as a family, 110–111
DISC-IV, 98
Discontinuous encopresis, 326
Discrimination, auditory, 248–249
Disengaged families, 353
Disintegrative psychosis, 294–295
    research on, 296
Disorder of written expression, 242
Disorders. *See also* specific disorders
    comorbid (or co-occurring), 12
    externalizing, 10. 12, 13
    internalizing, 10, 12, 13
    spectrum of, 289, 305
Disorganized attachment, 37
Diurnal enuresis, 327

Divorce
and antisocial behavior, 227–228
and anxiety, 155–156
and twins, 28
D-lysergic acid (LSD-25), 307
DNA, 24, 25. *See also* Genetics
Dolls, anatomically correct, 136–138, 347
Dominant genes, 25
Dominic-R, 97
Dopamine
and amphetamines, 115
and schizophrenia, 29–30, 305
Dopamine hypothesis, 305
Double depression, 178
Double helix, 25
Down syndrome, 26, 269–270, 278
Draw a Person, 89–90, 91
Dreaming, 329–330
Drinking. *See* Alcohol
Drug abuse, 4, 104, 108
cumulative risk model for, 113
and delinquency, 232, 233
prevention of, 117–119
and suicide, 191–192
treatment for, 8, 119–120
Drug Abuse Resistance Education (D.A.R.E.), 118
Drug Free Schools and Communities Act, 118
Drug treatments, 8, 356–358
for ADHD, 209–210
for anorexia nervosa, 318–319
for anxiety disorders, 169
for autism, 307, 308
for childhood schizophrenia, 307–308
for enuresis, 328
for learning disabilities, 255
for nightmares and night terrors, 332
for obsesive-compulsive disorder, 171, 172
for phobias, 169
Drugs
abuse of. *See* Drug abuse
antipsychotic, 307, 357
case study on use of illicit, 103, 120
diet, 323–324
effects of, 106
and family problems, 108–111
and poverty, 111–112
psychoactive, 356. *See also* Antidepressants; Neuroleptics;
Stimulants
and schools, 112–113
and teen employment, 107
DSM-IV-TR, 9, 80, 99
Duration recording, 94
Dysartia, 338
Dyskinesia, 307
Dyslexia, 239
Dysomnias, 329, 332–334
Dysthymic disorder, 178

E

Early intervention, 358–361
Eating disorders, 17, 313, 339, 340. *See also* Anorexia nervosa; Bulimia nervosa; Obesity
case studies on, 175, 195, 312, 340
Eating together, as a family, 110–111
Echolalia, 292
Eclectic approach, 344–345
Ecstasy, 115
Educational integration, 282
Educational neglect, 126, 140
Ego, 33
Ego identity, 34
Ego theory, 34–36
Elavil, 357
Elementary school children
abuse of, 141–142
and anxiety, 154–156
behaviors of, 12, 13–14, 16–18
and depression, 179, 181
and school refusal, 162
Emotional abuse, 126, 127, 140
Emotional factors, of learning disabilities, 250
Employment and teen drug use, 107
Encephalitis, 206
Encopresis, 326–327
Endocrine system, 31, 32
Enmeshed families, 353
Enuresis, 327–328
diurnal, 327
nocturnal, 327
Environmental factors
and ADHD, 208
and development, 24
and learning disabilities, 254
in mental retardation, 267, 269, 276–277
Epinephrine, 31
Equifinality, 4, 5, 39
Erikson's psychosocial stages, 35–36
Erogenous zones, 33
Error, in assessment, 81–82, 87
Erythroblastosis fetalis, 272
Ethics and research, 71–75
European Union, 129
Event recording, 94
Excitatory synapses, 29
Executive function, 202
Expectations, adults' unrealistic, 18
Experience deprivation, 336–337
Experimental matching, 70–71
Experimental research, 54–56
designs in, 60–65, 66
validity of, 67–70, 82
Experimental variable, 60–67
Expressive techniques, 88
External validity, 68–70

Externalizing behaviors, 216–217
Externalizing type of disorder, 10, 12, 13. *See also* Antisocial personality disorder; Conduct disorder; Oppositional defiant disorder
Extinction, 40–41, 185

F

Face validity, 82
Facilitated communication, 306
FAE, 114, 273
False Memory Syndrome Foundation, 134
False negative, 83
False positive, 83
Families and Schools Together model, 230
Family factors. *See also* Genetics; Parents; Twins
   in anorexia nervosa, 315, 317
   in antisocial behavior, 227–228
   in autism, 303
   and behavioral observation code, 96
   in child abuse, 129–131
   in delinquency, 233
   in drug use, 108–111, 119–121
   in mood disorders, 182–183
   in neglect, 140–141
   in suicide, 192
Family rules, covert, 353
Family skills-training interventions, 118–119
Family systems therapy, 120
Family therapies, 118–120, 318, 352–356
FAS, 114, 273
FAST Track model, 230, 359
Faulty learning, 43
Faulty self-reinforcement, 43
Fear hierarchy, 167, 350–351
Fear(s), 15, 153–156, 350–351. *See also* Anxiety; Phobias
   common, 154, 156
   definition of, 153
Feingold Diet, 208
Fetal alcohol effects (FAE), 114, 273
Fetal alcohol syndrome (FAS), 114, 273
Fetal development, 114, 268–277
Fictional reinforcement contingencies, 43
Figure-ground discrimination, 248
Fire-setting, chronic, 222
Flight or fight reaction, 15, 153–156, 350–351
Fluid reasoning, 238
Fluoxetine, 187, 318–319, 321, 332, 357
Fluvoxamine, 169, 172, 187, 328
Food, attitudes toward, 313, 322
"For the Children of the World," 148
Forebrain, 30–31. *See also* Cerebral cortex
Foster homes, 354–356
   for abused children, 145–146
   for juvenile delinquents, 236
Foster parents, 354–356

Fragile X syndrome, 26, 270, 305
Free association stage, of Rorschach, 89
Frequency recording, 94
Functional articulation disorders, 337
Functional behavior analysis, 100
Functional behavior assessment and classification system, 80, 99–100
Functional family therapy, 354
Functional nocturnal enuresis, 327

G

g factor, 86
GABA, 30
Galactosemia, 271
Gamma-aminobutyric acid (GABA), 30
Ganglia, basal, 171
Gangs
   case study on, 109
   and drug use, 108
   and juvenile delinquency, 43, 232–233
   research on, 233
   and suicide, 192
Gardner's multiple components of intelligence, 87, 88
Gay adolescents and suicide, 193
Gender differences, 25, 34
   in ADHD, 199
   in anorexia nervosa, 314
   in child abuse, 127–128, 135
   in conduct and oppositional defiant disorders, 223–224
   in problem behaviors, 16–18
   in depression, 17, 181–182
   in PTSD, 159
   in stuttering, 339
Gene-environment model, reciprocal, 28
Genes, 25–26
General ability factor, 86
General orientation, 19–20
Generalizability, 60, 68, 69
Generalized anxiety disorder, 158–159
Genetics. *See also* Family factors; Parents; Twins
   and abnormal behavior, 24–28
   and ADHD, 207–208, 209
   and anorexia nervosa, 315–316, 318
   and anxiety disorders, 165
   and autism, 303, 304–305
   behavioral, 26–27
   and childhood schizophrenia, 303, 305
   and depression, 185–186
   and learning disabilities, 253–254
   and mental retardation, 266, 267, 269–271
   and oppositional defiant disorder, 226–227
German measles. *See* Rubella
Gestational age, 275–276
GET IT strategy, 256
Group experimental studies, 65, 66, 67

Guided mastery treatment, 167–168, 350
Guided participation, 167–168, 350
Guns, 143

H

Haloperidol, 357
Hand-held computers, 95
Hand raising, 53
Hand regard, 302
Handwriting, and learning disabilities, 245–246, 249
Haptic perception, 249
Healthy Start Program, 144
Heller's syndrome, 294–295
    research on, 296
Hemispheres, of brain, 30–31
Hemp, 115
Heritability, 26. *See also* Genetics
Heroin, 116–117
Herpes simplex virus, 304
Hierarchy of fears, 167, 350–351
Hispanic American children
    academic achievement of, 14
    and schools, 113
    and suicide, 192–193
Home-visiting programs, 189
Homosexual adolescents and suicide, 193
Hormone(s), 29, 31
    antidiuretic, 327
Human Figure Drawing, 89–90, 91
Human participants committees, 71
Human rights, 147–148
Huntington's chorea, 26
Hydrocephalus, 273
HYPAC axis, 31
Hyperactivity
    in ADHD, 201, 202, 203–205
    and learning disabilities, 241, 243
    research on, 203–204
Hyperbilirubinemia, 272
Hyperkinesis, 200, 201, 202, 203–205, 243. *See also* Attention-deficit/hyperactivity disorder
Hypermasculinity, 226
Hyperplastic obesity, 322
Hypertrophic obesity, 322
Hypothalamic-pituitary-adrenalcortical (HYPAC) axis, 31
Hypothalamus, 31, 32

I

ICD-10, 80, 99
Id, 33
IDEA. *See* Individuals with Disabilities Education Act
Identity crisis, 14
Idiot savants, 301

Illicit drug use path, to juvenile delinquency, 232
Imipramine, 8, 186, 357
Imitation, 42–43, 104, 105
Immediate echolalia, 300
Immigrants, and drug use, 108
Impulsivity, in ADHD, 201, 202, 206
    research on, 203–204
In vivo desensitization, 167
Inappropriate reinforcement, 43
Inattention, in ADHD, 200, 201
Incidence, 267
Incidental learning, 250
Inconsistency, of parental discipline, 227
Independent variable, 60–67
Indian children, and suicide, 192
Indicated cases, of abuse, 132
Individuals with Disabilities Education Act (IDEA), 80, 99, 100
    and attention-deficit/hyperactivity disorder, 199
    and autism, 290
    and instruction, 281–282
    and learning disabilities, 240
    and mental retardation, 268
    and speech disorders, 334
Inequality, 6
Infants
    bonding of, with mother, 36–37
    and depression, 181
    and nonverbal motor tasks, 8–9
Influenza, 304
Informal observation, 50
Information
    for assessment, 79–80
    and consent to participate, 73, 74
Information subtest, of WISC-III, 87
Inhibitory synapses, 29
Inkblots, Rorschach, 89
Inpatient programs, for substance abusers, 119
Inquiry stage, of Rorschach, 89
Insecure attachment, 37
Insistence on sameness, and autism, 302
Insomnia, 328, 332–333
Institutional review boards (IRBs), 71
Instructional intervention
    for learning disabilities, 256–257
    for mental retardation, 280–282
Insufficent reinforcement, 43
Intelligence
    and autism, 300–301, 308
    and childhood schizophrenia, 301, 308
    definition of, 86
    heritability of, 27
    multiple components of, 87, 88
    and socioeconomic class, 83
    testing of, 83, 85–88
    triarchic theory of, 86–87
Intelligence quotient (IQ), 85

Interdisciplinary approach, 39
Intermittent reinforcement, 41
Internal consistency reliability, 82
Internal validity, 68–70
Internalization, 37
Internalizing behaviors, 216
Internalizing type of disorder, 10, 12, 13
International Classification of Diseases (ICD-10), 80, 99
Internet, resources on, 20
Interpersonal theory, 37–39
Interpretation, of events, 42
Inter-rater reliability, 82
Interval recording, 94
Interventions
   for anxiety disorders, 166–169
   early, 358–361
   family skills-training, 118–119
   for mental retardation, 278–279
   multimodal, 211–213
   for obesity, 324–325
Interviewing, 67, 79, 96–98
   in ABC system, 99
   of caretaker, 100
   and child abuse, 136–138
Intimate violence, 228
Introjection, 37, 38
IQ, 85
IRBs, 71

J

Jessness Personality Inventory, 91
Jigsaw Classroom program, 359–360
Juvenile delinquency, 43, 230–236

K

Kaufman Assessment Battery for Children (K-ABC), 86
Kidnapping, 152, 172
Klonopin, 169, 332

L

Labor, duration of, 275
Language
   and autism, 300, 308
   and brain, 30–31
   normal development of, 335
   system of augmented, 280
   and childhood schizophrenia, 300
Larry P. v. Riles, 87
Latency recording, 94
Lead, and brain damage, 208
Learned helplessness theory, 183, 184–185
Learning
   cooperative, 359–360
   faulty, 43

incidental, 250
operant, 40–42
vicarious, 42–43
Learning disabilities, 238–242. *See also* Academic achievement
   case studies on, 23, 48, 238, 259
   causes of, 252–254
   classifying, 241, 243–252
   developmental factors in, 252
   treatment of, 254–257
Learning disorders, 241–242. *See also* Learning disabilities
   diagnostic criteria for, 242
Least restrictive alternative, 282
Left hemisphere, of brain, 30
Legal rights, of children, 129, 147–148, 150
Leiter International Performance Scale (LIPS), 86
Lesbian adolescents, and suicide, 193
Letter reversals, 248
Life skills training programs, 119
LIPS, 86
Longitudinal designs, 61–63, 67
Low birth weight, 114
LSD-25, 307
Luvox, 169, 172, 187, 328

M

MADD, 156
Magnetic resonance imaging (MRI), 304
Mainstreaming, 282
Major depressive disorder, 177, 178, 187. *See also* Depression
Major depressive episode, 1, 177, 183. *See also* Depression
Maltreatment. *See* Abuse, child
Mandatory reporting, 124
Manic-depressive disorder, 26, 177–178
Maple syrup urine disease, 271
Marijuana, 106, 114–115
Matching, experimental, 70–71
Matching Familiar Figures Test, 202
Math anxiety, 242, 245
   case study on, 251–252
   research on, 246–247
Mathematics disorder, 242, 245, 246–247
   case study on, 251–252
   diagnostic criteria for, 242
   and self-instruction, 246–247
Mazes subtest, of WISC-III, 87
MBD, 200, 206
MDMA, 115
Mean score, 84
Media violence, 228–229
Mediating behaviors, 202
Medications. *See* Drug treatments
Medulla, 31
Megavitamin treatment, 307
Methodology, research, 54–65

Posttraumatic stress disorder (PTSD), 159–161
case studies on, 152, 160, 172
definition of, 141
Poverty
and academic achievement, 13
and anxiety, 155
and child abuse, 130
and child neglect, 140–141
and drug use, 111–112
and suicide, 192
Prazosin, 332
Precipitous birth, 275
Predictive validity, 82
Predominately hyperactive-impulsive type of ADHD, 201
Predominately inattentive type of ADHD, 201
Preschool children
abuse of, 141
behaviors of, 12
and depression, 181
Pretest-posttest study, 65, 66
Prevalence, definition of, 267
Prevention
of child abuse, 142–145
of drug abuse, 117–119
of mental retardation, 283, 285
of mood disorders, 189–190
of suicide, 193–195
Primary encopresis, 326
Primary insomnia, 332–333
Primary sleep disorders, 329
Privacy issues, in research, 73
Problem-solving skills training, 222, 351
Profound mental retardation, 266
Progressive muscle relaxation, 351
Projective tests, 88–91
Prozac, 187, 318–319, 321, 332, 357
Psychiatric classification, 99
Psychiatric interview, child, 97–98
Psychoanalytic theory/therapy, 32–34, 183, 184, 305–306
Psychodynamic theories/therapies, 32, 348
for antisocial disorders, 229
for anxiety disorders, 166
for autism and childhood schizophrenia, 303, 305–306
for depression, 187
for obsessive-compulsive disorder, 171
for phobias, 164
for toileting problems, 326, 327–328
Psychoeducational programs, 145
Psychological assessment, 81–98
Psychological treatment, 348–352. *See also* specific treatments
Psychopathology, child, 2, 9–20
causes of, 3
developmental, 39–40
theories of, 24. *See also specific theories*
Psychosexual personality development, 33–34

Psychosis, disintegrative, 294–295
research on, 296
Psychosocial factors in mental retardation, 276–277
Psychosocial stages, Erikson's, 35–36
Psychostimulants. *See* Stimulants
Psychotherapy
for abused children, 146
for depressed children, 187–188, 189
PTSD. *See* Posttraumatic stress disorder
Public Law 94–142, 281
Punishment, 41–42, 111, 127, 129
Purging type of bulimia nervosa, 319

Q

Qualitative research, 54–60
Quantitative research, 54–56, 60–67
Quasi-experimental designs, 61, 67
Questionnaire, research, 67
Questions, research
correlational, 52, 54
descriptive, 52
difference, 52, 59
relationship, 52, 54

R

Rain Man, 290
Random assignment, 70–71
Random error, 81–82
Random sampling, 70–71
Rating scales, for assessment of behavior, 91–94
Reactivity, 96
Reading disorder, 242, 243–244
case study on, 48, 75
Reasoning, commonsense, 52
Recapitulation, 38
Recessive genes, 25–26
Reciprocal gene-environment model, 28
Recording, 57, 94–96, 324
Recovered memories, 134
Rehabilitation Act of 1973, 80
Rehearsal, 354
Reinforcement, 40–43
differential, 203
inappropriate, 43
insufficient, 43
negative, 41–42
positive, 40–41, 207, 349
self-, 43
Reinforcement contingencies, 43, 349
Reinforcement-loss model, 183, 185
Reinforcer, 40, 349
Reinforcing consequences, 40
Rejection, 111, 323
Relationship research questions, 52, 54
Relaxation techniques, 167, 187, 222, 351

Sex chromosomes, 25, 226, 271
Sex differences, 25, 34
    in ADHD, 199
    in anorexia nervosa, 314
    in child abuse, 127–128, 135
    in conduct and oppositional defiant disorders, 223–224
    in problem behaviors, 16–18
    in depression, 17, 181–182
    in PTSD, 159
    in stuttering, 339
Sexual abuse
    case studies on, 123, 134, 149
    children's reports of, 138–139
    defining, 126, 132–133
    interviews concerning, 137
    prevention of, 145
    research on, 51
    victims of, 133–135
Sexual behavior, Samoan, 56
Sexual-minority youth, 193
Shoulder presentation, 275
Siblings, and child abuse, 131
Similarities subtest, of WISC-III, 87
Simple phobia, 157
Skill areas, adaptive, 264, 265
Skills, splinter, 301
Skills training
    case studies on, 53, 284–285
    and drug abuse, 119
    family, 118–119
    problem-solving, 222, 351
Sleep disorders, 328–334
    case study on, 175, 195
Sleep stages, 328–329
    and enuresis, 327
Sleep terror disorder, 328–332, 333
Sleep-walking disorder, 332
Social anxiety, 1, 21, 161
Social anxiety disorder, 1, 161
Social codes, 10
Social cognitive theory, 42–46, 350
    and conduct disorder, 230–231
    of depression, 183, 185
    and phobias, 164–165
Social development of autistic children, 298–300
Social factors
    and child abuse, 130
    and eating disorders, 313, 315
    and learning disabilities, 250
Social learning theory, 42–46, 350
    and conduct disorder, 230–231
    of depression, 183, 185
    and phobias, 164–165
Social phobia, 1, 161
Social services, and child abuse, 144
Social skills, and conduct disorder, 220–221
Social skills training, 53

Socially deviant models, 42–43, 108
Society of Clinical Psychology of the American Psychological
        Association, 352
Society to Prevent Cruelty to Animals (SPCA), 128
Socioeconomic class, and anorexia nervosa, 315
Socioeconomic integration, in schools, 113
Somatic nervous system, 29
Somnambulism, 332
Spanking, 127, 129
SPCA, 128
Specific phobia, 157
Spectrum of disorders, 289, 305
Speech, and brain, 30–31
Speech disorders, 334–339
Spelling, and learning disabilities, 245–246
Spina bifida, 273
Spinal cord, 31
Spirochete, 272
Splinter skills, 301
SSRIs, 8, 186–187, 318–319, 357
Standard deviation, 84
Standardization group, 83
Standardized measure, 83
Stanford-Binet Intelligence Test-Fourth Edition (SB-4th), 86
Starvation, self-inflicted. *See* Anorexia nervosa
Statistical analysis, of research results, 66–67
Stealing, 59–60
Stereotypic behavior, 29, 301–302, 306
Sternberg's triarchic theory of intelligence, 86–87
Stimulants, 115–117, 209–210, 328, 334, 356–357
Stimulus overselectivity, 302–303
Stress, 153. *See also* Posttraumatic stress disorder
    case studies on, 152, 155–156, 160, 163, 172
    and drug use, 111
    in families of children with autism, 303
    from participating in research, 71
    and somnambulism, 332
Structured interviews, 98
Study Group on Violence of the National Center for Clinical
        Infant Programs, 143
Stuttering, 338–340
Subclinical depression, 178
Substance abuse, 104, 105. *See also* Drug abuse
    diagnostic criteria for, 104
Substance dependence, 104, 105. *See also* Drug abuse
    diagnostic criteria for, 105
    Freud's explanation of, 33
Substance use, 103, 104
    reasons for, 106–113
Substantiated cases, of abuse, 132
Suicide, 176
    and family disturbance, 192
    prevention of, 193–195
    research on, 193
    statistics on, 190–191
    warning signs of, 191
Superego, 33

Vicarious learning, 42–43
Vicarious success, 44
Violence, 143, 148, 192, 228–229
  and anxiety, 154–155
  and delinquency, 232–233
  intimate, 228
  in media, 228–229
Virus, herpes simplex, 304
Visual perception problems, 248
Vitamin B, as treatment for autism or schizophrenia, 307
Vocabulary subtest, of WISC-III, 87
Voluntariness, in consent, 73, 74

W

Wechsler Intelligence Scale for Children—Third Edition
  (WISC-III), 86, 87
Wechsler Intelligence Scale for Children—Revised (WISC-
  III-R), 86

Wechsler Preschool and Primary Scale of Intelligence—
  Revised (WPPSI-R), 86
Word association, 88
World Health Organization, 99

X

Xanax, 117

Y

Yonkers Project, 112
Young Autism Project, 307

Z

Zoloft, 187
Zones, erogenous, 33